DIAGNOSTIC PROBLEMS IN BREAST PATHOLOGY

Frederick C. Koerner, MD

Associate Professor of Pathology
Harvard Medical School
Associate Pathologist
Massachusetts General Hospital,
Boston, Massachusetts

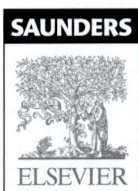

SAUNDERS

ELSEVIER

SAUNDERS
ELSEVIER

1600 John F. Kennedy Boulevard
Ste 1800
Philadelphia, PA 19103-2899

DIAGNOSTIC PROBLEMS IN BREAST PATHOLOGY   ISBN: 978-1-4160-2612-9

Notice

Knowledge and best practice in this field are constantly changing. As new research and experience broaden our knowledge, changes in practice, treatment, and drug therapy may become necessary or appropriate. Readers are advised to check the most current information provided (i) on procedures featured or (ii) by the manufacturer of each product to be administered to verify the recommended dose or formula, the method and duration of administration, and contraindications. It is the responsibility of the practitioner, relying on his or her own experience and knowledge of the patient, to make diagnoses, to determine dosages and the best treatment for each individual patient, and to take all appropriate safety precautions. To the fullest extent of the law, neither the publisher nor the author assumes any liability for any injury and/or damage to persons or property arising out of or related to any use of the material contained in this book.

The Publisher

Library of Congress Cataloging-in-Publication Data

Koerner, Frederick C.
    Diagnostic problems in breast pathology / Frederick C. Koerner. – 1st ed.
      p. ; cm.
    Includes bibliographic references.
    ISBN 978-1-4160-2612-9
  1. Breast–Cancer–Diagnosis. 2. Breast–Diseases. I. Title.
    [DNLM: 1. Breast–pathology. 2. Breast Diseases–pathology. WP 815 K78d 2009]
    RC280.B8K64 2009
    616.99′449075–dc22
                              2008038309

Publishing Director: Linda Belfus
Acquisitions Editor: William Schmitt
Developmental Editor: Katie DeFrancesco
Publishing Services Manager: Tina Rebane
Project Manager: Norm Stellander
Design Direction: Gene Harris

Working together to grow
libraries in developing countries

www.elsevier.com | www.bookaid.org | www.sabre.org

ELSEVIER   BOOK AID International   Sabre Foundation

Printed in China.
Last digit is the print number: 9 8 7 6 5 4 3 2 1

To my wife,

Doris Dewing,

whose belief in the value of this endeavor

never wavered

Preface

Readers will find the following work modest in its scope. It does not encompass the full range of clinical, pathological, and investigational information concerning diseases of the breast in encyclopedic detail, nor does it discuss the entire range of disorders that afflict the mammary gland. Several excellent texts of this type already exist, and I cannot improve upon them. Instead, I have set out three limited objectives. First, I have tried to record in both verbal and photographic format the morphologic characteristics of those mammary lesions commonly encountered in the practice of diagnostic surgical pathology. Second, I have endeavored to conceptualize lesions according to fundamental biologic processes and, in so far as possible, to categorize lesions according to these concepts. Identifying the underlying nature of a pathologic abnormality serves two purposes: it helps the diagnostician to shape the differential diagnosis, and it provides the context required to understand the origin and the significance of the morphologic characteristics. The analysis of these morphologic findings sometimes represents the most challenging element of the diagnostic process; therefore, I have set out a third objective: to offer a few lines of reasoning and points of general advice in the hope that they will assist pathologists when analyzing problematic cases. Drawn from the common wisdom and from personal experience, which includes occasional painful mistakes, these suggestions should serve as generalizations only, pertinent in certain situations but to be disregarded in others. I acknowledge that I have not met any of my goals completely. Nevertheless, I fervently hope that the information contained within these pages will make it easier for practicing pathologists to resolve certain of the diagnostic problems in breast pathology with confidence.

Many persons contributed to the creation of this book. I wish that I could acknowledge each of them by name and that I could recount the help that each of them offered, but space does not allow me this luxury. Nevertheless, with great pleasure and much appreciation I give credit to the following colleagues and collaborators.

Three eminent surgical pathologists of the latter part of the twentieth century inspired my study of mammary pathology. Dr. Robert E. Scully, Emeritus Professor of Pathology at Harvard Medical School and, until recently, the senior pathologist at the Massachusetts General Hospital, showed me the intellectual elegance and beauty inherent in the practice of academic surgical pathology. Dr. John G. Azzopardi, Emeritus Professor of Oncology at the Royal Postgraduate Medical School and formerly an Honorary Consultant in Pathology at the Hammersmith Hospital, demonstrated the power of detailed morphologic observation in the characterization of mammary lesions. Dr. Paul Peter Rosen, Professor of Pathology at Weill Medical College of Cornell University and Chief of Breast Pathology at New York Presbyterian Hospital-Cornell Medical Center, taught me the specific features of many mammary lesions and inspired me to try to discern the biologic mechanisms giving rise to these entities. From all three pathologists, I learned the importance of clear thinking and the need for critical reflection when evaluating both the common wisdom and one's personal observations, for, as Professor Azzopardi warned, "Experience can be merely the repetition of the same error often enough." It was the intellectual rigor in the pursuit of an understanding of mammary diseases shown by these scholars that inspired this young and callow pathologist to follow their lead.

The motivation to put these thoughts on paper came from many sources. Friends, family members, students, clinical colleagues, fellow pathologists, and trainees in the Department of Pathology at the Massachusetts General Hospital all encouraged me in many ways and at many times. Among the latter, Dr. Paula M. Arnell deserves special mention for her consistent and enthusiastic encouragement. Many ideas in these pages evolved during conversations with colleagues. Drs. Horacio M. Maluf and Melinda F. Lerwill listened to many off-beat ideas and unconventional notions with more patience and open-mindedness than one should expect even from friends. I must express my gratitude to these two intellectual companions for their interest, patience, generosity of spirit, and refusal to despair during our many exploratory discussions.

The text would never have materialized had Dr. Robert H. Young, Robert E. Scully Professor of Pathology at Harvard Medical School and Director of Gynecologic and Urologic Pathology at the Massachusetts General Hospital, not introduced me to the publishing staff at Elsevier and encouraged me at many points during my several years of writing. Mr. William Schmitt graciously but forcefully pried the manuscript from my hands, and Ms Katie DeFrancesco and Mr. Norman Stellander oversaw every detail of its transformation into the final text. To all, I express my heartfelt thanks.

FREDERICK C. KOERNER, MD

Contents

1

Introduction to the Diagnosis of Diseases of the Breast

Although diseases of the breast number relatively fewer than those affecting many organs, the field of mammary pathology challenges the histopathologist as much as any discipline in surgical pathology. The patient's signs and symptoms and the other clinical details of the case do not give the pathologist much more than general guidance regarding the nature of the lesion. The macroscopic examination might suggest a diagnosis in certain cases, but many of the most troublesome lesions cannot be seen with the unaided eye. Thus, it falls to the microscopist, and to the microscopist alone, to establish the diagnosis of the patient's disease. Guided primarily by one's knowledge of histopathology, one must distinguish the artifactual from the genuine, the reactive from the neoplastic, and the trivial from the life-threatening. This task requires a thoroughgoing understanding of the microanatomic structure of the mammary gland and the morphologic manifestations of mammary diseases. It takes patience, experience, and careful thought to develop this body of knowledge, but pathologists who undertake this endeavor will find themselves rewarded by an enhanced appreciation of the subtleties of mammary pathology.

One should begin one's study of diseases of the breast by mastering the microanatomy of the normal mammary gland. The author would encourage the reader to consult any standard textbook of histology to review the fundamentals of terminology and tissue organization. Neither poses much complexity, and experienced students will find them second-nature; yet even such basic principles as these play critical roles in the pathologist's study of breast tissue. Without knowledge of the composition of the breast, one will never detect the structural alterations that indicate the presence of a lesion. The nonspecialized stroma, for instance, usually consists of eosinophilic collagen, just a few fibroblasts, and rare chronic inflammatory cells. The presence of blue-gray myxoid material or a few unexpected cells within this stroma may represent the only clues to the presence of an invasive carcinoma.

Knowledge of mammary anatomy also allows one to understand the pathogenesis of certain lesions. For example, familiarity with the distribution of the glandular tissue and the organization of the glandular and stromal components make recognition of most hamartomas straightforward, and an understanding of the topologic relationships of the normal nonspecialized stroma allows one to comprehend the origin of the morphologic features of tumors derived from this tissue. Finally, once one understands the structure of the breast, one can appreciate the persistence of the normal organization in many benign alterations such as sclerosing and the obliteration of the normal relationships by malignant lesions such as cancers. Thus, the structures of the breast serve as a frame of reference that allows the pathologist to detect abnormalities, understand their development, and differentiate them from others showing superficial similarities.

Besides learning the anatomy of the gland, the pathologist must study the ways in which the normal gland changes with age. With the onset of ovulation, simple lobules sprout from small ductules, and each of these so-called *type I* lobules consists of little more than a coiled tubule with a few short stubby branches. Familiarity with the characteristics of these primitive lobules allows one to recognize them as the type of glandular tissue found in ectopic locations, such as the axilla and supernumerary nipples, as well as the variety of lobules that occasionally form in cases of gynecomastia. As the reproductive years come to an end and the menopause ensues, the glandular tissue shrinks, and the fibrous connective tissue turns to fat. These alterations leave acini embedded in adipose tissue in a pattern that superficially resembles the appearance of invasive well-differentiated carcinoma. Knowledge of the phenomenon of atrophy and its histologic features helps the pathologist from mistaking this age-related change as a carcinoma.

During the reproductive years, the breast undergoes a series of changes with each menstrual cycle, and pathologists will find it useful to become acquainted with these cytologic variations. The luteal phase brings about changes in scattered terminal duct–lobular units. The nuclei of the acinar luminal cells enlarge, and their nucleoli become especially prominent. A burst of mitotic activity takes place in the latter portion of the cycle, and a few days later, most of the newly created cells die. Pathologists can easily misinterpret the large nuclei and nucleoli, the increased nuclear-to-cytoplasm ratio, the division figures, and the apoptotic cells as evidence of carcinoma. The hormonal fluctuations that bring about these alterations of the normal cells also seem to affect other types of epithelial cells. Hyperplastic ductal cells and the epithelial cells of papillomas, for instance, can show unexpected nuclear enlargement, nucleolar prominence, and mitotic activity at this time of the cycle. One would have a difficult time disentangling the findings created by the superimposition of hormonal effects on other lesions without a secure appreciation of the appearance of the mammary epithelium at all stages of the menstrual cycle.

The information presented in histology texts serves the beginning pathologist well, but the experienced diagnostician requires a more detailed and nuanced understanding of the structure of the breast. Features such as the density of the glandular tissue, the ratio of ducts to lobules, the branching pattern and contour of the ducts, the size and shape of lobules, the cellularity of the stroma, the nature of the extracellular matrix, and the arrangement of the components of the gland, among others, serve as points of reference for the seasoned pathologist. Even subtle disturbances in the expected appearance of these attributes often signal the presence of an abnormality. For instance, an overly intimate positioning of epithelial cells and adipocytes or capillaries sometimes indicates the presence of an invasive carcinoma. Columns of malignant cells that look like distended ducts but branch in nonanatomic configurations probably represent invasive carcinoma, and fragmentation of collagen bundles or a disturbance in the pattern of their flow usually reflects the destructive growth of malignant cells. The discussions of diagnostic problems in the ensuing pages illustrate many examples of the way in which alterations in the fine points of mammary

structure contribute critical diagnostic information. The author cannot help the reader develop an understanding of these sophisticated aspects of mammary anatomy except to emphasize that such knowledge does not originate in a textbook. It comes only from untold hours at the microscope coupled with a constant reference to normal tissue and a conscious effort to nurture the growth of this understanding.

Although alterations in the structure of the breast indicate the presence of an abnormality, these anatomic deviations do not themselves provide much diagnostic information. An increase in the number of cells in the epithelium of a duct, for instance, could reflect an inflammatory process, a reaction to injury, a primary hyperplasia of ductal cells, or a neoplastic epithelial proliferation. To make specific diagnoses, pathologists must study the morphologic attributes of the cells in question. Because the resolution of many of the most difficult diagnostic problems requires an appreciation of subtle cellular characteristics, pathologists must work slowly and patiently and must make frequent use of high magnification. Diagnosticians attuned to the nuances of cytopathology will find themselves at home studying breast specimens. The remaining chapters of this work set out many of the specific cellular characteristics that serve as diagnostic criteria for certain common lesions; however, as a prelude, the author would remind the reader of a few well-known general points.

First, the comparison of pathologic structures or cells with their normal counterparts in the same specimen often makes subtle features, which might first appear minimal or perhaps even imaginary, stand out clearly. Most pathologists find it especially challenging to appreciate the slight enlargement of cells and their nuclei and the changes in chromatin texture that characterize neoplastic cells, but comparing the suspect cells with normal ones usually makes such findings clearer. The estimations of acinar size, lobular size, and glandular density all become easy if one follows this approach.

Second, pathologists must remain alert to the illusions created by off-center planes of section and by the structural disturbances caused by pathologic processes. As the intricately branching glands of the breast curve in and out of the tissue section, they can create the impression of epithelial stratification where none exists. Most pathologists have become so familiar with this artifact that they overlook it without noticing it, but the same phenomenon complicates the evaluation of the epithelium of fibroadenomas and papillomas. Disturbances of the stroma often distort the architecture of nearby glands, and alterations of glands can entrap stroma in ways that mimic the appearances of unrelated lesions.

The process of collagenous spherulosis can convert a lobule to a ductlike structure, and the distention of the peripheral acini of a lobule can reconfigure the intralobular stroma so that the focus looks like a papillary tumor growing in a small duct. Pathologists must not permit these illusions to interfere with their analysis of the pathologic changes.

Third, when studying cytologic characteristics, one must pay particular attention to the attributes of the nucleus, because no other subcellular structure offers a clearer insight into the nature of the cell. One should make note of the size and shape of the nuclei, their contours, the texture and staining qualities of their chromatin, the thickness of the nuclear membranes, and the characteristics of their nucleoli. These features vary somewhat from cell to cell, of course, so one must also study the variation of these properties within the population. Determining the average size of the nuclei and the range of their shapes elucidates important properties of an epithelial proliferation.

Fourth, the appreciation of subtle findings takes patient study. It sometimes requires the examination of many cells before one can conclude that the cytologic aberrations of a population of epithelial cells suffice for the diagnosis of malignancy, and the destructive relationship between the malignant cells of an invasive carcinoma and the underlying collagen may become evident only after the inspection of many clusters. Pathologists should not hesitate to examine additional sections of a suspicious focus, to submit additional tissue for histologic study, or to set aside uninterrupted time to study problematic cases. Furthermore, the fresh perspective that comes from a good night's sleep often helps clarify ambiguous cases.

Finally, immunohistochemical staining can provide critical information, but one must use this technique only in well-defined settings and one must interpret the results carefully. Antibodies to cytokeratin 5/6, for instance, have proved helpful in distinguishing conventional ductal hyperplasia from ductal carcinoma in situ, but one should restrict their use to foci in which the cells appear typical and grow in many layers. Especially florid forms of hyperplasia composed of large immature cells and flat proliferations of benign ductal cells both fail to express the protein. Staining with these antibodies in either situation invites an erroneous interpretation. Furthermore, pathologists must base their interpretation of immunohistochemical staining on experience rather than on expectation, no matter how well reasoned the latter.

Before relying on staining results to guide one in a difficult case, one must accumulate firsthand experience with the staining properties of normal mammary cells and well-characterized lesions. Assuming that all varieties of adenosis contain myoepithelial cells, one would misinterpret the absence of these cells in the glands of microglandular adenosis as proof of malignancy. On the other hand, the malignant cells of low-grade adenosquamous carcinomas typically express proteins present in myoepithelial cells, and ignorance of this characteristic could lead to an erroneous benign diagnosis in such a case. Pathologists may find that the use of panels of immunohistochemical stains permits more secure conclusions than staining for a single marker. When searching for myoepithelial cells, one might use a nuclear marker such as p63 protein in parallel with a cytoplasmic marker like myosin heavy chain; similarly, staining for keratin in conjunction with CD68 would allow one to distinguish invasive carcinoma cells from histiocytes.

Wise pathologists always integrate the results of immunohistochemical staining with the features observed in the conventional hematoxylin and eosin–stained sections, and the diagnosis suggested by the former must square with the interpretation of the latter. Immunohistochemical findings that seem to point in unexpected directions may represent spurious results or yet-undescribed phenomena. When the immunohistochemical features do not jibe with the conventional ones, this author bases his diagnosis on the traditional characteristics.

After detecting an abnormality and determining its characteristics, the pathologist must integrate the morphologic information to reach a diagnosis. When all the features of a case point in the same direction, their interpretation does not cause a problem; however, many specimens have inconclusive or conflicting findings, which bedevil even the most seasoned observer. Well-considered experience provides the best guide for resolving the ambiguous situations that so often arise in the practice of mammary pathology. Besides emphasizing the importance of experience, the author cannot do more than offer a few specific suggestions. For example, one should not expect all regions of a lesion to illustrate its diagnostic features equally. Ambiguous findings in one portion do not nullify convincing findings present in another, and one's diagnosis must rest on the characteristics of the most distinctive regions of the lesion. Moreover, cytologic features should probably carry more weight than structural or architectural ones. As a rule, malignant mammary cells display cytologic atypia, and one should usually refrain from making the diagnosis of malignancy unless one observes these aberrations. Developmental defects, pathologic processes, and iatrogenic forces can all displace benign epithelial cells into locations usually associated with carcinomas. One must not allow the unexpected position of these cells to over-rule their benign cellular attributes.

Pathologists must also keep their eyes on the entire context of the case, including the clinical details. The diagnosis of a small atypical ductal pro-liferation in an excision specimen might become obvious when compared with the remainder of the atypical population removed in a prior surgical pro-cedure. Marked nuclear enlargement and pleomor-phism of the type seen in high-grade carcinomas would not have the same significance in a patient who had undergone irradiation. Finally, pathologists learn a great deal from consultations with their col-leagues and discussions of difficult cases. Although pathologists base their diagnoses on more or less standardized criteria, they weight these observations differently and incorporate many other fine points of morphology derived from their own experiences into their analysis. Thus comparing thought processes and sharing personal wisdom about diagnostic problems will do more to enhance a pathologist's understand-ing of mammary pathology than any other single educational endeavor.

As a final point, the author would remind pathol-ogists that the histologic attributes of lesions do not represent random alterations of tissue and cellular structure. These features develop because the patho-logic processes that define the lesions alter the tissue in specific and characteristic ways. One can use the histologic findings to identify the underlying pro-cesses, and pathologists who master this ability will find that an appreciation of the fundamental nature of a lesion usually points to the proper diagnosis even in the presence of unexpected or conflicting evidence.

With these suggestions in mind, pathologists should feel well prepared to tackle the common diag-nostic problems of mammary pathology.

Selected Readings

Mills SE: Sternberg's Histology for Pathologists, 3rd ed. Philadelphia, Lippincott Williams & Wilkins, 2006.

Potten CS, Watson RJ, Williams GT, et al: The effect of age and menstrual cycle upon proliferative activity of the normal human breast. Br J Cancer 1988;58: 163-170.

Russo J, Rivera R, Russo IH: Influence of age and parity on the development of the human breast. Breast Cancer Res Treat 1992;23:211-218.

Part
I

EPITHELIAL PROLIFERATIONS

2

Concepts Basic to the Analysis of Epithelial Proliferations

The morphologic characteristics of epithelial proliferations arise from the interplay of several fundamental cellular properties. The ability to categorize these lesions depends on an understanding of these properties and of the histologic findings that spring from them. A thorough comprehension of the following five concepts provides pathologists with the foundation on which to develop their knowledge of the specific histopathologic features of epithelial proliferations.

CELLULAR PROLIFERATION

The histologic alterations produced by the proliferation of epithelial cells probably seem self-evident; nevertheless, two points merit elaboration. First, epithelial proliferation can lead to two different patterns. The more common and the more obvious pattern consists of an increase in the number of layers of cells, which causes filling of glandular lumens and distention of the glands (Fig. 2-1). The second, less commonly appreciated pattern of proliferation develops when the cells grow as a single layer rather than piling up (Fig. 2-2). This manner of growth causes enlargement of the structures without filling of their lumens; in fact, the lumens become distended and look like tiny cysts. The notion that such a pattern could reflect an increase in the number of cells strikes many observers as odd, but even an approximate calculation of the number of cells present on the walls of such structures makes clear that the epithelial cells have multiplied.

Of course, cellular proliferation does not underlie the formation of every distended gland. The microcysts that constitute a component of fibrocystic changes develop because of an imbalance in secretion and adsorption. One can recognize such cysts from the flat and inconspicuous appearance of their lining cells, features that contrast with those of cells lining proliferative glands (Fig. 2-3). The proliferative cells lining the latter crowd together, and this close packing causes them to assume columnar shapes. The nuclei become oval, and when extremely crowded, they sit at different positions in the cells, thereby creating a pseudostratified appearance. The cytoplasm collects at the apical pole of the cells and sometimes forms small blebs. When one observes cells with these characteristics lining distended glands, one can reliably identify the presence of cellular proliferation.

Second, pathologists must not misinterpret the apparent increase in the number of cell layers and the seeming compromise of the gland lumen created by an off-center plane of section of nonproliferative epithelium as evidence of cellular proliferation. The phenomenon often occurs at the ends of the profiles of longitudinally cut ducts as they curve out of the plane of section, at the points where ducts branch, and along the course of ducts distorted into unusual shapes (Fig. 2-4). Once one understands this artifact, its recognition becomes straightforward; however, attention to the following geometric principles will help inexperienced observers avoid this misimpression. Off-center sectioning cannot cause a duct or acinus to appear larger than its actual greatest dimension, whereas genuine proliferation usually leads to enlargement of the affected structure. Thus, an apparent accumulation of cells in a structure of normal size more often results from a tangential plane of section than from significant proliferation. Geometric considerations also make clear that one has a greater likelihood of cutting small structures tangentially than large ones. Thus, the recognition of proliferation rests most solidly on the evaluation of enlarged structures apparently cut in transverse section.

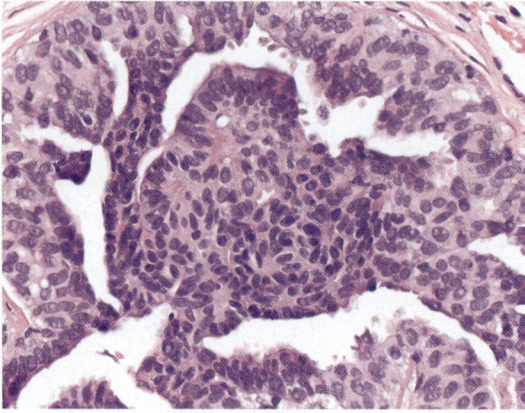

Figure 2-1 Stratification of these epithelial cells makes the presence of cellular proliferation obvious in this common pattern.

The phenomenon of cellular proliferation does not help distinguish among the forms of epithelial proliferations, because all of them represent proliferative processes. It stands to reason, though, that one should not consider any of these diagnoses in the absence of significant cellular proliferation except in specific, well-defined settings.

INTERCELLULAR COHESION

The property of intercellular cohesion refers to the adherence of cells to one another. Benign epithelial cells exhibit marked cohesion, whereas malignant ones stick together only loosely or not at all (Fig. 2-5). This difference in the level of adhesion accounts for certain differences in the morphologic characteristics of epithelial proliferations. For example, the marked

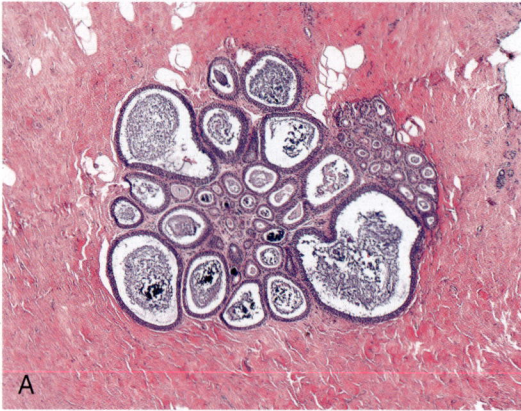

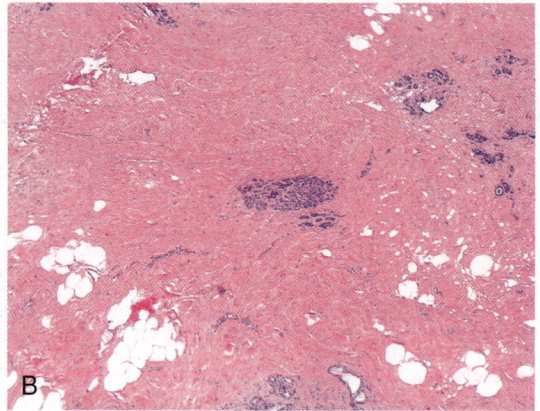

Figure 2-2 **A,** Pathologists may not recognize the presence of proliferation when the cells grow in a single layer. Comparison with an uninvolved lobule in **B,** however, highlights the increase in glandular size brought about by cellular proliferation.

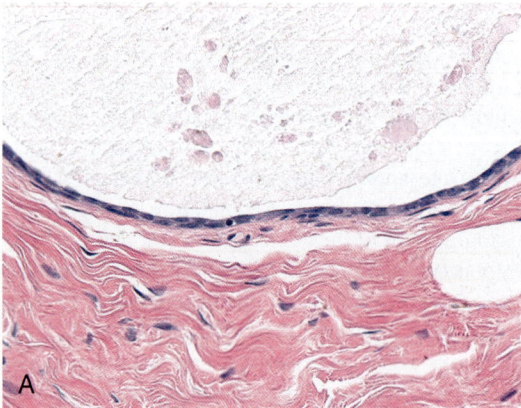

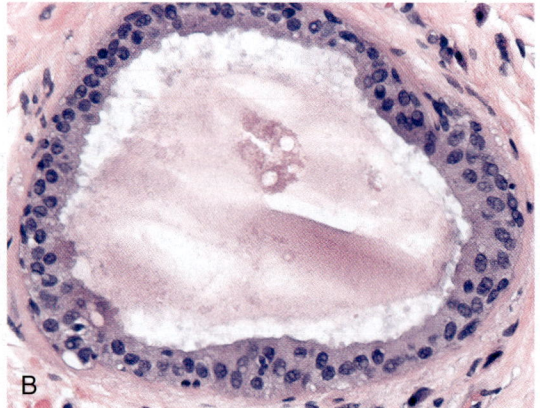

Figure 2-3 The morphologic attributes of the cells lining distended glands reveal the nature of the process causing the enlargement. **A,** The cells lining microcysts formed by an imbalance in secretion and absorption appear flattened. **B,** Cell lining glands distended because of cellular proliferation appear enlarged and closely packed.

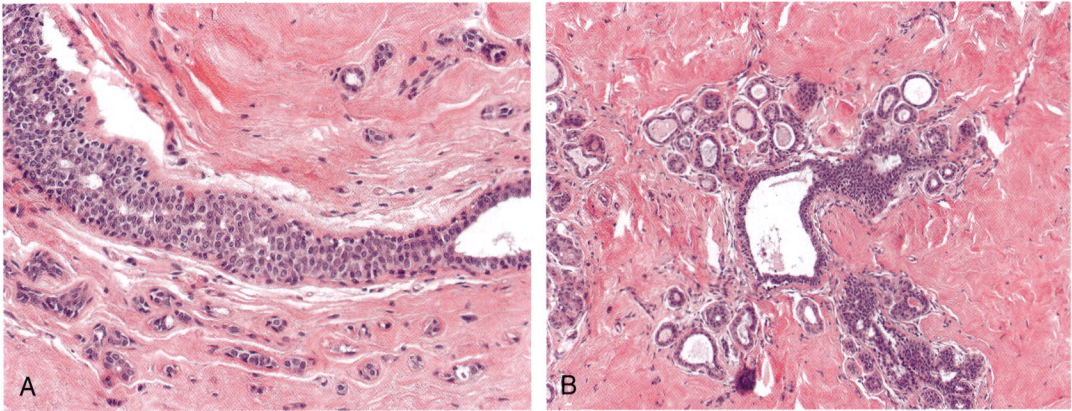

Figure 2-4 Off-center planes of section of transversely running ducts in **A,** branching ducts in **B,** and distorted ducts in **C** can create illusions of cellular stratification and filling of gland lumens.

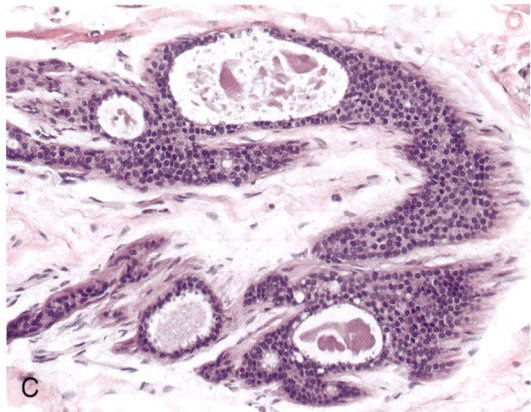

Figure 2-5 A, Benign cells form cohesive aggregates, in which the cells do not separate and the lumen appears free of individual cells and debris. **B,** Clusters of malignant cells tend to separate from one another and fall into the lumen.

cohesion of hyperplastic cells causes them to deform one another and thereby gives rise to variation in cell placement and cell and nuclear shape. This stickiness also prevents them from detaching from their neighbors and falling into the glandular lumen. Lacking this same level of cohesion, carcinoma cells cannot distort one another; therefore, their nuclei appear uniform and

regular in shape, and these dishesive cells frequently separate from one another.

The recognition of dishesion requires a bit of care. When cut in certain planes, tufts of epithelial cells look like separate groups of cells unattached to one another and to the wall of the affected gland (Fig. 2-6). One should not interpret such seemingly detached clusters

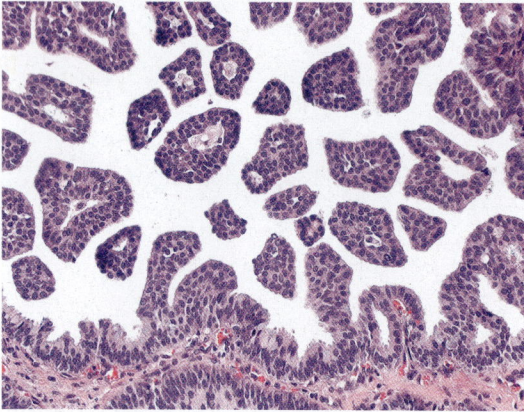

Figure 2-6 When cut in certain planes, micropapillary tufts can look like separate aggregates, but one must not regard this pattern as evidence of dishesion.

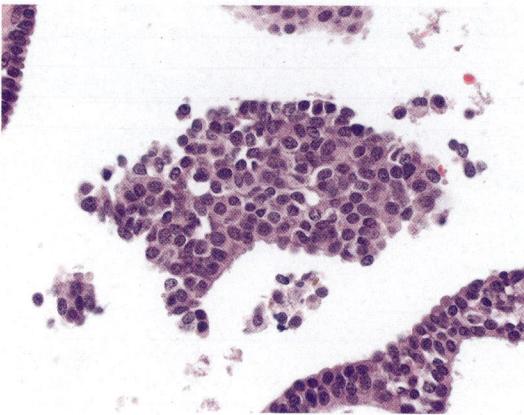

Figure 2-7 Fraying of the borders of cellular groups, separation of individual cells, and necrosis of detached cells reveal the loosely cohesive nature of these carcinoma cells.

as evidence of dishesion; instead, one should pay close attention to the cells at the edges of the cell clusters. Peripherally situated dishesive cells sometimes appear partially separated from adjacent cells or completely detached but still close to the cell cluster (Fig. 2-7). Once freed from their neighbors, the cells undergo degeneration. Cohesive, benign cells do not display these features.

CELLULAR POLARIZATION

The phenomenon of cellular polarization is a state of organization of a cell in which subcellular regions take on different functions and, therefore, different morphologic appearances. Polarization of a glandular cell causes the nucleus to occupy the region near the basement membrane (the basal pole) and the cytoplasm to collect at the opposite end (the apical pole), where it forms an apical cytoplasmic compartment. All normal luminal cells display polarization, and so do the cells of low-grade ductal carcinoma in situ (Fig. 2-8). Thus, the presence of polarization does not distinguish neoplastic cells from normal ones. Furthermore, the absence of polarization does not differentiate benign cells from malignant ones, either, because neither hyperplastic ductal cells nor neoplastic lobular cells appear polarized (see Fig. 2-8). Despite these limitations, the analysis of cellular polarization provides critical information for identifying the nature of an epithelial proliferation.

CYTOLOGIC ATYPIA

Cytologic atypia consists of a variety of cellular alterations that one observes in malignant cells but not in normal ones. The changes range from subtle, barely recognizable alterations of chromatin structure to obvious cellular pleomorphism. Although individual cases differ in their expression of specific atypical characteristics, the features of cytologic atypia tend to coexist in consistent clusters, which pathologists classify as low-grade (mild), intermediate-grade (moderate), or high-grade (severe). Common to almost all examples of cytologic atypia is the enlargement of the cell. An increase in the amount of cytoplasm accounts for part of this increase. In certain low-grade carcinomas, this phenomenon represents the only factor leading to the increase in cell size; however, more typically, an increase in the size of the nucleus also contributes to the cellular enlargement.

Cells showing low-grade atypia appear only slightly larger than normal and they possess smoothly contoured, oval or round nuclei of uniform size, homogeneous and finely dispersed chromatin, inconspicuous nucleoli, and ample amounts of eosinophilic cytoplasm (Fig. 2-9B). Cells characterized by high-grade atypia look obviously enlarged; the nuclei also appear enlarged and have irregular contours. The nuclear sizes and shapes typically vary considerably from one cell to the next, and the chromatin usually looks clumped and granular. Many nuclei contain one or more prominent nucleoli, which also look irregular and pleomorphic (Fig. 2-9D). Cells with high-grade atypia contain more cytoplasm than normal cells, but the nuclear changes often eclipse the cytoplasmic ones.

Between these two extremes lies intermediate-grade atypia (Fig. 2-9C). This degree of atypia does not display consistent characteristics, and this inconstancy makes it impossible to describe intermediate-grade atypia precisely. One typically observes cellular and nuclear enlargement; however, the nuclei can appear either regular or irregular in shape and either smooth

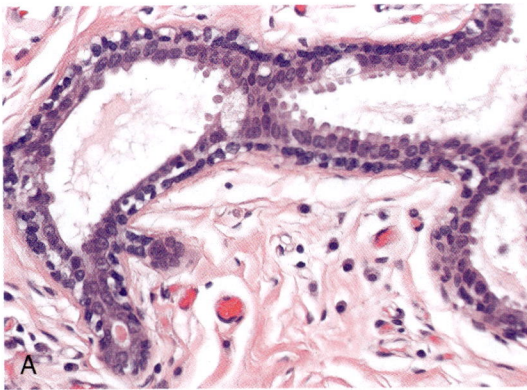
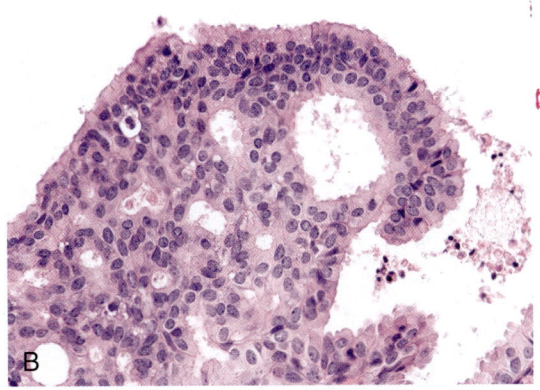

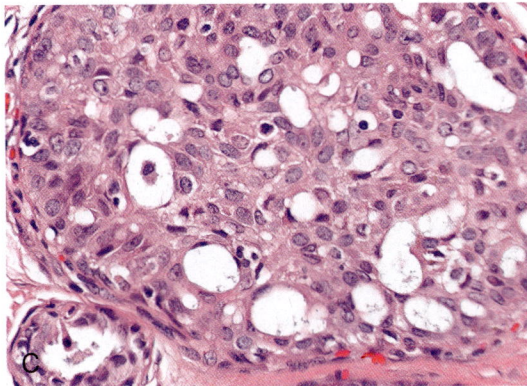
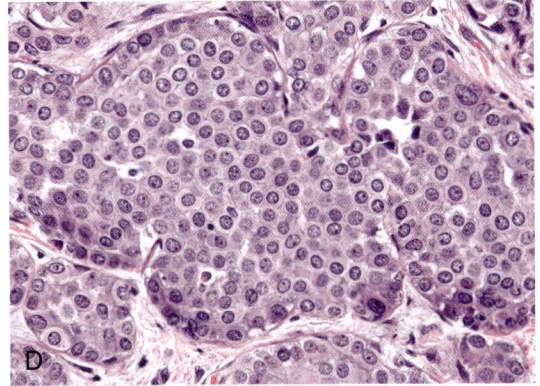

Figure 2-8 Luminal cells lining the small duct in **A,** exhibit polarization and so do the cells of the ductal carcinoma in **B.** The hyperplastic ductal cells in **C,** on the other hand, do not display this property, nor do neoplastic lobular cells in **D.**

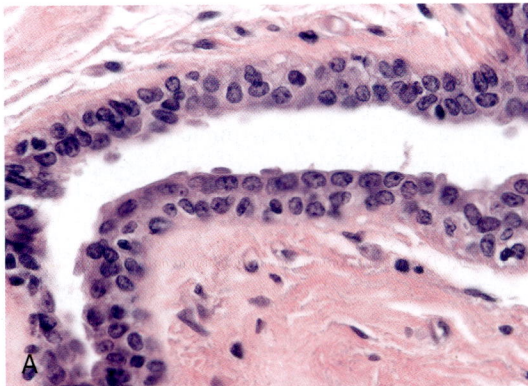
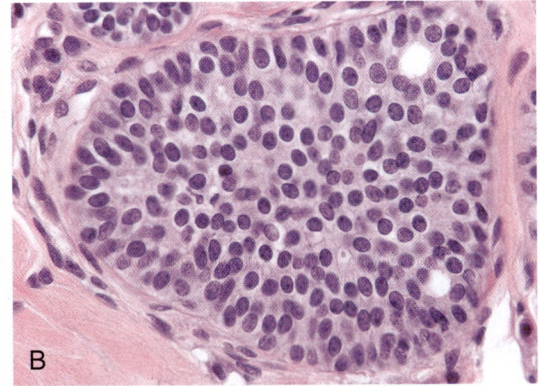

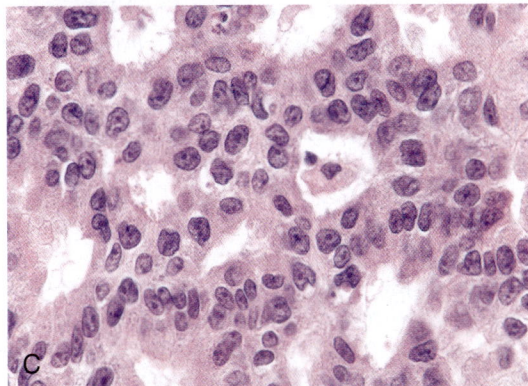
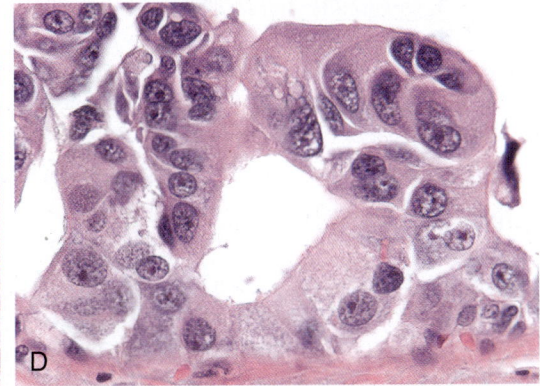

Figure 2-9 Contrast the characteristics of normal cells in **A** with the attributes of cells showing low-grade atypia in **B,** intermediate-grade atypia in **C,** and high-grade atypia in **D.**

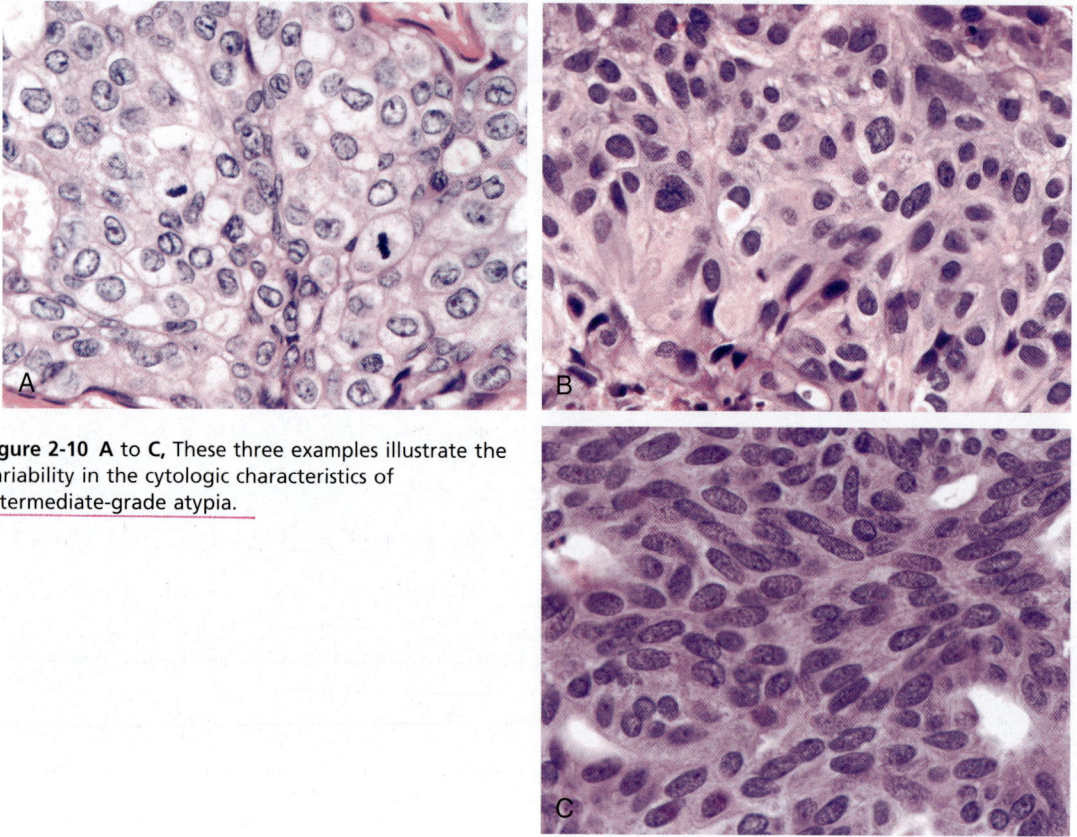

Figure 2-10 A to **C,** These three examples illustrate the variability in the cytologic characteristics of intermediate-grade atypia.

or jagged in contour, the chromatin either pale or dark in staining intensity and either granular or fine in texture, and the nucleoli either small or large (Fig. 2-10). Intermediate-grade atypia represents the most difficult form of cytologic atypia to learn to recognize.

Among the morphologic findings used in the analysis of ductal epithelial proliferations, cytologic atypia stands out as the most influential. One cannot classify an epithelial proliferation as either atypical or malignant in the absence of cytologic atypia. Students of breast pathology should therefore devote the necessary time and thought to the study of the many "faces" of cytologic atypia, for mastery of these features serves as the foundation of the analysis of mammary epithelial proliferations.

ARCHITECTURAL ATYPIA

The fifth phenomenon, architectural atypia, refers to deviation from the two-layered structure of the normal mammary epithelium. Multiplication of epithelial cells gives rise to varying structural patterns, which assume different forms depending on the degree of the proliferation, intercellular cohesion, and cellular polarization. Pathologists describe the architectural patterns produced by the proliferation of cohesive, nonpolarized, benign ductal cells as *typical, usual,* or *conventional* and those arising from the growth of dishesive, polarized cells as *atypical* (Fig. 2-11). Precision would probably favor regarding the former, conventional pattern as minimally atypical, for it does represent a deviation from the normal, two-layered structure of mammary epithelium; however, pathologists do not usually hew to this thinking. Instead, they reserve the concept of architectural atypia for only the more extreme examples of this phenomenon. Like the evaluation of proliferation, the assessment of architectural atypia requires constant guard against mistaking the appearance created by an off-center plane of section of normal epithelium as an atypical architectural pattern (Fig. 2-12). Evaluation of transversely sectioned, distended structures allows for the most secure assessment of architectural atypia.

The architectural patterns created by an epithelial proliferation provide important diagnostic information, but one must remember that the diagnostic significance of the architectural characteristics of a ductal proliferation never overrides the significance of the cytologic features.

Hyperplastic   *CA*

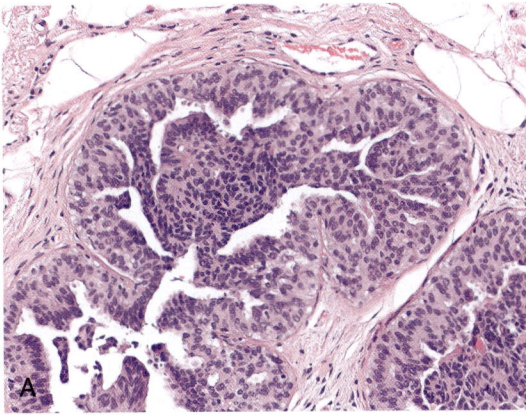

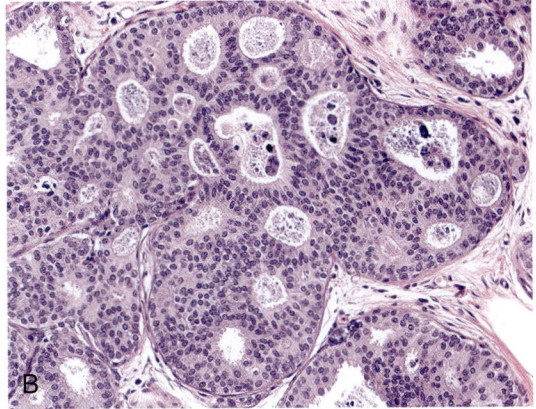

Figure 2-11 Pathologists regard the architectural pattern produced by hyperplastic ductal cells in **A** as typical and the one created by carcinoma cells in **B** as atypical.

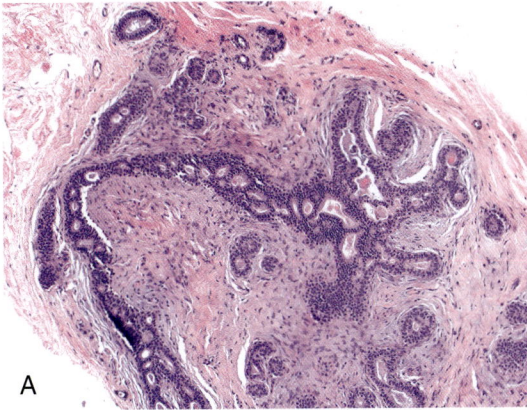

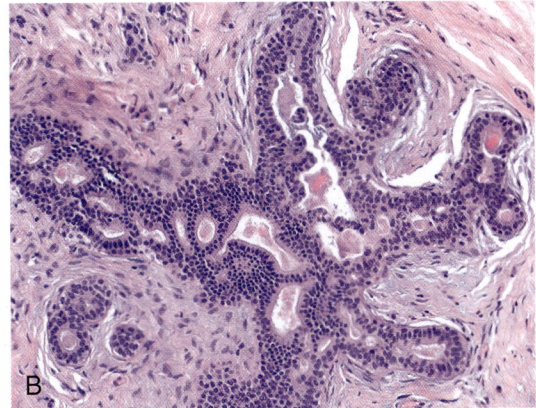

Figure 2-12 A and **B,** An off-center plane of section of the branching duct creates the false impression of architectural atypia.

Not atypical

CONCLUSION

Besides mastering these five concepts and learning how to apply them, pathologists would do well to keep in mind the following three practical observations derived from the experience of many observers:

- Individual microscopic fields of a case usually do not demonstrate all the characteristics of the lesion.
- One cannot depend on a single criterion or even a small group of criteria to classify all epithelial proliferations correctly.
- Tables of criteria cannot replace experience, reflection, and consultation.

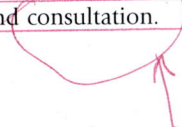

For these reasons, one must examine the entirety of the lesion, evaluate all its characteristics, and base the diagnosis on thoughtful consideration of the evidence, including the clinical details, rather than on slavish obedience to lists, algorithms, charts, or atlases.

Selected Reading

Azzopardi JG: Problems in Breast Pathology. (Major Problems in Pathology, vol 11.) London, WB Saunders, 1979.

3

Conventional Ductal Proliferations

DEFINITIONS AND CLINICOPATHOLOGIC CHARACTERISTICS

Usual Ductal Hyperplasia

Ductal hyperplasia represents a proliferation of primitive mammary epithelial cells. It occurs both as an isolated finding and in association with other lesions. As a component of the fibrocystic complex, ductal hyperplasia most commonly affects women during their reproductive years. One occasionally observes ductal hyperplasia in an older or younger woman, but such a situation should prompt the pathologist to search for an explanation. The use of hormone replacements, for example, could account for the presence of ductal hyperplasia in a postmenopausal woman, and the entity known as juvenile papillomatosis could explain its occurrence in women younger than 30 years. As a secondary phenomenon, conventional ductal hyperplasia also commonly coexists with pseudoangiomatous stromal hyperplasia, radial scars, and phyllodes tumors.

Conventional ductal hyperplasia does not commonly give rise to clinical signs or symptoms. Associated processes such as fibrosis and cyst formation can create palpable or radiologic abnormalities, but the proliferative ductal cells do not make themselves known to the patient or her physicians. Breast tissue harboring ductal hyperplasia also does not look or feel abnormal on macroscopic examination.

Ductal Carcinoma In Situ

Ductal carcinoma represents a neoplastic proliferation of malignant gland-forming cells. The cells recall their glandular heritage by displaying the phenomenon of polarization, and this property leads to glandular characteristics not evident in hyperplastic cells.

The observation that ductal carcinoma cells display greater glandular differentiation than hyperplastic cells strikes many beginning students of pathology as paradoxic. One must remember that ductal carcinoma develops from cells committed to luminal differentiation, whereas ductal hyperplasia arises from uncommitted, pluripotent epithelial cells. The hyperplastic cells never realize their potential to differentiate, but the carcinoma cells do so to varying degrees.

Ductal carcinoma in situ affects adult women of all ages; the mean age at the time of detection falls in the sixth decade. Before the institution of mammographic screening, the majority of cases came to clinical attention because of the presence of a mass. Today, mammographic calcifications disclose the lesion in many instances, and it represents an incidental finding in most of the rest. Unusual presentations include a mass, a discharge from the nipple, and Paget's disease of the breast. If untreated, most cases of ductal carcinoma in situ progress to invasive carcinoma.

Occasional examples of high-grade ductal carcinoma in situ incite marked periductal inflammation, which creates a palpable, firm mass evident to the patient, clinicians, and pathologist. Necrotic debris can accumulate in such massive amounts that the ducts exude pasty, yellow-white, or tan material upon being cut. Except in these circumstances, one cannot appreciate the presence of ductal carcinoma in situ with the naked eye.

Relationship between Ductal Hyperplasia and Ductal Carcinoma In Situ

The belief that conventional ductal hyperplasia represents an early step in the formation of ductal carcinoma in situ remained widely held and unquestioningly accepted throughout much of the twentieth century. A few eminent breast pathologists, such as Drs. McDivitt and Azzopardi, voiced skepticism about this view, but their objections largely went unnoticed. Newer studies of genetic alterations and cytokeratin profiles of conventional ductal hyperplasia and ductal carcinoma in situ have not disclosed evidence of a biologic continuum between these two lesions. It therefore seems that we should follow the lead of these earlier pathologists and abandon the concept of a continuum linking conventional ductal hyperplasia with ductal carcinoma in situ. Instead, it would seem that ductal hyperplasia represents a biologic dead end and that low-grade ductal carcinoma in situ usually arises from another setting.

HISTOLOGIC CHARACTERISTICS

Usual Ductal Hyperplasia

Usual ductal hyperplasia consists of a population of primitive mammary epithelial cells capable of both glandular and myoepithelial differentiation. They do not express this potential to any noticeable degree. The cells do not become polarized, for example, nor do they form glandular lumens or express the keratin molecules or other proteins characteristic of myoepithelial cells. Instead, the cells grow in tightly cohesive clusters and structureless, fenestrated sheets of bland and nondescript cells. The marked cohesion, lack of cellular polarization, and lack of cytologic atypia of the population give rise to architectural and cytologic characteristics that serve as the basis for the diagnosis.

Architectural Characteristics

Four architectural attributes characterize conventional ductal epithelial hyperplasia: ductular distention by central masses of cells surrounded by crescent-shaped spaces, irregular fenestrations within the cell masses, a streaming arrangement of the cells, and maturation (Box 3-1).

Ductular Distention by Central Masses of Cells Surrounded by Crescent-Shaped Spaces

Ductal hyperplasia seems to begin at independent points around the perimeter of a ductule. Accumulation of the hyperplastic cells leads to stratification and the formation of mounds and tufts (Fig. 3-1). As the level of proliferation increases, the cells form bands that traverse the lumen (Fig. 3-2). In more advanced examples, the cells form a mass in the center of the ductule, and the architectural pattern characteristic of ductal hyperplasia blossoms: a distended ductule containing a central mass of cells

---

Box 3-1

Architectural characteristics of conventional ductal epithelial hyperplasia:

- Central masses of cells surrounded by crescent-shaped spaces
- Irregular fenestrations
- A streaming arrangement of the cells
- Maturation

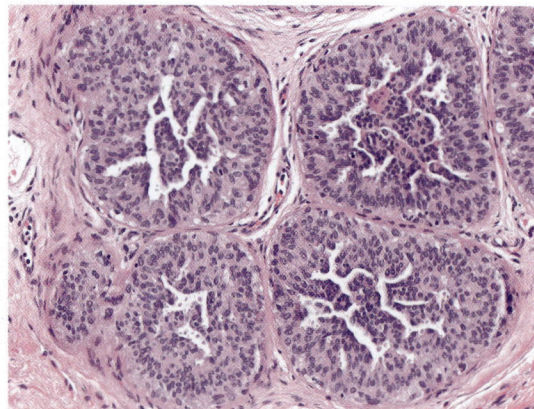

Figure 3-1 These hyperplastic ductal cells pile up and form mounds and tufts.

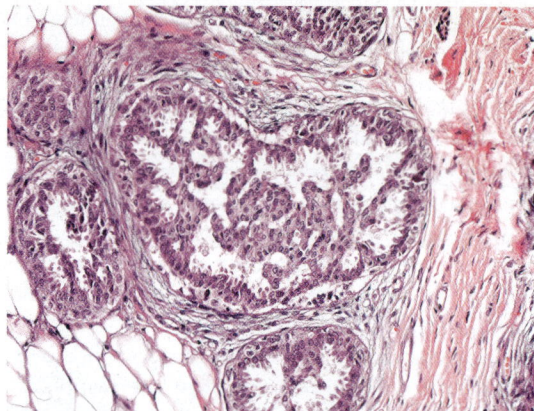

Figure 3-2 Hyperplastic ductal cells grow as bands traversing the lumen of the ductule.

---

supported by cellular struts and surrounded by curving, flattened spaces (Fig. 3-3). This architectural pattern so consistently indicates a benign proliferation that a diagnosis of carcinoma in situ for an epithelial proliferation showing this structure requires the presence of other incontrovertible evidence of malignancy.

The arrangement of the cells in the central mass offers important diagnostic clues. The cells usually form irregular spaces, and the cells occasionally

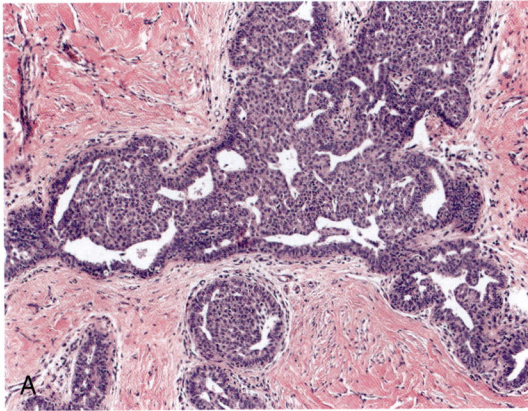

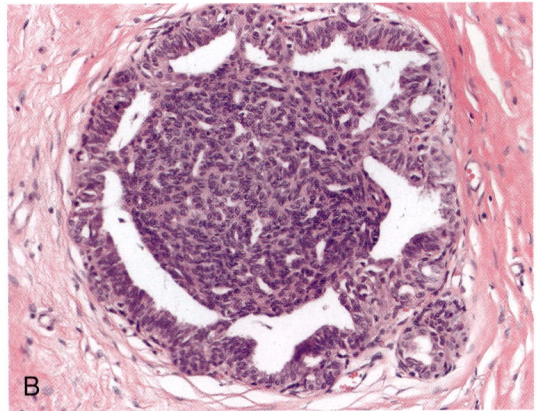

Figure 3-3 A to **C,** These three examples of florid ductal hyperplasia illustrate its fully developed architectural pattern: a mass of cells containing internal fenestrations, supported by struts, and surrounded by flattened, crescent-shaped spaces.

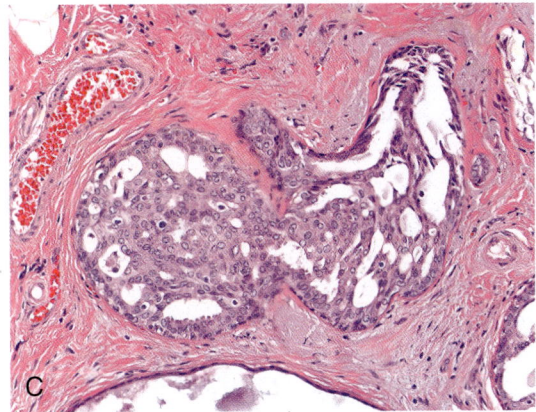

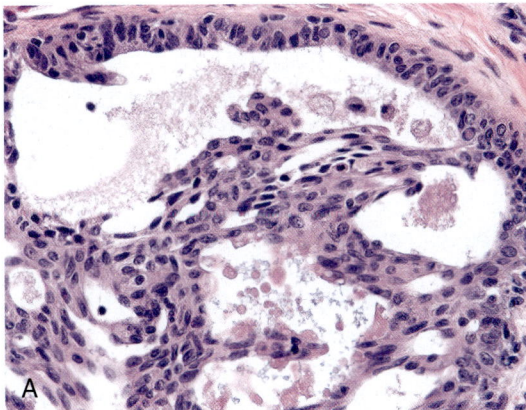

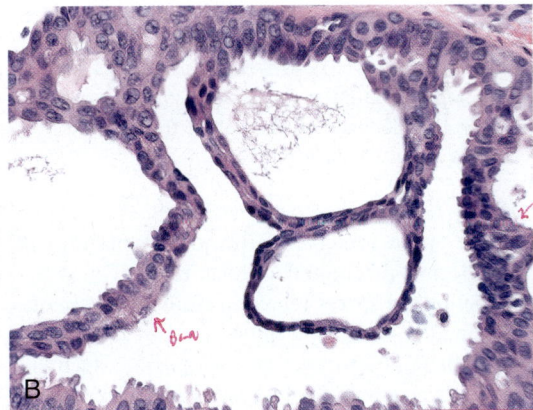

Figure 3-4 A, The long axis of the nuclei in these spindle cell bridges run in the direction of the bridge. **B,** The carcinoma cells in the center of the field form a few bands that closely resemble benign spindle cell bridges; however, the bars at either side reveal the malignant nature of the proliferation.

display patterns referred to as streaming and maturation; subsequent paragraphs elaborate on both of the latter features in detail. The struts supporting the mass and the strands of cells traversing the ductule can also yield information. Because of their cohesion, the cells in these structures become stretched and attenuated as they multiply, and their nuclei tend to adopt an orientation parallel to the long axis of the structure.

The struts and strands often taper so that their centers become thinner than their ends. Cellular bars showing these characteristics go by the name *spindle cell bridges*. Their presence usually indicates a hyperplastic proliferation, but rare ductal carcinomas exhibit similar structures (Fig. 3-4).

Findings at the periphery of an involved ductule or acinus usually provide several diagnostic clues.

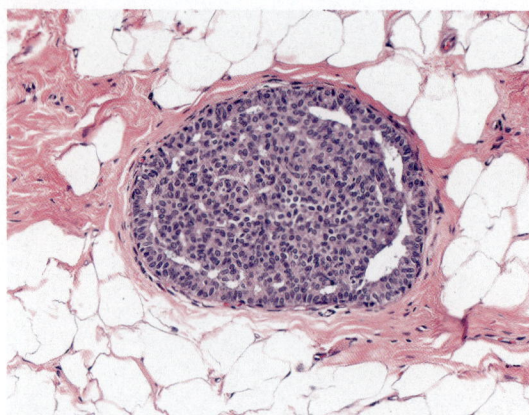

Figure 3-5 A series of flattened, curving spaces surround this mass of hyperplastic cells.

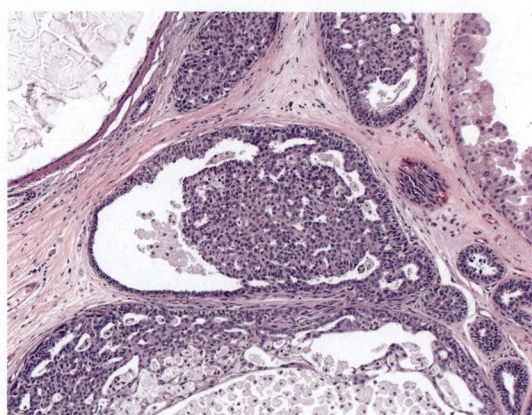

Figure 3-6 The space at the left of this mass of hyperplastic cells clearly represents the lumen of the affected ductule, and so do the compressed spaces to the right of the mass.

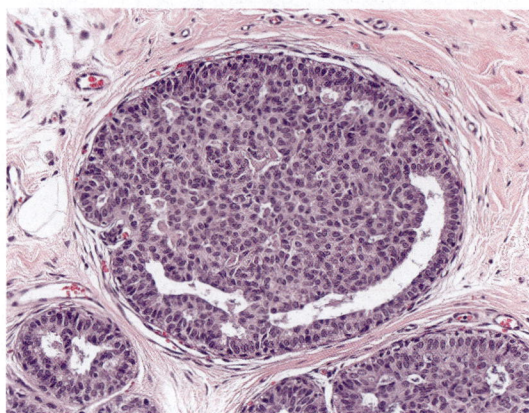

Figure 3-7 A few residual, polarized, columnar luminal cells form a single layer on the wall of this ductule overrun by hyperplastic ductal cells.

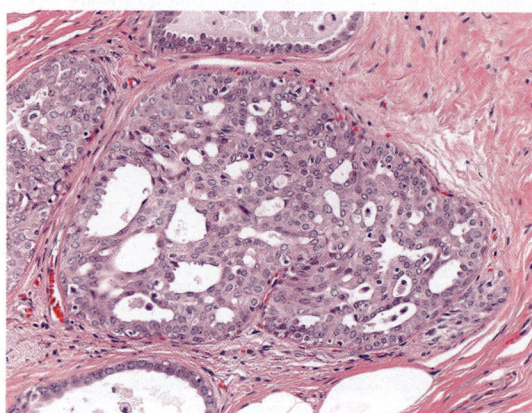

Figure 3-8 This mass of hyperplastic cells contains irregular fenestrations often referred to as secondary spaces.

Flattened spaces frequently form an interrupted ring enclosing the central cellular mass (Fig. 3-5). These peripheral spaces represent residual fragments of the ductular lumen still unoccupied by the hyperplastic cells (Fig. 3-6). At times, preexisting ductular epithelial cells remain on the basement membrane of these spaces (Fig. 3-7). One can recognize these preexisting cells from their arrangement in a single layer and their polarized appearance. This orderly arrangement and polarized nature can lead the inexperienced observer to regard these cells as polarized atypical ductal cells or even ductal carcinoma. To avoid this mistake, one must remember that residual luminal cells do not possess the atypical nuclei present in atypical or malignant ductal cells. In most foci of ductal hyperplasia, the preexisting ductular epithelial cells do not persist. The hyperplastic ductal cells spread along the basement membrane and obliterate the indigenous population.

Irregular Fenestrations

The central masses of hyperplastic cells usually contain fenestrations or spaces commonly referred to as *secondary* (Fig. 3-8). Pathologists adopted this term because they mistakenly believed that the spaces represent newly formed lumens, which do not communicate with the lumen of the involved ductule, the *primary space*. In fact, reconstruction studies have shown that the spaces within the cell masses do communicate both with the lumen of the ductule and with one another. Like the crescentic spaces surrounding the cell masses, the fenestrations within the masses represent regions of the primary (ductular) lumen unoccupied by the hyperplastic population. Originating as haphazardly preserved remnants of the ductular lumen, these spaces have inconsistent and irregular shapes. Many exhibit a slitlike configuration in which the sides of the spaces run approximately parallel to each other (Fig. 3-9). The compressed, narrow configuration arises because

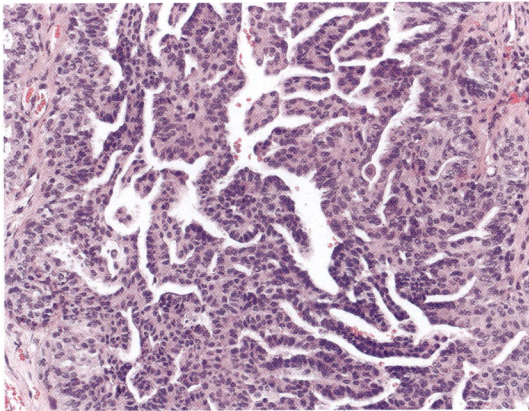

Figure 3-9 Because the aggregates of cells tend to run parallel to one another, the spaces have slit-like shapes, and these serpentine spaces give the masses an appearance often described as collapsible.

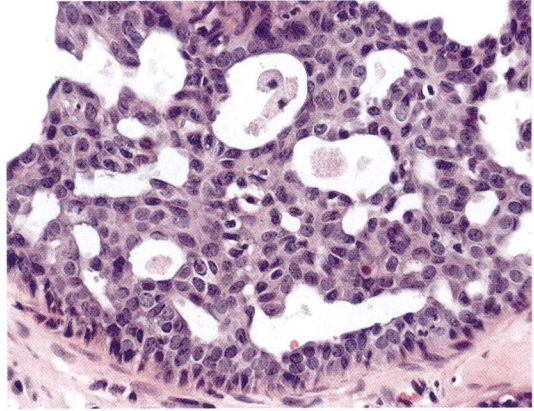

Figure 3-10 Hyperplastic cells do not display the phenomenon of polarization. Their nuclei do not occupy the base of the cells, nor does cytoplasm collect near the lumen.

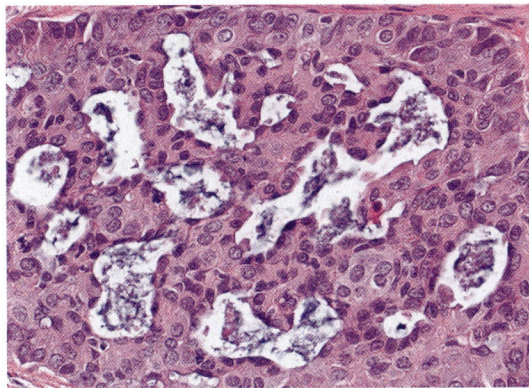

Figure 3-11 Hyperplastic nuclei appear compressed against the cell membranes without deforming the contours of the cells or bulging into the spaces. The long axes of the nuclei run parallel to the perimeter of the spaces.

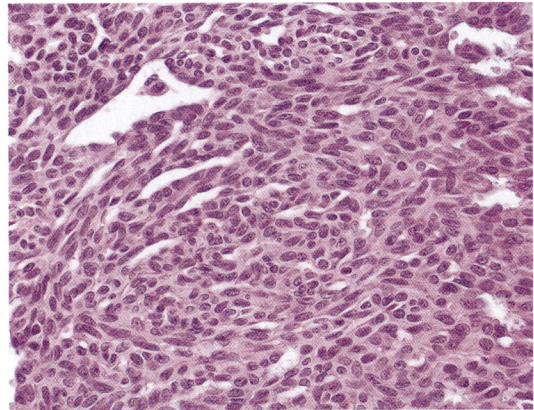

Figure 3-12 The nuclei of these hyperplastic ductal cells run parallel and thereby create a streaming pattern.

the cell clusters accommodate to the shapes of their neighbors as they enlarge. This molding of the groups narrows the space between them to thin, serpentine channels, which look like slits in tissue section.

Although the inconsistency and irregularity in the shapes of the spaces represent an important architectural feature of hyperplasia, the lack of polarization of the cells surrounding the spaces provides the most powerful and reliable information about the nature of the proliferative cells. Unlike normal luminal cells and those of low-grade ductal carcinoma in situ, hyperplastic cells do not display polarization (Fig. 3-10). They do not have basal nuclei or well-developed apical cytoplasmic compartments, nor do their nuclei sit with their long axes radially oriented with respect to the spaces. Instead, the nucleus of such a cell most often resides just beneath the luminal aspect of the cell membrane, sometimes pressed against the

membrane yet not deforming it (Fig. 3-11). If the nucleus has a long axis, it commonly runs around the perimeter of the space rather than in a radial orientation. This flattening of the nucleus against the cell membrane requires solid anchoring of the cell to its neighbors; less cohesion among the cells would allow their nuclei to bulge into the lumen, thereby deforming the contour of the cells while preserving the round shape of the nucleus.

Streaming

Cells within the hyperplastic masses and the supporting struts sometimes exhibit an appearance known as *streaming*. The term refers to an arrangement in which elongate cells containing fusiform nuclei run roughly parallel to one another, an appearance resembling a school of fish (Fig. 3-12). Often, the streaming arrangement appears focal or subtle, and it can take several forms, depending on the structure of

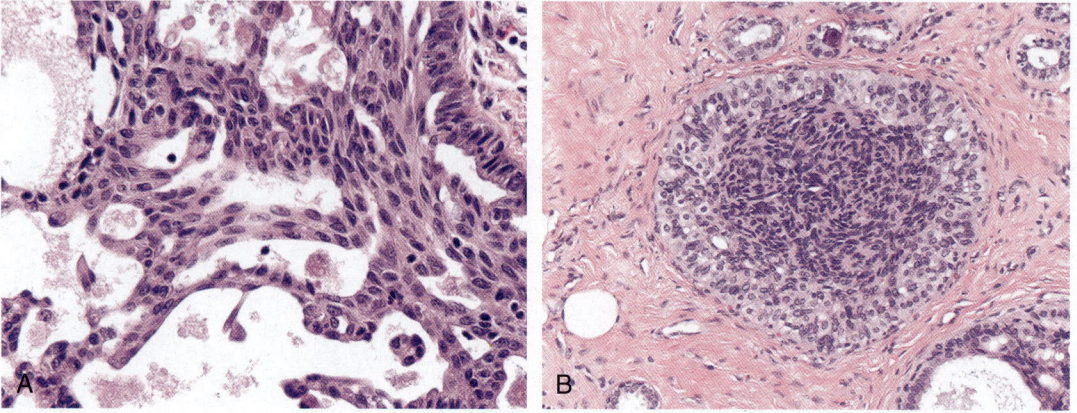

Figure 3-13 A, The nuclei in certain of these bridges stream in the direction of the bridge. **B,** The nuclei in the solid aggregate stream in a circular direction.

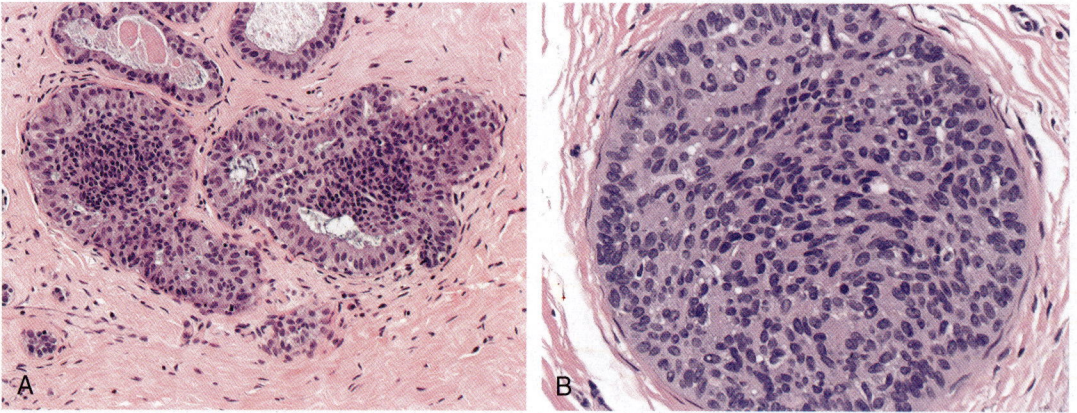

Figure 3-14 A and B, The cells in these ductules display the pattern of maturation. The cells in the center appear smaller and closely packed, and they contain small dark nuclei and dense, eosinophilic cytoplasm.

the underlying cell mass. In bridges and struts, the long axis of the cells parallels the long axis of the structure, and the cells seem to flow in the direction of the bridge (Fig. 3-13A). If the cells grow in mounds or solid aggregates, the cells tend to stream in a circular direction, producing concentric layers suggesting the appearance of a cut onion (Fig. 3-13B).

Maturation

The cells within the central masses of hyperplastic cells occasionally display a characteristic gradient of morphologic changes termed *maturation*. In this pattern, the cells along the basement membrane, which constitute the proliferative population of the mammary epithelium, appear large and active. They possess large pale nuclei, prominent nucleoli, and abundant pale cytoplasm, and they sometime show division figures. As the cells move toward the center of the ductule, they become smaller and more closely packed; their nuclei smaller, darker, and more irregular; and their cytoplasm reduced in amount and more

deeply eosinophilic (Fig. 3-14). Observers have suggested that these alterations arise because the cells lose their proliferative potential and mature, but the literature does not contain direct evidence to support this suggestion.

Whatever the nature of these changes, the presence of maturation generally indicates a benign ductal proliferation, but the interpretation of this pattern requires careful consideration and certain qualifications. First, one observes the obvious and fully developed appearance in only a minority of cases of ductal hyperplasia, so the absence of this finding does not exclude that diagnosis. Second, rare carcinomas simulate maturation because their central cells appear smaller and possess smaller, darker nuclei than the peripheral ones. These central cells do not look completely mature, however; they lack the irregular nuclear spacing, the very dense chromatin, and the deeply eosinophilic cytoplasm seen in genuine examples of the phenomenon (Fig. 3-15). With these cautions kept in mind, one can regard the

Figure 3-15 The appearance of this example of low-grade ductal carcinoma in situ resembles the pattern of maturation. Although the central cells have smaller and darker nuclei than the peripheral cells, the central nuclei do not appear as condensed as the nuclei seen in genuine maturation.

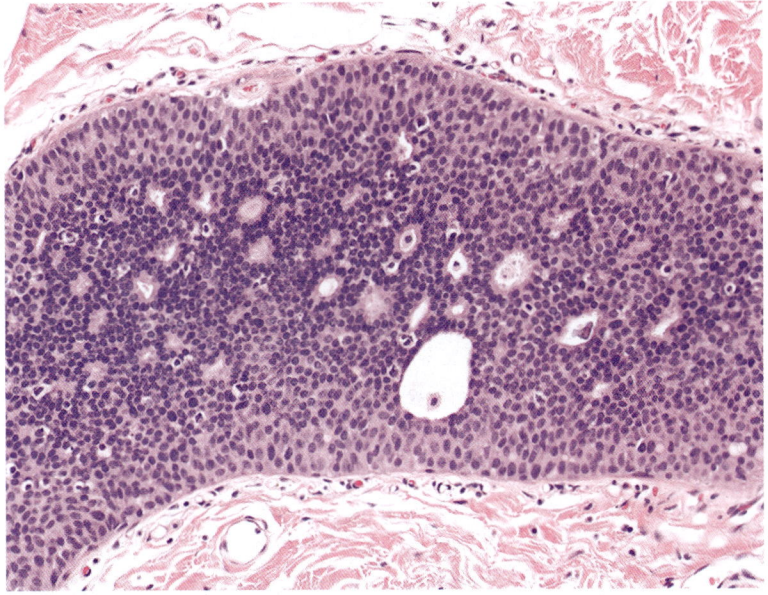

presence of maturation as strong evidence of the benign nature of a proliferation.

Cytologic Characteristics

Most hyperplastic cells do not show convincing evidence of either glandular or myoepithelial differentiation; therefore, they appear nondescript (Box 3-2). One cannot usually see cell membranes, so the cell masses have a syncytial appearance (Fig. 3-16). The nuclei display an irregular distribution, and they cluster and overlap even in 5-µm sections (Fig. 3-17). Their shapes vary from elongate through oval to reniform, folded, or convoluted; they usually do not appear round, nor do they look uniform (Fig. 3-18).

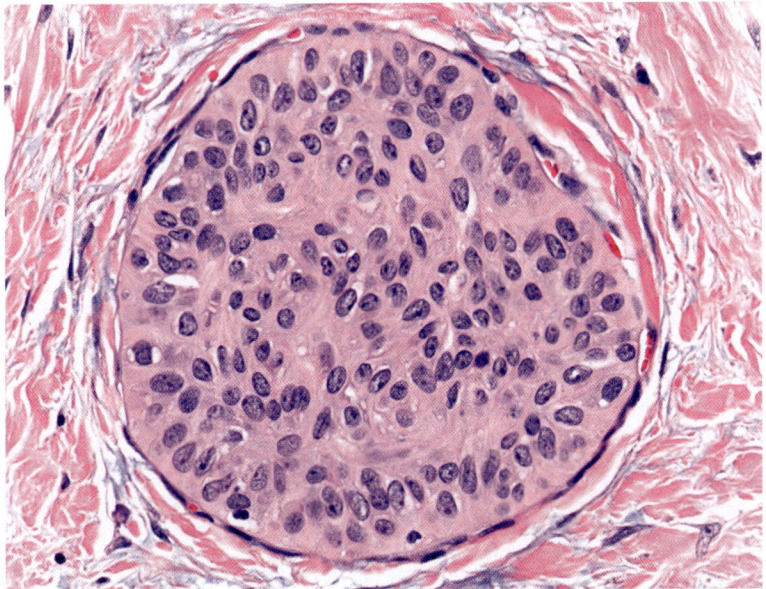

Using high magnification, one can identify folds, notches, and grooves in the nuclei (Fig. 3-19). The nuclear membranes appear uniform in thickness. The chromatin pattern varies from nucleus to nucleus. Many nuclei have granular chromatin, which often shows some clearing, whereas others, usually constituting a small minority, have finely dispersed chromatin. Most nuclei contain a single, easily seen, round or oval nucleolus.

The nuclei sometimes contain eosinophilic inclusion bodies of an unknown nature (Fig. 3-20). Only extremely rarely does one observe these so-called *helioid bodies* in conventional low-grade carcinoma cells. The nuclei of high-grade carcinoma cells,

Figure 3-16 Because one has difficulty identifying the cells' membranes, foci of ductal hyperplasia take on a syncytial appearance.

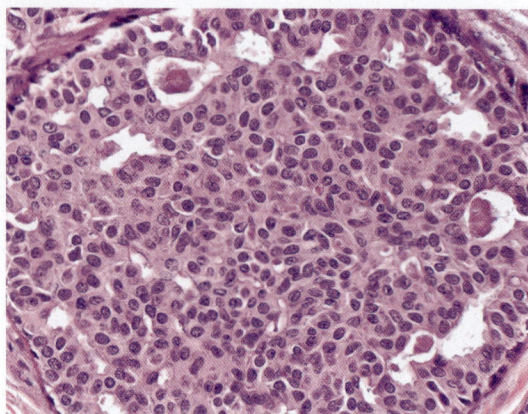

Figure 3-17 The nuclei in this focus of ductal hyperplasia appear unevenly distributed.

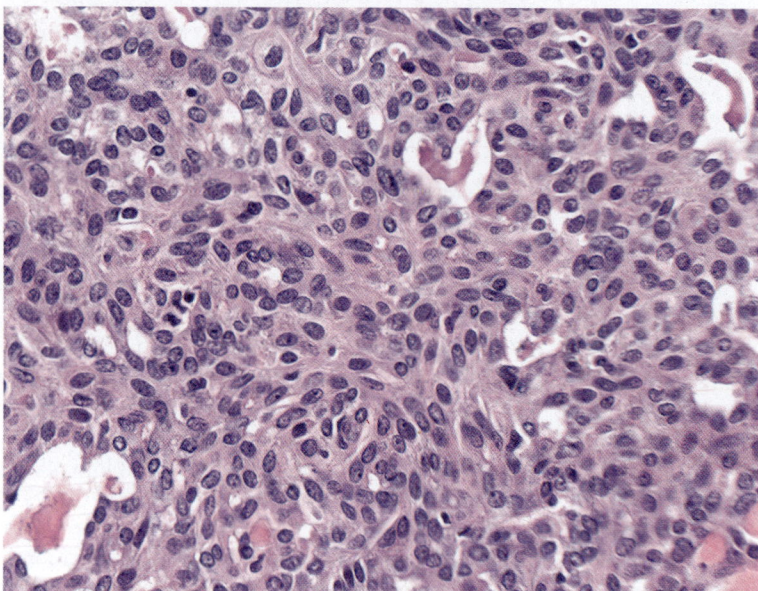

Figure 3-18 These hyperplastic nuclei vary in both their shape and the staining intensity of their chromatin.

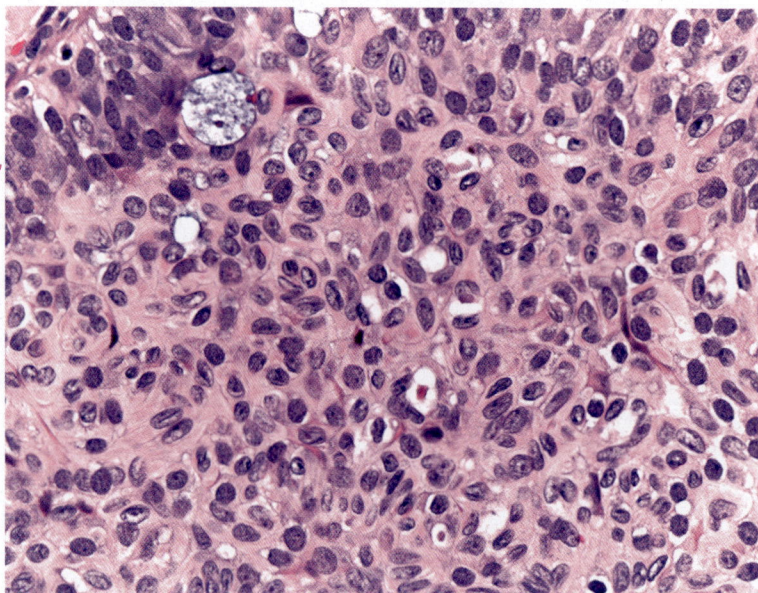

Figure 3-19 The presence of folds, notches, and groves gives the nuclei of these hyperplastic cells irregular contours.

Figure 3-20 Several hyperplastic nuclei in **A** contain eosinophilic pseudoinclusions; two atypical apocrine cells in **B** and one irradiated luminal cell in **C** do, also.

See p. 324
Complex spear
in malignant cells.

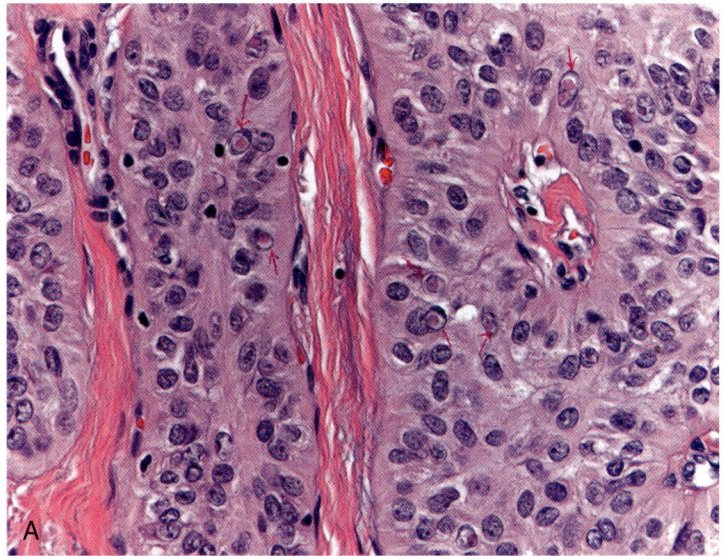

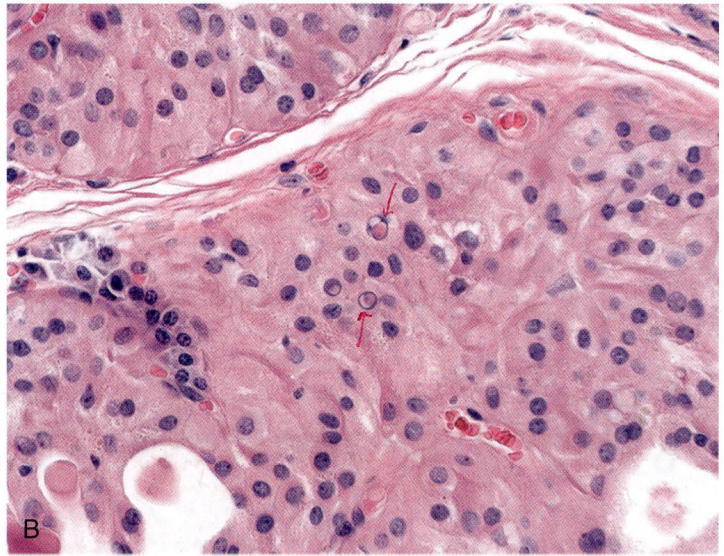

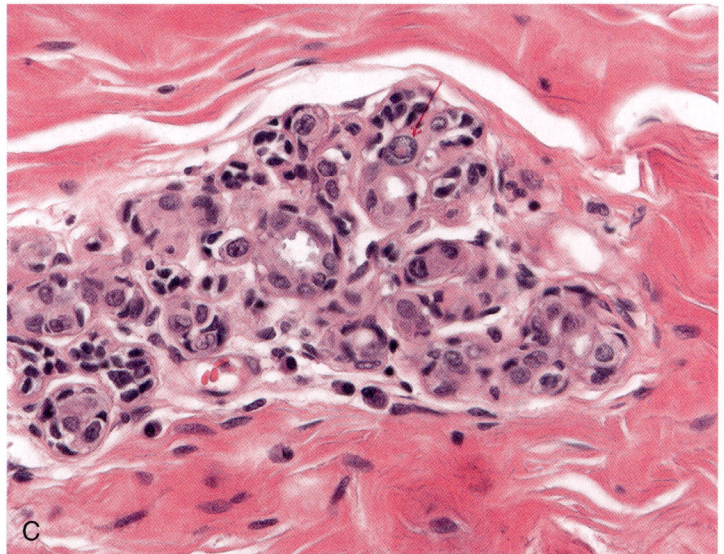

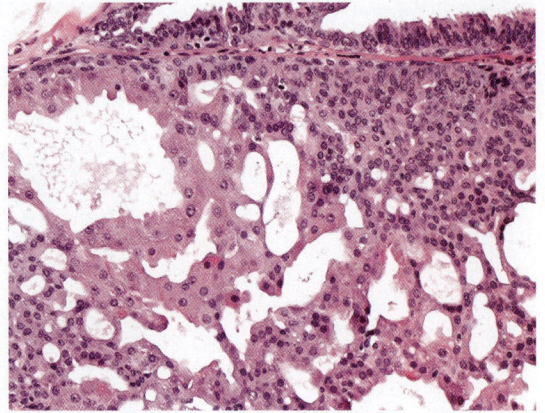

Figure 3-21 The intermingling of apocrine cells with ductal cells usually identifies the latter as benign.

endocrine carcinoma cells, neoplastic apocrine cells, and irradiated benign cells can all display similar intranuclear inclusions, but their presence in a proliferation of bland ductal cells strongly favors a benign diagnosis. Especially florid examples of ductal hyperplasia can show normal-appearing mitotic figures in cells near the basement membrane, but one does not observe atypical mitotic figures in cases of conventional ductal hyperplasia. The cytoplasm varies from eosinophilic to amphophilic; almost never does it appear clear.

A few hyperplastic cells sometimes have features suggestive of glandular or myoepithelial differentiation. Those with glandular features have polygonal shapes and eccentric, round, pale nuclei, whereas cells with myoepithelial attributes look fusiform and contain oval, hyperchromatic nuclei and densely eosinophilic cytoplasm. Cell exhibiting these characteristics should constitute a tiny proportion of a hyperplastic population. An epithelial proliferation containing a noticeable fraction of well-developed glandular or myoepithelial cells probably does not represent conventional ductal hyperplasia.

Ancillary Characteristics
Three findings not intrinsic to the hyperplastic cells can provide diagnostic clues: intermixed apocrine metaplasia, calcifications, and necrosis.

Intermixed Apocrine Metaplasia
Foci of ductal hyperplasia sometimes mingle with foci of apocrine metaplasia. Although the absence of this finding does not carry significance, the intermingling of proliferative ductal cells and conventional apocrine cells provides strong evidence supporting the diagnosis of ductal hyperplasia (Fig. 3-21). Pathologists must keep two cautions in mind when evaluating the significance of this finding. First, the apocrine cells must mingle with the proliferative ductal cells intimately. Ductal carcinoma in situ can abut foci of apocrine metaplasia, of course, and one would not want to dismiss the presence of the malignant cells in this situation. Second, uncommon ductal carcinomas have apocrine features; thus, the intermixed apocrine cells must look like conventional apocrine cells rather than atypical apocrine cells. Acknowledging these two

limitations, pathologists will find that the commingling of conventional apocrine cells and proliferative ductal cells usually indicates the benign nature of the latter.

Calcifications
Calcifications, especially those of the psammomatous type, do not usually form in ductal hyperplasia. One observes calcium precipitates in benign lesions that do not show epithelial stratification, such as sclerosing adenosis, microcysts, papillomas, and fibroadenomas, and in many cases of ductal carcinoma in situ. Rare cases of conventional ductal hyperplasia do contain calcium crystals. Because one observes such cases so infrequently, one might wonder how conventional ductal hyperplasia could ever come to contain calcifications. It seems possible that certain examples arise from the engulfment of preexisting calcifications, which originally formed in association with another process, such as microcyst formation or adenosis (Fig. 3-22). Such exceptional cases notwithstanding, the presence of calcifications that seem to arise within an epithelial proliferation should lead one to suspect the presence of an atypical or malignant ductal proliferation.

Necrosis
Most examples of conventional ductal-type epithelial hyperplasia do not exhibit necrosis, although one can see it in radial scars, nipple adenomas, and juvenile papillomatosis. Since carcinomas frequently show necrosis, the presence of this finding in an epithelial proliferation always requires an explanation. If the lesion in question displays the characteristics of one of these three benign lesions and the proliferative cells display the characteristics of benign cells, then one can make one of these benign diagnoses confidently. Much more often, the cells exhibit features of

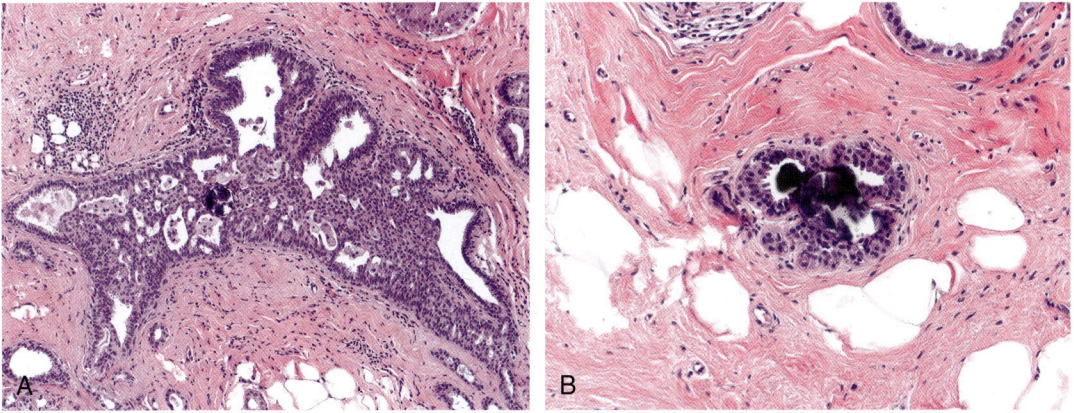

Figure 3-22 The focus of hyperplasia seen in **A** contains a calcification. This finding probably originated when hyperplastic ductal cells engulfed a preexisting calcification like the one shown in **B**.

malignancy and thereby lead to the diagnosis of carcinoma.

Uncommon Characteristics

Cases of conventional ductal hyperplasia do not vary a great deal in their morphologic characteristics, but rare examples exhibit unexpected findings and thereby create diagnostic uncertainty. For example, one occasionally observes a few round spaces, a bit of luminal mucin, or cells with signet ring morphology in a proliferation showing other characteristics of conventional ductal hyperplasia.

Round Spaces

The spaces formed by hyperplastic cells exhibit a wide range of sizes and shapes. Because of this variability, one occasionally encounters a few round or nearly round spaces (Fig. 3-23). Such spaces do catch the eye when one is working at medium power, and

they do require careful study to determine the characteristics of the cells surrounding the spaces. If these cells display the morphologic features of hyperplastic cells, the presence of a rare round space need not detract from the diagnosis of conventional ductal hyperplasia.

Mucin

Hyperplastic ductal cells do not produce mucin as frequently as carcinoma cells, therefore, the presence of mucin should alert the pathologist to the possibility of malignancy. This finding serves an especially helpful role in the recognition of solid papillary carcinoma, a type of low-grade carcinoma commonly misinterpreted as ductal hyperplasia or atypical ductal hyperplasia. Without wishing to diminish the value of the general practice of regarding the presence of mucin with suspicion, one must acknowledge that occasional bona fide cases of ductal hyperplasia do show slight mucin production. Figure 3-24 illustrates

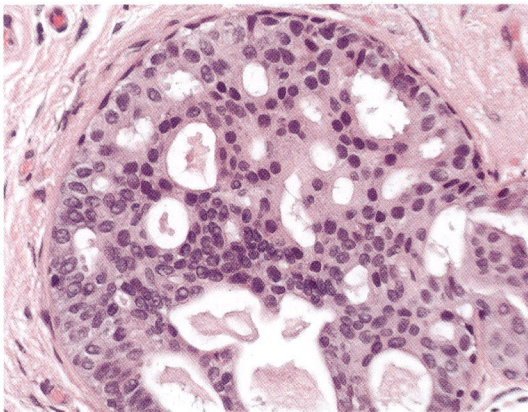

Figure 3-23 The presence of round spaces like those formed by these hyperplastic ductal cells should not dissuade one from making a benign diagnosis.

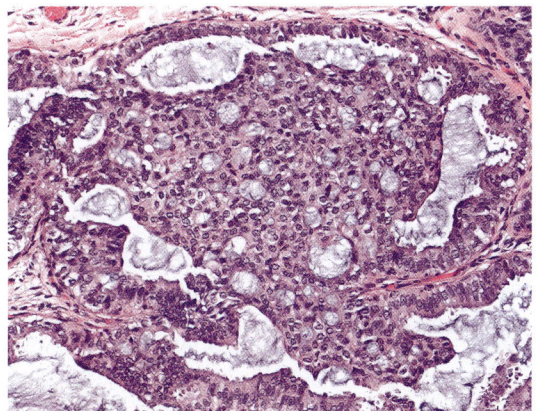

Figure 3-24 Mucin fills the fenestrations in this focus of ductal hyperplasia.

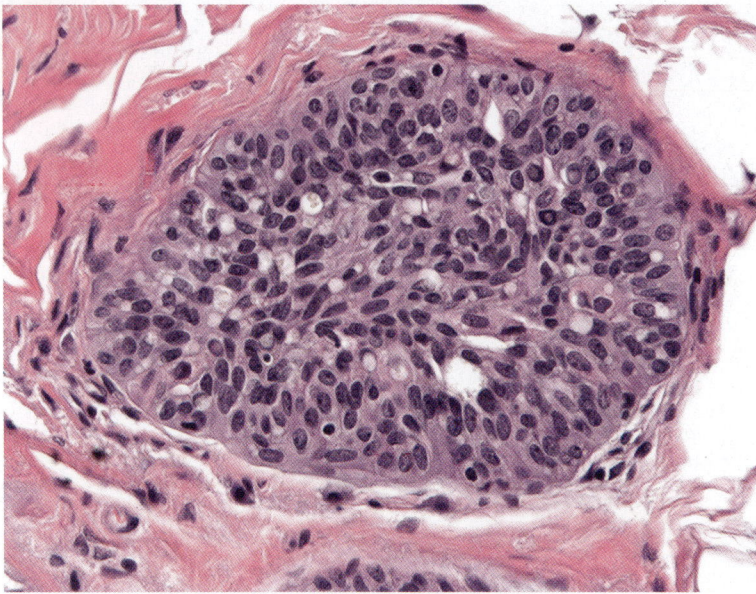

Figure 3-25 The presence of vacuoles in these hyperplastic cells has created signet ring cells.

such a case. Thus, the finding of mucin in an epithelial proliferation should prompt a careful consideration of the other histologic findings. If they favor the diagnosis of hyperplasia, the presence of a modest amount of luminal mucin should not alter this impression.

Signet Ring Cells

Benign epithelial cells do not commonly take on a signet ring appearance. Infrequently, apocrine cells can accumulate a large, subluminal cytoplasmic vacuole; even less commonly, hyperplastic ductal cells can do so (Fig. 3-25). Although these cells superficially resemble genuine signet ring cells, the nuclear characteristics of these signet ring—like cells indicate their benign nature. Like the presence of mucin in an epithelial proliferation, the observation of cells with large vacuoles should provoke a thorough search for other features of malignancy. If the results of such an investigation fail to disclose other sinister findings and instead indicate a benign diagnosis, then one can make it without qualification.

Low-Grade Ductal Carcinoma In Situ

Low-grade ductal carcinoma consists of a proliferation of mammary epithelial cells exhibiting the characteristics of ductular luminal cells. Because of their polarized nature, these carcinoma cells consistently display better-developed glandular characteristics than hyperplastic cells; moreover, the carcinoma cells lack the marked intercellular cohesion of hyperplastic cells. This loosely cohesive property and the tendency of

---

Box 3-3

Architectural characteristics of low-grade ductal carcinoma in situ:

- Formation of cribriform spaces and their variants
- Regular placement of cells

---

the cells to recapitulate the structure of glands or ductules give rise to characteristic architectural and cytologic features.

Architectural Characteristics

The architectural atypia of low-grade ductal carcinoma in situ takes two forms, the formation of cribriform spaces and their variants, and the regular placement of the cells and their nuclei (Box 3-3). The former arises because of the polarized state of the neoplastic cells, and the latter develops because of their dishesive nature.

Cribriform Spaces and their Variants

Cribriform spaces represent neoplastic glands formed by the malignant population. Observers usually describe them as uniform, round, and punched-out. Although mostly accurate, these three adjectives overlook the most important characteristic of a cribriform space: the polarization of the cells creating the space. It is this phenomenon of polarization of the cells around the space, rather than the characteristics of the space itself, that defines it as cribriform. Polarized glandular cells have basally positioned nuclei and apical cytoplasmic compartments. When a group of polarized cells forms a cribriform space, the consistent basal position of the nuclei and the formation of apical cytoplasmic compartments create a rosette configuration. If the cell has a columnar shape, the nucleus usually appears oval, and the long axes of the cell and its nucleus exhibit a radial orientation with respect to the space (Fig. 3-26). The nuclei seem to sit on the spokes of a wheel that converge on the center of the cribriform space.

One must take care not to regard spaces formed by cells growing in a single layer on a basement membrane as cribriform (Fig. 3-27). Normal ductal cells and, possibly, certain carcinoma cells use basement membrane proteins as a point of reference when establishing a polarized configuration. The region of the cell in contact with these molecules becomes the base of the cell, and the opposite side takes on luminal characteristics such as the formation of tight junctions and microvilli. Cribriform spaces arise when cells establish a polarized state in the absence of recognizable basement membrane proteins; therefore, one must search for cribriform spaces in regions of cellular stratification. This ability to establish cellular polarity and thereby to create cribriform spaces in the absence of the organizing influences of basement membrane proteins distinguishes malignant ductal cells from all other cells of the breast. Thus, the formation of genuine cribriform spaces within masses of cells represents an especially

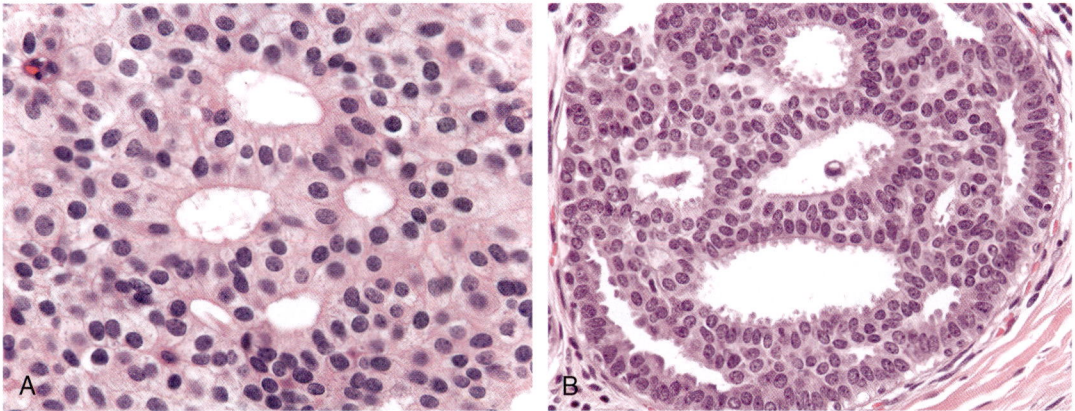

Figure 3-26 **A,** The nuclei of the cells forming the cribriform space in the center of the field have basal nuclei and apical cytoplasmic compartments. **B,** The long axes of the nuclei exhibit a radial orientation with respect to the spaces.

Figure 3-27 The cells growing on the basement membrane of the wall of the duct display polarization; nevertheless, one must not regard the space created by these cells as cribriform. The spaces in the upper right corner of the field represent genuine cribriform spaces.

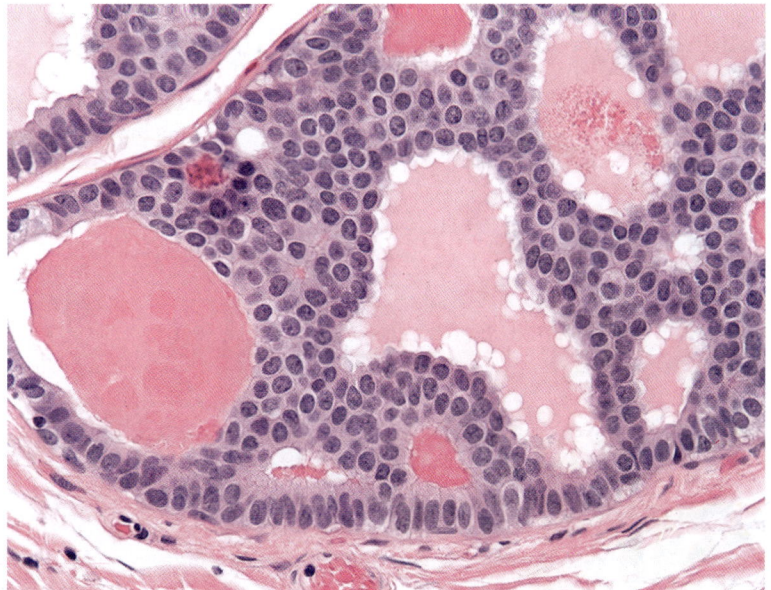

important architectural characteristic of low-grade ductal carcinoma in situ.

Three other architectural patterns, each also arising as a result of cellular polarization, represent variants of cribriform spaces; they are trabecular bars, cartwheel formations, and Roman bridges. A *trabecular bar* consists of a column of cells in which the long axes of the nuclei lie perpendicular to the long axis of the bar (Fig. 3-28). If one determined the nuclear orientation in reference to the adjacent space, however, one would see that the nuclei of a trabecular bar have a radial orientation with respect to the space. Thus, trabecular bars represent cribriform spaces viewed from a different point of reference. The same line of reasoning allows one to recognize the *cartwheel* pattern (Fig. 3-29) as a series of peripheral, especially large, cribriform spaces, and the *Roman bridge* pattern (Fig. 3-30) as trabecular bars arching around the periphery of a distended duct. As variations on the concept of a cribriform space, these three other patterns carry the same diagnostic implications.

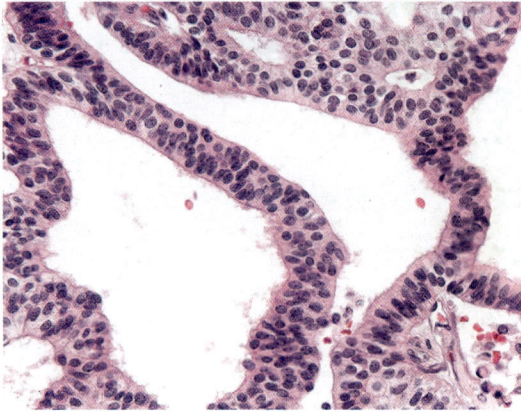

Regular Placement of Cells

Regularity in the placement of the cells and their nuclei, the second manifestation of architectural atypia, reflects the loosely cohesive property of the neoplastic cells. Because they stick together only slightly and cannot deform one another, carcinoma cells tend to grow as smoothly contoured, spherical units with round, central nuclei. When sectioned, the cells therefore appear uniform, evenly spaced, and round or polygonal, and the nuclei, too, appear uniform, centrally located, smoothly contoured, and round or oval (Fig. 3-31). One observes this regularity in most conventional patterns of low-grade ductal carcinoma in situ. It plays a secondary role in the recognition of carcinomas with cribriform and micropapillary architectures, because these proliferations exhibit other evidence of architectural atypism; however, regularity of cell and nuclear placement represents the only evidence of significant architectural atypia in the solid variety of ductal carcinoma in situ.

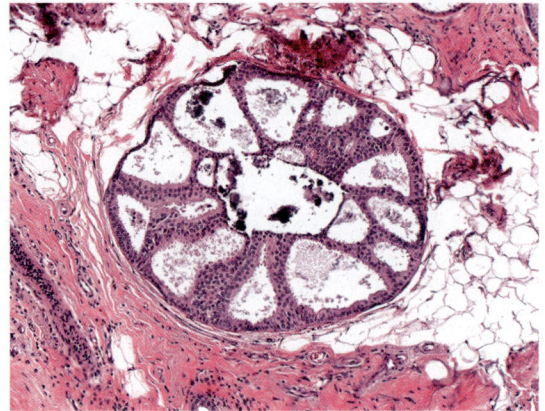

Figure 3-28 The nuclei of this trabecular bar run perpendicular to the long axis of the bar.

Figure 3-29 This structure resembles a cartwheel. The central calcification marks the position of the axle, and the radiating trabecular bars represent the spokes.

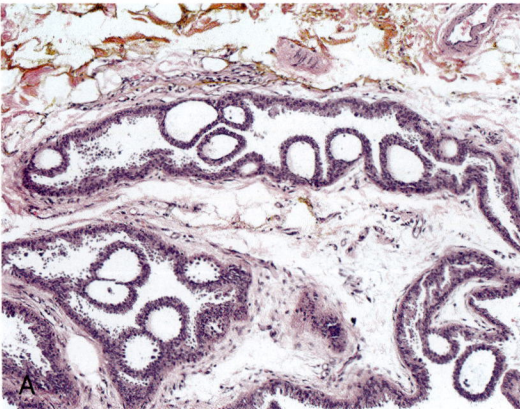

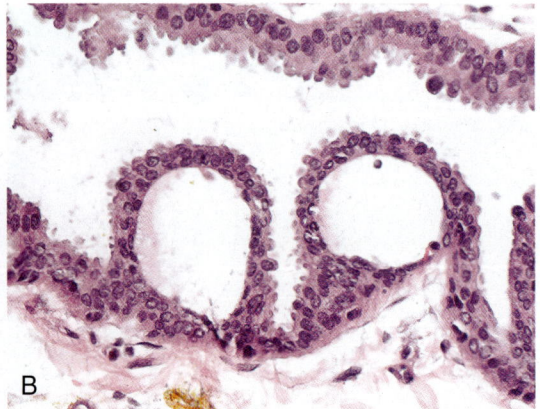

Figure 3-30 A and **B,** The bars creating these peripheral cribriform spaces look like the stone arches supporting bridges and aqueducts built in Roman times.

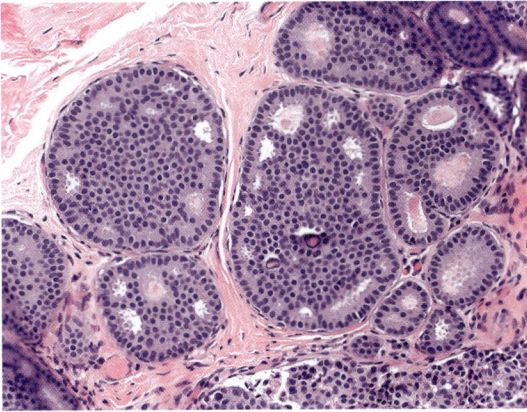

Figure 3-31 The cells in this focus of ductal carcinoma in situ appear evenly spaced.

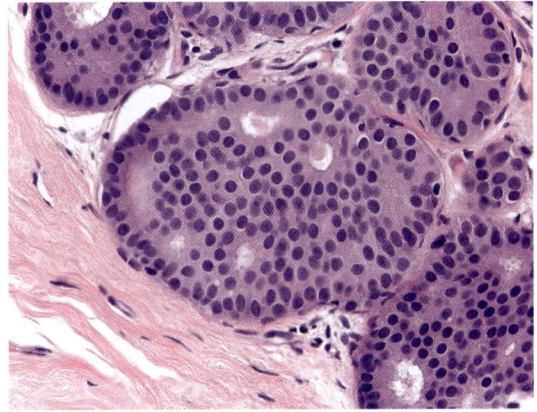

Figure 3-32 The nuclei of low-grade ductal carcinoma in situ have similar round or oval shapes.

Cytologic Characteristics

Uniformity is the dominant feature of the cells of low-grade ductal carcinoma in situ (Box 3-4). Unlike the variably shaped nuclei seen in conventional ductal hyperplasia, those of low-grade ductal carcinoma in situ have remarkably similar shapes, which vary from round to oval (Fig. 3-32). Furthermore, the nuclei of the malignant cells have smooth contours, which contrast with the irregularities, notches, and folds of benign nuclei (Fig. 3-33). The appearance of the chromatin does not usually vary much among the nuclei of a low-grade carcinoma, and this consistency of chromatin texture differs from the slight variability seen in the nuclei of hyperplastic cells. Many low-grade carcinomas exhibit finely dispersed chromatin (Fig. 3-34A), which stains more intensely than the chromatin of hyperplastic nuclei; less commonly, the chromatin has a finely granular texture (Fig. 3-34B). Prominent granularity of the chromatin often indicates nuclei of an intermediate grade of atypia. Without resorting to extremely high magnification, one usually has difficulty detecting nucleoli in low-grade carcinoma cells, whereas the nuclei of hyperplastic cells typically contain a single nucleolus of modest size and smooth contour.

Cytoplasmic characteristics do not play an important role in the recognition of most malignant ductal cells; nevertheless, two properties occur so infrequently in hyperplastic cells that their presence should alert pathologists to the possibility of malignancy: fine, eosinophilic granularity and pronounced clarity. Finely granular, eosinophilic cytoplasm characterizes the cells of many low-grade ductal carcinomas in situ (Fig. 3-35), and in uncommon cases, the granularity and eosinophilia become so pronounced that the cytoplasm takes on a dense, pink color. The cytoplasm of hyperplastic ductal cells can appear eosinophilic, but it usually does not contain such fine granules, nor do hyperplastic cells contain as much cytoplasm as carcinoma cells. Apocrine cells have eosinophilic and granular cytoplasm; however, the amount of cytoplasm in these cells vastly exceeds the quantity in carcinoma cells. Furthermore, the nuclei of apocrine cells have prominent nucleoli, which low-grade carcinoma cells lack. These two differences allow one to distinguish apocrine cells from those of low-grade ductal carcinoma without difficulty. The cytoplasm of cells showing low-grade atypia often appears somewhat pale (Fig. 3-36). In rare cases, the cytoplasm becomes almost clear, and this phenomenon gives the cells a delicate, almost fragile appearance. Except in their immature forms, hyperplastic cells do not have clear cytoplasm, so the presence of this feature should bias one in favor of a diagnosis of malignancy. Finally, the cell membranes of malignant cells often stand out clearly, whereas one usually has difficulty detecting the membranes of hyperplastic cells. Distinct cell membranes do occur in occasional examples of ductal hyperplasia, so if other features of a ductal proliferation fit with the diagnosis of hyperplasia, then one can probably disregard the presence of distinct cell membranes.

Figure 3-37 contrasts the features of conventional ductal hyperplasia and low-grade ductal carcinoma in situ.

Box 3-4

Cytologic characteristics of low-grade ductal carcinoma in situ include uniformity in:

- Cellular distribution
- Nuclear shape
- Chromatin texture

See Case S13-508 for
extensive DCIS low to intermediate grade
solid, cribiform + micropapillary types

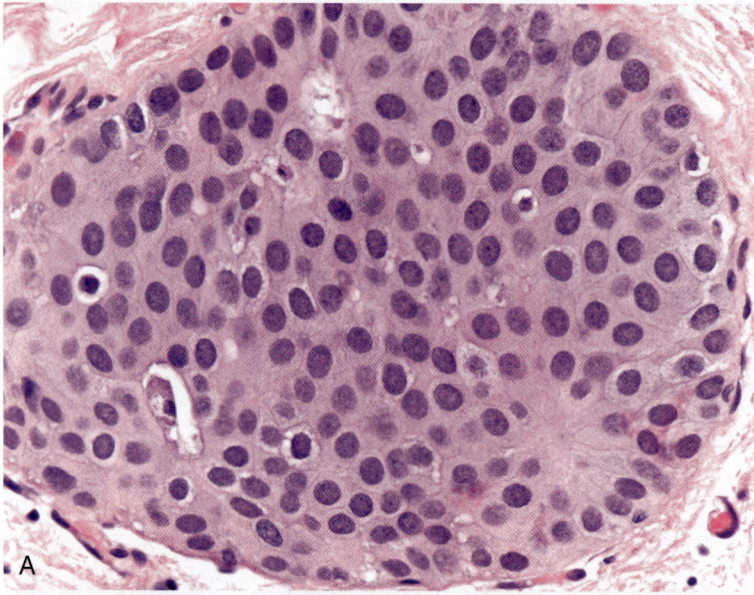

Figure 3-33 Contrast the smooth contours of the nuclei of carcinoma cells in **A** with the irregular contours of hyperplastic nuclei in **B**.

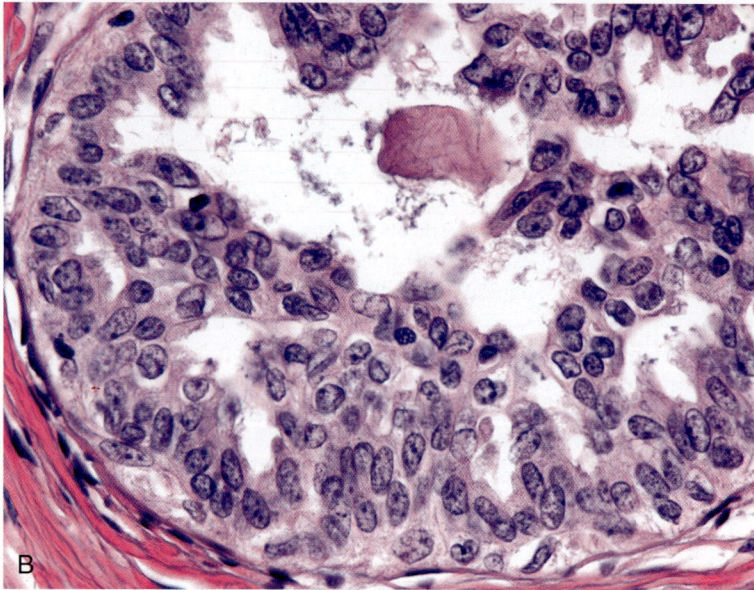

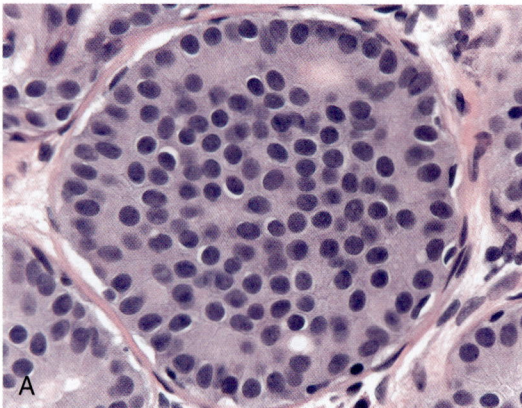

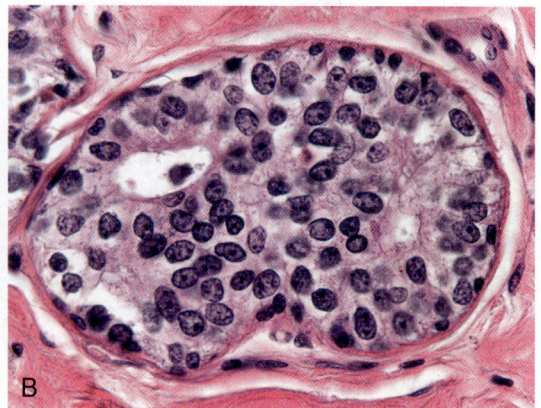

Figure 3-34 A, The chromatin of low-grade ductal carcinoma in situ often appears finely dispersed and darkly staining. **B,** Less commonly, it looks slightly granular.

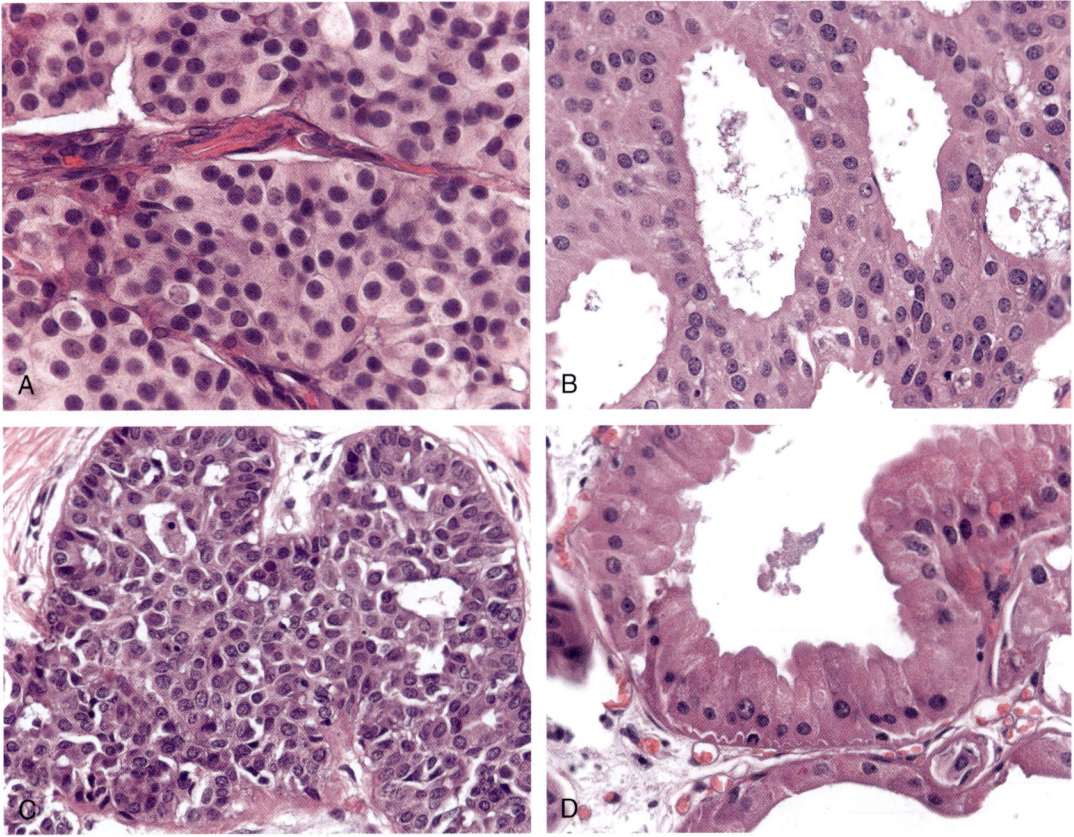

Figure 3-35 A, The cytoplasm of ductal carcinomas often exhibits an eosinophilic tint and a fine granularity. **B,** In rare carcinomas, both attributes become accentuated. **C,** Uncommon cases of ductal hyperplasia consist of cells with eosinophilic cytoplasm, but the hyperplastic cells contain less cytoplasm than the carcinoma cells. **D,** Eosinophilic carcinoma cells do not possess as much cytoplasm as apocrine cells, which also contain eosinophilic and granular cytoplasm.

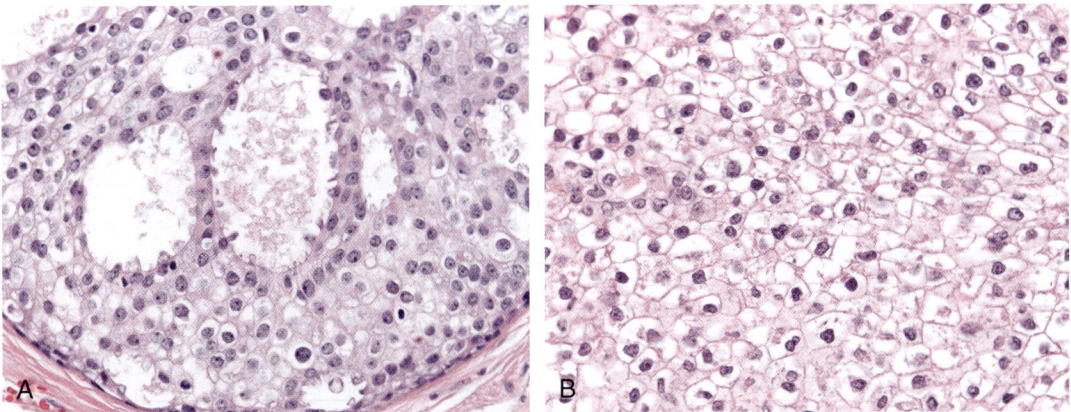

Figure 3-36 A and B, The cytoplasm of carcinoma cells often appears pale and sometimes looks extremely pale.

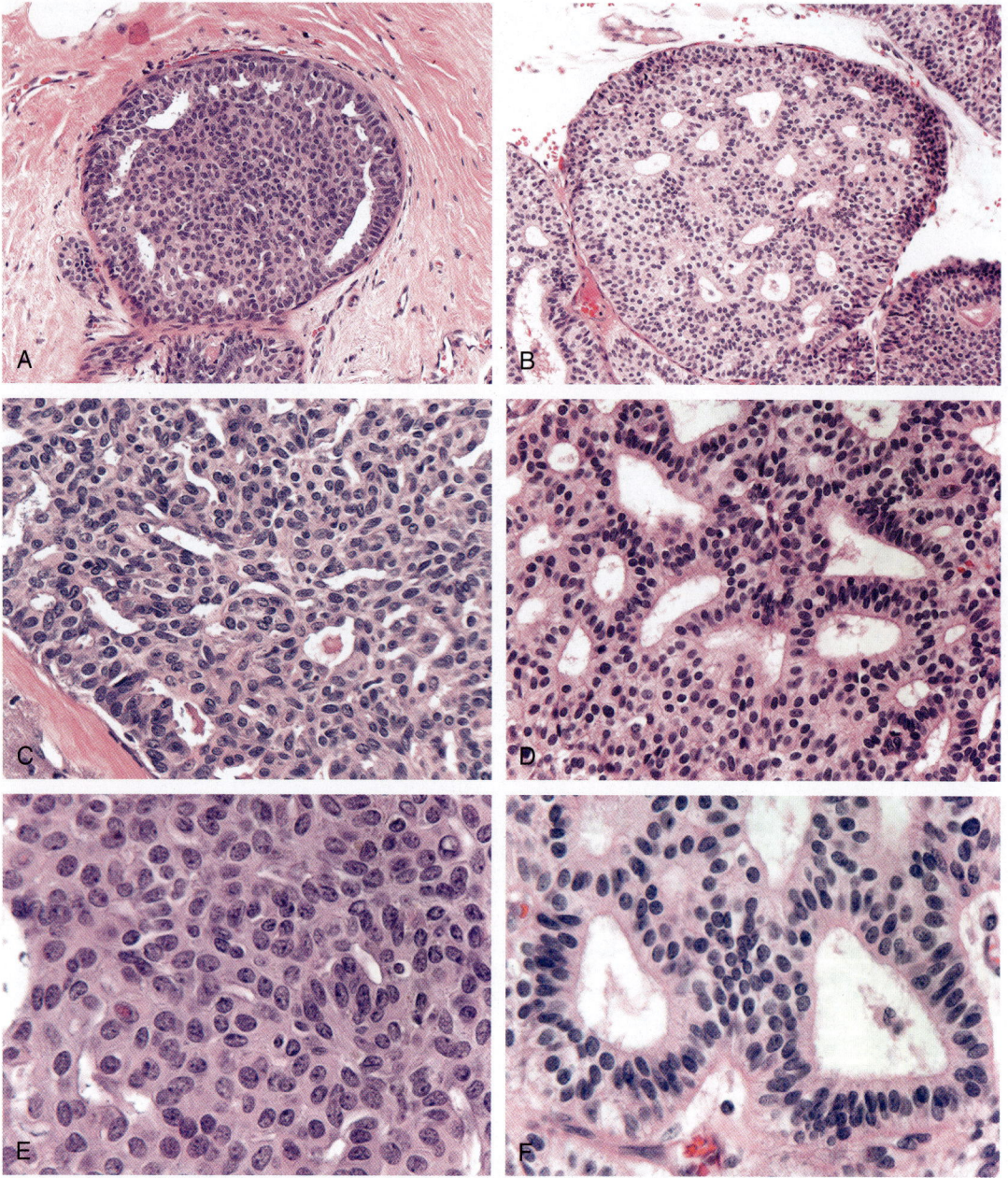

Figure 3-37 A, Hyperplastic ductal cells form masses centrally supported by struts and surrounded by flattened, curving spaces. **B,** Ductal carcinoma cells do not preferentially grow in the center of the ductule. **C,** The fenestrations in ductal hyperplasia appear irregular in size and shape, many have slit-like configurations, the cells appear irregularly disposed, and those surrounding the spaces do not display polarization. **D,** Evenly distributed, polarized cells give rise to the cribriform spaces in ductal carcinomas. **E,** Hyperplastic nuclei have irregular contours, small nucleoli, and slightly granular chromatin. **F,** Carcinoma cells appear uniform; most have oval or round nuclei, homogeneous, dark chromatin, inconspicuous nucleoli, and ample, eosinophilic cytoplasm.

High-Grade Ductal Carcinoma In Situ

Architectural Characteristics

The cells of high-grade ductal carcinoma in situ look so anaplastic that one can recognize their malignant nature without regard to the architectural properties of the proliferation. The cells most often form solid or fenestrated sheets; however, they can also create cribriform spaces, trabecular bars, and Roman bridges. The cells sometimes form micropapillae, and they can grow in just one or two layers, also. Although pathologists occasionally make note of them, these patterns of growth need not play a role in the diagnosis of high-grade ductal carcinoma in situ.

Cytologic Characteristics

High-grade ductal carcinoma in situ consists of cells showing the archetypal characteristics of malignancy. The cells appear greatly enlarged and pleomorphic, and the nuclei and nucleoli usually look large, irregular, and pleomorphic. The nucleus-to-cytoplasm ratios appear increased. One can usually observe signs of cellular dishesion, necrosis, and cell division. The irregularities of nuclear contour and the prominence of the nucleoli contrast with the characteristics of the nuclei of low-grade ductal carcinoma in situ, which exhibit smoothly contoured nuclei and inconspicuous nucleoli, and the marked pleomorphism of high-grade ductal carcinoma in situ distinguishes it from conventional ductal hyperplasia, which shows only slight cellular variation.

Intermediate-Grade Ductal Carcinoma In Situ

Architectural Characteristics

Like high-grade ductal carcinoma in situ, intermediate-grade ductal carcinoma in situ consists of cells with malignant cytologic characteristics. These proliferations form solid sheets, cribriform spaces and their variants, and micropapillary tufts. When present, the latter two manifestations of architectural atypia aid in the recognition of malignancy, but one must sometimes rely solely on cytologic findings to make the diagnosis of intermediate-grade ductal carcinoma.

Cytologic Characteristics

By definition, the cytologic characteristics of the cells of intermediate-grade ductal carcinoma in situ fall between those of low-grade ductal carcinoma in situ and high-grade ductal carcinoma in situ; however, these intermediate-grade proliferations do not exhibit a consistent set of cytologic characteristics. The constellations of cytologic findings vary from case to case. This lack of consistency of cellular attributes makes it impossible to describe the cytologic characteristics of intermediate-grade ductal carcinoma in situ precisely. Enlargement of the cells and their nuclei represents the most consistent feature of this lesion, but irregularities of the nuclear membranes, hyperchromasia, extreme clumping of the chromatin and pallor of the nuclei, enlargement and irregularity of nucleoli, and mitotic activity also occur. Because certain of these attributes also occur in hyperplastic cells, the differentiation of intermediate-grade ductal carcinoma in situ from conventional ductal hyperplasia represents one of the greatest challenges and most vexing problems in the evaluation of epithelial proliferations. A later section addresses this problem.

Atypical Ductal Hyperplasia

Occasional ductal epithelial proliferations do not fall squarely into either the benign or the malignant category. This ambiguity can stem from a failure to meet either qualitative criteria or size criteria for malignancy.

Qualitative Criteria

For many years, pathologists referred to borderline ductal proliferations as *atypical ductal hyperplasia* despite the lack of both a definition of the term and a clear description of the lesion. Most agreed that atypical ductal hyperplasia consists of cells displaying some features of malignancy but not all of them. Although conceptually accurate, this definition does not specify either the required features (if any) or the optional features, nor does it guide the pathologist in integrating the cytologic features with the architectural ones. A more explicit definition would state that atypical ductal hyperplasia represents a proliferation of ductal cells showing cytologic atypia but lacking architectural atypia. Stated in other words, lesions classified as atypical ductal hyperplasia must demonstrate cytologic atypia of a low or intermediate grade and cannot exhibit significant architectural atypia (Fig. 3-38). It also follows that lesions composed of cells showing the cytologic characteristics of hyperplastic cells do not represent atypical ductal hyperplasia no matter what the architectural pattern.

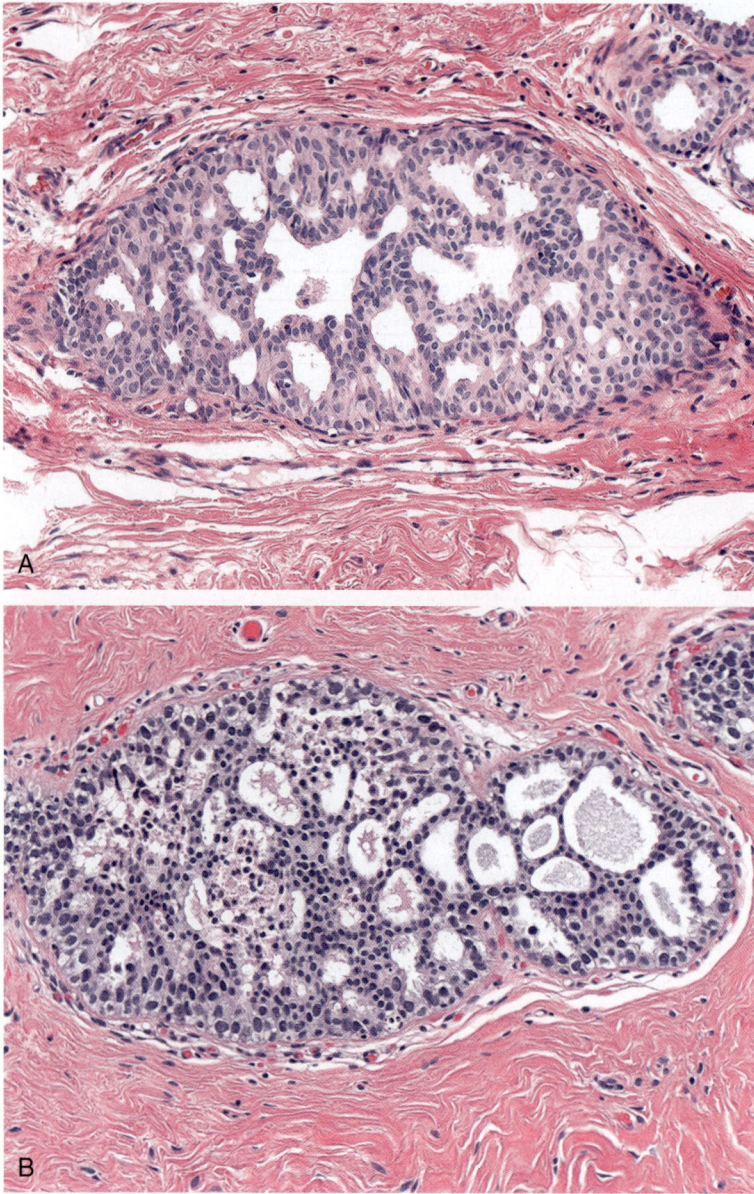

Figure 3-38 A and **B,** These two ductal proliferations display cytologic atypia but lack convincing architectural atypia.

Size Criteria

Although most pathologists incorporate an assessment of the size of a focus in their analyses of ductal proliferations showing low-grade cytologic atypia, certain observers have formalized the use of this parameter. One approach uses the involvement of two glandular profiles to distinguish atypical ductal hyperplasia from low-grade ductal carcinoma in situ; another one employs an aggregate diameter of 0.2 cm. Although these approaches have the benefits of simplicity and practicality, they run the risk of leaving this distinction in the hands of the histotechnologist (Fig. 3-39). Furthermore, surgical pathologists do not commonly employ quantitative criteria

as the deciding factor to distinguish benign from malignant lesions. Observers do incorporate quantitative findings, such as the size of a lesion and the number of mitotic figures, to name just two, in the analysis of tumors, and at times, pathologists used these findings as the sole criterion to distinguish benign lesions from malignant ones. In earlier days, for instance, the diameter of a renal cortical tumor distinguished an adenoma from a carcinoma, and the mitotic count of a uterine smooth muscle tumor differentiated a leiomyoma from a leiomyosarcoma; however, contemporary thinking has overturned these specific examples, and one must search extensively to discover others. It therefore seems that the

Figure 3-39 The atypical ductal proliferation shown in **A** occupies just one duct profile, so some would classify it as atypical ductal hyperplasia. The deeper section depicted in **B** reveals involvement of two ducts, changing the diagnosis from atypical ductal hyperplasia to ductal carcinoma in situ.

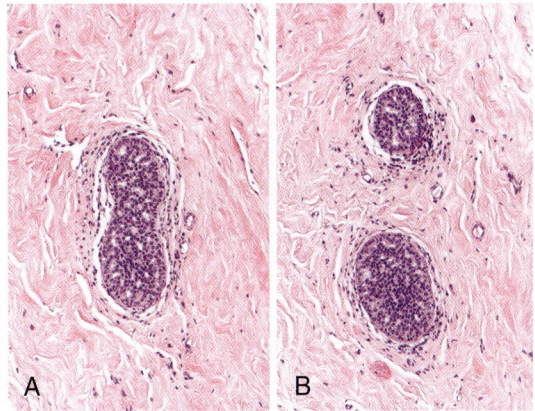

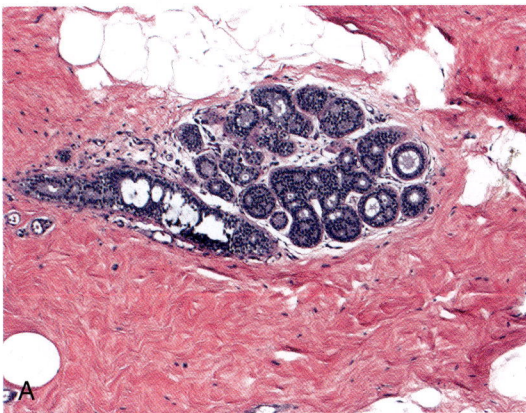

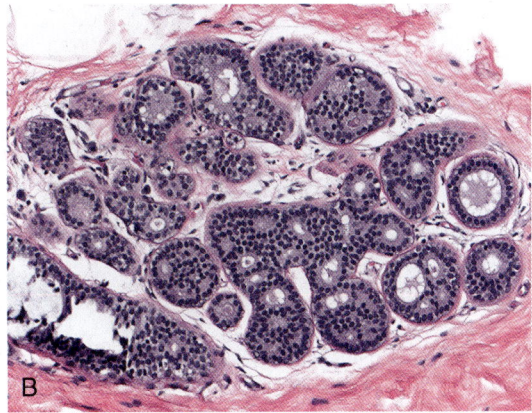

Figure 3-40 A and **B,** Certain pathologists would classify the focus as atypical ductal hyperplasia, others as a microscopic focus of ductal carcinoma in situ.

reliance on quantitative findings to establish the diagnosis of malignancy does not have a strong foundation. It may seem more sensible to make diagnoses purely on the basis of morphologic findings and to describe the size of the focus as a separate attribute. One could use a diagnosis such as *ductal carcinoma in situ, microscopic focus,* for a ductal proliferation that shows both convincing cytologic and architectural atypia but fails to meet certain quantitative thresholds (Fig. 3-40).

Biologic Significance of Atypical Ductal Hyperplasia

Despite refinement of the criteria and the approach to the diagnosis of atypical ductal hyperplasia, the term still encompasses a motley collection of abnormalities that probably do not result from a single biologic process. In fact, one can identify three types of lesions commonly assigned to the category atypical ductal hyperplasia (Fig. 3-41). First, certain cases probably represent foci of genuine carcinoma in situ that fail to demonstrate the morphologic features needed to

justify an outright diagnosis of malignancy for one reason or another. Extremely small proliferations of atypical ductal cells would fall in this category, and so would foci of carcinoma compromised by artifacts of either specimen handling or tissue processing. Another form of atypical ductal hyperplasia probably represents an intermediate stage in the evolution of ductal carcinoma. This lesion displays the cytologic characteristics of malignancy but lacks sufficient architectural complexity. Cases of conventional ductal hyperplasia showing unexpected cytologic features, perhaps the results of medications or iatrogenic intervention, constitute the third group of lesions classified as atypical ductal hyperplasia.

Pathologists have begun to consider the topic of atypical ductal hyperplasia in greater detail. By making careful morphological observations and studying these lesions with advanced genetic methods, investigators will probably come to recognize the biologic processes that underlie the formation of these different types of atypical ductal hyperplasia and thereby place them in more specific diagnostic categories. We will, for

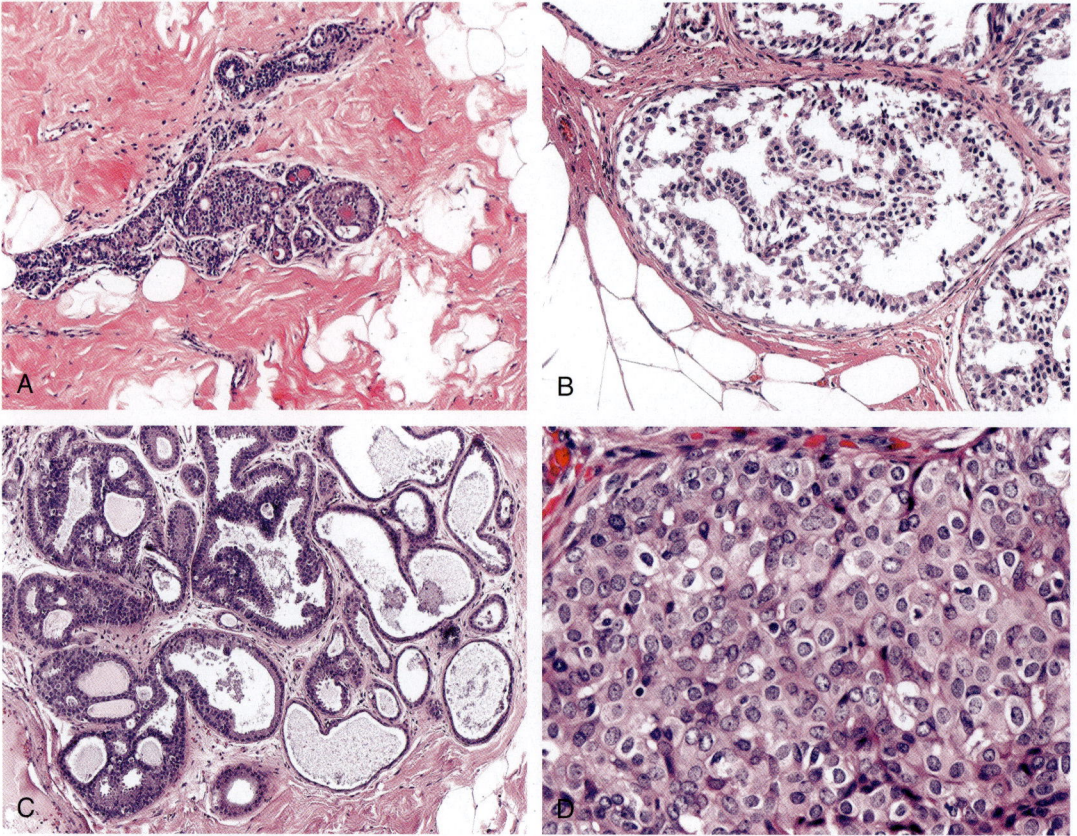

Figure 3-41 A, The ductule in the center contains atypical cells, but they number so few that one cannot evaluate their characteristics fully. **B,** Handling artifacts impede the recognition of this carcinoma. **C,** The focus shown here has the cytologic attributes of ductal carcinoma in situ but lacks sufficient architectural atypia, in part because of an off-center plane of section. **D,** Hormonal influences have caused the cells in the conventional hyperplasia to appear larger than normal.

example, come to recognize tiny carcinomas in situ as such rather than as atypical ductal hyperplasia and to regard conventional ductal hyperplasia showing reactive cytologic atypia as a benign proliferation rather than a preneoplastic one. This ability to classify lesions more precisely will reduce the number of cases classified as atypical ductal hyperplasia; at the same time, it will restrict the diagnosis to lesions representing intermediate stages in the formation of a carcinoma. Many of these more precisely defined cases of atypical ductal hyperplasia will fall into the category discussed next, flat epithelial atypia.

Flat Epithelial Atypia

Histologic Characteristics

During the past decade or so, several groups of pathologists have called attention to a form of atypical proliferation composed of columnar ductal cells. The cells of this lesion do not pile up to fill terminal duct–lobular units, as one sees in conventional ductal proliferations; instead, the atypical cells grow in a single layer, which enlarges the glands and gives them a cystic appearance. Each group of investigators has proposed a different name for the lesion, and representatives of the World Health Organization currently favor the term *flat epithelial atypia*. Whatever the terminology, many writers consider the lesion a preneoplastic proliferation closely related to low-grade micropapillary/cribriform ductal carcinoma in situ. Studies have begun to elucidate the pathologic and clinical features of this type of atypical ductal proliferation, but many of its characteristics remain undefined. It seems prudent to regard our current understanding as provisional and somewhat fluid and to acknowledge that we require additional studies to develop a secure knowledge of the biologic properties of this lesion.

Although experts in mammary pathology disagree about certain fine points of flat epithelial atypia, these observers have reached a consensus regarding its basic properties. Four attributes characterize well–developed examples of flat epithelia atypia. First, the acini and terminal ductules appear greatly enlarged

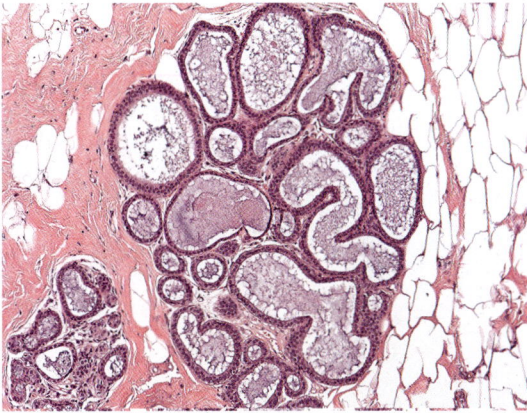

Figure 3-42 The ductules and acini of this terminal duct–lobular unit altered by flat epithelial atypia appear greatly distended.

Figure 3-43 A single layer of luminal cells line the distended acini in flat epithelial atypia. The cells exhibit either cuboidal shapes in **A** or columnar shapes in **B**.

(Fig. 3-42). The distended glands often span one or two millimeters each, but smaller, perhaps earlier, examples of the lesion exhibit lesser degrees of distention.

Second, a single layer of ductal cells lines the distended glands. In glands showing minimal proliferation, the cells have cuboidal shapes; more advanced lesions consist of tall cuboidal cells, whose height measures several times their width (Fig. 3-43). The columnar shape of the cells reflects the crowding that results from their proliferation while they remain attached to the basement membrane. When the cells become especially closely packed, their nuclei can occupy different positions within the cells and thereby create a pseudostratified appearance (Fig. 3-44). Pathologists disagree about the presence of genuine stratification; certain ones allow a limited amount,

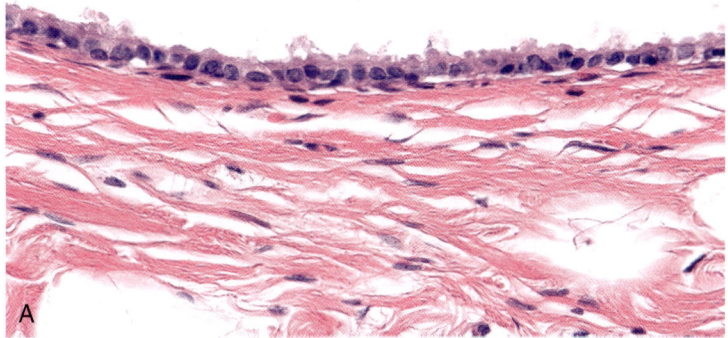

A

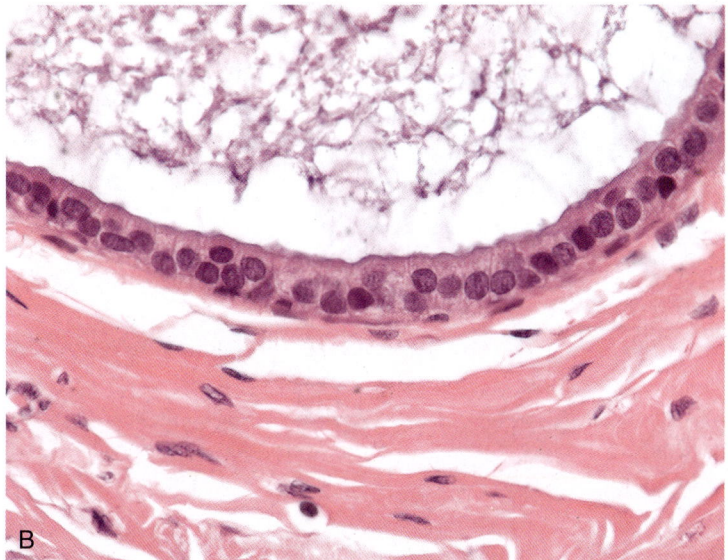

B

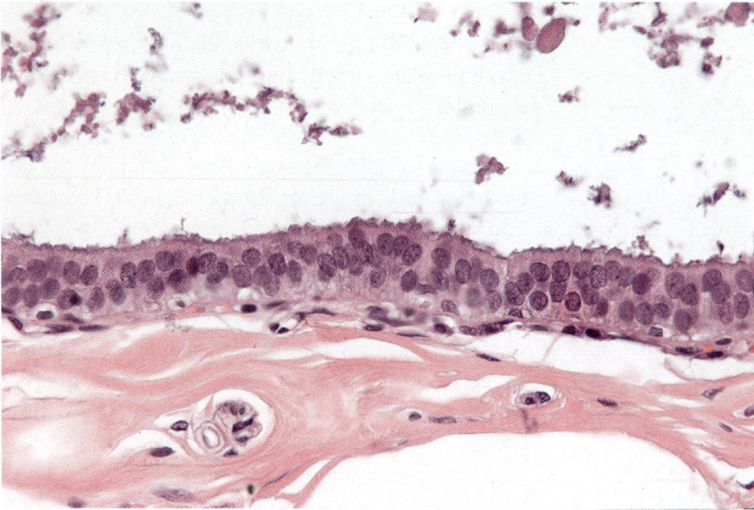

Figure 3-44 Crowding of these columnar cells on the basement membrane causes their nuclei to sit at different positions within the cells, thereby producing a pseudostratified pattern.

Flat epithelial atypia (Text, p. 37)

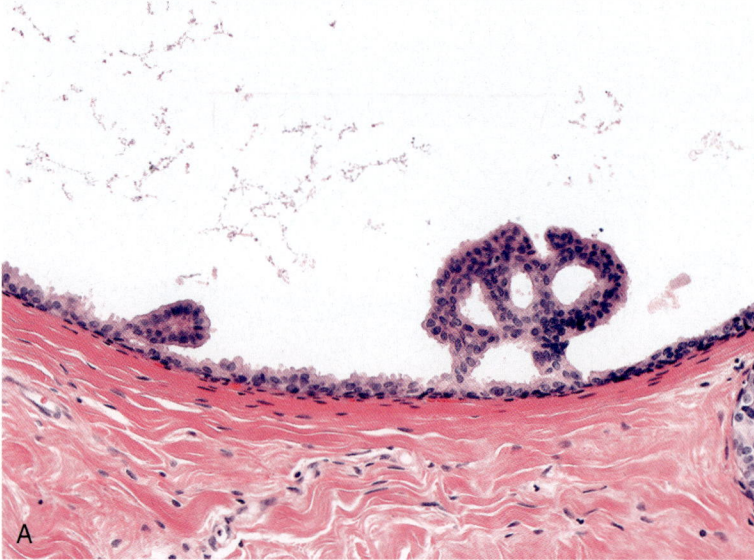

Figure 3-45 A, Certain pathologists would classify this proliferation as carcinoma, others as flat epithelial atypia. **B,** The marked stratification would lead most to classify this proliferation as carcinoma.

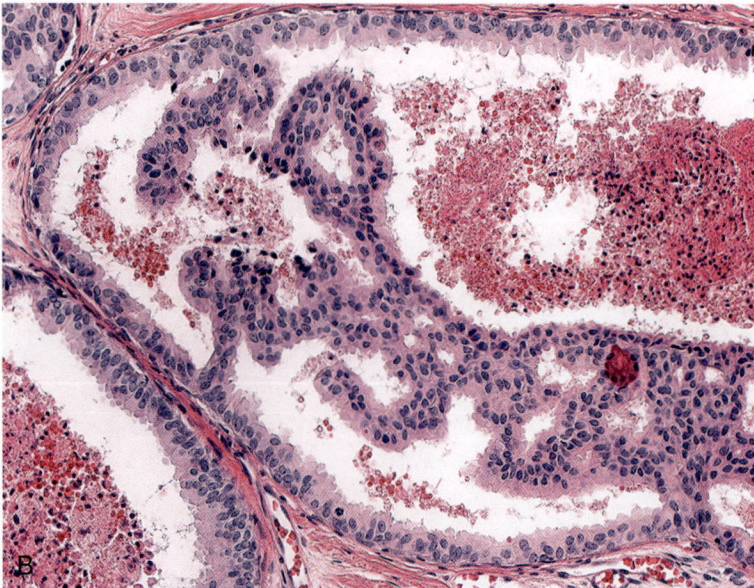

Figure 3-46 The cells of flat epithelial atypia display low-grade cytologic atypia.

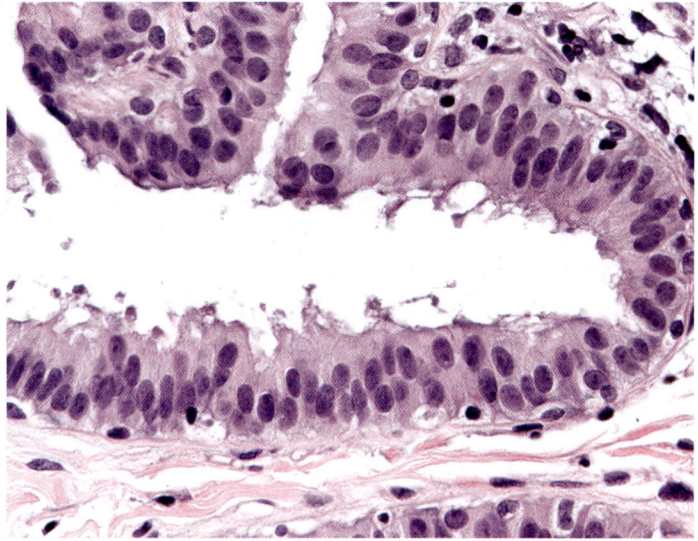

Figure 3-47 In this variety of flat epithelial atypia, the chromatin has a granular quality, and one can see small nucleoli.

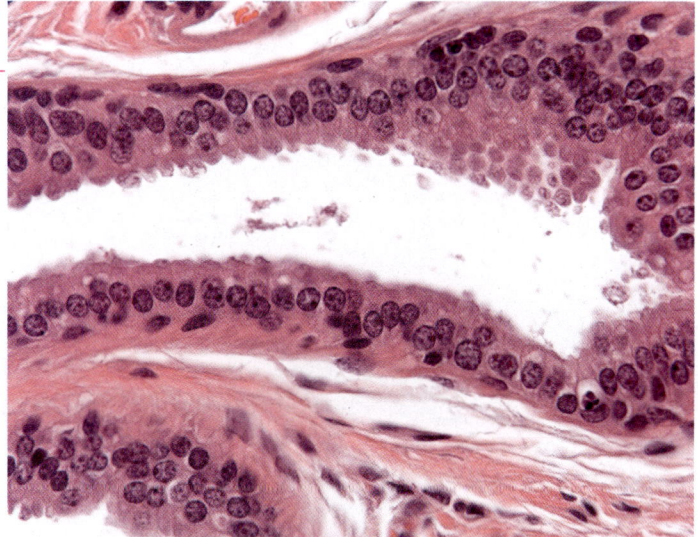

whereas others classify proliferations showing stratification as ductal carcinoma in situ (Fig. 3-45).

Third, the ductal cells display low-grade cytologic atypia (Fig. 3-46). Like the nuclei of low-grade ductal carcinomas, the nuclei of atypical columnar cells look slightly enlarged, smoothly contoured, and round or oval. Crowding of the cells causes the nuclei to take on especially long, fusiform shapes. The chromatin most often appears homogeneous and hyperchromatic, and the nucleoli indistinct, but these aspects can vary. In one variation, the chromatin appears finely granular, and one can detect nucleoli (Fig. 3-47). The nuclei sit along the basement membrane, and

eosinophilic cytoplasm collects at the apical poles to create well-developed apical cytoplasmic compartments. The cytoplasm usually has an eosinophilic hue and a finely granular texture, and the atypical cells contain more cytoplasm than normal cells (Fig. 3-48). Occasionally, the cytoplasm looks deeply eosinophilic and dense (Fig. 3-49); although these features give the cells an apocrine look, the volume of cytoplasm never equals the amount seen in conventional apocrine cells. The cytoplasm can form apical blebs, but this feature does not appear in all cases.

Finally, the proportion of the epithelium represented by myoepithelial cells seems reduced (Fig. 3-50).

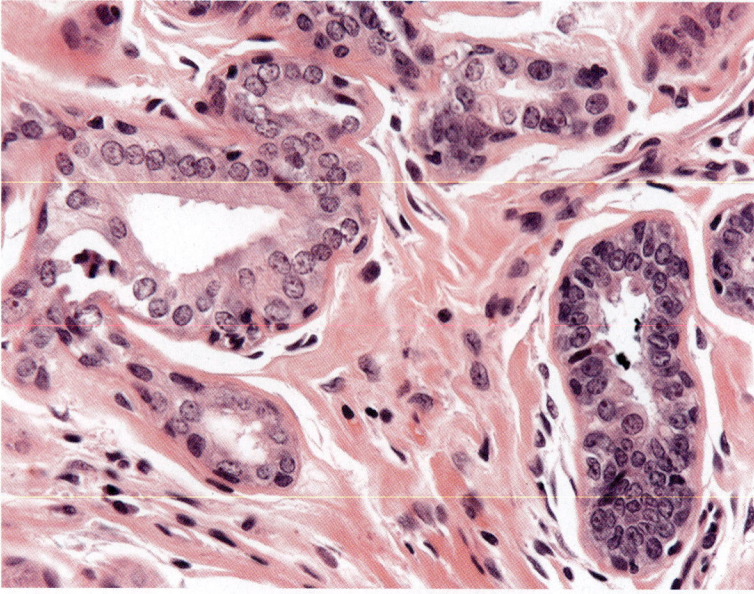

Figure 3-48 The acini in the left of the field show very early changes of flat epithelial atypia. Note the increase in the amount of cytoplasm compared with the normal cells present in the right.

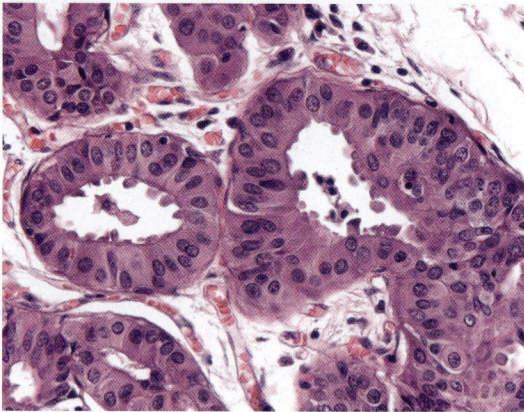

Figure 3-49 The cells in this example of flat epithelial atypia have unusually eosinophilic and dense cytoplasm.

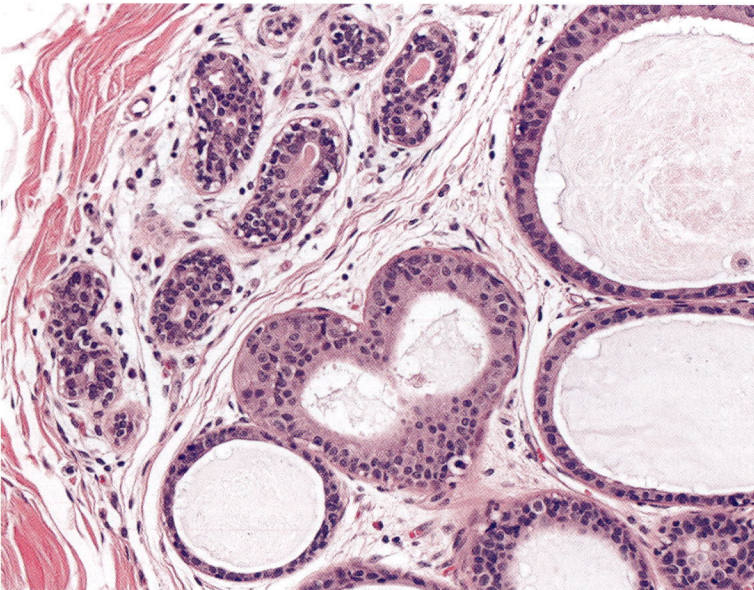

Figure 3-50 Myoepithelial cells make up a smaller proportion of the epithelium in the acini showing flat epithelial atypia compared to the epithelium in the normal acini.

It appears that luminal cells constitute the proliferative component and that the indigenous myoepithelial cells become diluted as the atypical luminal cells accumulate. One should probably require the presence of the first three characteristics to establish the diagnosis of flat epithelial atypia; the final one seems important but not essential.

Calcifications often occupy the lumen of a distended gland or sit in the adjacent stroma. The specialized stroma usually appears unremarkable, but one occasionally observes reactive fibroblastic changes.

Differential Diagnosis

One must differentiate flat epithelial atypia from the following three benign conditions: the microcysts seen in fibrocystic changes, blunt duct adenosis, and flat ductal hyperplasia.

The spectrum of fibrocystic changes encompasses two types of microcysts, those lined by conventional apocrine cells and those lined by flattened cells. Both types of microcysts superficially resemble acini distended by flat epithelial atypia, but one can easily differentiate the lesions by studying the characteristics of the epithelial cells. The columnar cells of flat epithelial atypia lack the voluminous cytoplasm of conventional apocrine cells; furthermore, the nucleoli of the former usually look inconspicuous, whereas those of the latter appear prominent. The atypical columnar cells do not show the flattening and attenuation that characterize the cells lining microcysts (Fig. 3-51).

Pathologists have used the term *blunt duct adenosis* to refer to two different lesions. When they introduced the term, Drs. Foote and Stewart applied it to an abnormality that most would now consider conventional ductal hyperplasia involving ductules and acini. Because this alteration consists of a filling rather than a dilatation of the ductules, one would not confuse this entity with flat epithelial atypia. Most contemporary pathologists use the diagnosis *blunt duct adenosis* to refer to a lesion different from the one described by the originators. In current usage, this designation refers to a form of lobular hypertrophy in which the glands become dilated. This lesion can closely mimic flat epithelial atypia. In the early, proliferative phase of blunt duct adenosis, the luminal cells take on a columnar shape and possess abundant apical cytoplasm and slightly enlarged, round nuclei. Such characteristics bring to mind the atypical columnar cells of flat epithelial atypia, but

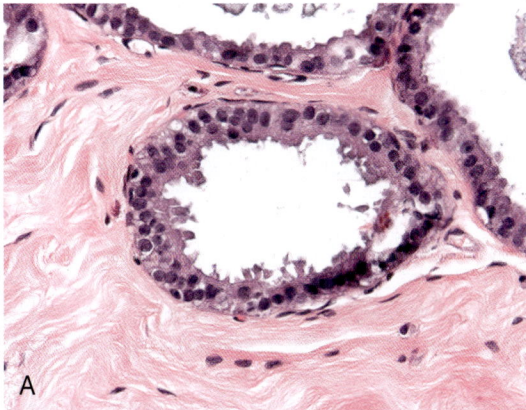

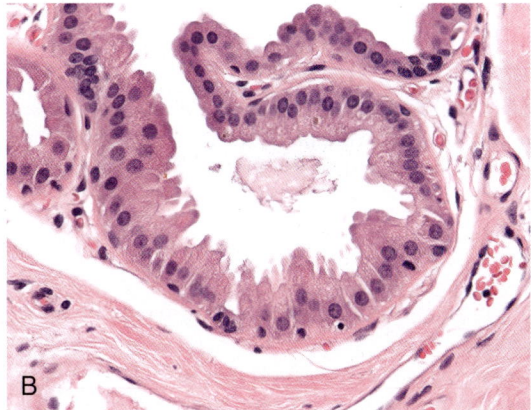

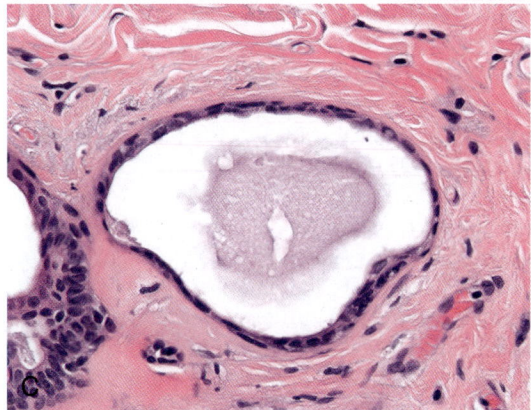

Figure 3-51 Contrast the characteristics of the atypical cells lining the distended acinus in **A** with the plump apocrine cells in **B** and the flattened cells in **C**.

Flat epithelial atypia

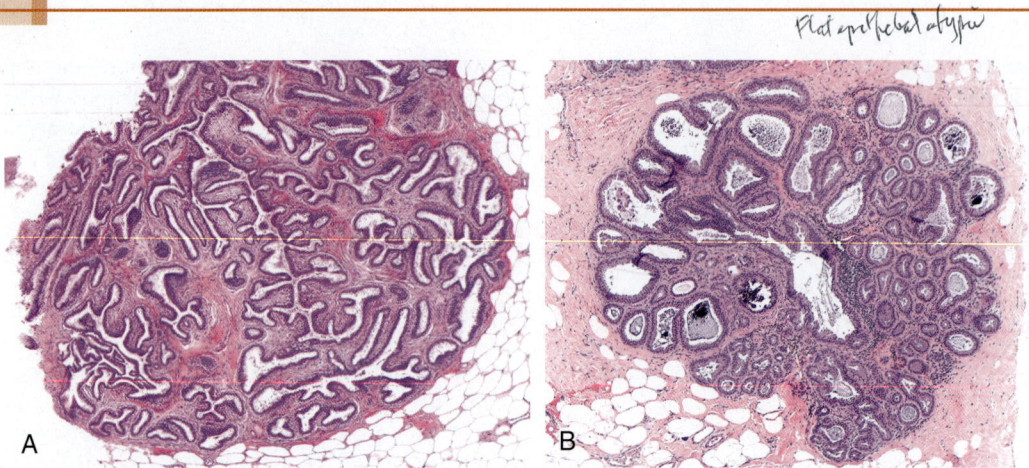

Figure 3-52 A, The glands in the focus of blunt duct adenosis shown here have branching, staghorn shapes. **B,** The acini distended by flat epithelial atypia look globular.

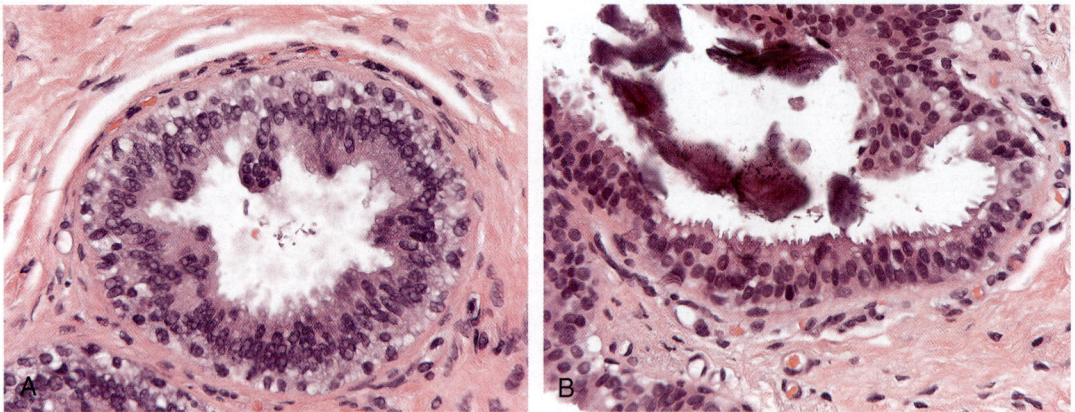

Figure 3-53 A, A prominent layer of myoepithelial cells containing abundant, pale cytoplasm underlies the columnar luminal cells in this region of blunt duct adenosis. **B,** One has difficulty detecting myoepithelial cells in this example of flat epithelial atypia.

the following three findings help differentiate these two lesions.

First, the glands of early blunt duct adenosis have flattened, branching configurations in contrast to the round, globular shapes seen in flat epithelial atypia (Fig. 3-52). Second, in early blunt duct adenosis, the myoepithelial cells appear especially prominent and often form an obvious, continuous ring between the luminal cells and the basement membrane (Fig. 3-53). The myoepithelial cells of flat epithelial atypia, on the other hand, seem reduced in number and do not form a continuous layer. Third, the stroma of early blunt duct adenosis consists of numerous fibroblasts and abundant myxoid ground substances. The stroma of most examples of flat epithelial atypia does not exhibit these reactive features. As blunt duct adenosis evolves, the stromal changes disappear, and the blunt ducts take on round

configurations, furthering the superficial resemblance to acini involved flat epithelial atypia (Fig. 3-54). During this evolution, though, the luminal cells become cuboidal or even flattened, and this lack of a columnar configuration, together with the presence of myoepithelial cells, permits one to distinguish the inactive stage of blunt duct adenosis from flat epithelial atypia.

Although hyperplastic ductal cells usually grow in a stratified pattern, they can also grow in a flat sheet. This form of ductal hyperplasia, sometimes called *columnar cell hyperplasia*, can arise either as an isolated finding or as a component of another lesion, such as pseudoangiomatous stromal hyperplasia (Fig. 3-55). The resulting lesions sometimes resemble flat epithelial atypia, but attention to several cellular characteristics allows the pathologist to distinguish the two (Fig. 3-56). First, the cells of flat

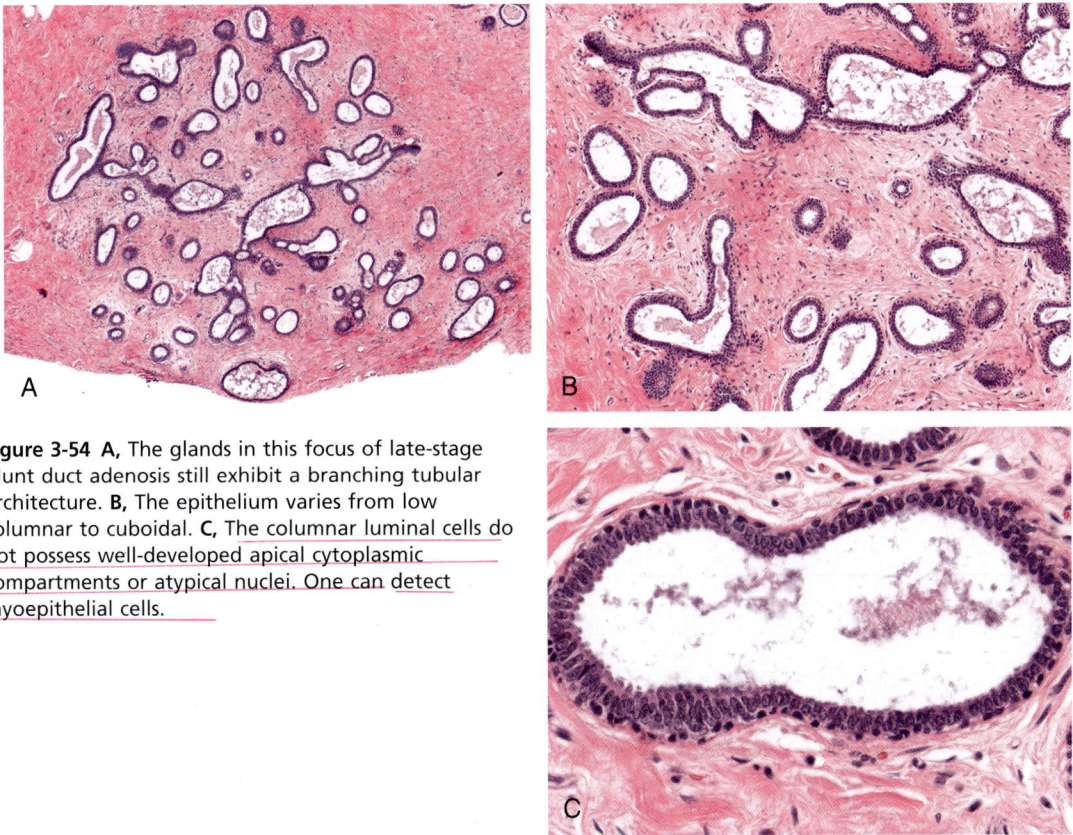

Figure 3-54 A, The glands in this focus of late-stage blunt duct adenosis still exhibit a branching tubular architecture. **B,** The epithelium varies from low columnar to cuboidal. **C,** The columnar luminal cells do not possess well-developed apical cytoplasmic compartments or atypical nuclei. One can detect myoepithelial cells.

ductal hyperplasia do not show the regular placement and even spacing seen in flat epithelial atypia. Hyperplastic ductal cells look crowded and jumbled, and the cells point in different directions, rather than running parallel to each other as atypical columnar cells do. Second, the hyperplastic cells do not have atypical nuclei. Like those seen in conventional hyperplastic cells, the nuclei in the flat variety have irregular and variable shapes, granular chromatin, and small nucleoli. The nuclei of flat epithelial atypia display low-grade atypia. Third, one often spots a few flattened cells sitting on top of the columnar cells in examples of flat hyperplasia. Finally, hyperplastic ductal cells growing in a predominantly flat pattern often pile up a bit in a few areas. The merging of the flat pattern of growth with the conventional stratified pattern helps identify the proliferations as a variety of conventional ductal hyperplasia.

Flat Epithelial Lesions Showing Intermediate- or High-Grade Atypia

Contemporary discussions of flat epithelial atypia usually emphasize the low-grade nature of the cytologic atypia, yet cells with more advanced degrees of anaplasia can also grow in a single layer. Contemporary usage does not place proliferations characterized by either intermediate-grade or high-grade cytologic atypia in the category of flat epithelial atypia, because by decree, this term refers only to ductal proliferations showing low-grade cytologic atypia. Instead, pathologists often use the diagnosis introduced by Dr. Azzopardi, *clinging carcinoma*, for carcinomas of intermediate- or high-grade that are growing in just one or two layers of cells. The section devoted to this topic considers problems related to the recognition and differential diagnosis of clinging carcinomas.

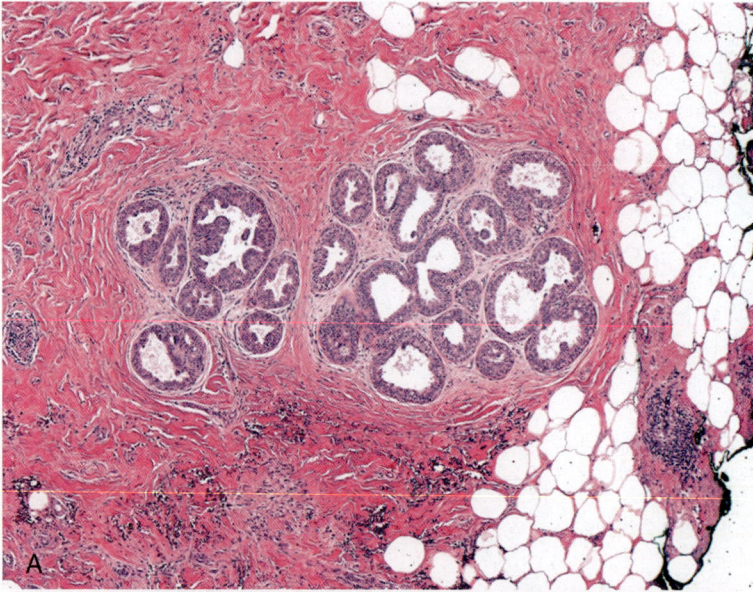

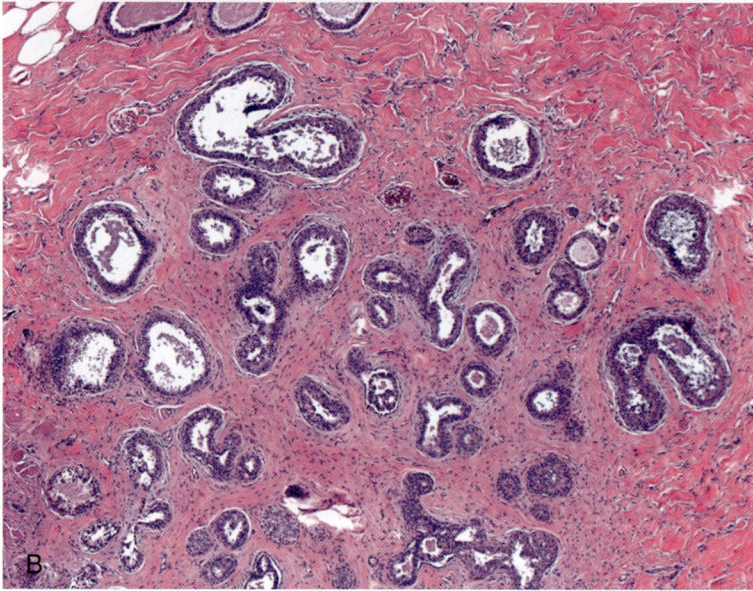

Figure 3-55 Flat hyperplasia occurs as a solitary lesion in **A** and as part of a focus of pseudoangiomatous stromal hyperplasia in **B**.

Columnar cell hyperplasia

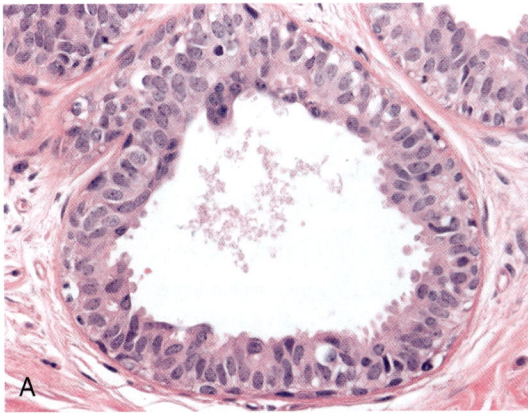

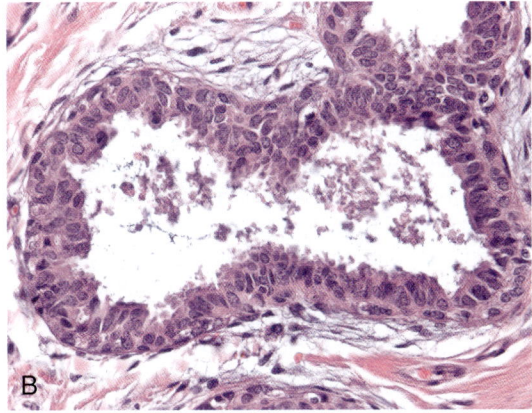

Figure 3-56 A, The cells of flat hyperplasia appear disheveled in their arrangement, and they point in different directions. **B,** The hyperplastic nuclei show the features of usual hyperplasia. **C,** The nuclei of flat epithelial atypia demonstrate atypia.

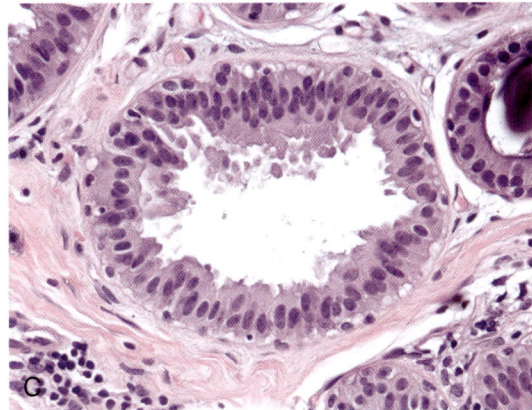

IMMUNOHISTOCHEMICAL CHARACTERISTICS OF DUCTAL PROLIFERATIONS

Studies have demonstrated that usual ductal hyperplasia and ductal carcinoma in situ differ in their expression of cytokeratins and many other proteins, and several researchers have suggested that this difference in cytokeratin profile may represent a helpful point of differentiation. Practical considerations suggest that staining for cytokeratin 5/6 is the most useful approach currently available for the study of cytokeratin expression, but the successful interpretation of the immunohistochemical staining results requires knowledge of the staining properties of both normal and abnormal cells. When interpreting stains for these proteins, pathologists should keep the following two points in mind. First, the distribution of positive cells varies markedly within the breast. Terminal duct-lobular units containing many positive cells sit side-by-side with other units without so much as a single reactive cell. Myoepithelial cells of ducts and ductules usually stain intensely, and a fraction of the columnar luminal cells lining small ducts often stain. Many normal luminal cells within lobules do not stain, whether of polygonal or columnar shape, and the acinar myoepithelial cells often do not stain either. Second, the expression of this type of keratin by normal cells depends on their state of differentiation. Epithelial cells having the capability to differentiate into either luminal or myoepithelial cells express keratin 5/6 until they take on specific characteristics of either luminal or myoepithelial cells.

Most of the cells in examples of minimal usual ductal hyperplasia, the peripheral cells of florid usual ductal hyperplasia, the columnar cells of flat epithelial atypia, and the cells of lobular neoplasia and ductal carcinoma fail to stain for cytokeratin 5/6. Thus, this technique serves best in the evaluation of proliferations that consist of several layers of cells and in which the diagnostic problem involves distinguishing conventional ductal hyperplasia from intermediate-grade ductal carcinoma in situ, papilloma with conventional ductal hyperplasia from solid papillary carcinoma, or micropapillary ductal hyperplasia from micropapillary ductal carcinoma in situ.

APPROACH TO THE DIAGNOSIS OF CONVENTIONAL DUCTAL PROLIFERATIONS

The preceding considerations suggest the following approach to the diagnosis of epithelial proliferations composed of conventional ductal cells. After assessing the level of proliferation, one should analyze the cytologic characteristics. If they exhibit marked atypia, then one can make the diagnosis of high-grade ductal carcinoma in situ without regard to other findings. If the cells exhibit low-grade atypia, then one must evaluate the architectural features. The formation of cribriform spaces, trabecular bars, or Roman bridges and the regular placement of cells constitute evidence of architectural atypia. Proliferations showing low-grade cytologic atypia and well developed architectural atypia merit the diagnosis of low-grade ductal carcinoma in situ. Lesions characterized by low-grade cytologic atypia but lacking well-established architectural atypia usually belong in the category of atypical ductal hyperplasia. One would classify proliferations showing low grade cytological atypia growing in a flat pattern as flat epithelial atypia. The diagnosis of conventional ductal hyperplasia would apply to proliferations that do not demonstrate cytologic atypia.

In the absence of clear-cut proliferation, one must think carefully before making a diagnosis of either atypical ductal hyperplasia or ductal carcinoma in situ. In such cases, the diagnosis necessarily rests entirely on cytologic findings, so one must have a well-founded understanding of the range of unusual cytologic features that benign cells can exhibit. With experience, one can occasionally make a diagnosis of atypical ductal hyperplasia or ductal carcinoma in situ in the absence of proliferation, but such cases arise only rarely.

Summary

Ductal hyperplasia develops from multipotent epithelial cells having the capacity to differentiate into both luminal and myoepithelial cells. The cells do not express either potential to a noticeable degree; instead, they grow in cohesive masses. The marked cohesion and lack of luminal differentiation give rise to characteristic architectural patterns. The cells do not display atypical cytologic features. Ductal carcinomas do not typically emerge from a background of ductal hyperplasia. They originate from a different type of cell, probably one committed to luminal differentiation. These cells lack the cohesion of hyperplastic cells and display cellular polarization, and these phenomena result in the formation of dishesive masses containing cribriform spaces. Carcinoma cells exhibit a constellation of atypical cytologic features. The malignant properties of a ductal carcinoma develop in graded steps classified as flat epithelial atypia and atypical ductal hyperplasia. Pathologists continue to attempt to define the limits of these stages, but the boundaries remain imprecisely marked.

PROBLEMS IN THE DIAGNOSIS OF CONVENTIONAL DUCTAL HYPERPLASIA

Mastering the architectural and cytologic features of conventional ductal hyperplasia makes it easy to recognize most examples with confidence, because the histologic findings do not vary much from one case to the next; however, the cytologic features deviate from the expected on occasion, and when they do, one's confidence can wane. For example, the nuclei of hyperplastic cells sometimes contain dark and finely dispersed chromatin similar in its staining properties to the chromatin of low-grade carcinoma cells, and hyperplastic nuclei from women in their perimenopausal years sometimes appear large

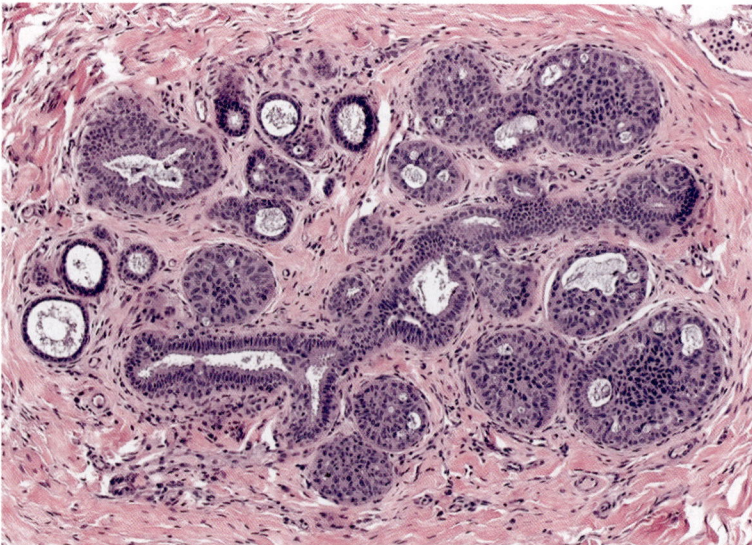

Figure 3-57 Hyperplastic cells with dark nuclei expand several acini.

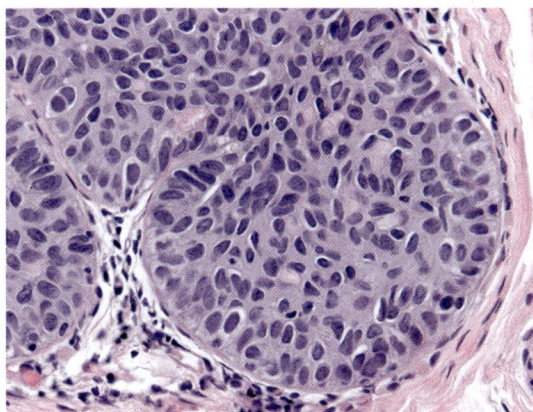

Figure 3-58 Although the chromatin of these hyperplastic cells appears dark and finely distributed, the nuclei exhibit irregularity of both shape and contour.

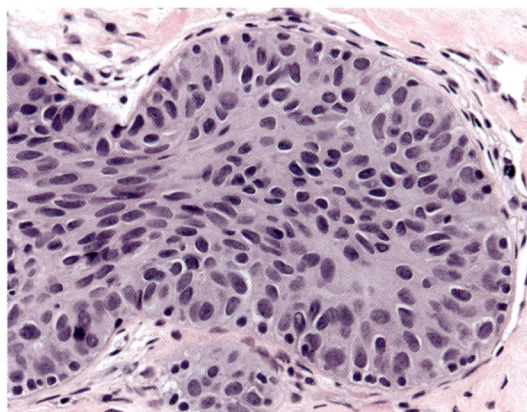

Figure 3-59 This population of hyperplastic cells displays the phenomenon of maturation.

enough to suggest the presence of cytologic atypia. In cases showing intense proliferation, the hyperplastic cells may fail to develop their usual cellular characteristics; the presence of these large, uniform, immature cells brings to mind the diagnosis of carcinoma growing in an intraepithelial position. Pathologists must not assume that every cell showing unusual features represents a neoplastic cell. Irradiation of the breast alters the appearance of the glandular cells, and so do degenerative processes; one must not misinterpret these unusual cells as neoplastic. Finally, most pathologists have little firsthand knowledge of the cellular characteristics of the adolescent mammary gland; consequently, we do not know how to apply experience derived from the study of specimens from adults to those from teenagers. In the face of this ignorance, caution seems prudent. The discussion that follows elaborates on these problems.

Ductal Hyperplasia with Hyperchromatic Nuclei

One occasionally encounters focal proliferations of ductal cells containing homogeneous, finely dispersed dark chromatin (Fig. 3-57). The homogeneity and hyperchromasia of the chromatin differ from the variable staining and granular nuclear material typically seen in hyperplastic nuclei, and these features recall the appearance of the nuclei of low-grade ductal carcinoma in situ; however, other attributes of the proliferative cells and their nuclei match those of hyperplastic ductal cells. For example, the nuclei appear irregularly disposed; they have folds and notches in their contours; and one can observe small nucleoli in the paler nuclei (Fig. 3-58). The population displays subtle evidence of maturation, and the cytoplasm tends to shrink from the nuclei

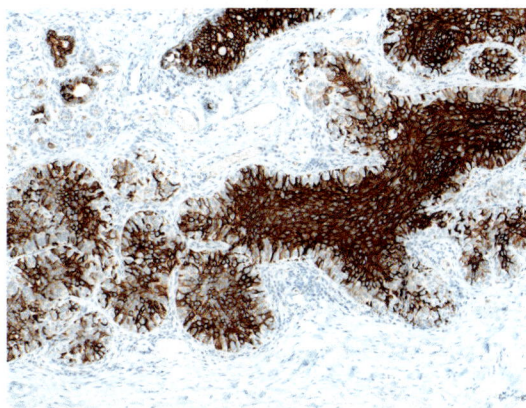

Figure 3-60 These hyperplastic cells stain intensely for cytokeratin 5/6.

to create perinuclear halos (Fig. 3-59). A stain for cytokeratin 5/6 often stains all the cells intensely (Fig. 3-60). These findings suggest that this type of proliferation represents a variety of conventional ductal hyperplasia. The hyperchromasia remains unexplained.

Ductal Hyperplasia in Perimenopausal Women

During the years surrounding menopause, hyperplastic ductal cells can take on characteristics that make the cells appear slightly atypical. One sees this phenomenon in premenopausal women in their late forties and early fifties and in postmenopausal women taking certain types of ovarian hormone medications and other compounds with similar endocrine effects. These hyperplastic cells appear larger than those in cases of ordinary ductal hyperplasia (Fig. 3-61). This cellular enlargement tends to catch the eye of the

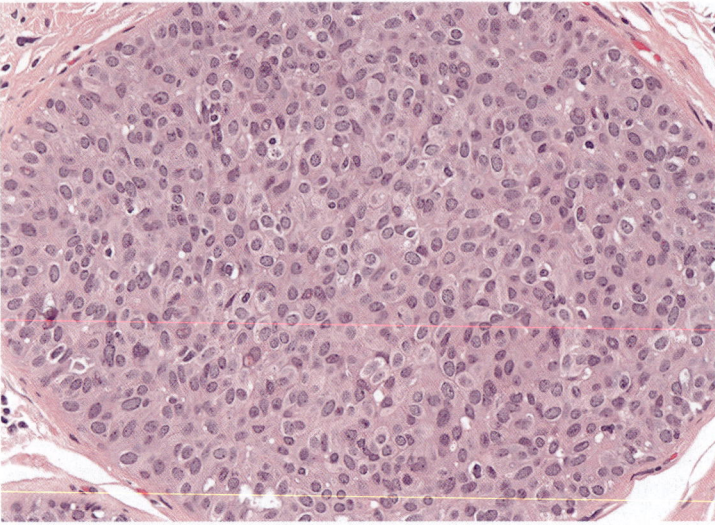

Figure 3-61 The large size of the nuclei in these hyperplastic cells suggests the presence of atypia.

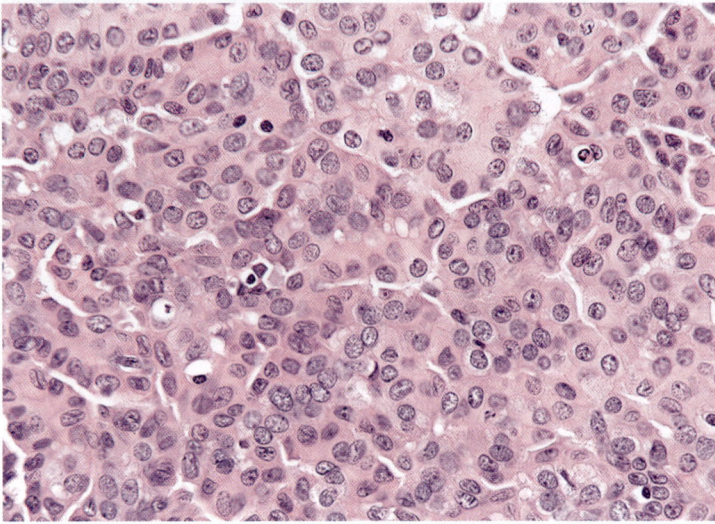

Figure 3-62 Although these large nuclei seem atypical, they appear irregularly distributed, and the spaces between the cells have irregular, slit-like shapes.

pathologist and to suggest the presence of neoplastic atypia, but consideration of other findings establishes the benign nature of the cells. Like conventional hyperplastic cells, these "atypical" ones appear irregularly distributed (Fig. 3-62), and despite their larger size, they sometimes show the phenomenon of maturation (Fig. 3-63). Careful inspection of the nuclei demonstrates nuclear folds and grooves, pale granular chromatin, and occasional pseudoinclusions (Fig. 3-64). The spaces have the slitlike configurations characteristic of hyperplasia, and the nuclei of the cells abutting the spaces tend to sit just beneath the luminal aspect of the cell membrane (Fig. 3-65).

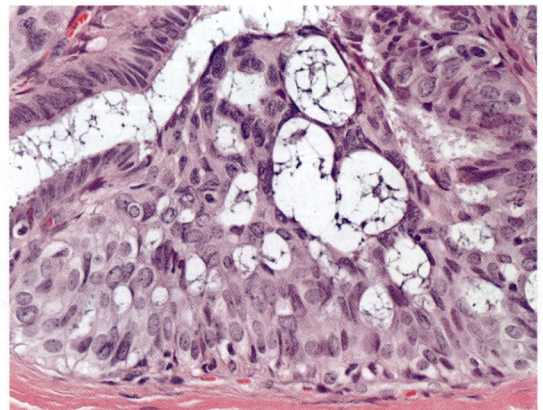

Figure 3-63 The peripheral nuclei seem unexpectedly large, but the population displays the phenomenon of maturation.

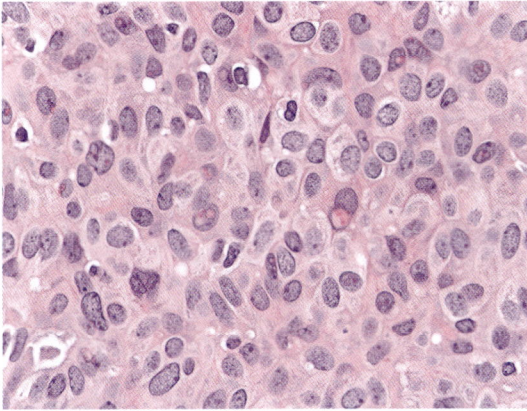

Figure 3-64 These large nuclei have folds, grooves, irregular shapes, and nuclear pseudoinclusions.

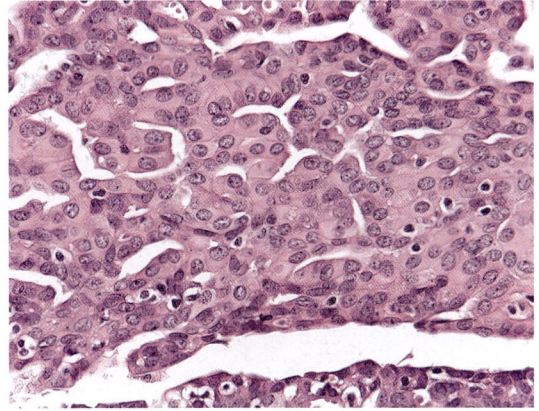

Figure 3-65 The nuclei of these proliferative cells occupy the region adjacent to the lumen, and the spaces look like slits.

Researchers have not determined the clinical significance of this variety of ductal proliferation. Because most of the characteristics of these cells match those of conventional hyperplastic cells, it seems prudent to take a conservative view of such foci and to regard the cellular and nuclear enlargement as a reactive phenomenon rather than a neoplastic one.

Immature Hyperplasia

If one studies cases of early conventional ductal hyperplasia, one usually observes a few large cells containing large nuclei along the basement membrane (Fig. 3-66), and in certain examples, these cells become conspicuous (Fig. 3-67). The nuclei of such cells vary in shape and contain homogeneous chromatin. In cases most easily recognized as hyperplastic, the chromatin appears pale and slightly granular, somewhat similar in quality to the chromatin of conventional hyperplastic nuclei, and such nuclei often contain a single nucleolus. The chromatin in more problematic cases often looks hyperchromatic and finely dispersed, making it difficult to appreciate the presence of nucleoli. The cytoplasm typically has an amphophilic hue, but it can appear pale. One can find a mitotic figure or two; these dividing cells typically sit near the basement membrane but not on it (Fig. 3-68). The large cells usually merge with smaller, centrally situated cells that display the typical morphologic features of ductal hyperplasia; however, in uncommon circumstances, the large peripheral cells do not demonstrate this morphologic evolution obviously. They retain their large

Figure 3-66 The cells along the basement membrane in this focus of slight conventional ductal hyperplasia appear large and they possess large nuclei and prominent nucleoli.

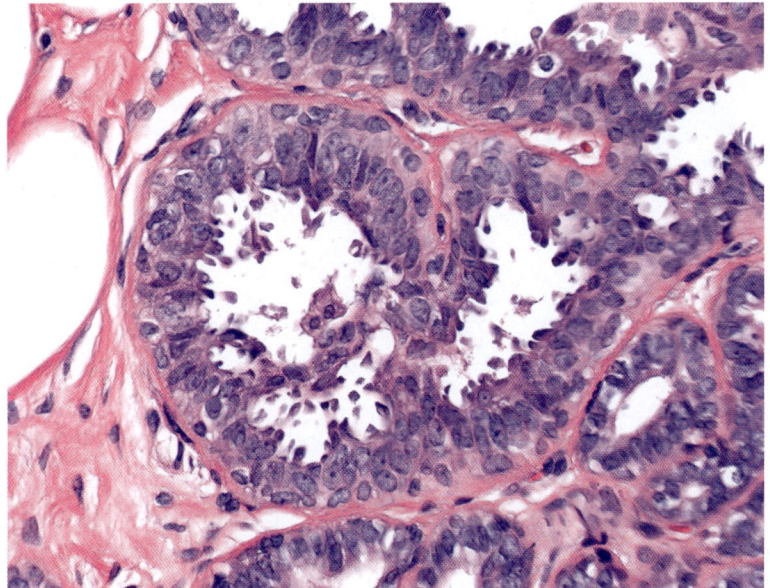

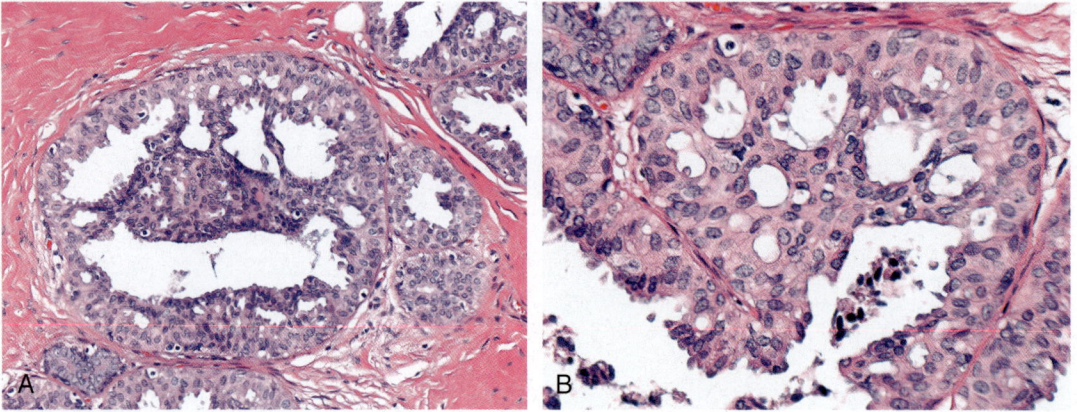

Figure 3-67 A and **B,** The peripheral, immature cells constitute a noticeable fraction of the cells in this focus of ductal hyperplasia. Although the cells appear large and possess large nuclei, their subtle variability bespeaks their benign nature.

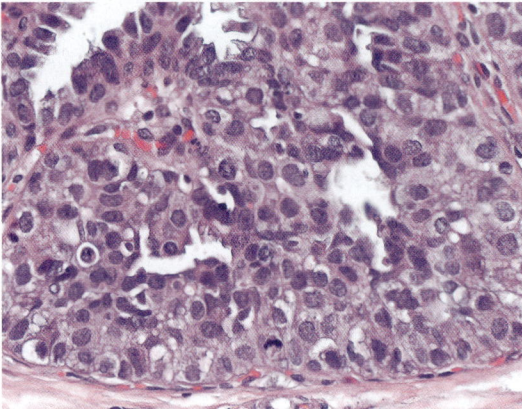

Figure 3-68 These immature hyperplastic cells have finely dispersed, dark chromatin, which makes them look atypical. One cell near the basement membrane contains a mitotic figure.

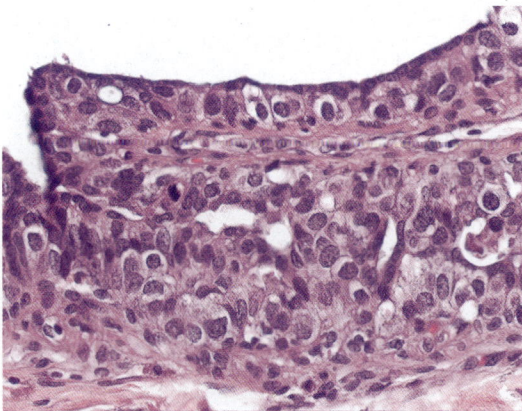

Figure 3-69 The abrupt transition between these immature hyperplastic cells and the flattened luminal cells on the surface and the trapping of intact small glands combine to simulate the appearance of the pagetoid spread of carcinoma cells.

size as they accumulate and dominate the population. Furthermore, these large cells often undermine preexisting benign luminal cells and entrap acinar cells, and the resulting pattern simulates the appearance of the pagetoid growth of malignant cells (Fig. 3-69).

Because of the large size of the cells and this manner of growth, pathologists unfamiliar with immature hyperplasia may worry that it represents a form of atypical ductal hyperplasia or even ductal carcinoma in situ, especially when the large, immature cells swamp their conventional counterparts. Attention to several features helps allay these worries and prevents misinterpretation. First, the cells of immature hyperplasia grow in cohesive masses, which do not resemble the dishesive cells of many carcinomas (Fig. 3-70). Second, immature hyperplasia usually displays an orderly appearance. The proliferative cells typically form a uniform layer encircling the duct lumen and symmetrically narrowing it (Fig. 3-71); furthermore, the degree of proliferation seems constant from gland to gland, and the glands have similar diameters and similar round, oval, or bosselated contours (Fig. 3-72). This uniformity and symmetry bespeak a physiologic process and contrast with the haphazard and irregular appearance of carcinomas. Third, despite the unexpectedly large size of the cells and their nuclei, both continue to exhibit many of the features of hyperplastic cells in subtle form. The nuclei display an irregular distribution and irregular shapes; usually, at least a few nuclei show the notches and folds characteristic of hyperplastic ductal cells (Fig. 3-73). If the cells form spaces, the cells outlining the spaces do not display polarization, and one can usually spot a hint of maturation if the cells form a mass occupying the duct lumen. Fourth, one can often observe preexisting benign cells entrapped within

Figure 3-70 The neoplastic lobular cells within the epithelium of the duct in the left of the field demonstrate dishesion. The immature hyperplastic ductal cells thickening the epithelium of the duct in the right appear cohesive.

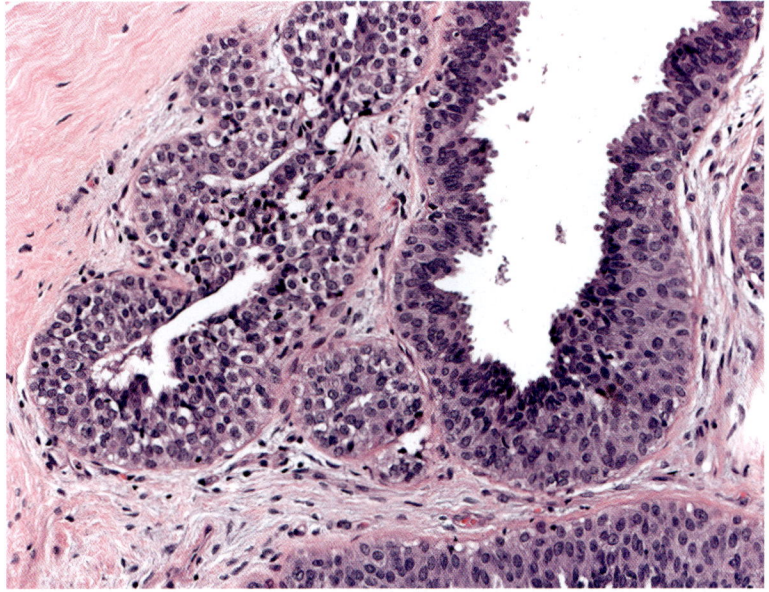

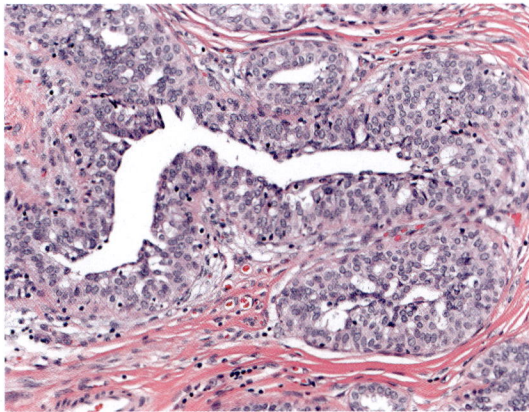

Figure 3-71 In this example of immature hyperplasia, the hyperplastic cells thicken the epithelium to form a uniform layer around the perimeter of this ductule.

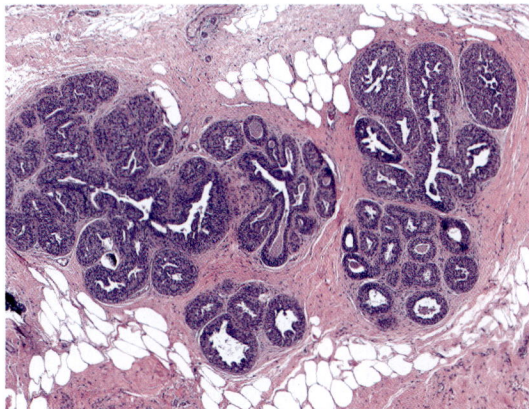

Figure 3-72 Immature hyperplasia has distended these glands to a uniform extent.

the hyperplastic population. The former can persist as attenuated cells sitting on the surfaces of the proliferative ones or even as intact small glands composed of bland, polarized, acinar cells (Fig. 3-74). In foci showing only modest proliferation, these preexisting cells remain as periodically spaced, radially oriented, attenuated cells that seem to tether flattened superficial luminal cells to the basement membrane (Fig. 3-75). A careful search often turns up foci in which the immature cells form a continuum with smaller, conventional hyperplastic cells (Fig. 3-76). Finally, immature hyperplasia typically involves a discrete collection of glands, and the stroma surrounding them frequently appears hypercellular or proliferative. Sometimes the stroma displays pseudoangiomatous stromal hyperplasia (Fig. 3-77); in other cases it looks hamartomatous (Fig. 3-78). This confinement of such an epithelial proliferation to a nodule showing stromal proliferation should caution the pathologist against making a diagnosis of malignancy.

Staining for keratin 5/6 does not offer much help in the diagnosis of immature hyperplasia. Mostly, the immature cells fail to stain, although entrapped benign cells do stain, and one sometimes observes faint staining of cells located near the surface of the cellular mass (Fig. 3-79).

Because of their unfamiliarity with this form of hyperplasia, pathologists may prefer to classify it as atypical ductal hyperplasia. This preference seems reasonable until we have gained more understanding of its biologic potential.

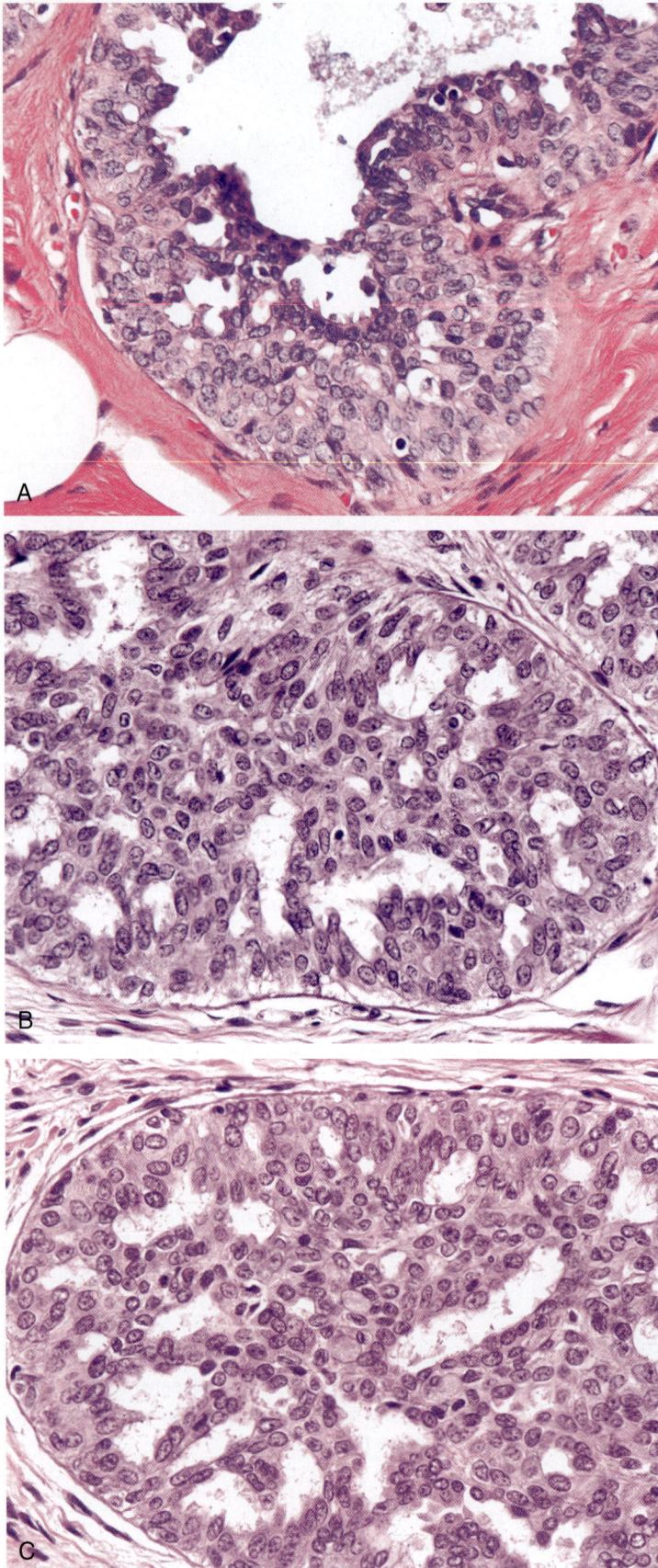

Figure 3-73 A, These immature cells show the irregularity in their placement characteristic of hyperplastic ductal cells. **B,** The chromatin varies in its staining qualities and so do the nuclear shapes and contours. **C,** The cells forming the spaces do not display polarization, and one can recognize a suggestion of maturation in the central cells.

Figure 3-74 The population of immature hyperplastic ductal cells with pale cytoplasm has entrapped a few preexisting luminal cells. Most of the latter persist as intact lumens.

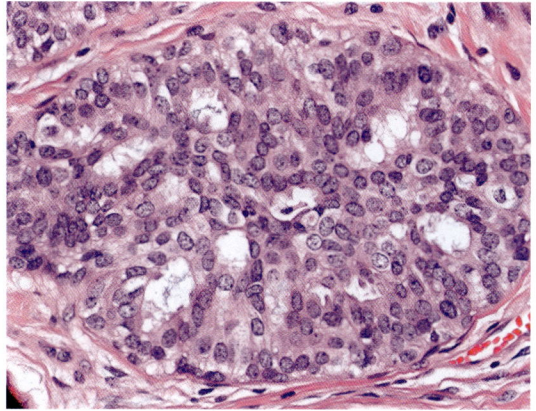

Figure 3-75 Benign epithelial cells remain as periodically spaced, attenuated cells stretching from the flattened luminal cells to the basement membrane.

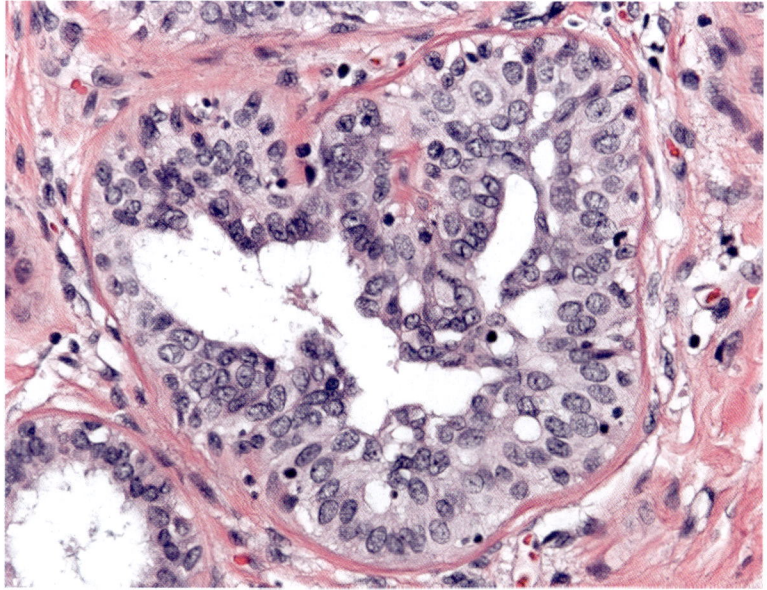

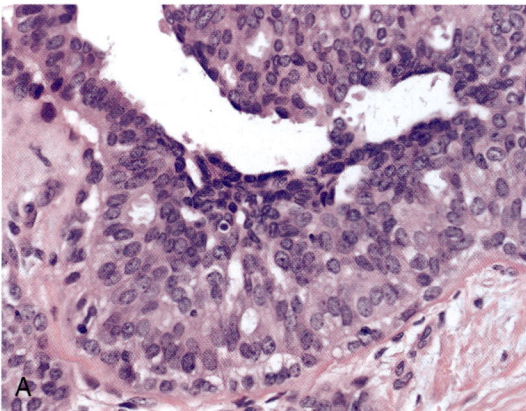

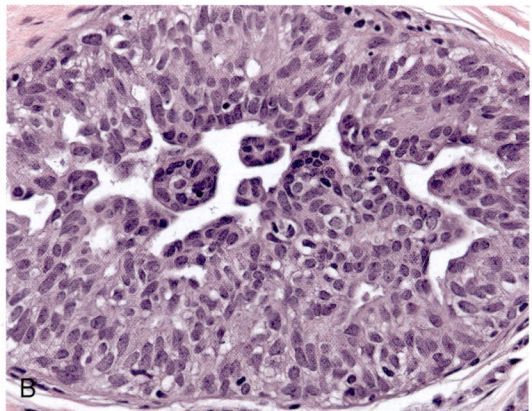

Figure 3-76 A, In the center of the field, the large cells form a continuum with others that look like mature hyperplastic cells. **B,** The immature hyperplastic cells display maturation of the centrally situated cells.

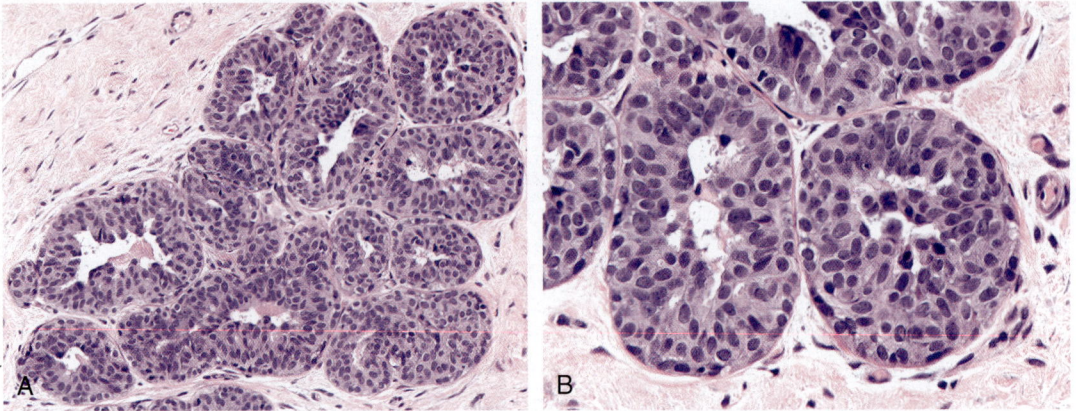

Figure 3-77 A, This focus of immature hyperplasia has developed in a region of pseudoangiomatous stromal hyperplasia. **B,** The predominance of the large cells and the homogeneity and hyperchromasia of their chromatin make the proliferation look like atypical ductal hyperplasia or, possibly, ductal carcinoma.

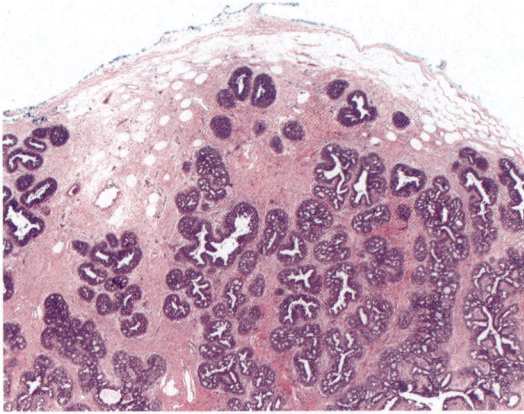

Figure 3-78 This nodule, composed of oddly structured glands and collagenous stroma, looks like a hamartoma. The glandular tissue within it displays the orderly proliferation of immature hyperplasia.

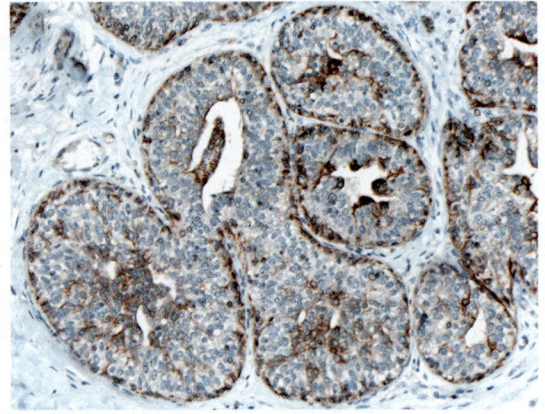

Figure 3-79 A stain for cytokeratin 5/6 shows that a few central cells in this focus of immature hyperplasia express the protein strongly, and a few others near the center stain faintly. Many cells do not stain at all.

Unusual Forms of Cytologic Atypia

The cellular alterations that constitute cytologic atypia tend to coexist in certain repetitive constellations, but one occasionally observes abnormal cells whose features do not fit the usual patterns of atypia. Such cells sometimes represent examples of rare types of neoplastic proliferations; more often, these uncommon patterns of cytologic atypia reflect an unusual benign process. Pathologists must take care not to label every proliferation showing unusual cellular features as atypical, because clinical colleagues commonly regard atypical proliferations as neoplastic phenomena and react accordingly. One finds unusual, atypical cells in two apparently benign conditions.

Effects of Irradiation

Irradiation leads to marked alteration of mammary tissues. Although the specific findings vary in degree from case to case, the changes in the tissue result from two phenomena, the development of cytologic atypia and atrophy of the terminal duct–lobular units. The cytologic alterations usually attract the most attention, because irradiated benign epithelial cells can mimic anaplastic carcinoma cells. The most conspicuous changes occur in the luminal cells, which appear enlarged. Increases in the size of the nucleus and the amount of the cytoplasm explain the genuine enlargement of the cells, and atrophy of nearby cells exaggerates, the degree of these increases. The altered cells typically exhibit cuboidal

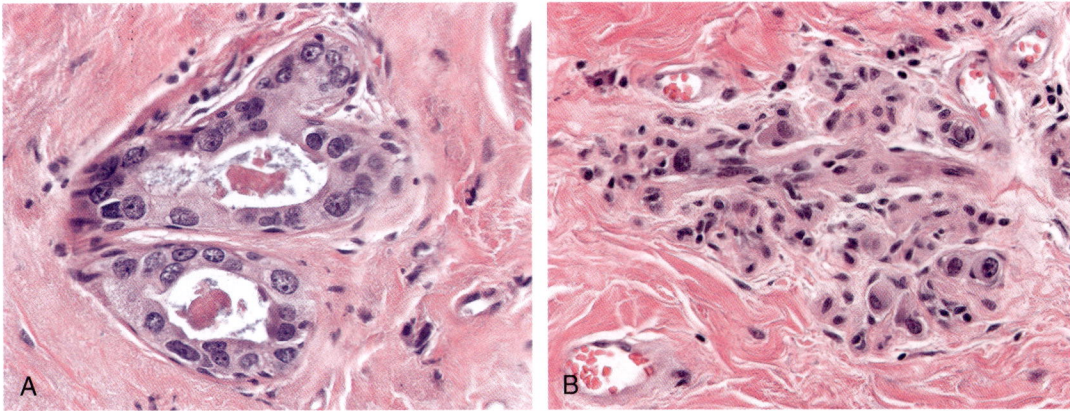

Figure 3-80 A and **B,** Cells showing the effects of irradiation appear larger than normal cells. They contain large nuclei and abundant cytoplasm. Atrophy of neighboring cells exaggerates the apparent enlargement of the altered cells.

or polygonal shapes, but a few cells appear flattened and arch around the acinar lumen (Fig. 3-80). Most of the altered cells contain enlarged, irregular, folded, or notched nuclei with pale, homogeneous, and washed-out chromatin, but occasional nuclei appear hyperchromatic (Fig. 3-81). The nuclei often possess nucleoli, which frequently look especially prominent. The cytoplasm has a dense quality and often a deeply eosinophilic color, and many cells contain cytoplasmic vacuoles. The nucleus-to-cytoplasm ratio of most cells falls within the normal range, although rare cells have an increased ratio. The basal cells show less pronounced alterations (Fig. 3-82). Their nuclei have an oval shape and folded contour, and the larger ones contain a small nucleolus. Although the nucleoli vary somewhat in size and shape, they do not demonstrate the pleomorphism shown by the luminal cell nuclei. The smallest basal cells have scant, eosinophilic cytoplasm, whereas the larger ones contain pale cytoplasm in an amount proportional to the size of the nucleus.

To recognize the atypia of radiation and to avoid misinterpreting the cells as malignant, one must search for evidence of the second radiation-induced phenomenon: atrophy of the glandular tissue. Terminal duct–lobular units show the most obvious effects. The altered lobules appear small. Comparison of irradiated lobules with unirradiated ones makes the extent of atrophy obvious (Fig. 3-83). The radiation-induced death of epithelial cells and the resulting loss of acini cause the lobules to collapse. Some of them consist of tiny, closely packed acini, many of which lack lumens (Fig. 3-84). This absence of glandular spaces can create the mistaken impression of cellular proliferation unless the pathologist realizes that this appearance results from a combination of the enlargement of the epithelial cells and the coalescence of the

cells as the acini shrink rather than from filling of acinar lumen because of cellular proliferation. Attention to the diameter of the acini helps avoid this mistake. In more severely affected lobules, the acini disappear entirely, leaving only nodules of dense collagen in their places. This disappearance of acini seems to begin at the periphery of the lobules, so that in some, only the central acini and the intralobular terminal ductule remain (Fig. 3-85). The basement membranes of the acini usually appear thickened (Fig. 3-86). The specialized stroma comes to consist of dense, sometimes hyalinized, collagen in most cases; however, the intralobular stroma can remain virtually unaltered.

One sometimes also observes hyalinization, endothelial prominence, or intimal thickening of blood vessels and atypia of fibroblasts (Fig. 3-87). The intralobular plasma cells often appear numerous and plump (Fig. 3-88).

Two other factors influence the histologic characteristics of the irradiated breast. First, irradiation does not affect the tissue uniformly. Markedly altered lobules often sit next to unaffected ones (Fig. 3-89). Pathologists must not expect to observe a uniform distribution to the histologic changes, nor should they let this variation in the extent of the changes dissuade them from ascribing these findings to irradiation. Because of this variability, detection of radiation changes sometimes requires a conscious and determined search. Second, the extent of the changes varies according to the interval between the treatment and the tissue examination. With the passage of time and the death of irradiated cells, the epithelial changes become less evident, especially at low magnification. This seeming disappearance of radiation effects does not occur because the cytologic alterations of individual cells abate; instead, it arises because the number of affected cells decreases. The disappearance of

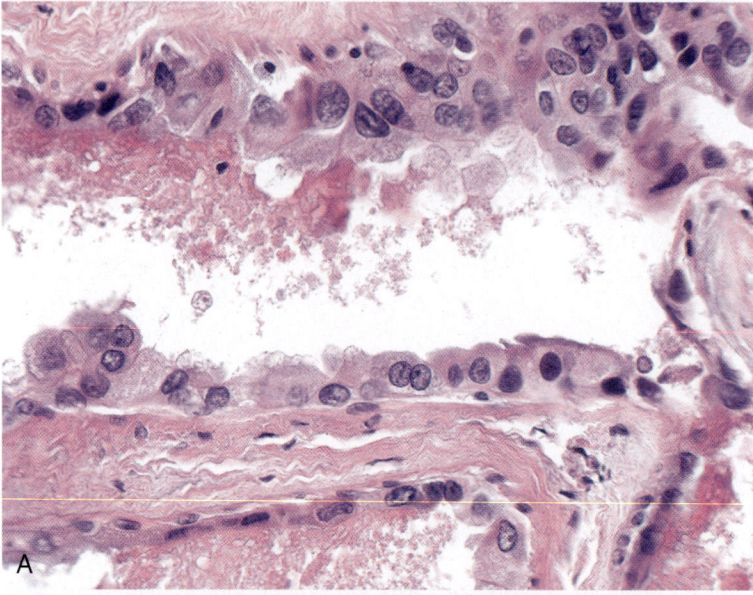

Figure 3-81 A, The nuclei of irradiated luminal cells often appear irregular and their chromatin pale. **B,** One can also observe smoothly contoured nuclei containing homogeneous dark chromatin.

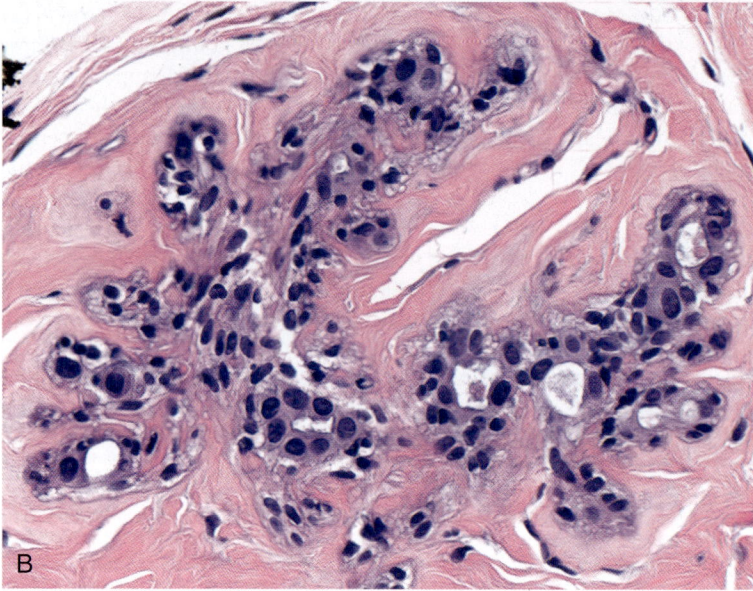

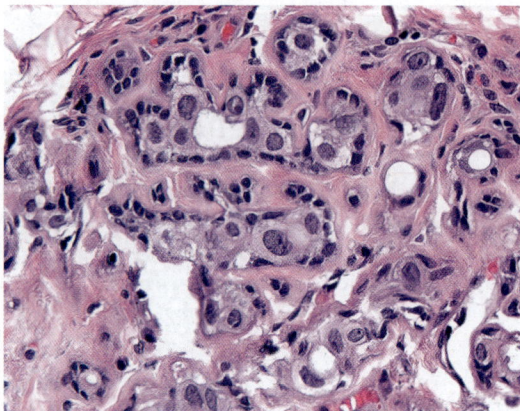

Figure 3-82 The large cells harboring large nuclei represent luminal cells; the basal cells display only slight enlargement.

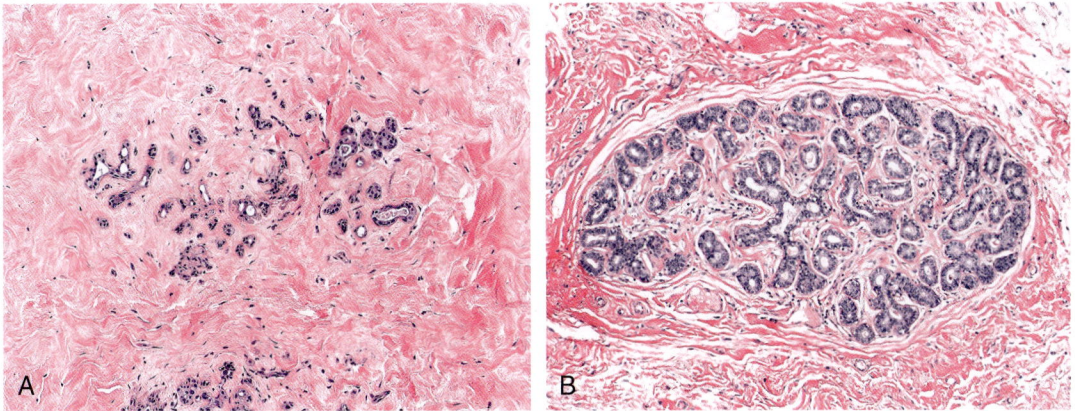

Figure 3-83 Compare the size of the irradiated lobule shown in **A** with the size of a similar lobule from the same patient resected prior to the radiation treatment, shown in **B**.

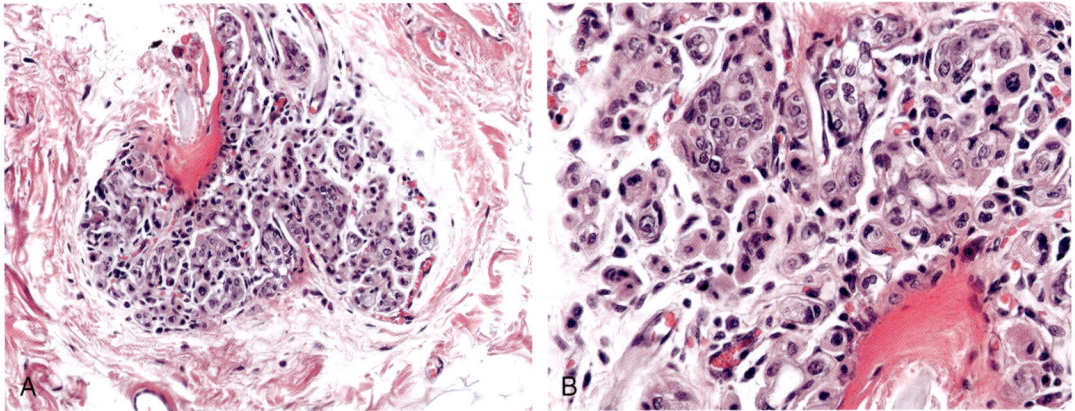

Figure 3-84 A, Radiation has caused the acini to shrink and this lobule to collapse. **B,** The absence of lumens and the close packing of the glands can create the false impression of cellular proliferation.

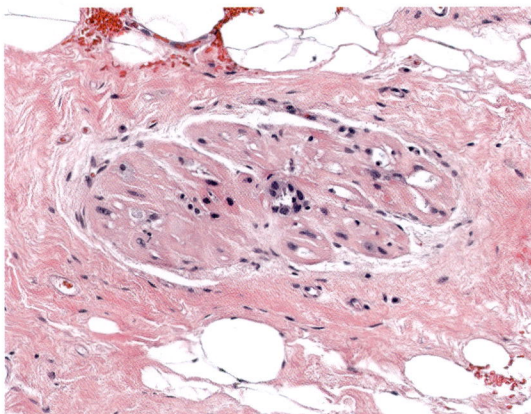

Figure 3-85 This irradiated lobule consists of only the intralobular terminal ductule and the ghosts of a few acini.

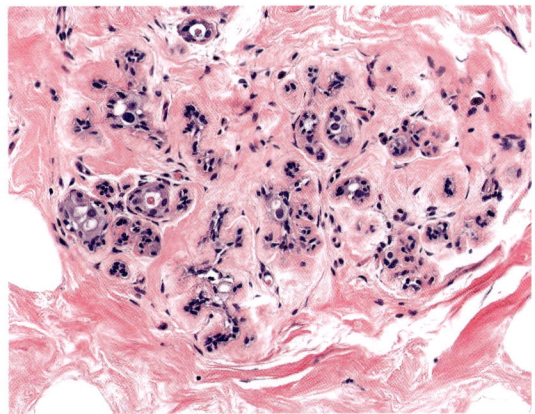

Figure 3-86 Note the thickened basement membranes of these radiation-damaged acini.

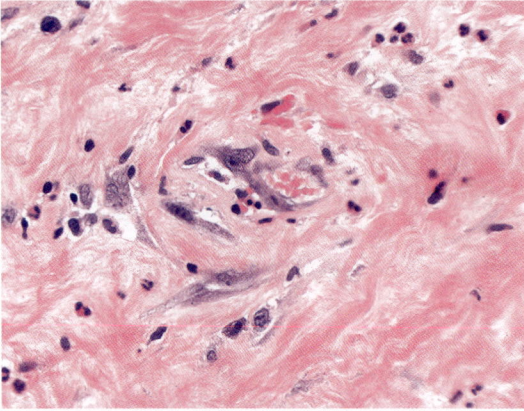

Figure 3-87 The nuclei of these irradiated fibroblasts appear large and somewhat atypical, and the cells have unusually elongated configurations.

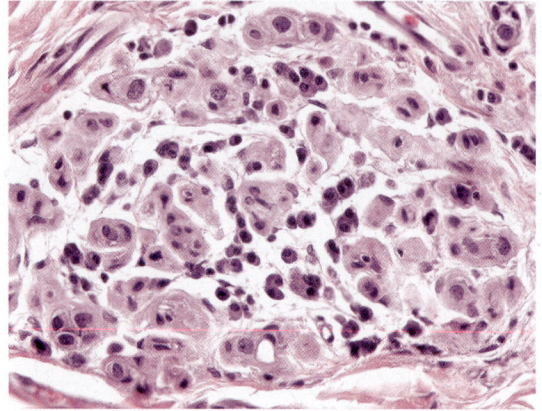

Figure 3-88 Many plasma cells remain in this irradiated lobule.

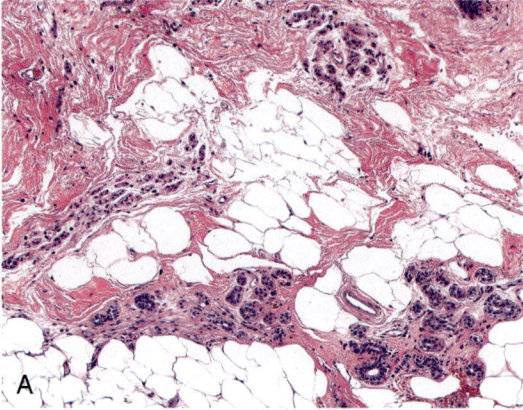

A

Figure 3-89 A, An atrophic lobule in the center left of the field sits among others of nearly normal size. The cells of the atrophic lobule in **B** demonstrate the typical features of irradiation, but those in a neighboring lobule in **C** do not.

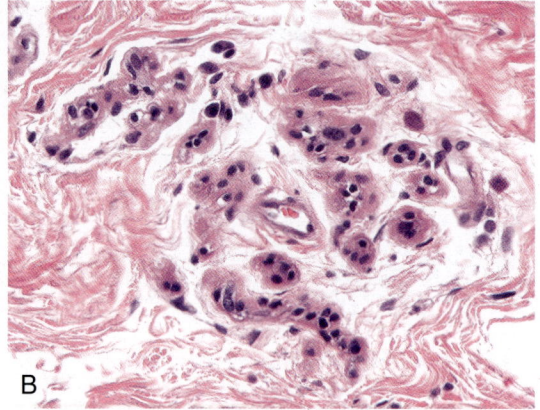

B

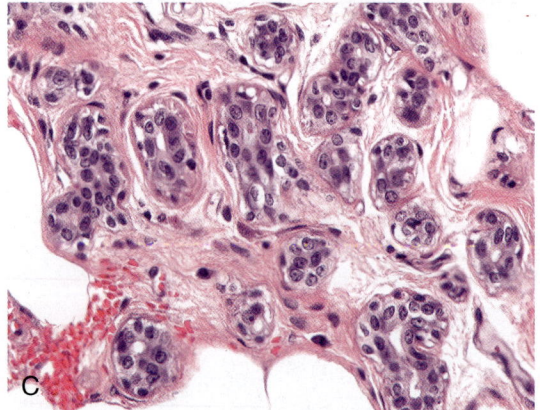

C

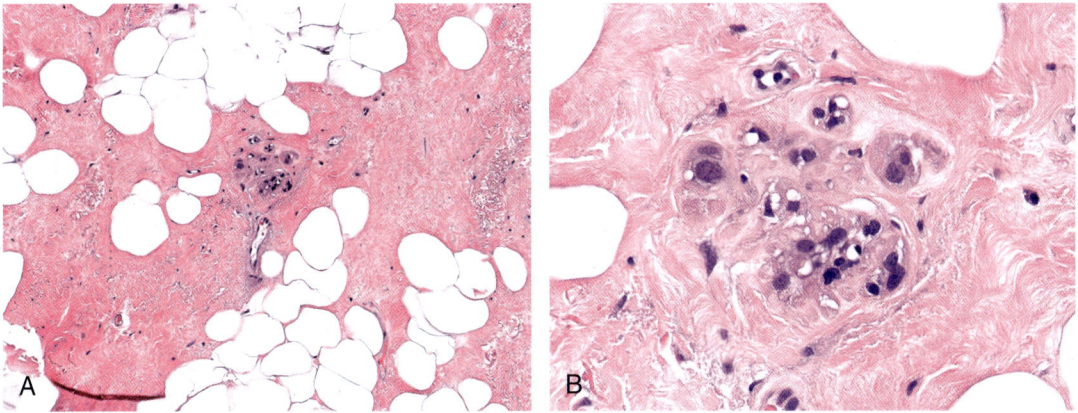

Figure 3-90 A, Twenty-five years after treatment with radiation, one tiny lobule, a mere shadow of its former self, remains. **B,** It still contains a few cells displaying the typical alterations caused by irradiation.

damaged epithelial cells accounts for the unimpressive low-power appearance. Despite the extensive loss of irradiated cells, one can still find a few showing the typical features even as long as 25 years after treatment (Fig. 3-90).

In specimens resected a decade or so after the irradiation, the stromal changes tend to eclipse the glandular ones. In fact, so much of the glandular tissue disappears that only a few epithelial cells exhibiting radiation changes remain. The stroma, on the other hand, continues to appear greatly altered.

"Apocrine-Like" Atypia

An especially rare form of cytologic atypia consists of large cells containing large, folded nuclei and smudgy, hyperchromatic chromatin (Fig. 3-91). The cells most often occupy acini and terminal ductules, where they form a single layer abutting the lumen.

The only information about this change in the commonplace literature comes from a caption to Figure 12.20 in the textbook, *Diagnostic Histopathology of the Breast*, by Dr. David Page.[1] He writes, "Very rarely, lobular units with cytology suggestive of apocrine type will have foci with greatly enlarged and hyperchromatic nuclei without much internal detail. Although unusual, the foci cannot be recognized as atypical in the sense of indicating heightened risk of subsequent carcinoma development at this time."

On the basis of this description and personal experience, it would seem that this lesion consists of small groups of cells within terminal duct–lobular units. Although the cells look bizarre, they do not show necrosis or mitotic activity, and the level of proliferation appears minimal. Pathologists should probably keep an open mind about the significance of this lesion. It may well represent a degenerative phenomenon, and one can probably overlook it when it occurs in a patient without a history of carcinoma or in an excision specimen

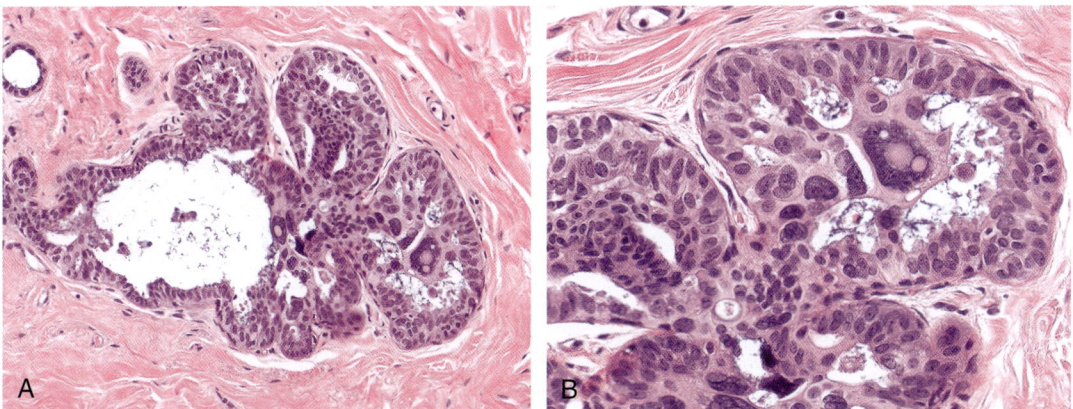

Figure 3-91 The small terminal duct–lobular unit in **A** contains a few extremely unusual cells as seen in **B**, which probably arose through a degenerative process rather than a neoplastic one.

that does not contain evidence of malignancy. On the other hand, one must think carefully before disregarding such a focus in a core biopsy specimen or in any sample from a patient with carcinoma, because small foci of high-grade carcinoma can mimic this lesion.

Atypia in the Adolescent

The criteria for the evaluation of ductal epithelial proliferation have evolved primarily from the examination of specimens taken from women older than 30 years, yet pathologists must also interpret changes present in tissues removed from younger patients. Although the same principles of analysis seem to apply, one should probably take an especially cautious approach to the diagnosis of malignancy in adolescents, especially in girls with only minimally developed glandular tissue and in boys. During active growth of the gland, the epithelial cells become crowded and even slightly stratified, and their nuclei can sometimes show characteristics similar to those seen in atypical ductal cells of middle-aged women (Fig. 3-92). Furthermore, the small size of the glandular structures makes it easy to section them in off-center planes, creating the appearance of architectural atypia (Fig. 3-93). Thus, to make a diagnosis of ductal carcinoma in situ in an adolescent, one should insist on the presence of all three components of ductal carcinoma in situ: well-established cytologic atypia, clear-cut architectural atypia, and substantial proliferation.

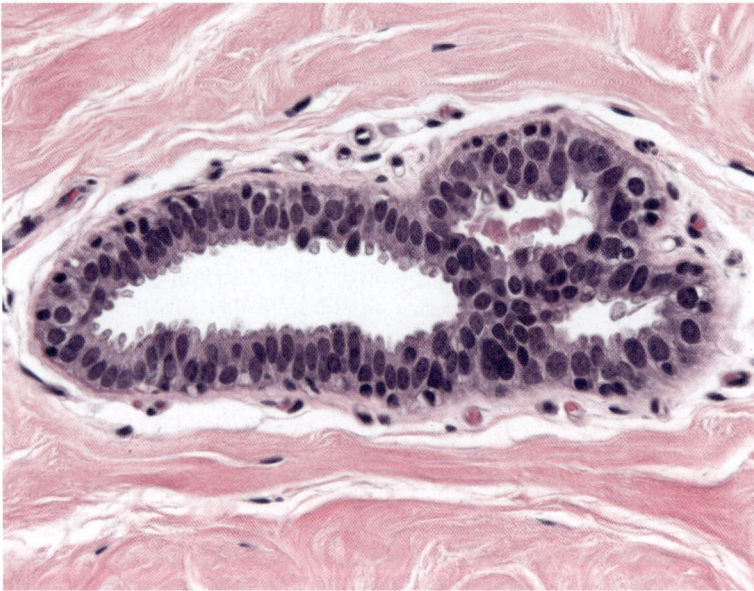

Figure 3-92 These apparently normal epithelial cells from a 17-year-old woman have large, smoothly contoured, oval or round nuclei and homogeneous dark chromatin. These features would constitute cytologic atypia in many situations.

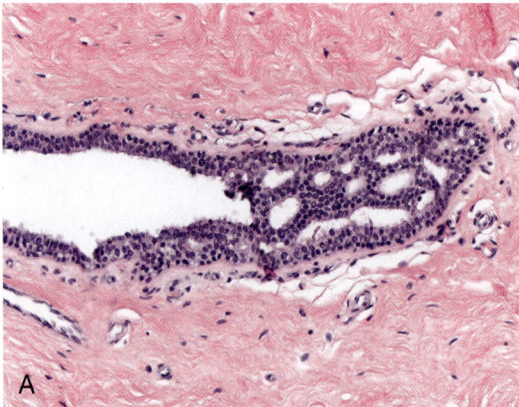

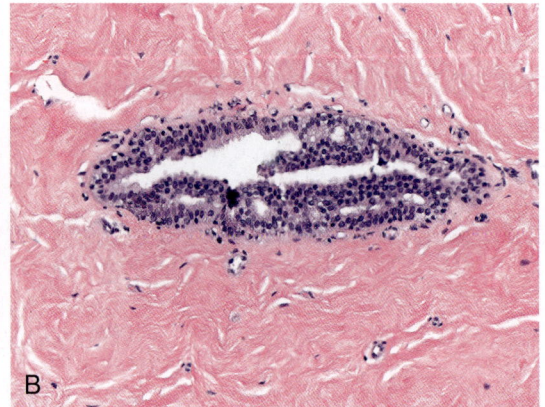

Figure 3-93 Off-center planes of section of the end of a curving duct in **A** and the edge of another in **B** create the impression of proliferation and architectural atypia where neither exists.

PROBLEMS IN THE DIAGNOSIS OF DUCTAL CARCINOMA IN SITU

Unlike cases of ductal hyperplasia, which resemble one another to a great extent, examples of ductal carcinoma in situ present varied appearances. Many of these variations do not pose diagnostic problems once pathologists familiarize themselves with their characteristics, but a few varieties cause persistent headaches. The differentiation of intermediate-grade ductal carcinoma in situ from conventional ductal hyperplasia, for instance, often proves extremely difficult, and the presence of malignant cells with differing morphologic features (dimorphic carcinoma) can complicate one's analysis. Carcinomas growing in a flat pattern present problems in detection and diagnosis.

Reaching a diagnosis of ductal carcinoma in situ does not end the pathologist's potential problems, because invasive carcinomas can closely mimic the pattern of ductal carcinoma in situ, and so can carcinoma growing in lymphatic vessels. To distinguish these situations, pathologists carry out immunohistochemical staining to detect proteins present in myoepithelial cells. This technique is a powerful tool, but one must interpret the results carefully to avoid incorrect conclusions. Finally, the detection of ductal carcinoma in situ in uncommon settings requires special consideration. Specimens exhibiting the effects of irradiation and gynecomastia represent two common situations of this type. The following discussion offers a few suggestions as solutions to these problems.

Distinction of Intermediate-Grade Ductal Carcinoma In Situ from Conventional Ductal Hyperplasia

Pathologists expect to have difficulty distinguishing conventional ductal hyperplasia and atypical ductal hyperplasia from low-grade ductal carcinoma in situ; however, they usually do not imagine having to struggle to differentiate ductal hyperplasia from intermediate-grade ductal carcinoma in situ. Nevertheless, this problem in differential diagnosis often proves especially difficult, because the two lesions can share several cytologic characteristics. For example, like the nuclei of hyperplastic cells, those of intermediate-grade ductal carcinoma in situ can display irregular contours, granular chromatin, and nucleoli of a modest size (Fig. 3-94). The polarity of the cells of intermediate-grade carcinomas may not appear obvious, and the cells may not form well-developed cribriform spaces. This absence of both cellular and architectural evidence of polarization furthers the resemblance to ductal hyperplasia.

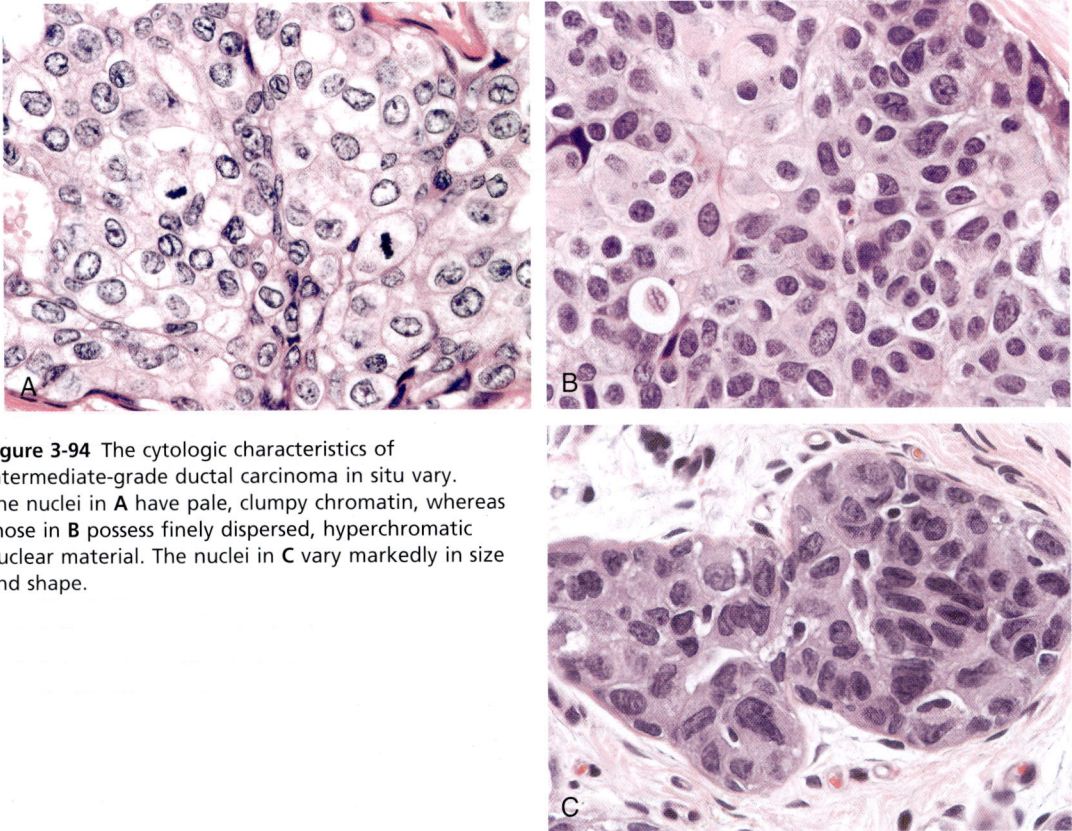

Figure 3-94 The cytologic characteristics of intermediate-grade ductal carcinoma in situ vary. The nuclei in **A** have pale, clumpy chromatin, whereas those in **B** possess finely dispersed, hyperchromatic nuclear material. The nuclei in **C** vary markedly in size and shape.

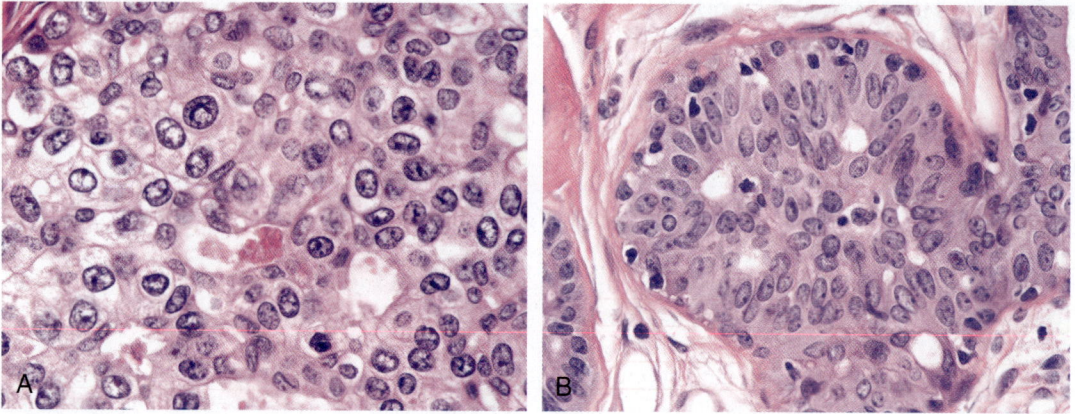

Figure 3-95 The nuclei of the intermediate-grade carcinoma illustrated in **A** appear larger than those of the hyperplastic cells present in the same specimen, shown in **B**.

Several features allow one to distinguish most cases of intermediate-grade ductal carcinoma in situ from those of ductal hyperplasia, although no single feature will differentiate these two lesions in every instance. The size of the cells and their nuclei probably represents the most consistent and most helpful feature to separate the entities, because the cells of intermediate-grade ductal carcinoma in situ typically appear larger than those of ductal hyperplasia. The larger size of the malignant cells arises because they possess larger nuclei than hyperplastic cells and they usually contain more cytoplasm, also. One must remember that proliferative cells exhibit a range of sizes and that the largest cells in a hyperplastic population can look larger than the smallest carcinoma cells. The presence of these exceptional cells does not invalidate the observation that the average size of the cells of intermediate-grade ductal carcinoma in situ noticeably exceeds the average size of hyperplastic ductal cells. Juxtaposition of the two populations highlights these differences and helps solidify one's tentative diagnosis (Fig. 3-95).

The evaluation of other nuclear characteristics also helps differentiate intermediate-grade ductal carcinoma in situ from ductal hyperplasia. Although the features of the nuclei tend to overlap in these two entities, the attributes often appear exaggerated in the nuclei of the carcinoma cells. For example, the nuclei of hyperplastic ductal cells typically exhibit slight pleomorphism, but the degree of pleomorphism shown by the population in Figure 3-94C goes beyond that seen in hyperplasia. A proportion of the cells of hyperplasia typically have granular chromatin and slight clearing. The extent of chromatin clumping and nuclear clearing pictured in Figure 3-94A surpasses the amount seen in hyperplastic cells. Folds and notches in the nuclear contours give hyperplastic nuclei irregular shapes, but never ones as irregular as those seen in the carcinoma cells shown in Figure 3-94B. Thus, the presence of nuclei showing exaggeration of the typical morphologic features of hyperplastic nuclei should suggest the diagnosis of carcinoma, and so would the presence of dishesion, necrosis, or mitotic figures. Immunohistochemical staining for cytokeratin 5/6 helps establish the diagnosis in many of these problematic cases; however, one must keep in mind that ductal carcinoma in situ of the basal-like type shows staining for cytokeratin 5/6.

Dimorphic Ductal Carcinoma

When studying breast cancers, pathologists first applied the term *dimorphic* to a variety of papillary carcinoma in which the malignant cells exhibit two distinctly different morphologic forms. The cells growing on the basement membrane usually appear larger and possess clearer cytoplasm and larger nuclei than those adjacent to the lumen. Although many pathologists have come to appreciate that this phenomenon occurs in papillary carcinomas, fewer observers recognize that one can observe cellular dimorphism in ductal carcinomas growing in conventional patterns, also. In fact, careful scrutiny reveals frequent examples of this occurrence.

The dimorphic cells in conventional ductal carcinomas display the same pattern as their counterparts in papillary carcinomas. Cells along the basement membrane appear larger than the centrally located cells, and the former have larger and paler nuclei and a greater amount of cytoplasm than the latter (Fig. 3-96). Because of their presence in a single layer and their cytoplasmic pallor, these basally positioned ductal carcinoma cells simulate the appearance of prominent myoepithelial cells and neoplastic lobular cells growing in a pagetoid pattern.

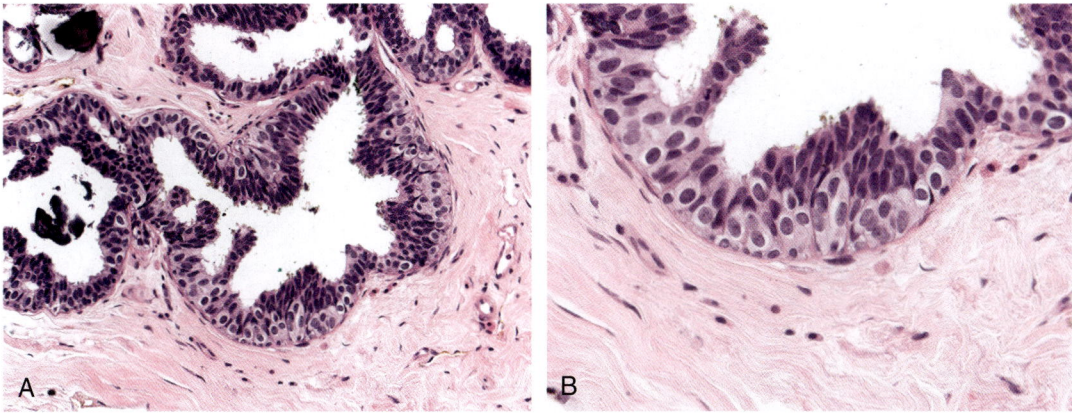

Figure 3-96 A, This dimorphic ductal carcinoma illustrates the characteristic appearances of the malignant cells. The basally situated carcinoma cells appear larger than the superficial carcinoma cells, and the former possess larger and paler nuclei than the latter. **B,** The nuclei of the two types of cells appear atypical, and both types of nuclei contain homogeneous, dark chromatin. Cells in the upper left form a continuum linking the two populations of carcinoma cells.

There are two strategies to distinguish dimorphic ductal carcinoma from these entities.

First, one can determine whether the cells constitute a single population or a mixture of two types of cells. Like the dimorphic cells of papillary carcinomas, those in dimorphic ductal carcinomas represent a single neoplastic population displaying two appearances. One recognizes this common heritage by noting the similarities in the fundamental properties of the nuclei in the two types of cells and by detecting regions containing transitional forms. Although the nuclei of the superficial cells most often appear somewhat smaller and darker than those of the basal cells, the nuclei of both types of cells look atypical, and the texture of the chromatin in both types of cells appears similar. These similarities of nuclear characteristics strongly suggest a common origin for the two types of carcinoma cells, and a careful search often reveals foci in which cells with intermediate features bridge the dimorphic populations. This finding cements the impression of a single population of carcinoma cells. Specimens showing prominent myoepithelial cells or lobular neoplasia, on the other hand, consist of two distinct populations of cells, which lack transitional forms. Prominent myoepithelial cells usually have grooved or folded nuclei, pale chromatin, and relatively abundant cytoplasm, features that contrast with the small, bland nuclei and modest amounts of cytoplasm of the overlying luminal cells. Neoplastic lobular cells also have larger nuclei than their benign counterparts, and the former display dishesion not shown by the latter. In neither of these lesions does one observe cells showing intermediate features and thereby uniting the basal cells with the superficial ones (Fig. 3-97).

Second, in addition to looking for signs of a common origin of the two types of cells, one should evaluate the morphologic characteristics of the different types of cells. In specimens showing prominent myoepithelial cells, neither the basal cells nor the luminal cells appear atypical. The former usually have pale, folded nuclei, and the latter small round or oval nuclei. In glands containing lobular neoplasia, only the basally situated, neoplastic lobular cells look atypical; the overlying luminal cells possess small, bland nuclei and usually display flattened shapes. All the cells of dimorphic ductal carcinoma, in contrast, contain atypical nuclei, which usually look enlarged and smoothly contoured and contain homogeneous chromatin.

Recognizing the proliferative cells as a single population does not establish the diagnosis of dimorphic ductal carcinoma, for the phenomenon of dimorphism of the malignant population brings to mind the appearance of maturation seen in hyperplastic ductal proliferations. Although the central cells in both conditions appear smaller and have smaller nuclei and darker chromatin than the peripheral cells, attention to other characteristics of the central cells allows one to differentiate these two lesions. The central cells of carcinomas do not display the crowding, overlapping, or molding that the maturing cells of ductal hyperplasia display. Central carcinoma cells appear larger than mature hyperplastic cells, because the former have larger nuclei and more abundant cytoplasm than the latter. Finally, the chromatin of the central carcinoma cells exhibits a finely dispersed texture, which contrasts with the condensed, clumpy nuclear material seen in mature hyperplastic cells (Fig. 3-98).

Clinging Carcinoma

In his textbook *Problems in Breast Pathology,* Dr. Azzopardi introduced the term *clinging carcinoma* to refer to an uncommon pattern of growth of

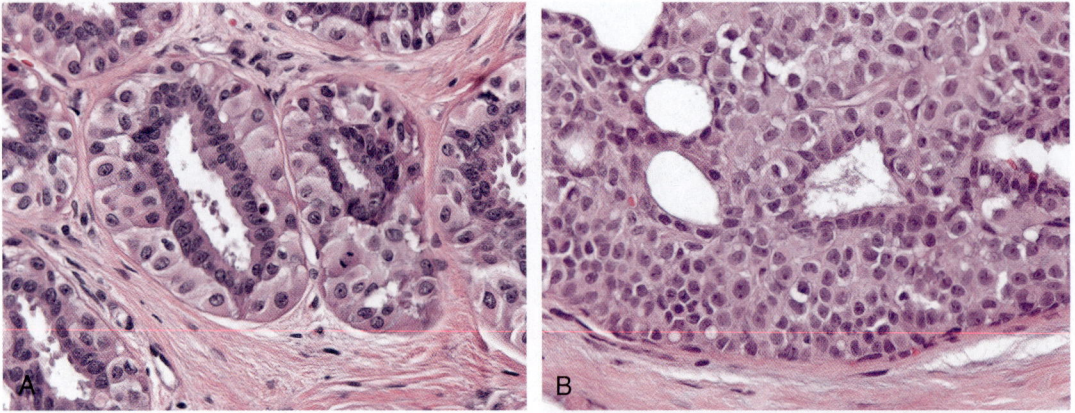

Figure 3-97 A, A ring of prominent myoepithelial cells underlies the luminal cells. Neither type of cell appears atypical. **B,** Dishesive neoplastic lobular cells spread beneath the luminal cells of these acini. The neoplastic cells display atypia, but those lining the lumens do not. **C,** Similarities in nuclear characteristics indicate that the cells in the dimorphic carcinoma represent a single malignant population.

carcinomas in which the malignant cells "are limited to the periphery of the containing structures, in the sense that they do not fill the lumen in solid or cribriform fashion nor do they show the numerous cells layers usually seen in comedo cancer."[2] Dr. Azzopardi went on to recognize the following two types of clinging carcinoma: (1) a type showing marked nuclear pleomorphism, which he regarded as a variant of comedocarcinoma, and (2) the more common, low-grade type characterized by monomorphic nuclei. Both types of clinging carcinoma present the pathologist with two diagnostic problems: detection of the lesion, and the recognition of its malignancy.

The detection of foci of clinging carcinoma can represent the greatest challenge in the diagnosis of this form of carcinoma. At scanning magnification, the

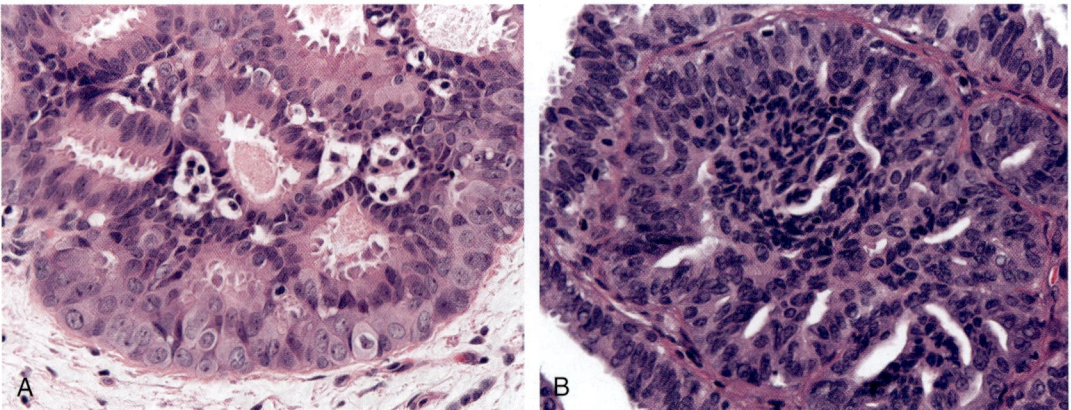

Figure 3-98 The appearance of the dimorphic ductal carcinoma in **A** resembles the pattern of maturation seen in ductal hyperplasia, but the central cells do not display the crowding, the condensed nuclei, or the scant cytoplasm seen in the mature hyperplastic ductal cells shown in **B**.

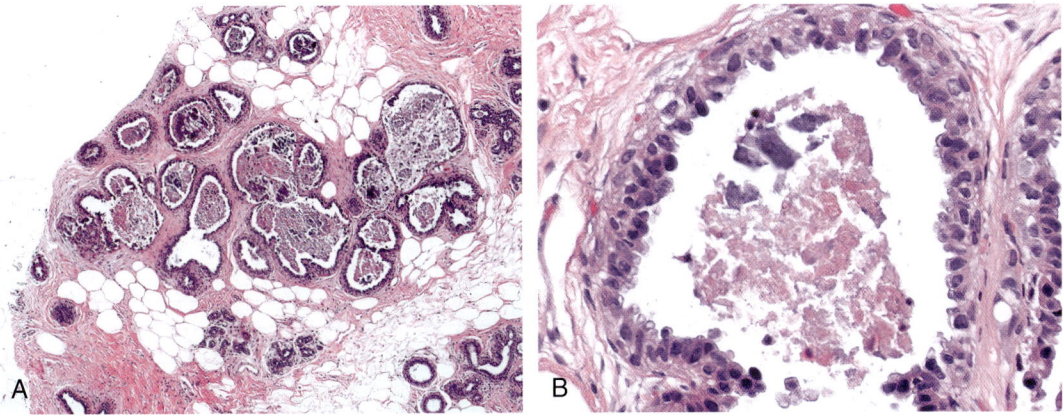

Figure 3-99 A, The large dimensions of the glands, the thickness of their epithelium, and the proteinaceous debris and calcifications in their lumens make it easy to spot this focus of clinging carcinoma using low magnification. **B,** High-magnification reveals the presence of necrotic epithelial cells and cytologic atypia.

altered glands might not differ appreciably from the microcysts of fibrocystic changes, so an inexperienced observer could fail to recognize the malignant foci entirely. Attention to the height of the epithelial cells lining distended ducts and acini helps to avoid this mistake. The cells lining cysts usually appear flattened and stretched around the perimeter of the space, whereas the cells of clinging carcinoma have polygonal, cuboidal, or columnar shapes and appear closely packed. The epithelium of clinging carcinoma therefore appears thicker and more prominent than the epithelium lining cysts, and one can usually appreciate this difference at even low magnification (Fig. 3-99).

The nature of contents of the glands also provides diagnostic clues. Examples of high-grade clinging carcinoma often contain sloughed, degenerating cells and cellular detritus in the lumens, and this debris often alerts the pathologist to the malignant cells growing on the wall of the gland. Small cysts can contain secretory material and histiocytes; however, this type of proteinaceous material exhibits a smooth and uniform texture different from the granular quality of cellular debris, and the nuclear characteristics and nucleus-to-cytoplasm ratios of histiocytes usually differ from those of detached carcinoma cells. Calcium crystals can also precipitate in the lumens of gland lines by clinging carcinoma, either within the proteinaceous material or as independent calcifications. Microcysts, sclerosing adenosis, and blunt duct adenosis commonly contain calcium deposits, too, so this finding does not establish a diagnosis of malignancy. Nevertheless, the presence of large acini and ducts that are lined by a prominent epithelial layer and that contain cellular debris or calcifications, all features evident at low magnification, should prompt pathologists to examine the cytologic characteristics of such foci carefully.

Having detected a region that makes one suspect the diagnosis of clinging carcinoma, one must investigate one's suspicion by studying the cytologic properties of the cells, because the diagnosis of malignancy rests entirely on the cytologic characteristics of the cells. When they display marked nuclear pleomorphism, chromatin aberrations, and high nucleus-to-cytoplasm ratios, the diagnosis of high-grade clinging carcinoma becomes virtually self-evident (Fig. 3-100); however, an especially difficult problem arises when the degree of anaplasia falls short of that required for a secure cytologic diagnosis of malignancy. One cannot solidify a diagnosis of carcinoma by detecting cellular stratification or other manifestations of architectural atypia, because clinging carcinoma lacks these features. Furthermore, the histologic characteristics of clinging carcinomas composed of cells with monomorphic nuclei blend with those of flat epithelial atypia so imperceptibly

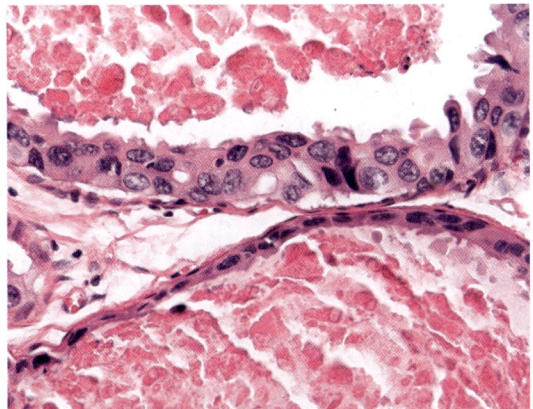

Figure 3-100 This example of high-grade clinging carcinoma displays anaplastic nuclei.

that one wonders whether one can ever distinguish the two lesions.

Most contemporary scholars of mammary pathology seem to believe that one cannot make this distinction, for they use the terms *flat epithelial atypia* and *clinging carcinoma, monomorphous type*, synonymously; however, a careful consideration of the histogenesis of flat epithelial atypia exposes a flaw in this usage. Flat epithelial atypia seems to arise when luminal cells of small ducts and terminal duct–lobular units develop cytologic aberrations and thereby gradually transform into atypical cells. Thus, the morphologic features of the slightest examples of flat epithelial atypia deviate only minimally from those of normal structures. What diagnosis should one use for the early stages in this process, such as the one pictured in Figure 3-101? Acknowledging that the cells display low-grade cytologic atypia and grow in a flat pattern, one could classify the focus as flat epithelial atypia; however, one could never endorse the use of the diagnosis of clinging carcinoma for such a minimal lesion. This example leads one to conclude that one cannot regard these two terms as synonymous. Instead, it seems preferable to reserve the term *clinging carcinoma, monomorphous type*, for well developed proliferations composed of atypical ductal cells growing in a flat pattern and the term *flat epithelial atypia* for less developed examples of the same type of proliferation.

Pathologists will have trouble following this line of reasoning, for neither the literature nor common experience enumerates criteria that allow one to identify the line separating clinging carcinoma from flat epithelial atypia. This author cannot write authoritatively about the solution to this diagnostic dilemma; however, in the spirit of helpfulness, he would offer the following opinions. First, extreme enlargement of the cells and their nuclei suggests the diagnosis of malignancy. A patient examination of the cellular characteristics sometimes reveals nuclei so large or so unusually shaped that one simply cannot accept them as benign or atypical (Fig. 3-102). Second, extreme crowding of the cells also suggests the diagnosis of carcinoma (Fig. 3-103). Especially dense packing of the cells can cause them to take on very tall, slender, columnar shapes and their nuclei to become somewhat spindly or pseudostratified. Finally, the presence of necrosis would probably clinch a diagnosis of cancer. It can appear minimal and consist of just a tiny bit of granular, eosinophilic material and a nuclear fragment or two (Fig. 3-104). Pathologists will find it profitable to search diligently for necrotic debris and, if found, to weigh its presence heavily. Because of the subtleties of these findings and the imprecision in their evaluation, pathologists often disagree about the diagnosis of such specimens, a few making the diagnosis

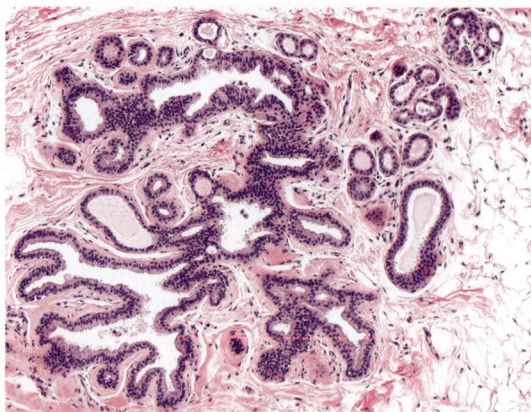

Figure 3-101 The small ducts in this focus of early flat epithelial atypia harbor slightly atypical columnar cells. One would not want to classify such a proliferation as low-grade clinging carcinoma.

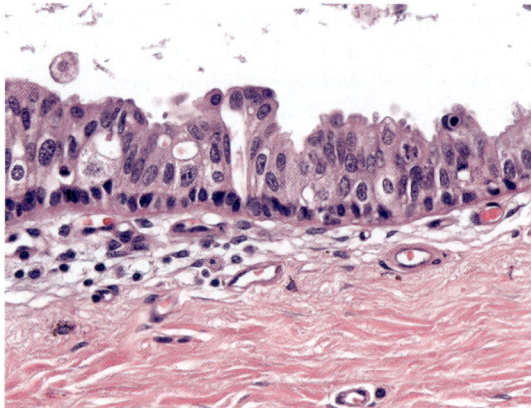

Figure 3-102 These nuclei look so large that one would have difficulty considering them benign.

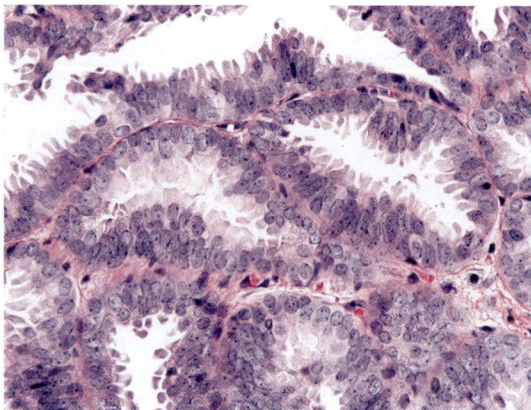

Figure 3-103 The dense packing of these cells suggests the diagnosis of malignancy.

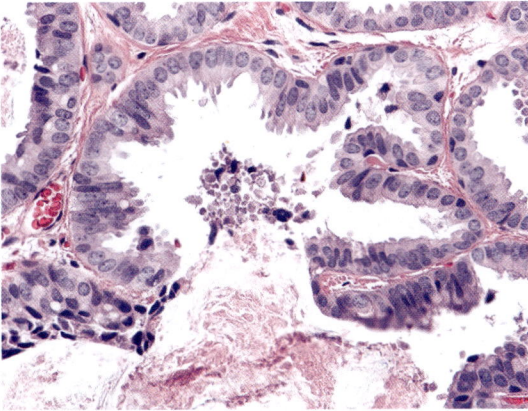

Figure 3-104 These few necrotic cells provide strong evidence to support a diagnosis of malignancy.

of carcinoma, whereas most favoring a diagnosis of severely atypical ductal hyperplasia. In light of this poor interobserver reproducibility and pathologists' tradition of refraining from making a diagnosis of malignancy in uncertain cases, pathologists may find it prudent to render a diagnosis of atypical ductal hyperplasia unless these worrisome findings dominate the histologic sections.

Recognition of Stromal Invasion

Pathologists do not have much trouble detecting the presence of stromal invasion in most cases, but the following four settings regularly create problems of this type: microinvasion by single cells or small groups that escape detection, invasion of well-differentiated carcinomas in groups that simulate lobules or foci of adenosis, invasion by small groups that simulate glands distorted by benign processes, and invasion in the form of nests that look like ducts distended by carcinoma in situ.

Microinvasion

In the first setting, pathologists do not even see the invasive cells, for they grow as individual cells or small clusters that do not provoke a stromal reaction. Invasive lobular carcinoma stands out as a notorious example of a carcinoma that creates this difficulty, but ductal carcinomas, too, can give rise to the same problem. Treatment of certain cancers eliminates nearly all the malignant cells, making it hard to detect the lone survivors, for instance, and the inflammatory reaction accompanying high-grade carcinomas can mask small invasive nests. Spotting the cells in question represents the most challenging aspect of this diagnostic problem; thereafter, the diagnosis of invasive carcinoma becomes relatively straightforward.

The author cannot offer any specific techniques to help pathologists recognize these invasive groups except to maintain a high level of alertness, especially in cases likely to create this problem. When studying specimens resected after neoadjuvant chemotherapy, pathologists must look especially carefully for isolated, bizarre cells (Fig. 3-105). The liberal use of immunohistochemical stains for keratin (Fig. 3-106) facilitates this search. On more occasions than the author cares to admit, the abundance of the cytoplasm and the irregular shape of the nucleus in cells like those pictured in Figures 3-105 have led him to wonder whether they represent histiocytes; almost all have been carcinoma cells. It therefore seems prudent to maintain a bias that large cells

Figure 3-105 A and **B,** One might find it difficult to detect these isolated carcinoma cells. Furthermore, degenerative changes can alter the cytologic characteristics of the cells and thereby call into question their malignant nature.

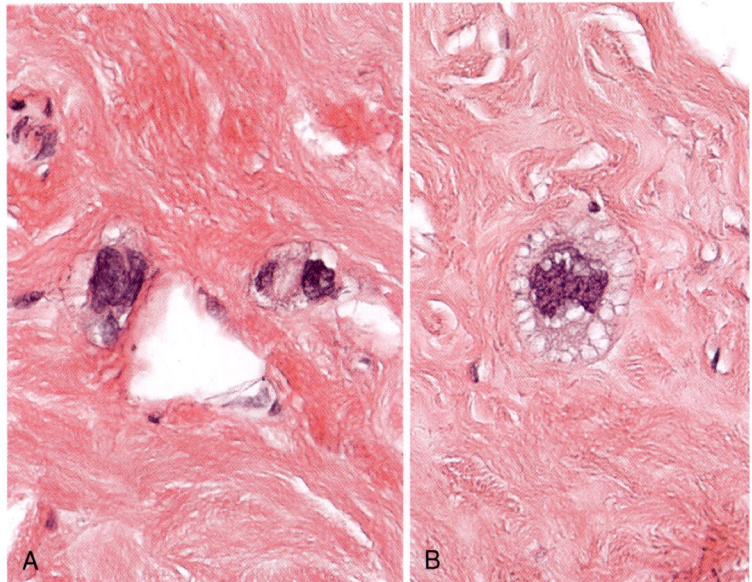

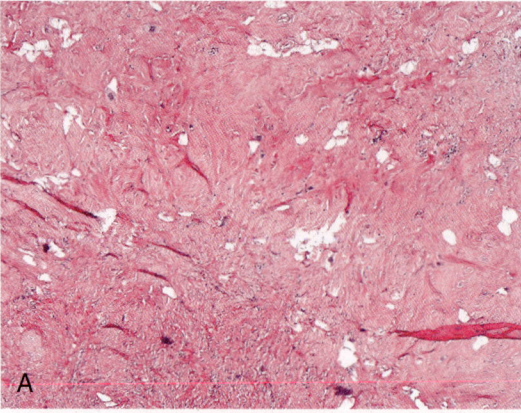

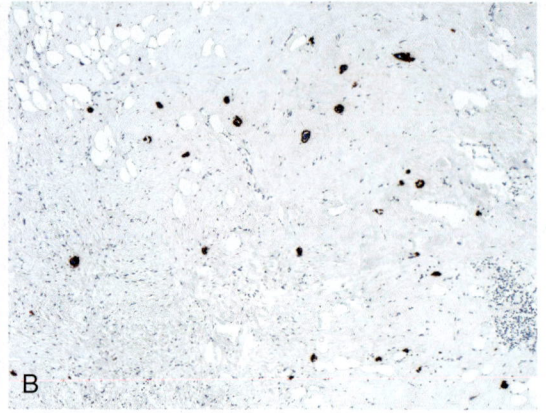

Figure 3-106 A, This field contains several carcinoma cells; however, one can only suspect their presence in the section stained with hematoxylin and eosin. **B,** An immunohistochemical stain for keratin makes the job seem like child's play.

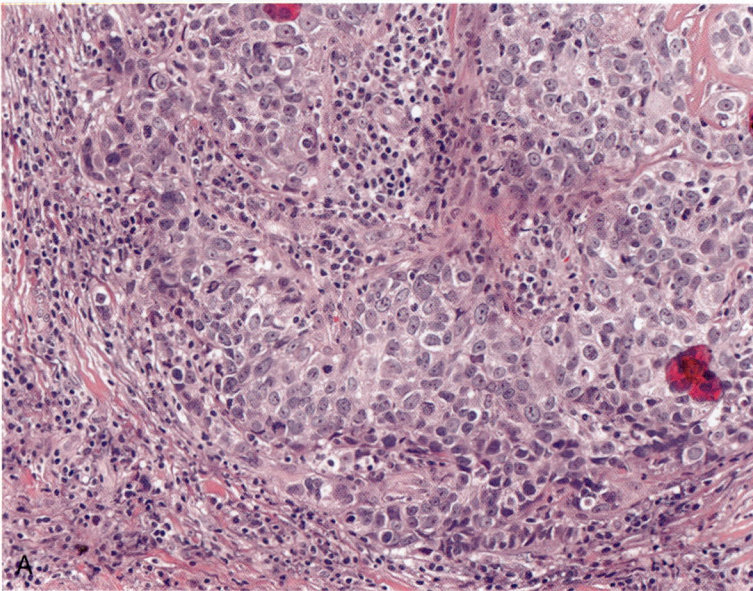

Figure 3-107 A, The marked inflammation makes it difficult to appreciate the irregularity in the contour of this aggregate of carcinoma cells. **B,** Staining using a mixture of antibodies, including those to keratin (*red*), myosin heavy chain (*brown*), and p63 protein (*brown*) reveals the lack of myoepithelial cells along one border of the aggregate and thus the presence of invasion.

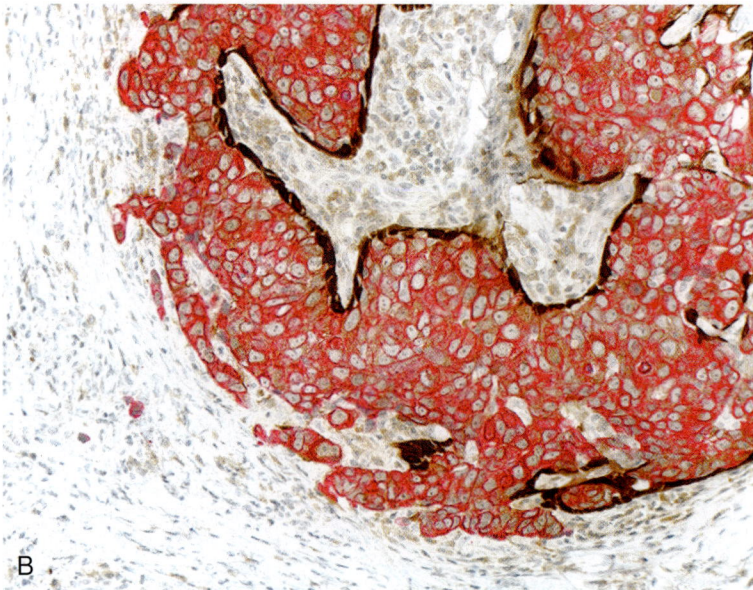

with atypical features in the setting of recent chemotherapy probably represent malignant cells unless one demonstrates another nature.

The dense inflammatory infiltrate surrounding ducts involved by ductal carcinoma in situ can obscure the interface between the epithelium and the stroma and thereby impair one's ability to recognize the irregularities in the contour of the aggregates, which often signal the presence of invasion. In Figure 3-107, for example, the nests of carcinoma cells appear rather smooth and well-defined, but an immunohistochemical stain using a mixture of antibodies to keratin, myosin heavy chain, and p63 protein reveals the lack of myoepithelial cells and thus the invasive nature of the cells. The numerous lymphoid cells can also mask individual carcinoma cells and small groups of cells (Fig. 3-108). On the other hand, the mere presence of cells with large nuclei

does not establish the diagnosis of invasive carcinoma, because activated lymphocytes and histiocytes can resemble carcinoma cells and so can endothelial cells (Fig. 3-109). Immunohistochemical staining for keratin offers the obvious solution to all these difficulties, but one must remember to carry out such procedures.

Mimicry of Benign Lobules

In the second problematic instance, foci of well-differentiated invasive ductal carcinomas form small, easily seen aggregates. Pathologists undoubtedly visualize the groups but run the risk of ignoring them because the cells appear bland and the aggregates resemble lobules or foci of adenosis. For example, Figure 3-110 illustrates a cluster of glands that looks a bit like a lobule; however, the group has an irregular shape and a poorly defined perimeter, the glands

Figure 3-108 This field contains both noninvasive (lower left and center) and invasive carcinoma. The invasive cluster in the upper center appears obvious, but the four small, individual carcinoma cells in the open circle hide among the inflammatory cells.

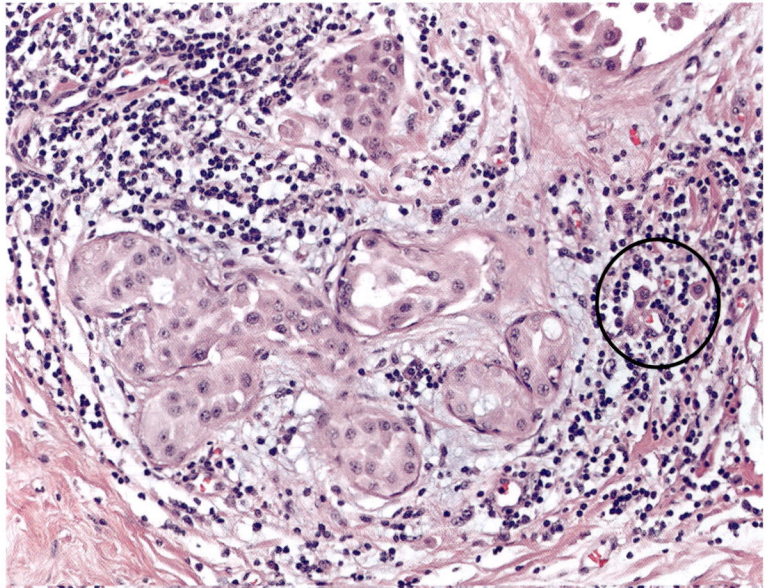

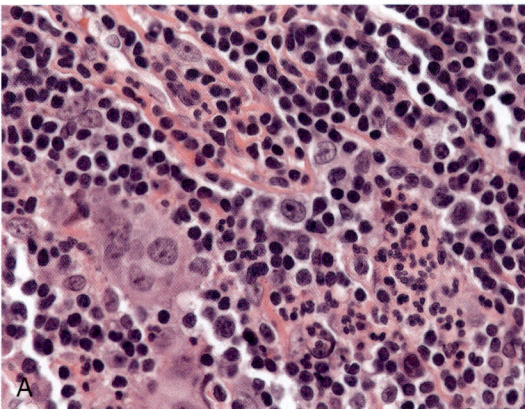

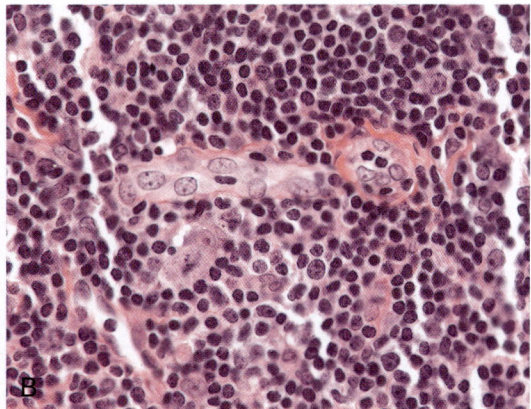

Figure 3-109 A, The large lymphocytes in the center of the photograph share certain features with the carcinoma cells in the lower left. **B,** One could mistake these endothelial cells for carcinoma cells, also.

within it appear loosely and haphazardly disposed, and the nodules lack specialized stroma. Taken together, these findings identify the region as invasive carcinoma. One might interpret the glands shown in Figure 3-111 as a focus of adenosis; however, the collection does not display the organization characteristic of any form of adenosis, and the presence of the tubules within the adipose tissue requires an explanation. The tubules constitute invasive carcinoma. A strong visual sense of the anatomic arrangement of normal mammary ducts and lobules and the internal structural organization of benign alterations of the glands represents the pathologist's most important tool in preventing these oversights. Furthermore, one must always keep a sharp eye out for out-of-place glands in the setting of lesions likely to generate well-differentiated invasive carcinoma. One must remember that tubular carcinomas often coexist with lobular neoplasia, flat epithelial atypia, and low-grade micropapillary ductal carcinoma in situ and that well-differentiated adenosquamous carcinoma frequently emerges from an underlying sclerosing lesion.

Involvement of Altered Tissue

In the third group of problematic settings, pathologists identify the cells in question and recognize their malignant nature, but alterations in the architecture of the parenchyma make it difficult to decide whether the cells represent invasive carcinoma or carcinoma in situ growing in altered glands. Damage to the tissue from crushing or cauterization, for example,

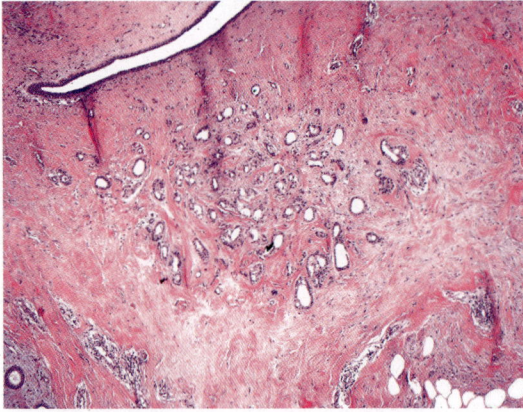

Figure 3-110 Despite a superficial resemblance to a lobule, this cluster of glands represents a focus of well-differentiated invasive ductal carcinoma.

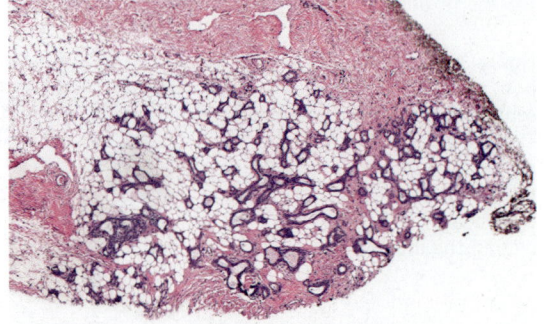

Figure 3-111 One might regard this collection of tubules as a focus of adenosis, but they do not display the structure seen in that lesion. The glands represent well-differentiated invasive ductal carcinoma.

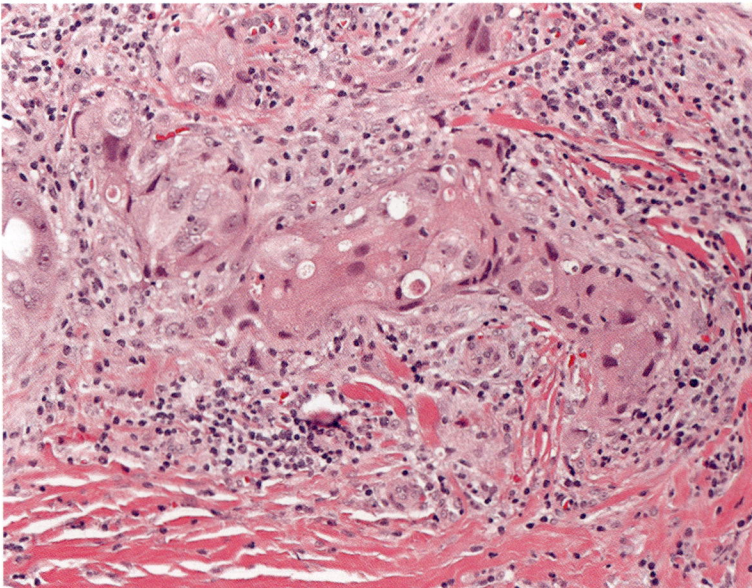

Figure 3-112 Although the nests look vaguely like interconnected acini, they do not display the anatomic arrangement of a genuine lobule. Furthermore, their irregular contours and odd, lumpy shapes should prompt one to consider the presence of invasion.

can create this problem, and so can distortion of the tissue by pathologic lesions such as sclerosing adenosis, radial scars, and papillomas. The scarring and inflammation associated with high-grade ductal carcinoma in situ commonly makes it especially difficult to detect small foci of invasion. A few clues can help pathologists recognize invasion in distorted tissue. Observers should first examine the cytologic characteristics of the cells, for invasive carcinoma cells should always display cytologic atypia. Second, pathologists should study the shape and arrangement of the clusters. Those with irregular or angular contours or situated in an arrangement that does not resemble the architecture of the mammary glandular tree (Fig. 3-112) should raise the suspicion of invasion, and so should the presence of isolated cells or linear chains. Third, microscopists may find it useful to examine the boundaries of these irregular or oddly placed groups carefully, looking for

disruption of the pattern of the collagen bundles (Fig. 3-113) and the lack of a basement membrane, which usually stands out as a distinct and well-defined eosinophilic band of uniform thickness. The absence of this layer of collagen leads to an intimate juxtaposition of malignant cells and stroma (Fig. 3-114). Finally, the presence of myxoid changes in the stroma often calls attention to foci of microinvasion.

Taken together, these signs steer pathologists toward the correct diagnosis in many cases, but these clues do not provide foolproof evidence of invasion. Sclerosing lesions sometimes distort glands to form small clusters or even short chains, and they frequently give rise to a reactive, myxoid stroma that looks like the stroma associated with invasive cancers. Ductal carcinoma in situ, too, sometimes causes a pronounced reaction of the surrounding specialized stroma. The dense inflammation that accompanies certain high-grade carcinomas can disrupt the

Figure 3-113 Notice the disarray in the arrangement of collagen bundles around this focus of invasive carcinoma.

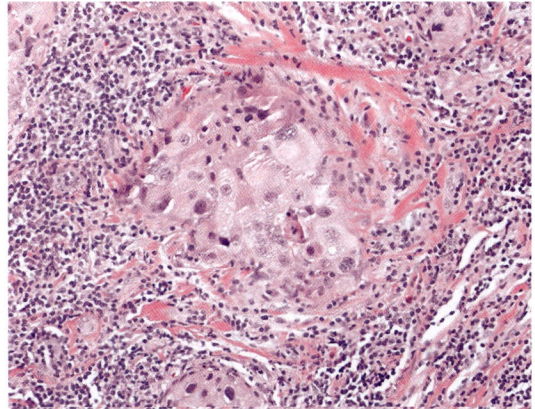

Figure 3-114 The cluster of cells in the right of the field represents invasive carcinoma; the one in the left, noninvasive carcinoma. The former has an irregular, notched contour, which contrasts with the smooth outline of the latter. The invasive cells appear naked, but one can appreciate the eosinophilic basement membrane and a few myoepithelial cells covering the noninvasive carcinoma cells.

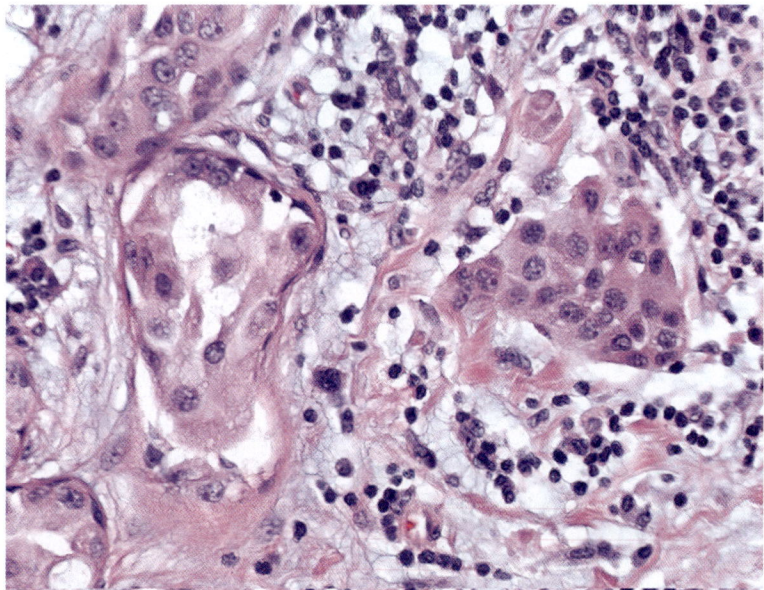

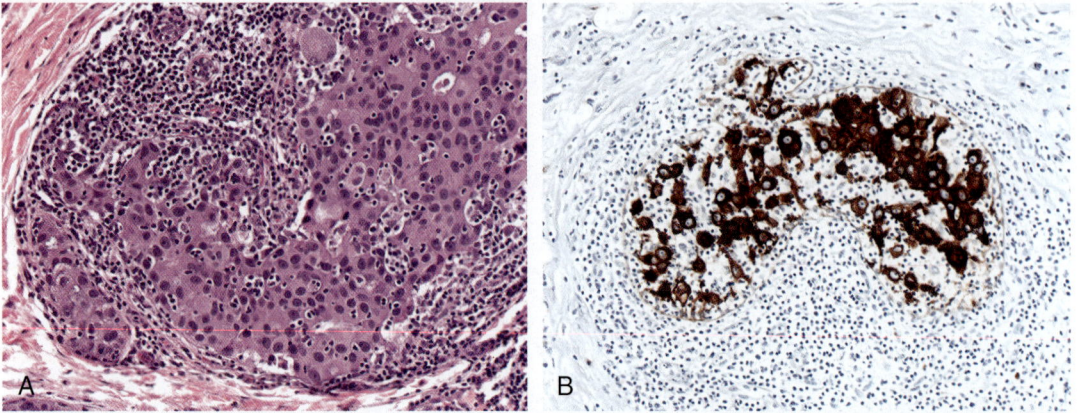

Figure 3-115 A, Alterations resulting from marked inflammation create the look of microinvasion. **B,** A stain for keratin highlights the disruption of the epithelium by inflammatory cells. **C,** A stain for myosin heavy chain demonstrates an intact myoepithelial layer.

epithelium in a way that produces irregularities in the outlines of the cell clusters, and these irregular groups look just like invasive cells (Fig. 3-115). Thus, these signs can only suggest the presence of invasion. Once detected, these findings should prompt pathologists to carry out the special studies needed to confirm or exclude the presence of invasion.

As a final point, one must realize that these slight deviations in shape and structural pattern represent especially subtle findings. It takes a great deal of experience and repeated correlations between appearances at low and high magnification and in sections stained with conventional and immunohistochemical techniques to learn to detect these signs of invasion. The nonspecific nature and the subtlety of these worrisome findings notwithstanding, the failure to search consciously and diligently for them constitutes the greatest impediment to their use.

Blunt Invasion

The final situation that presents a problem in the recognition of invasion arises when carcinomas infiltrate as round or linear nests that simulate ducts distended by carcinoma in situ. The aggregates of the carcinoma cells can mimic comedocarcinoma, solid ductal carcinoma in situ, cribriform ductal carcinoma in situ, and papillary ductal carcinoma in situ. In fact, the so-called intracystic papillary carcinoma seems to represent an extreme example of the phenomenon. Because published writings have not illustrated this pattern of blunt invasion, ignorance of its existence stands as the most significant barrier to recognizing such foci as invasive.

Knowledge of this phenomenon does not eliminate the diagnostic difficulties, for the foci may not display obvious histologic features of invasion. Nonetheless, several findings should cause a pathologist to wonder about the presence of blunt invasion. First, the formation of extremely large masses of cells displaying shapes that do not resemble those of ducts or terminal duct–lobular units should raise the suspicion of invasion (Fig. 3-116). Second, the distribution of groups in an arrangement that does not resemble the architecture of the mammary glandular tree also brings up the possibility of invasion. Glandular tissues distended by carcinoma cells typically retain the proportion, the distribution, and the branching pattern of normal ducts and lobules. Distended ducts typically appear either as aggregates of round or polygonal structures, which fit together in a geometric fashion, or as longitudinally sectioned structures, which branch dichotomously, and

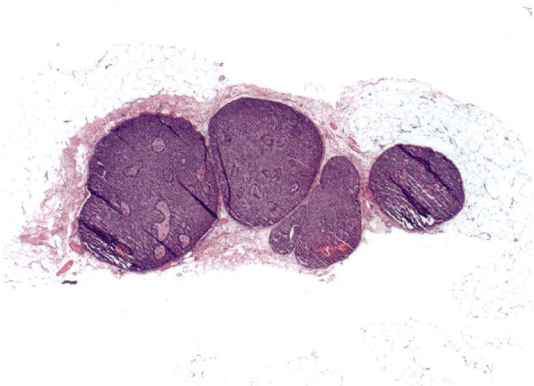

Figure 3-116 These aggregates look like ducts distended by carcinoma, but the sheer size of the groups should make one reconsider this interpretation.

enlarged acini cluster in rounded aggregates at the ends of ducts (Fig. 3-117). The distended ducts and acini have smooth, flowing contours, the structures seem to connect with one another, and the obviously involved glands coexist with others showing partial filling, less distention, or only limited proliferation. Thus, the presence of aggregates that seems to represent ducts cut only in transverse section, dispersed aggregates that do not seem to connect, or aggregates with irregular contours or odd angles of branching should lead one to suspect that the groups represent invasive carcinoma rather than ductal carcinoma in situ (Fig. 3-118).

Finally, the tissue immediately surrounding invasive nests does not display the histologic structure of a duct wall nor does it look like specialized stroma.

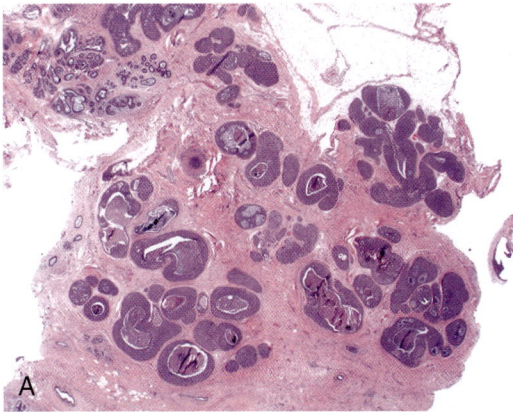

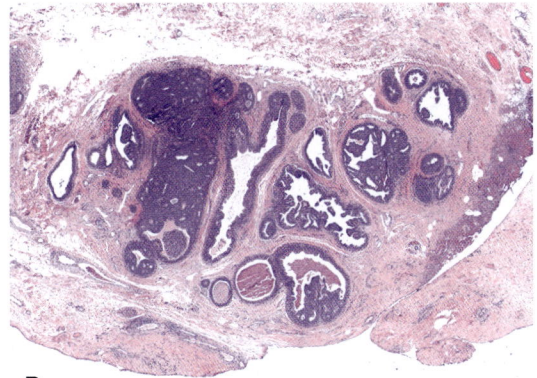

Figure 3-117 A, The ducts and lobules occupied by carcinoma cells retain the anatomic architecture of the mammary glandular tree. Note the similarity in the anatomic pattern of the uninvolved glands in the upper left and the involved one along the right of the photograph. **B,** Gland filled with ductal carcinoma in situ connects with others showing incomplete filling and less distention.

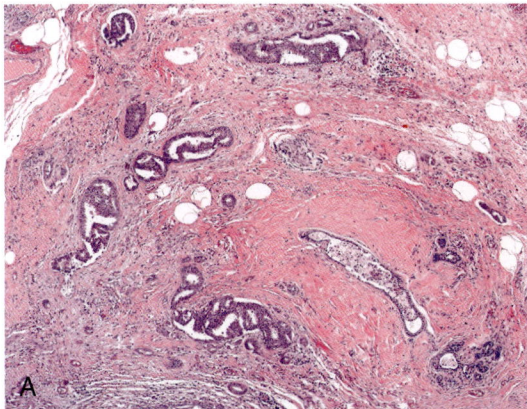

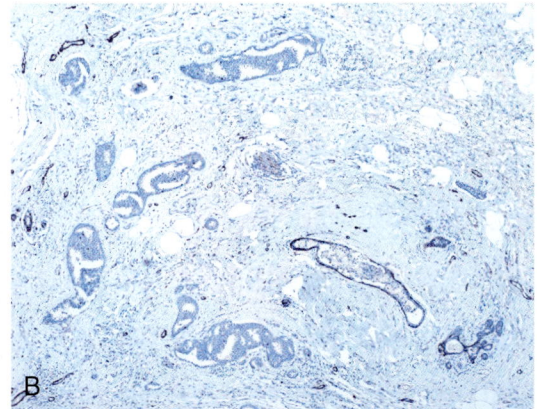

Figure 3-118 A, Although these groups look like ducts distended by carcinoma, the discontinuous arrangement, the lack of branching, the irregular contours of the groups, and the interspersed uninvolved structures suggest that the clusters represent invasive carcinoma. **B,** A stain for myosin heavy chain demonstrates the presence of myoepithelial cells around the uninvolved ducts and the lack of these cells around the invasive nests.

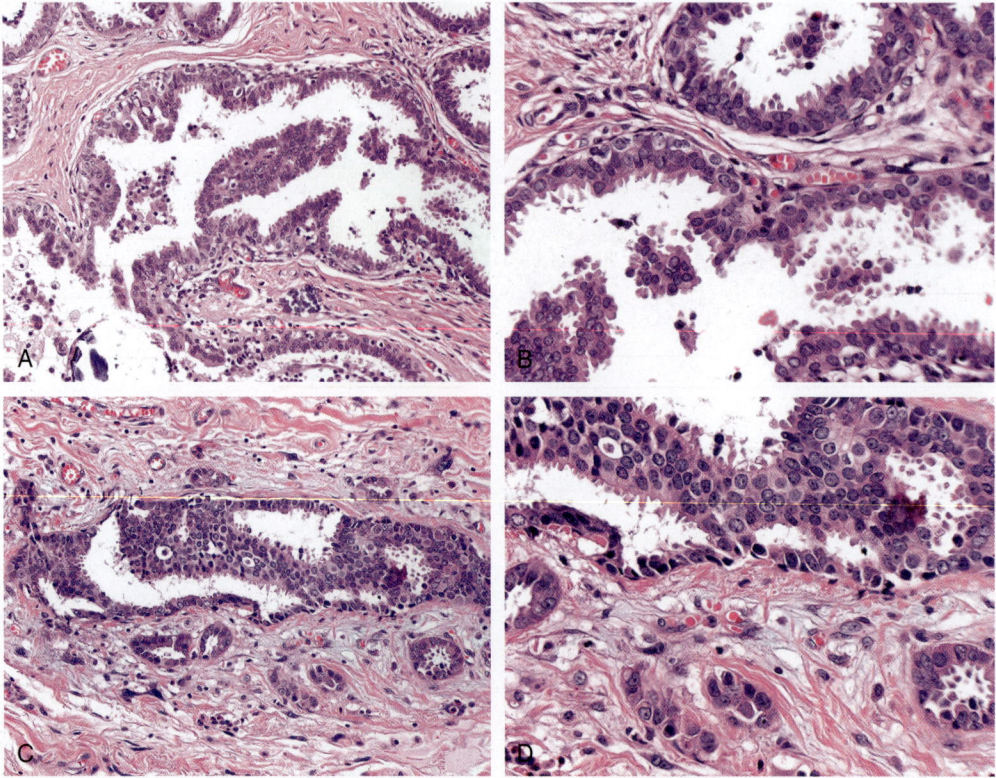

Figure 3-119 A, The collagenous tissue surrounding the duct involved by carcinoma in situ displays an orderly arrangement with respect to the duct. **B,** At high magnification, one can detect myoepithelial cells, basement membrane, and a layer of specialized stroma containing ground substances, fibroblasts, and capillaries. **C,** The stroma surrounding the large nest of invasive carcinoma does not appear organized, nor does it display an orderly relationship with the cells. **D,** One cannot appreciate myoepithelial cells or basement membrane, and the collagen bundles look disorganized.

Beneath the basement membrane of a normal small duct sits a thin layer of collagen bundles and a few fibroblasts and, external to that layer, a band of specialized stroma, which consists of loose fibrous connective tissue, capillaries, lymphatic vessels, lymphocytes, and plasma cells. Nonspecialized stroma composed of dense collagen surrounds the duct and its specialized stroma in a graceful, orderly arrangement. In many cases of ductal carcinoma in situ, certain of these structural elements persist in the tissue surrounding the involved glands, whereas foci of blunt invasion lack such findings (Fig. 3-119). In the latter circumstance, the orderly flow of the collagen bundles can appear disrupted, or the dense collagen can abut the carcinoma cells without an intervening layer of loose stroma and capillaries (Fig. 3-120). While inspecting this interface between the nests of cells and the stroma, the pathologist should look for focal fraying of the smooth contour of the nests, which may indicate subtle permeation by malignant cells. The presence of just a few of them among the collagen bundles and fibroblasts would cement the diagnosis of invasion. One must

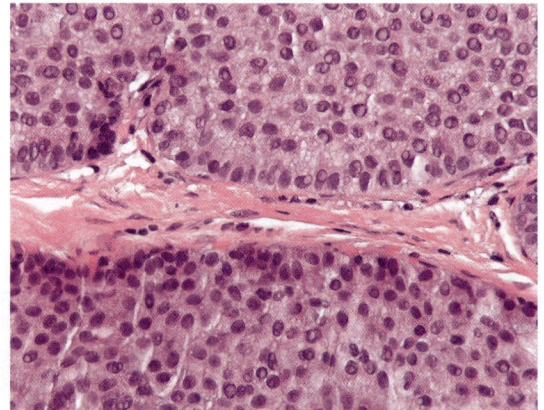

Figure 3-120 The cells in this large, round nest of invasive carcinoma abut the collagen directly. One cannot detect the structures of a ductal wall or the components of the specialized, periductal stroma.

acknowledge that extreme distention of the ducts by the carcinoma, periductal inflammation and scarring, and the presence of preexisting sclerosing lesions or other processes all can conspire to make it impossible to

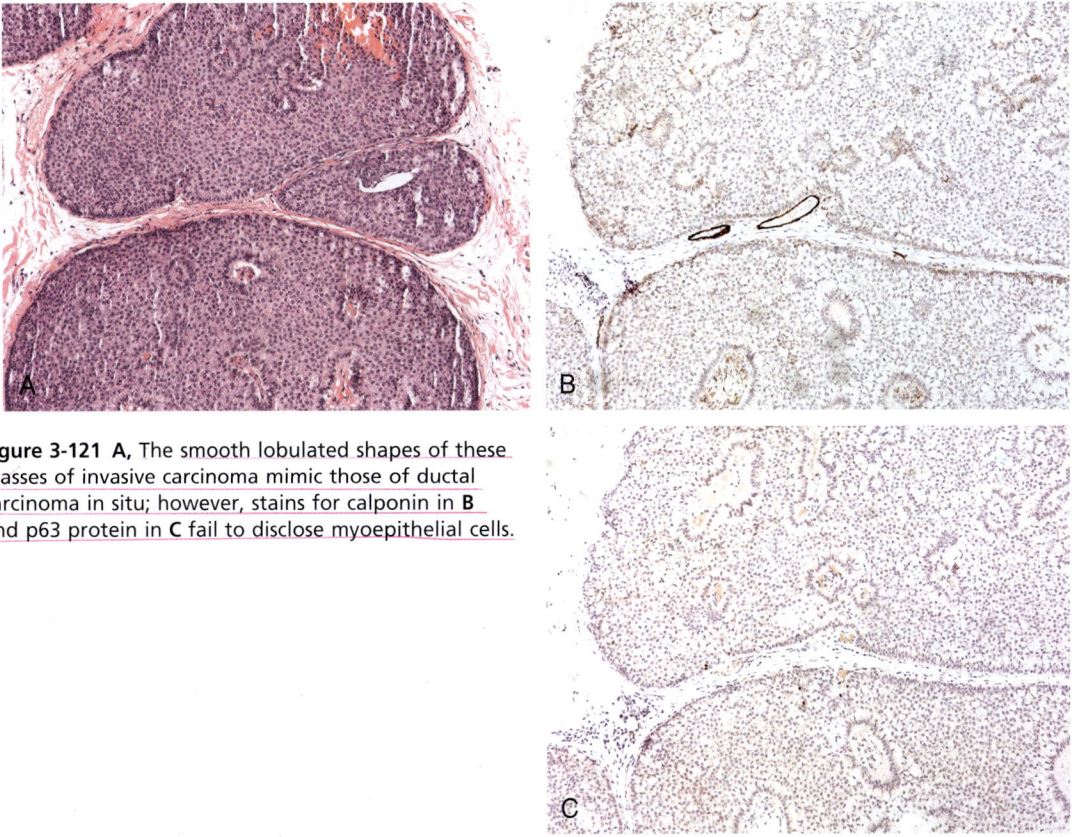

Figure 3-121 A, The smooth lobulated shapes of these masses of invasive carcinoma mimic those of ductal carcinoma in situ; however, stains for calponin in **B** and p63 protein in **C** fail to disclose myoepithelial cells.

recognize the structural elements of a duct wall or specialized stroma; nevertheless, a diligent search for these structures around large nests with irregular shapes may lead one either to favor or to dismiss the diagnosis of blunt invasion. Once a suspicion of blunt invasion has surfaced, staining for markers of myoepithelial cells usually resolves the uncertainty (Fig. 3-121).

Summary

An ever-present and keen awareness of the problem of recognizing stromal invasion and patient study of problematic foci represent the most important defenses against overlooking microinvasion, mistaking invasive glands for adenosis, confusing invasion with involvement of distorted glands by invasive carcinoma and misinterpreting invasive carcinoma as carcinoma in situ.

Distinction between Ductal Carcinoma In Situ and Carcinoma in Lymphatic Vessels

All practicing pathologists have firsthand experience with the difficulty of distinguishing stromal invasion with retraction artifacts from carcinoma within lymphatic vessels. Although a mistake of this type can have implications for patient care, the widespread awareness of this diagnostic problem and of the strategies for resolving it prevents most errors. Pathologists have much less appreciation for the situation in which complete filling of a lymphatic vessel by carcinoma cells creates a pattern that nearly duplicates the appearance of ductal carcinoma in situ (Fig. 3-122). Furthermore, carcinoma cells growing in lymphatic vessels can display central necrosis, and the cells at the periphery of the masses can grow in a single layer of columnar cells. Both phenomena enhance the similarity with ductal carcinoma in situ. Confusion of these two entities can lead to a failure to recognize the presence of invasive carcinoma, an oversight of significant clinical importance, but consideration of several distinguishing features helps to prevent this mistake.

First, invasion of lymphatic vessels often produces a spotty, discontinuous involvement of mammary tissues, in which nests of carcinoma cells sit in a seemingly haphazard distribution among the background, unaltered glands (Fig. 3-123). Ductal carcinoma in situ does not usually involve the glandular tree in this interrupted fashion. Ducts and acini greatly distended by carcinoma cells usually connect with others showing lesser involvement, and the latter, in turn, merge with minimally altered glands. One usually observes ducts cut in longitudinal

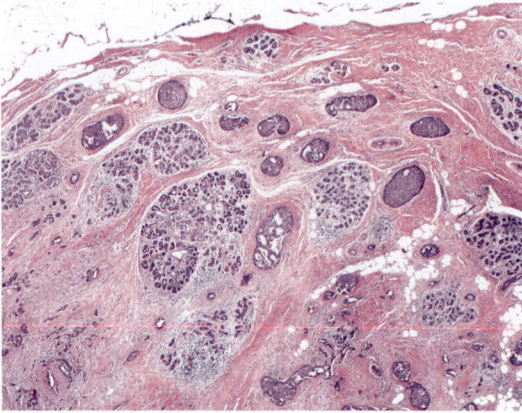

Figure 3-122 Growth of carcinoma in lymphatic vessels produces a pattern that superficially mimics the appearance of ductal carcinoma in situ.

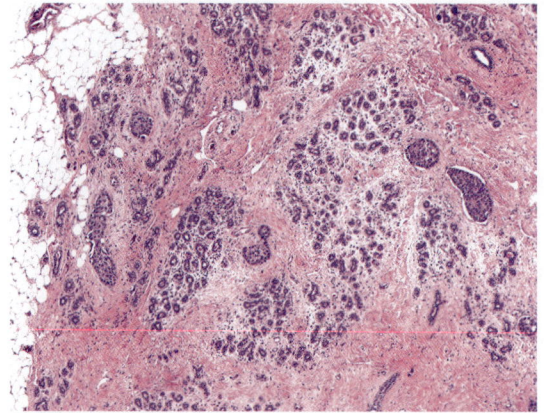

Figure 3-123 The presence of aggregates that look like ducts distended by ductal carcinoma in situ widely interspersed among normal glandular tissue suggests the diagnosis of lymphatic vessel invasion.

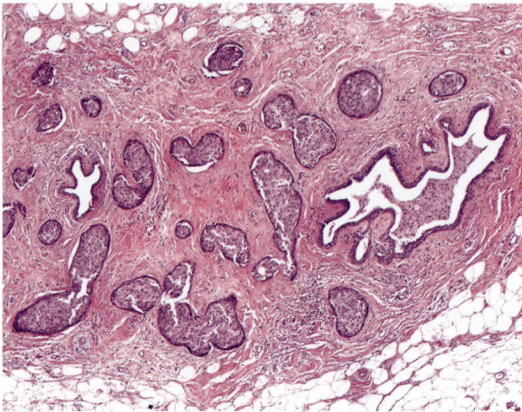

Figure 3-124 These aggregates of carcinoma cells do not interconnect to form a pattern characteristic of mammary ducts and terminal duct–lobular units; furthermore, the presence of uninvolved ducts would not fit with a diagnosis of ductal carcinoma in situ.

section and others that branch, and together, the involved glands display the architecture of the mammary ductal and lobular tissue. One would not expect to see isolated, carcinoma-filled ducts sprinkled among glands uninvolved by the carcinoma or clusters of malignant cells that do not branch or aggregate in an anatomic pattern (Fig. 3-124).

Second, the location of the suspect clusters of carcinoma cells often provides an important clue. Lymphatic vessels travel in the specialized stroma around large ducts and next to small arteries and veins; ducts, in contrast, only rarely occupy these positions. The presence of nearby large ducts or vascular bundles often serves as an important clue that a cluster of carcinoma cells occupies a lymphatic vessel rather than a glandular structure (Fig. 3-125).

Third, when carcinoma cells invade and fill lymphatic vessels, the cells usually also invade the stroma,

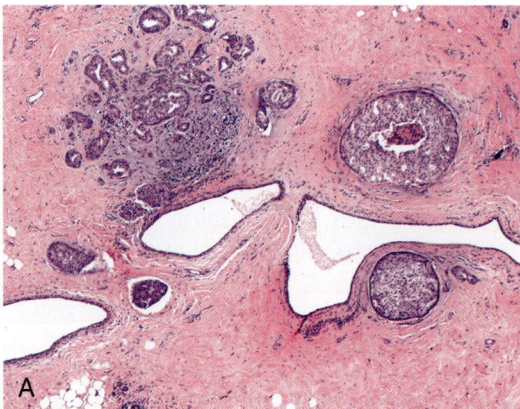

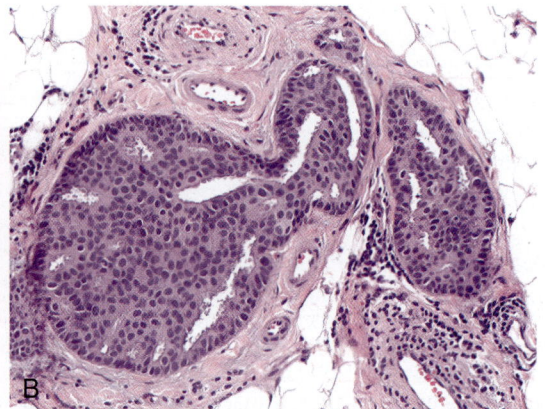

Figure 3-125 These large groups of carcinoma occupy lymphatic vessels that course around ducts in **A** and blood vessels in **B**.

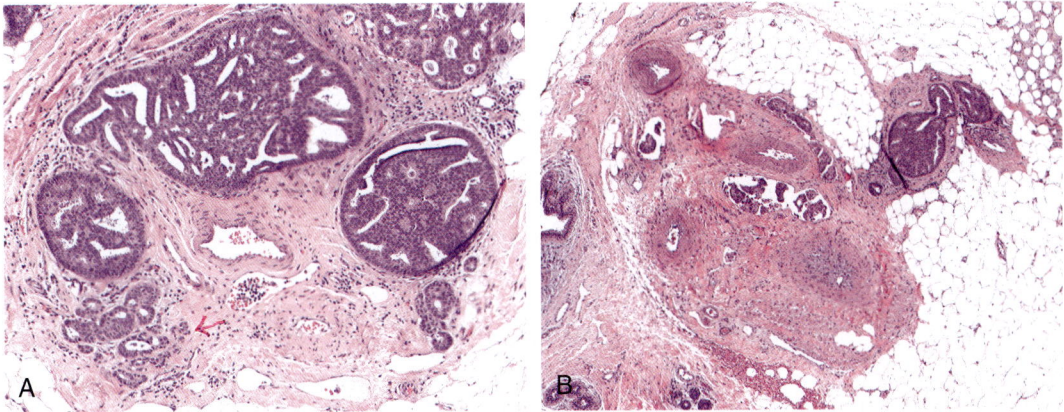

Figure 3-126 A, Small clusters of carcinoma cells invade the stroma adjacent to carcinoma-filled lymphatic vessels. **B,** Other sections display typical examples of lymphatic vessel invasion.

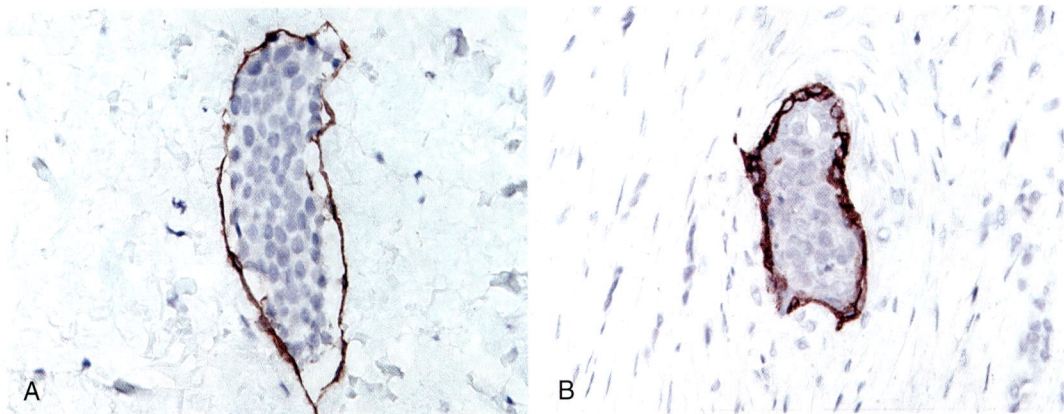

Figure 3-127 Immunohistochemical staining for D2-40 protein reveals a positive reaction in lymphatic endothelial cells in **A** and myoepithelial cells **B**. The former shows a linear staining pattern and the latter a granular one.

myoepithelial – Not vessel.

and they frequently involve other lymphatic vessels in a less exuberant and more traditional morphologic pattern. Thus, a careful search for foci of conventional stromal invasion and lymphatic vessels containing only small clusters of malignant cells often exposes the true nature of a focus of intralymphatic carcinoma masquerading as ductal carcinoma in situ (Fig. 3-126).

Finally, one can use the results of immunohistochemical stains to resolve problematic cases and to confirm the impression reached after study of hematoxylin and eosin—stained sections. One must choose immunohistochemical reagents carefully. For example, both myoepithelial cells and lymphatic endothelial cells contain the D2-40 protein (Fig. 3-127). Although the former usually exhibit a granular pattern of staining and the latter a linear distribution, one may not wish to rely on the results of staining for this antigen alone. A panel consisting of a stain for D2-40 and another for p63 protein provides more secure results.

Interpretation of Immunohistochemical Stains for Myoepithelial Cells

Because the histologic findings apparent in conventional, hematoxylin and eosin—stained sections sometimes only suggest the presence of invasion, pathologists turn to immunohistochemical staining for markers of myoepithelial cells to help to establish the diagnosis of invasive carcinoma. The success of this approach depends on care in the choice of the markers and experience in the interpretation of the results. The nuclear localization of the p63 protein, for instance, makes it nearly impossible to interpret stains for this molecule in foci of sclerosing adenosis; stains for antigens such as calponin and myosin heavy chain, which mark the cytoplasm of the myoepithelial cells, provide a much clearer picture of their distribution and the relationship between the myoepithelial cells and carcinoma cells.

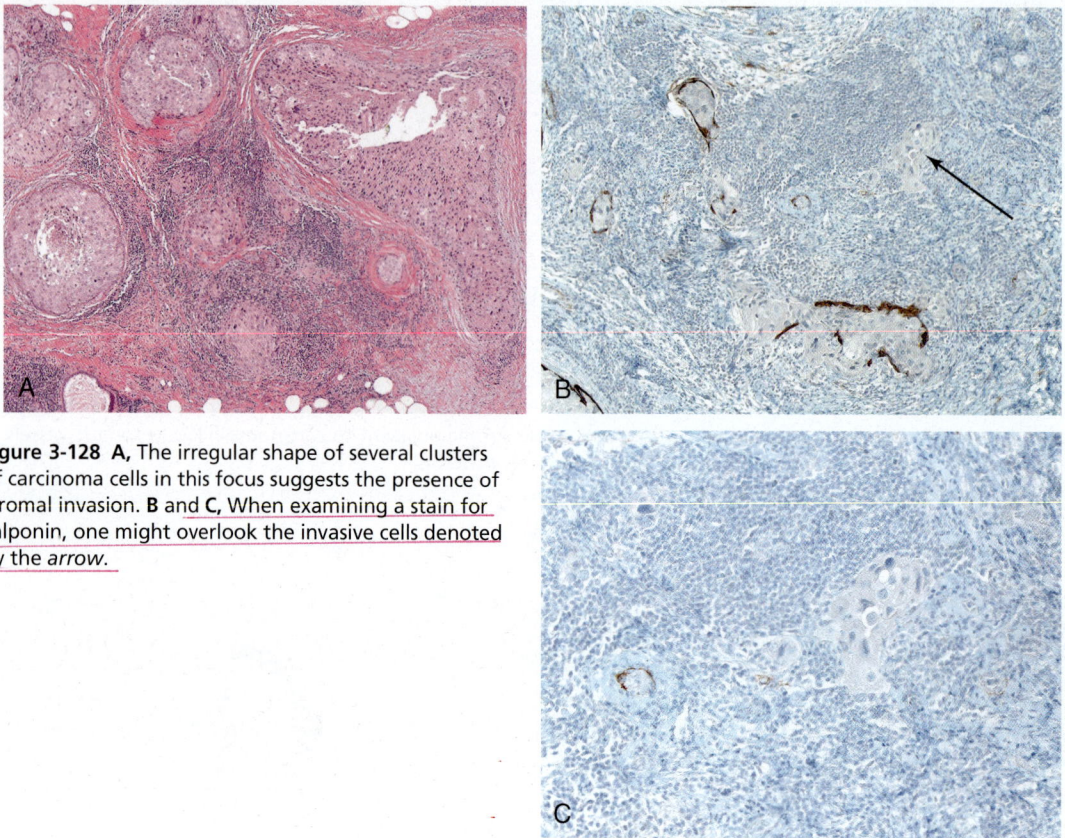

Figure 3-128 A, The irregular shape of several clusters of carcinoma cells in this focus suggests the presence of stromal invasion. **B** and **C,** When examining a stain for calponin, one might overlook the invasive cells denoted by the *arrow.*

When examining sections stained for myoepithelial markers, pathologists can fail to identify invasive carcinoma for two reasons, failure to notice the invasive cells and misinterpretation of myofibroblasts as myoepithelial cells. The former error merits special attention, because it represents an understandable and easily made mistake. In the examination of sections stained for calponin, myosin heavy chain, or other proteins found in the cytoplasm of myoepithelial cells, the ducts and lobules outlined by positively staining cells attract immediate attention and tend to distract from the search for cell clusters lacking myoepithelial cells. Pathologists must train themselves to look in the regions of the tissue that show only background staining to identify malignant cells lacking a rim of myoepithelial cells. To illustrate, Figure 3-128 depicts a case of high-grade ductal carcinoma in situ stained with hematoxylin and eosin and for calponin. The intense staining for calponin of the myoepithelial cells catches one's eye, and so does the focal discontinuity of the myoepithelial layer in a few structures. Because of these distractions, one could easily fail to notice the cluster of invasive carcinoma cells seen on high magnification.

Misinterpretation of staining of myofibroblasts accounts for the second common way of failing to recognize invasive carcinoma in sections stained with immunohistochemical techniques. Depending on the antibody used and the nature of the tissue, myofibroblasts can stain for proteins present in myoepithelial cells. Calponin antibodies tend to stain myofibroblasts more than myosin heavy chain antibodies, for example, and reactive myofibroblasts show more staining than resting ones. When myofibroblasts abut clusters of carcinomas, one can easily mistake them for myoepithelial cells (Fig. 3-129). To avoid this mistake, one must pay attention to the morphology of the stained cells. The nuclei of myoepithelial cells typically bulge toward the lumen of the gland, creating a triangular blob of cytoplasm enclosing the unstained nucleus. Myofibroblasts, on the other hand, have long and attenuated shapes, and their nuclei do not protrude toward the glandular lumen. Figure 3-130 illustrates the difference in the staining patterns of the two types of cells.

Attention to the choice of stains and careful analysis of the results of staining allow one to interpret these preparations confidently.

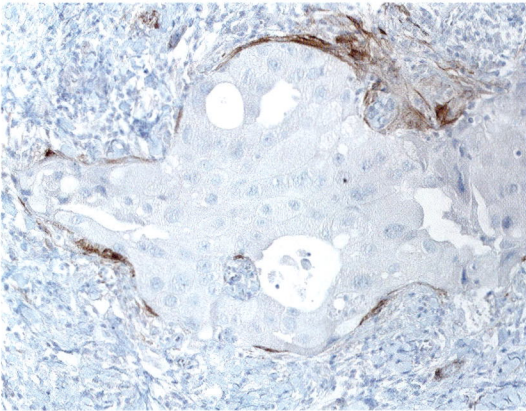

Figure 3-129 When studying this section stained for calponin, one could mistake the staining of myofibroblasts adjacent to this nest of invasive carcinoma for staining of myoepithelial cells.

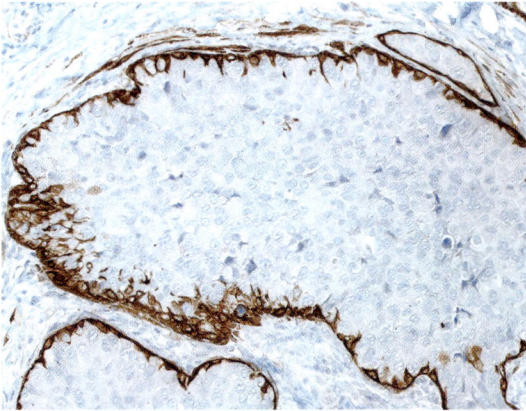

Figure 3-130 Myoepithelial cells outline the perimeter of this duct harboring ductal carcinoma in situ. A few myofibroblasts in the upper region of the field also stain for calponin. *See nuclei buldging toward lumen*

Recognition of Ductal Carcinoma In Situ in the Irradiated Breast

The cytologic alterations introduced by irradiation of the breast can make it difficult to recognize the presence of carcinoma in situ, because the atypia induced by irradiation mimics the anaplasia of malignancy. Pathologists can guard against this misinterpretation by keeping several points in mind. First, careful attention to the clinical details of a specific case minimizes the potential for mistakes. In the presence of a history of irradiation, one should adopt a circumspect approach to the diagnosis of malignancy when examining a sample from the treated breast. One cannot depend on one's clinical colleagues to supply such details consistently, so the careful pathologist keeps a sharp eye out for a record of a previously treated carcinoma when studying every biopsy specimen. Treatment of a breast cancer almost always consists of either a mastectomy or an excision of the carcinoma followed by irradiation. Therefore, if one receives a breast biopsy specimen from a patient with a history of a prior carcinoma in the ipsilateral breast, one should probably assume that the patient has received radiation therapy.

Second, carcinomas that recur after radiation therapy do not display the effects of radiation. In fact, the cells of the recurrence closely resemble those of the original carcinoma: High-grade carcinomas recur as high-grade carcinomas (Fig. 3-131), and low-grade carcinomas as low-grade carcinomas. Knowledge of this consistency of morphologic features coupled with direct examination of the primary carcinoma usually prevents mistaking benign, irradiated cells for cells of carcinomas of low or intermediate grade. Distinguishing high-grade carcinomas from irradiated normal cells poses a more difficult problem; both lesions consist of large cells with large,

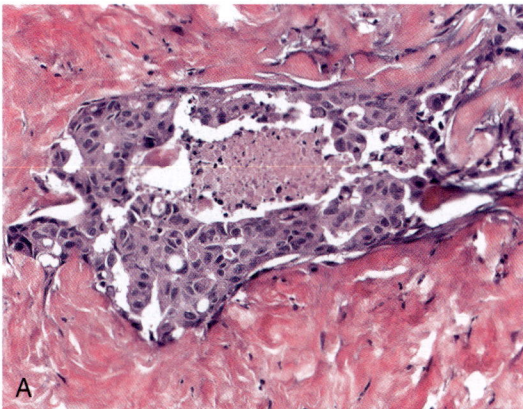

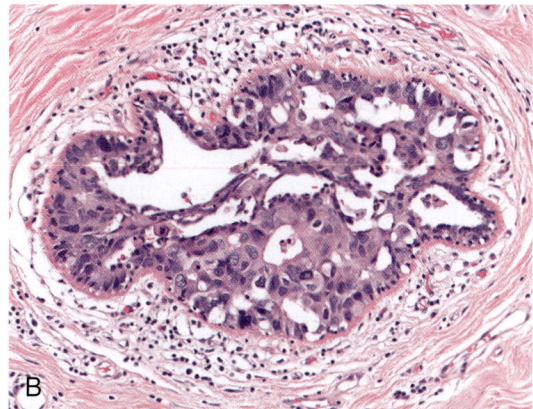

Figure 3-131 The recurrence of this high-grade ductal carcinoma in situ seen in **A** appears identical to the primary carcinoma in **B**.

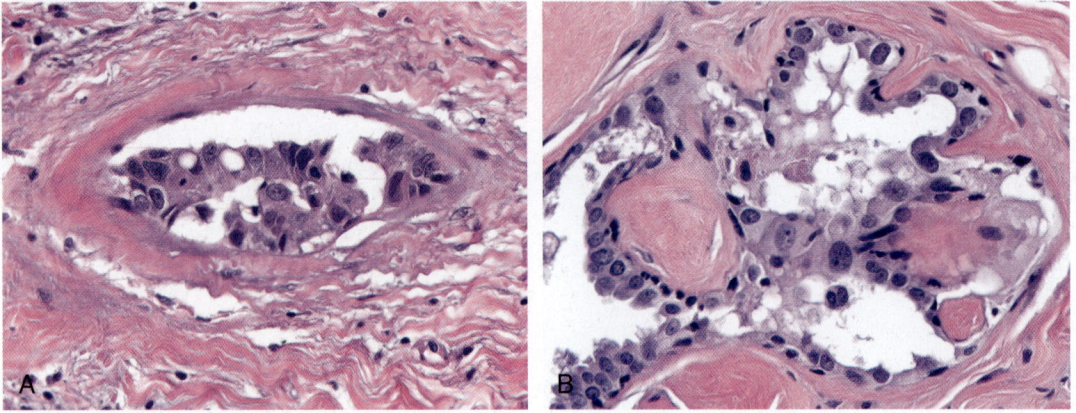

Figure 3-132 The recurrent high-grade ductal carcinoma in **A** resembles the irradiated benign cells in **B**.

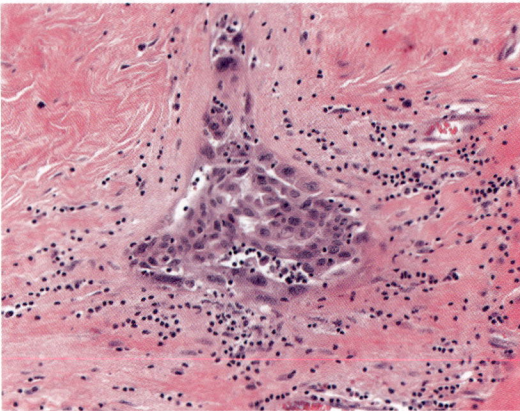

Figure 3-133 An off-center plane of section has created the false impression of proliferation of these irradiated begin ductal cells.

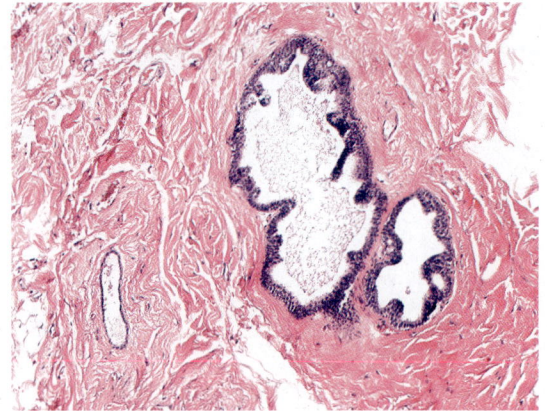

Figure 3-134 The atypical ductal cells growing in this irradiated breast look identical to other examples of severely atypical ductal hyperplasia. Contrast the size of the atypical cells, their crowded arrangement, and the diameter of the duct in which they grow with the corresponding features of the uninvolved duct in the lower left.

pleomorphic nuclei (Fig. 3-132). Attention to the presence of cellular proliferation and the composition of the cellular population allows one to distinguish the lesions in most cases. Pathologists should remember that irradiation induces an atrophy of lobules and small ducts, whereas the cellular proliferation characteristic of carcinomas usually enlarges these structures. Thus, irradiated glands appear small, and the atypical cells do not usually fill their lumens, although one must guard against interpreting cells cut off-center as a focus of epithelial proliferations (Fig. 3-133). Carcinoma cells, on the other hand, typically fill the lumens partially or completely and expand the dimensions of the glands. The nature of the cellular population also offers important diagnostic information. One can usually discern both luminal and myoepithelial cells in irradiated epithelium,

and the number and arrangement of the two types of cells appear normal. Carcinomas, in contrast, do not usually maintain such an orderly structure. Finally, cells showing radiation changes do not divide; thus, the presence of mitotic figures and necrotic cells strongly favors a diagnosis of malignancy.

Finally, carcinomas that arise after radiation treatments seem to evolve along the same pathways as carcinomas arising in an untreated breast. Neither the premalignant proliferations arising in the irradiated breast nor the carcinomas that develop from them display the cellular changes associated with radiation treatment (Figs. 3-134 to 3-136). One can

Figure 3-135 A, Flat epithelial atypia occupies the duct in the right of the field and irradiated normal cells the duct in the left. **B,** High magnification allows one to contrast the large size and pleomorphism of the irradiated nuclei with the smaller size and uniformity of the atypical cells.

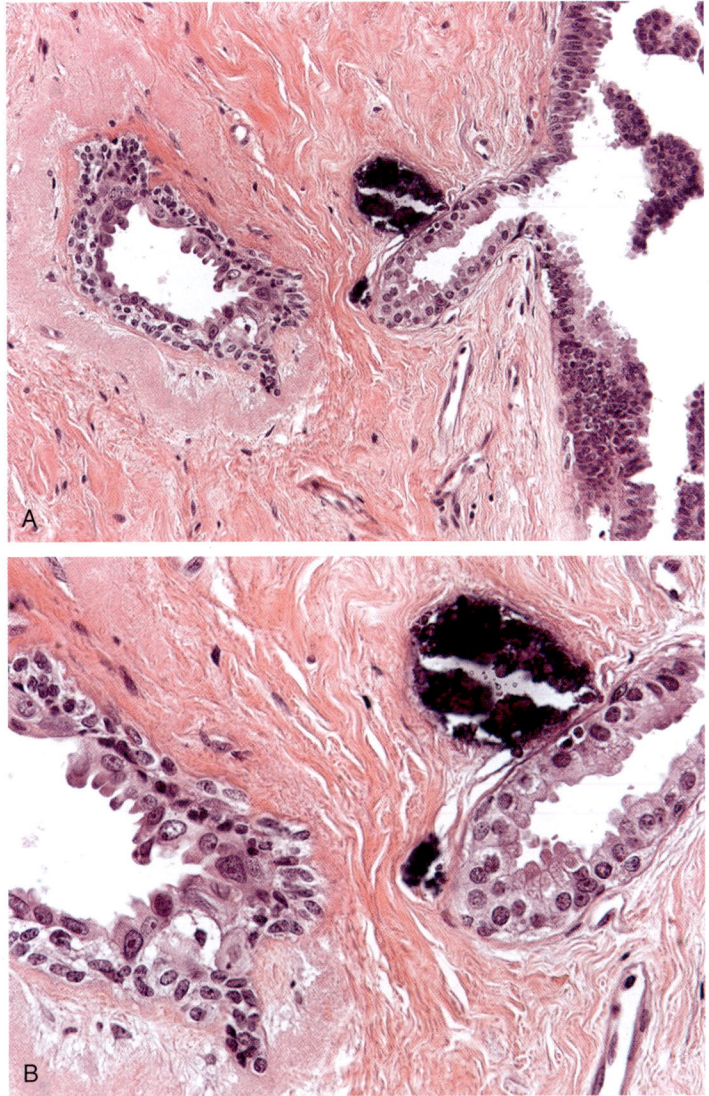

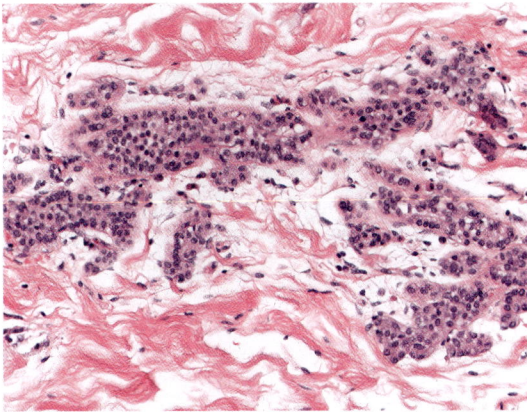

Figure 3-136 The lobular neoplasia arising in these irradiated glands looks completely conventional.

therefore rely on the usual morphologic criteria and diagnostic approach when evaluating epithelial proliferations in irradiated breast tissue.

Ductal Carcinoma In Situ in Gynecomastia

The diagnosis of ductal carcinoma in situ in the male breast rests on the same principles as it does in the female breast, and it usually seems more straightforward, because men's breast tissue does not commonly harbor the confounding benign conditions that complicate the diagnosis in women's breasts. Many cases of carcinoma seen in men arise in the setting of gynecomastia, and pathologists can feel insecure about distinguishing the pronounced ductal hyperplasia seen in the florid phase of gynecomastia from low-grade ductal carcinoma in situ.

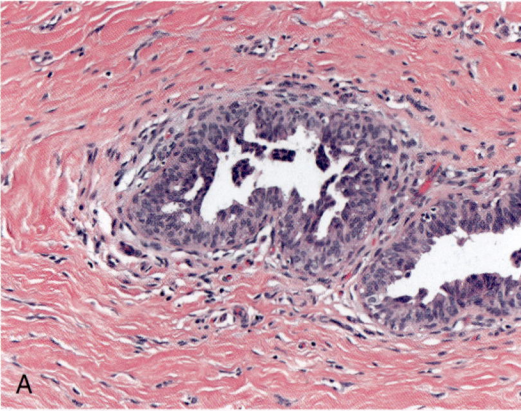

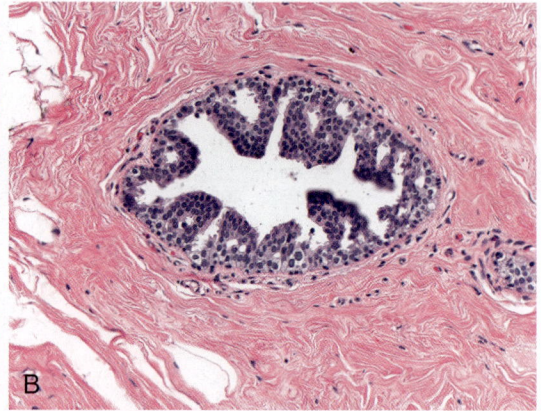

Figure 3-137 A, This specimen from a young man contains florid gynecomastia. The duct in B lacks the expected periductal stromal changes and the cells within it displays cytologic and architectural atypia, seen in **C**.

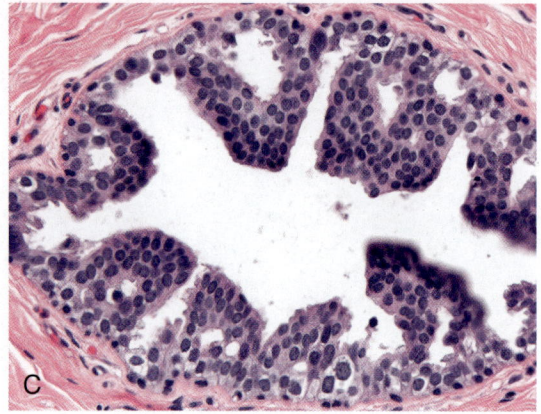

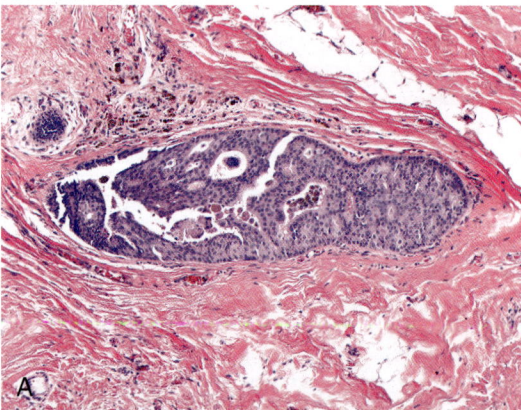

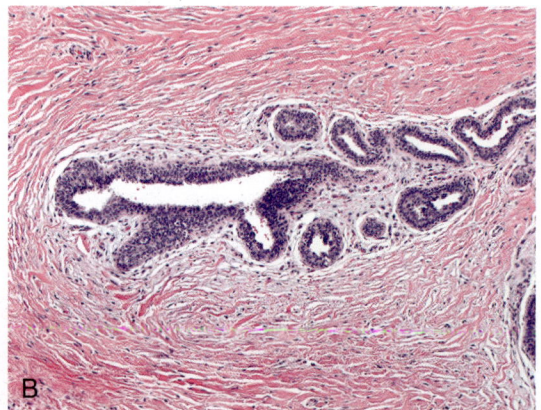

Figure 3-138 A, Both the cytologic atypia and the architectural atypia of the proliferative cells occupying this duct appear convincing. Furthermore, the periductal stroma does not show the cellularity and edema seen in the stroma surrounding this uninvolved duct in **B**.

The hyperplasia of gynecomastia most often assumes a micropapillary configuration, at least in part, and the criteria set forth in the discussion of micropapillary proliferations allow one to distinguish this form of ductal hyperplasia from micropapillary low-grade carcinomas. To summarize that discussion, the presence of cytologic atypia, convincing architectural atypia, and the absence of maturation of the micropapillary tufts represent the most important findings in reaching a diagnosis of carcinoma. Moreover, carcinomas arising in men rarely grow in a purely micropapillary architecture; they usually produce a cribriform pattern or grow as papillary carcinomas. Pathologists should also remember that ducts harboring atypical ductal hyperplasia and ductal carcinoma in situ generally do not display the edema or hypercellularity of the periductal stroma characteristic of gynecomastia (Figs. 3-137 and 3-138).

References

1. Page DL, Anderson TJ: Diagnostic Histopathology of the Breast. Edinburgh, Churchill Livingstone, 1987.
2. Azzopardi JG: Problems in Breast Pathology. (Major Problems in Pathology, vol 11). London, WB Saunders, 1979.

Selected Readings

Abdel-Fatah TM, Powe DG, Hodi Z, et al: High frequency coexistence of columnar cell lesion, lobular neoplasia, and low-grade ductal carcinoma in situ with invasive tubular carcinoma and invasive lobular carcinoma. Am J Surg Pathol 2007;31: 417-426.

Azzopardi JG: Problems in Breast Pathology. (Major Problems in Pathology, vol 11). London, WB Saunders, 1979.

Azzopardi JG: Benign and malignant proliferative epithelial lesion of the breast: a review. Eur J Cancer Clin Oncol 1983;19:1717-1720.

Bodian CA, Perzin KH, Lattes R, et al: Prognostic significance of benign proliferative breast disease. Cancer 1993;71:3896-3907.

Boecker W, Buerger H, Schmitz K, et al: Ductal epithelial proliferations of the breast: A biologic continuum? Comparative genomic hybridization and high-molecular-weight cytokeratin expression patterns. J Pathol 2001;195:415-421.

Boecker W, Moll R, Dervan P, et al: Usual ductal hyperplasia of the breast is a committed stem (progenitor) cell lesion distinct from atypical ductal hyperplasia and ductal carcinoma in situ. J Pathol 2002;198:458-467.

Dabbs DJ, Carter G, Fudge M: Molecular alterations in columnar cell lesions of the breast. Mod Pathol 2006;19:344-349.

Dupont WD, Page DL: Risk factors for breast cancer in women with proliferative breast disease. N Engl J Med 1985;312:146-151.

Eusebi V, Feudale E, Foschini MP: Long-term follow-up of in situ carcinoma of the breast with special emphasis on clinging carcinoma. Semin Diagn Pathol 1994;11:223-235.

Leibl S, Regitnig P, Moinfar F: Flat epithelial atypia (DIN 1a, atypical columnar cell change): An underdiagnosed entity very frequently coexisting with lobular neoplasia. Histopathology 2007;50:859-865.

London SJ, Connolly JL, Schnitt SJ, et al: A prospective study of benign breast disease and the risk of breast cancer. JAMA 1992;267:941-944.

McDivitt RW, Holleb AI, Foote FW: Prior breast disease in patient treated for papillary carcinoma. Arch Pathol 1968;85:117-124.

McDivitt RW, Stevens JA, Lee NC, et al: Histologic types of benign breast disease and the risk for breast cancer. The cancer and steroid hormone study group. Cancer 1992;69:1408-1414.

McDivitt RW, Stewart FW, Berg JW: Tumors of the Breast. Washington, DC, Armed Forces Institute of Pathology, 1950.

Moinfar F, Man YG, Bratthauer GL, et al: Genetic abnormalities in mammary ductal intraepithelial neoplasia-flat type ('clinging ductal carcinoma in situ'): A simulator of normal mammary epithelium. Cancer 2000;88:2072-2081.

Oyama T, Maluf H, Koerner F: Pathologic findings after therapeutic irradiation of mammary tissues and carcinomas. Anat Pathol 1998;3:181-193.

Otterbach F, Bánkfalvi A, Bergner S, et al: Cytokeratin 5/6 immunohistochemistry assists the differential diagnosis of atypical proliferations of the breast. Histopathology 2000;37:232-240.

Page DL, Anderson TJ: Diagnostic Histopathology of the Breast. Edinburgh, Churchill Livingstone, 1987.

Raju U, Crissman JD, Zarbo RJ, et al: Epitheliosis of the breast: An immunohistochemical characterization and comparison to malignant intraductal proliferations of the breast. Am J Surg Pathol 1990;14:939-947.

Schnitt SJ, Connolly JL, Harris JR, et al: Radiation-induced changes in the breast. Hum Pathol 1984;15:545-550.

Simpson PT, Gale T, Reis-Filho, et al: Columnar cell lesions of the breast: The missing link in breast cancer progression? A morphologic and molecular analysis. Am J Surg Pathol 2005;29:734-746.

Tavassoli FA, Norris HJ: A comparison of the results of long-term follow-up for atypical intraductal hyperplasia and intraductal hyperplasia of the breast. Cancer 1990;65:518-529.

4

Apocrine Proliferations

Even the greenest of pathologists has become accustomed to observing apocrine cells in mammary specimens. Their origin remains undiscovered and their significance unknown, so observers usually dismiss them with little more than a shrug. One can understand this indifference, because apocrine cells contribute to the evolution of fibrocystic changes much more often than they do to the growth of neoplasms. Nevertheless, apocrine cells can proliferate, and when they do, they give rise to perplexing lesions.

The diagnostic problems associated with these lesions arise in two settings, one inconsequential and the other significant. The former situation develops when obviously atypical or malignant cells possess such abundant, eosinophilic, and granular cytoplasm and such large, pleomorphic nuclei that pathologists wonder whether they should subclassify the lesion as a type of apocrine proliferation. The literature does not contain data to suggest that apocrine lesions have clinical features different from those of similar lesions composed of conventional ductal cells; however, this topic remains largely unexplored, in part because of the lack of widely accepted and validated criteria for establishing the apocrine nature of a cell. Pathologists find the usually cited morphologic features somewhat vague and difficult to evaluate reproducibly, and immunohistochemical staining for gross cystic disease fluid protein-15, a protein produced in high amounts by apocrine cells, lacks specificity. Most cells that exhibit the morphologic features of apocrine cells express the protein, but so do many cells that look like conventional ductal cells. Because of these limitations, one need not fret about whether to classify a neoplastic proliferation as apocrine. One could do so when the cells display many of the following features: abundant, eosinophilic, granular cytoplasm; large nuclei; pale and clumpy chromatin; thick nuclear membranes; and prominent nucleoli. When cells display just one or two of these findings, one can

probably ignore them and classify the cells as conventional ductal cells.

The significant diagnostic difficulty develops when cells of an obviously apocrine nature exhibit atypical cytologic or architectural characteristics and thereby suggest the presence of a neoplastic proliferation, such as atypical ductal hyperplasia or ductal carcinoma in situ. Unlike the preceding situation, which does not have clinical implications, this one has obvious ramifications for patient care.

BASIC CONCEPTS

The literature does not offer much guidance for the evaluation of apocrine proliferations. Lacking a suitable alternative, pathologists must return to first principles and analyze these lesions by using the concepts that underlie the evaluation of proliferations composed of conventional ductal cells—the phenomena of proliferation, intercellular cohesion, cellular polarization, cytologic atypia, and architectural atypia. Although these same processes and morphologic alterations play out in the creation of apocrine lesions, certain of them manifest themselves in somewhat different ways. Consequently, the assessment of these basic phenomena sometimes requires either a shift in emphasis or outright alteration when one is examining apocrine proliferations.

The phenomenon of proliferation does not require modification. One gauges the extent of cellular proliferation of apocrine cells by the same measures that one uses with conventional ductal cells. Stratification of the cells and filling and distention of the glands serve as reliable indications of proliferation. Cellular polarization, on the other hand, does not manifest itself in neoplastic apocrine cells as clearly as in neoplastic ductal cells of the low-grade type. In fact, the absence of the well-established and obvious cellular polarization displayed by conventional

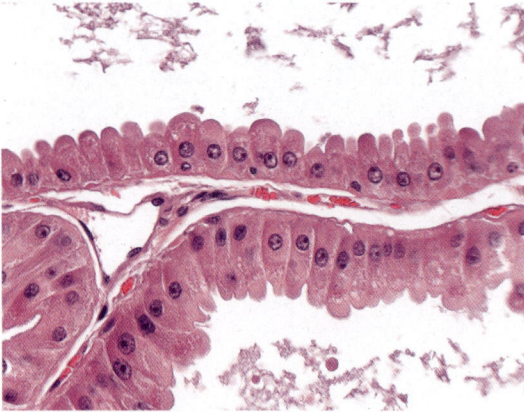

Figure 4-1 These conventional apocrine cells grow in a single layer; they possess abundant, eosinophilic cytoplasm, basal nuclei, and prominent nucleoli.

Box 4-1

Features of architectural atypia of apocrine cells:

- Cellular crowding
- Cellular stratification
- Formation of micropapillary tufts, glandular spaces, and cellular bars

---

Box 4-2

Features of cytologic atypia of apocrine cells:

- Cytoplasmic pallor
- Lack of basal position of nuclei
- Nuclear pleomorphism
- Nucleolar prominence
- Nucleolar pleomorphism

---

apocrine cells typifies neoplastic apocrine lesions. Like neoplastic conventional ductal cells, neoplastic apocrine cells lose their cohesive properties, so the signs of cellular dishesion can call attention to the atypical nature of certain apocrine proliferations; however, benign apocrine cells do not display the marked cohesion evidenced by hyperplastic ductal cells. Consequently, the streaming arrangement of the cells and the formation of spindle cell bridges do not develop in benign apocrine lesions.

Just as they do in the study of conventional ductal proliferations, the evaluations of architectural atypia and cytologic atypia form the foundation for the diagnosis of apocrine lesions. Both phenomena take different forms in this setting. To understand the origin of these differences and to derive the criteria of atypia, one should begin by studying the properties of conventional apocrine cells (Fig. 4-1). In their commonplace forms, apocrine cells look generally similar and they display the following properties:

1. Evenly spaced columnar or cuboidal cells grow in a cohesive single layer.
2. The nucleus sits at the base of the cell and abundant cytoplasm collects near the lumen.
3. The cytoplasm looks homogeneous and eosinophilic; occasionally, it contains a large supranuclear vacuole.
4. The nuclei and nucleoli appear uniform.
5. The cells do not display necrosis or noticeable mitotic activity.

Deviations from these characteristics represent manifestations of atypia of apocrine cells. Alterations of the first attribute reflect architectural atypia (Box 4-1), and deviations in the next four constitute cytologic atypia (Box 4-2).

Because neoplastic apocrine cells lose their polarized nature, they cannot form the architectural structures that spring from this property. Thus, neoplastic apocrine cells do not commonly form obvious, classic cribriform spaces, trabecular bars, or Roman bridges; instead, architectural atypia expresses itself as crowding of cells, cellular stratification, and the formation of loose, micropapillary tufts (Fig. 4-2). When they pile up, neoplastic apocrine cells do create spaces and bars of cells, but the cells bordering the spaces do not appear fully polarized (Fig. 4-3). Cytologic atypia arises when the cytoplasmic or nuclear characteristics deviate from the expected. Aberrations in the position of the nucleus, disarray in the location of the cytoplasmic granules, and loss of cytoplasmic eosinophilia and granularity usually indicate mild degrees of atypia, whereas alterations in the characteristics of the nuclei and nucleoli represent serious deviations from the conventional characteristics.

Besides studying the fundamental properties of the cells, pathologists can sometimes find diagnostic clues by looking for ancillary findings (Box 4-3). The presence of necrosis represents one such finding and a particularly worrisome one, because lesions composed of conventional apocrine cells do not demonstrate cell death. One can find dead cells in apocrine lesions showing minimal cytologic atypia, but the necrotic cells typically number only a few. Proliferations composed of markedly atypical cells tend to display a greater level of necrosis. Most lesions showing necrosis probably have a neoplastic nature. The presence of cellular dishesion, the second ancillary finding, usually parallels the presence of necrosis and, like the latter, probably indicates a neoplastic proliferation. Finally, noticeable mitotic

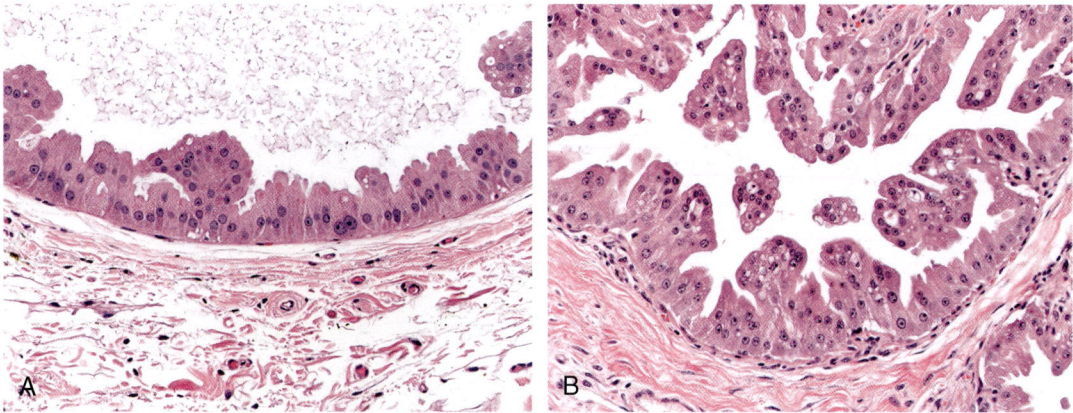

Figure 4-2 A, These proliferative apocrine cells apparently grow in just one layer, but they look crowded. **B,** These cells exhibit genuine stratification and the formation of tufts. The latter findings constitute architectural atypia.

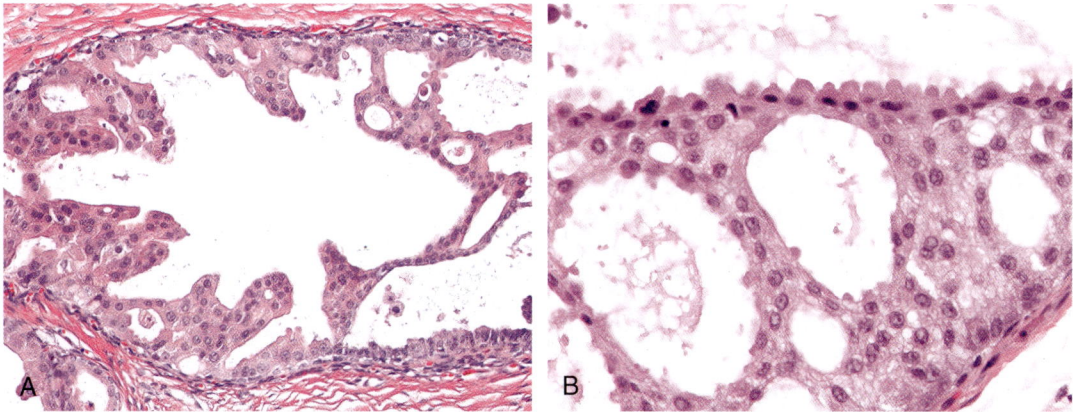

Figure 4-3 A, Although the cells pile up and form internal spaces and cellular bars, the cells abutting the lumen do not consistently display well-developed polarization. **B,** Certain cells surrounding these spaces exhibit polarization, but many do not.

Box 4-3

Ancillary features of atypia of apocrine cells:

- Necrosis
- Cellular dishesion
- Mitotic activity

activity does not occur commonly in conventional apocrine cells. Seemingly benign apocrine lesions sometimes contain a few dividing cells, so the presence of division figures by itself does not identify apocrine cells as neoplastic. When one observes mitotic activity in conjunction with cytologic and architectural atypia, on the other hand, one should probably favor the diagnosis of malignancy.

These atypical features and ancillary findings do not emerge in consistent clusters, and the variability in their expression makes it difficult to establish grades of atypia for apocrine lesions as clearly as one can for proliferations of ductal cells. Nevertheless, one can make the following generalizations. Characteristics of low-grade apocrine atypia are: crowding and stratification of cells, loss of the basal position of the nucleus, pallor or vacuolization of the cytoplasm, mild enlargement of the nuclei or nucleoli, and mild pleomorphism of the nuclei or nucleoli (Fig. 4-4). Characteristics of high-grade apocrine atypia are: crowding and stratification of cells, loss of the basal position of the nucleus, pallor or vacuolization of the cytoplasm, marked enlargement of the nuclei or nucleoli, and marked pleomorphism of the nuclei or nucleoli (Fig. 4-5). The ancillary finding of necrosis, dishesion, and mitotic activity can occur in conjunction with either low-grade or high-grade atypia, but they occur more commonly in the latter setting (Fig. 4-6).

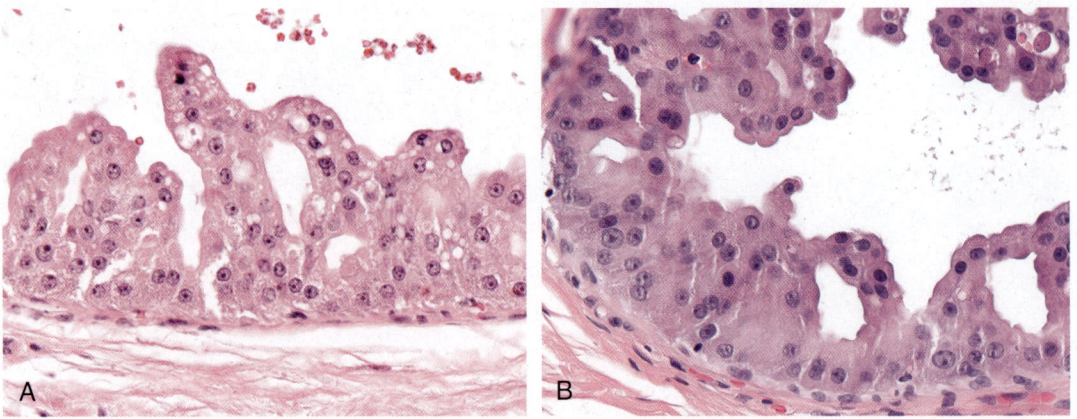

Figure 4-4 Low-grade cytologic atypia of apocrine cells takes the form of cytoplasmic vacuolization, loss of the basal position of the nucleus in **A**, and mild nuclear pleomorphism in **B**.

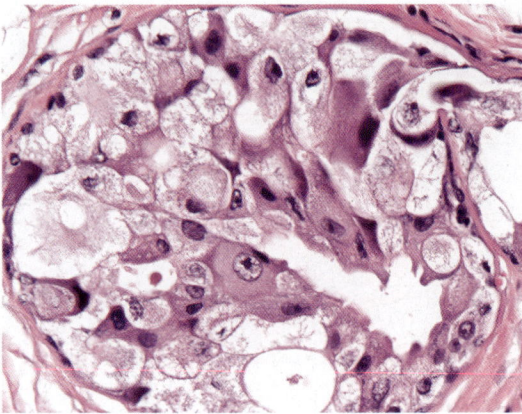

Figure 4-5 High-grade cytologic atypia of apocrine cells consists of marked nuclear and nucleolar enlargement and pleomorphism.

Application of the basic concepts of epithelial proliferations modified in these ways should provide pathologists with a basis for their study of apocrine lesions.

DEFINITIONS AND CLINICOPATHOLOGIC CHARACTERISTICS

Genuine apocrine lesions consist of a type of luminal cell possessing abundant, eosinophilic, and granular cytoplasm, granular or clumped chromatin, thick nuclear membranes, and easily seen nucleoli. Pathologists must keep a firm rein on their willingness to consider every cell with eosinophilic cytoplasm apocrine, because cytoplasmic attributes alone do not constitute sufficient grounds to identify this type of cell. For example, one occasionally encounters ductal cells with copious eosinophilic cytoplasm,

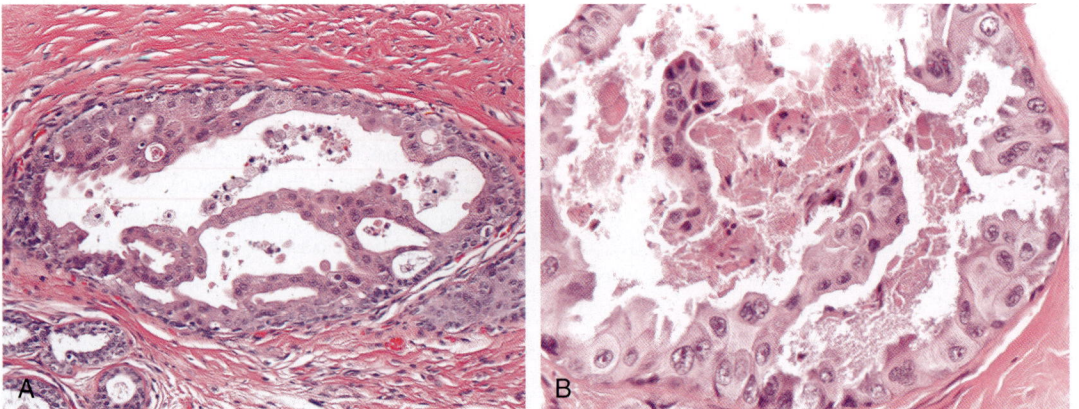

Figure 4-6 Necrosis, dishesion, and mitotic activity constitute ancillary evidence of cellular atypia. They can occur in conjunction with both low-grade in **A** and high-grade in **B** proliferations.

and carcinomas regularly contain finely granular, eosinophilic cytoplasm (Fig. 4-7), yet neither represents a type of apocrine cell. Bona fide apocrine cells possess characteristic nuclei, and these nuclear attributes seem to develop before the eosinophilic and granular cytoplasm accumulates in abundance (Fig. 4-8). Thus, one must observe the appropriate features in both the nucleus and the cytoplasm to establish the apocrine nature of a cell.

Although apocrine lesions represent a form of ductal epithelial proliferation, they do not seem to originate from established proliferations of conventional ductal cells. Apocrine proliferations probably develop from their own seeds. They might emerge from the nonproliferative foci of apocrine change, which constitute a common component of fibrocystic change, or sprout de novo from conventional luminal cells. This point requires specific study. The multiplication of apocrine cells can take several forms. Growth in a single layer of well-organized, conventional cells can simply expand the duct or acinus to create a cyst. Less commonly, the cells seem to unfold a terminal duct–lobular unit and thereby create a frondlike architecture and the lesion referred to as *papillary apocrine metaplasia.* When the proliferative apocrine cells exhibit atypical cytologic or architectural features, lesions in the atypical hyperplasia–ductal carcinoma in situ spectrum develop.

Apocrine proliferations do not exhibit distinctive clinicopathologic characteristics. They affect women of all ages, and they do not give rise to unique

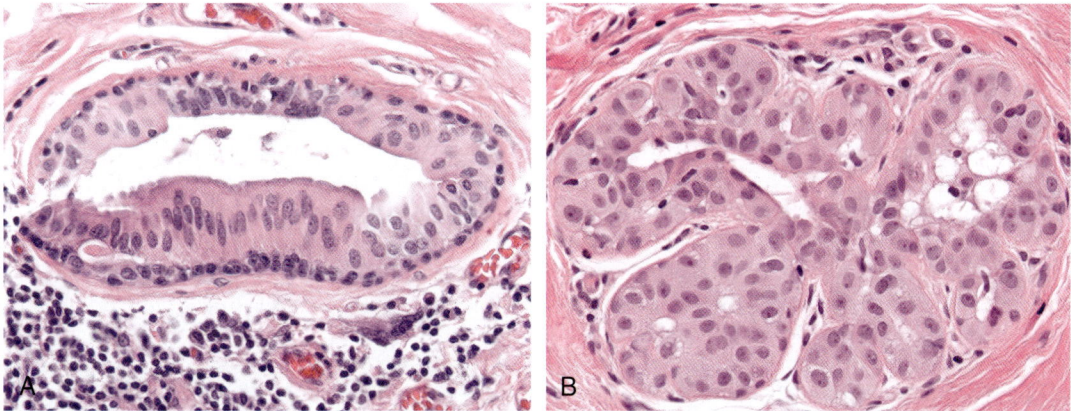

Figure 4-7 A, These ductal cells have copious, eosinophilic cytoplasm, but their nuclei do not have the attributes of apocrine cells. **B,** One can make the same points about these carcinoma cells.

Figure 4-8 Apocrine cells arise from luminal cells. One can detect the point of origin of the apocrine population in the center of the field. One can observe characteristic apocrine nuclei in cells containing only scant eosinophilic cytoplasm.

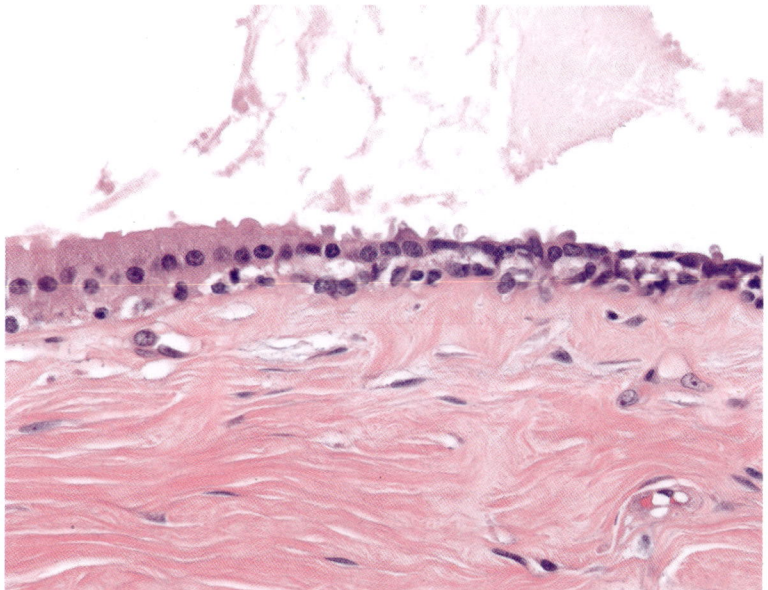

complaints or clinical signs. Like other entities derived from ductal cells, proliferations of apocrine nature can lead to the precipitation of calcium salts, and the pleomorphism of the resulting calcifications sometimes startles radiologists. Only apocrine cells cause the formation of calcium oxalate crystals, and the conventional wisdom asserts that only benign apocrine cells cause this variety of calcification. The jury is still out concerning this latter point, because pathologists' ability to classify apocrine proliferations lacks sophistication.

One cannot detect most apocrine proliferations during a macroscopic examination. Certain examples create small, complex cystic masses, but most lesions are invisible.

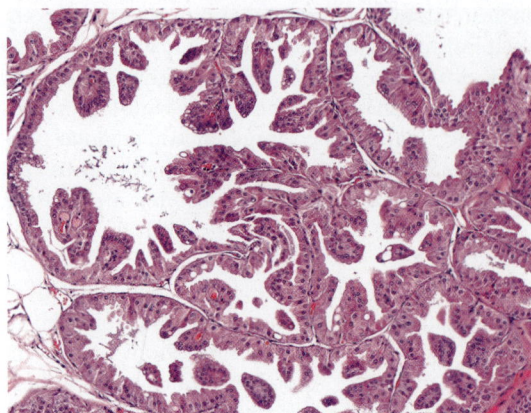

Figure 4-9 In this example of papillary apocrine metaplasia, the apocrine cells grow in an orderly single layer that unfolded a terminal duct–lobular unit.

HISTOLOGIC CHARACTERISTICS

Papillary Apocrine Metaplasia

Conventional apocrine metaplasia (apocrine change) does not involve significant proliferation of the apocrine cells, but one can encounter foci that seem to include a component of proliferation superimposed on the metaplastic process. They usually consist of small regions in which distended acini contain papillary infoldings of stroma covered by a single, somewhat crowded layer of tall, otherwise conventional apocrine cells (Fig. 4-9). Pathologists must take care not to mistake this lesion for a form of atypical apocrine proliferation, because the architecture resulting from off-center planes of section of this lush, folded epithelium can simulate the appearance of genuine cellular stratification, and the pseudo-stratification of the nuclei can make it look like they no longer sit in their normal basal position (Fig. 4-10).

Recognizing that these apocrine cells grow in a single layer represents the first step toward avoiding this misinterpretation. The congested capillaries that usually underlie foci of apocrine changes can serve as a marker of the stromal network supporting the apocrine cells and thereby allow one to appreciate the single-layered arrangement of the cells. Experience with the artifacts of histologic sectioning enables one to realize that small tufts represent off-center sections of micropapillae. Both insights help guard against the conclusion that the apocrine cells display architectural atypia in the form of stratification. Furthermore, the cells of papillary apocrine metaplasia do not exhibit cytologic features of atypia: the nuclei and nucleoli appear uniform, and the cytoplasm does not look pale or foamy. On rare occasion, this change can involve large regions of the gland (Fig. 4-11).

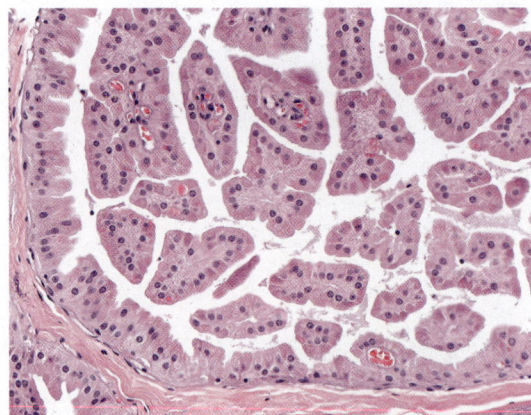

Figure 4-10 The engorged capillaries mark the stromal cores of the papillary frondlets. Despite the apparent complexity of the architecture, the cells form just one layer. The cells on one segment of the wall look crowded and possibly slightly stratified, a small deviation, which one can, perhaps, overlook.

Atypical Ductal Hyperplasia and Ductal Carcinoma In Situ of Apocrine Type

The classification of lesions characterized by atypical apocrine cells remains mostly unexplored, a terra incognita of mammary pathology in which pathologists must chart their own paths. Nevertheless, working from first principles and common sense, one can establish a few points of reference in this landscape. First, it stands to reason that to classify an apocrine proliferation as either atypical ductal hyperplasia or ductal carcinoma in situ, one must observe cytologic atypia in all cases and evidence of proliferation in most. Second, the proportions of the two phenomena needed to establish a diagnosis vary according to the degree of cytologic atypia. Proliferations showing high-grade atypia, for example, require signs of only

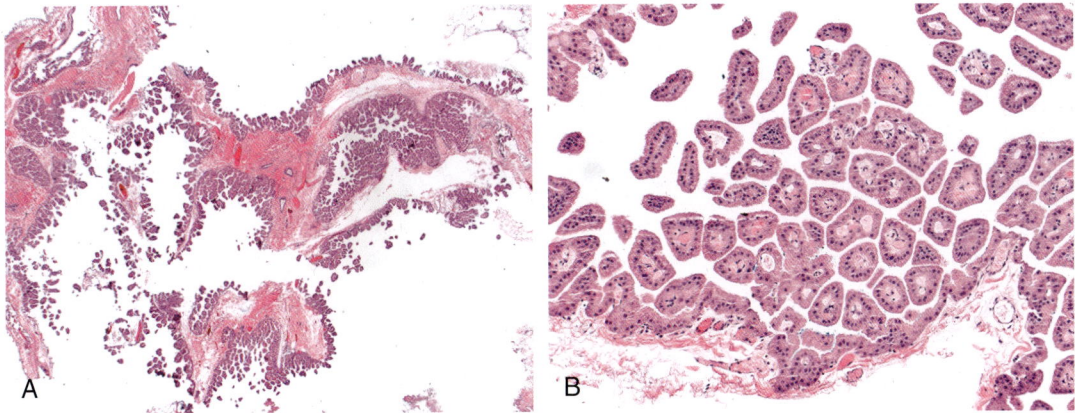

Figure 4-11 **A** and **B,** Papillary apocrine metaplasia involves an unusually large region of the gland.

minimal proliferation to make the diagnosis of malignancy, whereas those displaying low-grade atypia must appear more extensive to warrant that diagnosis. Third, pathologists do not know how to separate low-grade ductal carcinoma in situ of apocrine type from atypical ductal hyperplasia of apocrine cells.

Our ignorance about the nature of proliferations of apocrine cells with slightly atypical features stems, in part, from the belief that conventional apocrine cells vary considerably in their cytologic characteristics and their pattern of growth. According to the popular wisdom, classifying a slightly atypical cell as apocrine eliminates the possibility that it has a neoplastic nature. Consequently, when confronted with an apocrine lesion demonstrating slight cytologic atypia and minor architectural abnormalities, most pathologists would think of it as a form of benign hyperplasia of apocrine cells. This interpretation does not seem well founded, because no other type of mammary luminal cell gives rise to benign proliferations. Furthermore, recent studies suggest that cells showing low-grade apocrine atypia carry mutations commonly seen in breast cancer.

Perhaps the time has come to reconsider the significance of these deviations in cellular attributes. The author cannot offer more than personal opinions about this matter, but two come to mind. First, pathologists might find it worthwhile to place more significance on deviations from the usual single-layered manner of growth. Genuine stratification of cells, the formation of cellular bars or micropapillary tufts, and the creation of spaces all indicate architectural atypia even in the absence of clear-cut polarization of the proliferative cells. If encountered in the setting of a conventional ductal proliferation, these formations would merit careful study; one should do the same when they are created by apocrine cells.

Second, mild alterations in the cytologic properties should not go unnoticed. Malpositioning of the nucleus, nuclear and nucleolar enlargement, and cytoplasmic pallor should alert the pathologist to the possible presence of cytologic atypia. Having detected atypical features, the pathologist might not find it straightforward to reach a final diagnosis. In this circumstance, one might find it helpful to incorporate an estimate of the extent of cellular proliferation in one's analysis. One could evaluate this phenomenon by noting the size of the lesion, the extent of glandular distention, and the amount of cellular stratification. Researchers have proposed other, better defined, and standardized systems for integrating the size of a lesion in the analysis of apocrine lesions, but these systems require clinical validation.

By integrating the cytologic and architectural properties of an apocrine proliferation and, in certain cases, the extent of the lesion, one can usually reach a reasonable diagnosis. Small regions showing minimal atypia (Fig. 4-12) could probably go unmentioned, depending on the clinical circumstances. Larger regions and those showing more cellular proliferation probably require comment (Fig. 4-13), and a diagnosis such as *atypical ductal hyperplasia of apocrine type* offers a reasonable choice. Lesions showing architectural atypia, low-grade cytologic atypia, and an ancillary finding such as necrosis, dishesion, or mitotic activity in noticeable amounts might warrant a diagnosis of ductal carcinoma in situ of apocrine type (Fig. 4-14). The presence of high-grade cytologic atypia, even in the absence of extensive proliferation and architectural atypia, establishes the diagnosis of apocrine ductal carcinoma in situ without controversy (Fig. 4-15).

Pathologists should realize that other types of atypical epithelial proliferation, both ductal and lobular in nature, frequently accompany atypical

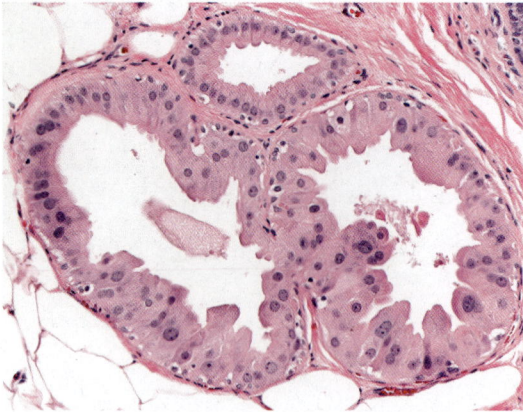

Figure 4-12 The apocrine cells lining the gland at the top of the field exhibit conventional characteristics. Those lining the other two glands display crowding, malposition of the nuclei, and pleomorphism of a few nuclei. One might reasonably overlook this miniscule focus if encountered in the appropriate setting.

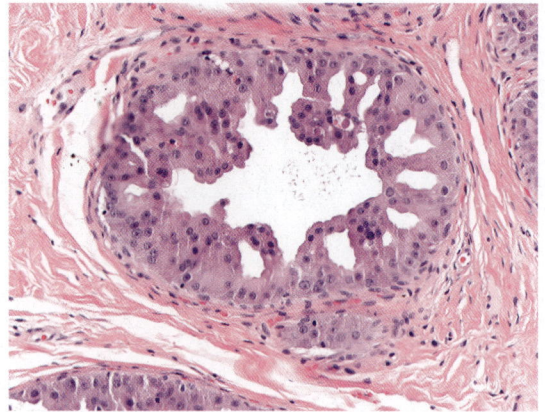

Figure 4-13 This focus of mild apocrine atypia probably deserves a mention. It features malposition of the nuclei, genuine cellular stratification, architectural complexity, and mild nuclear pleomorphism.

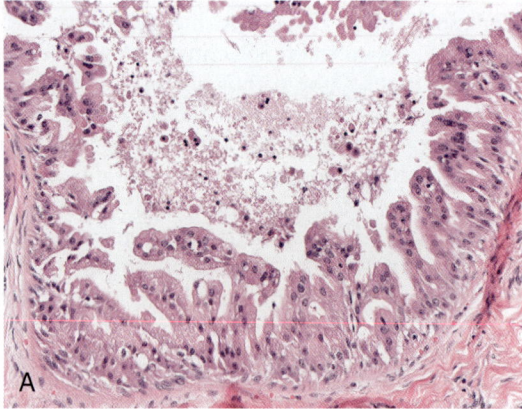

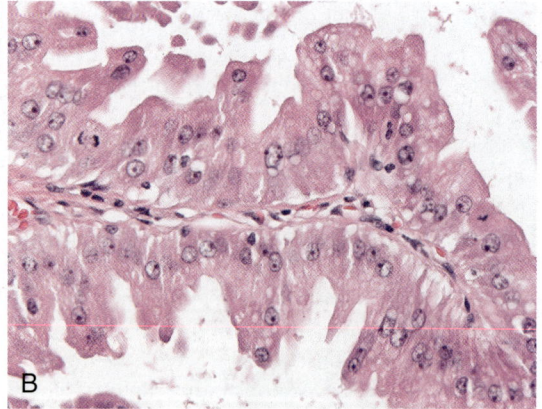

Figure 4-14 A and **B,** This apocrine proliferation represents low-grade apocrine ductal carcinoma in situ. The cells exhibit obvious stratification and architectural complexity, mild nuclear pleomorphism, dishesion, necrosis, and mitotic activity.

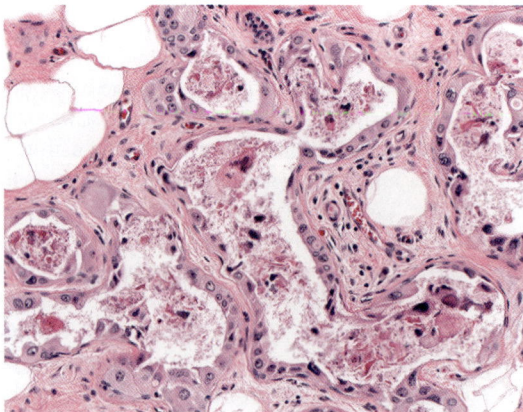

Figure 4-15 The extreme cytologic atypia of these apocrine cells would allow one to recognize their malignant nature from a mile away. The presence of dishesion and necrosis only makes the job easier.

apocrine proliferations. After discovering an atypical apocrine lesion, the savvy pathologist conducts a careful search for these conventional types of atypia. Their presence may render the classification of the atypical apocrine focus less important for patient care.

Atypical Apocrine Sclerosing Lesion

This unusual lesion features the elements of adenosis, fibrosis, and apocrine atypia. Densely packed compressed glands sit in a fibrous stroma (Fig. 4-16). When the abnormality affects older women, as it often does, fat may have replaced the nonspecialized fibrous connective tissue, so the outermost glands can appear to extend into adipose tissue (Fig. 4-17). The tiny acini are home to slightly atypical apocrine cells. Reflecting their apocrine heritage, these cells appear larger than normal luminal cells and possess

Figure 4-16 A and **B,** The nodule of sclerosing adenosis contains atypical apocrine cells.

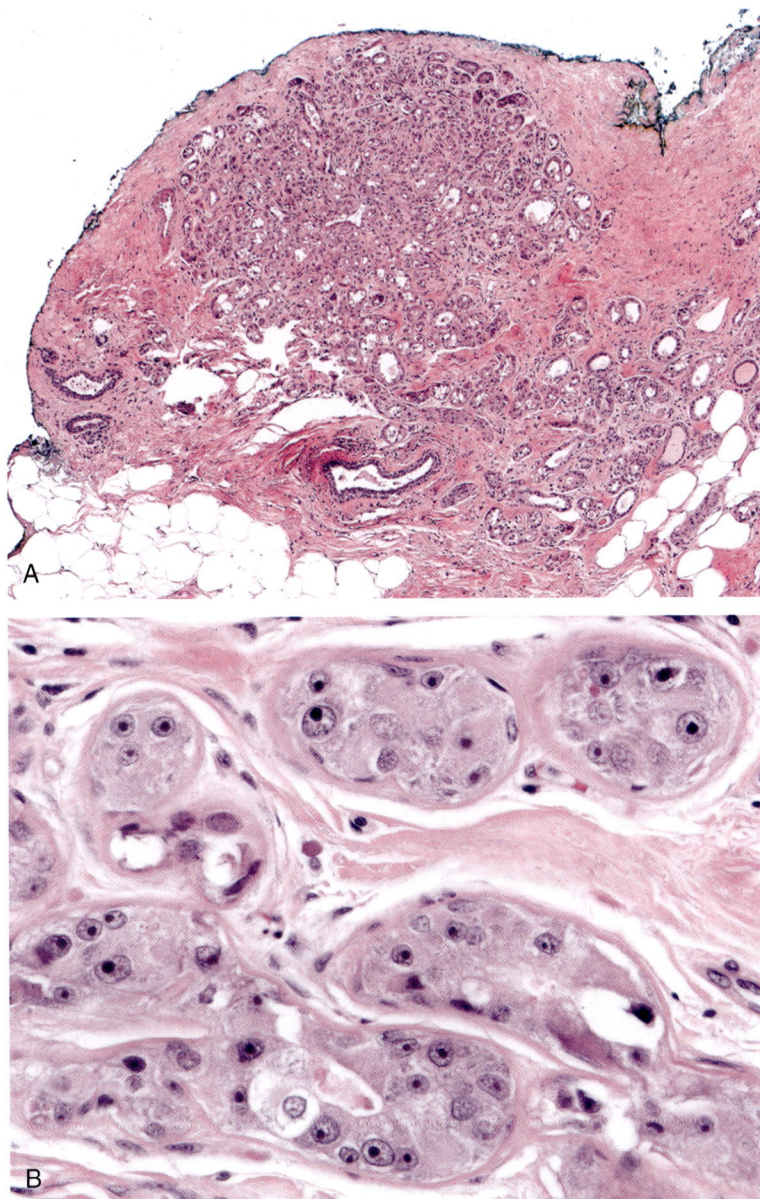

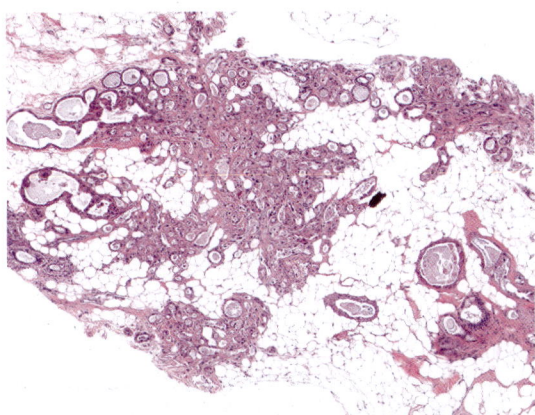

Figure 4-17 Stromal atrophy makes it seem that the sclerotic lobules extend into the adipose tissue.

the characteristic apocrine nuclei; however, in other respects, the cells look atypical (Fig. 4-18). The nuclei vary somewhat in size, the nucleoli can appear modestly enlarged, and the cytoplasm usually looks pale and frothy (Fig. 4-19). Despite the presence of cytologic atypia, the lesion does not appear proliferative. No more than a few cells occupy each acinus, and accumulation of cytoplasm within individual cells, rather than an increase in their number, can account for the increase in the diameter of the glands.

Researchers have not determined the clinical significance of this lesion. Like other forms of apocrine atypia, atypical apocrine sclerosing lesions often coexist with atypical or malignant proliferations of conventional ductal or lobular cells, so the prudent

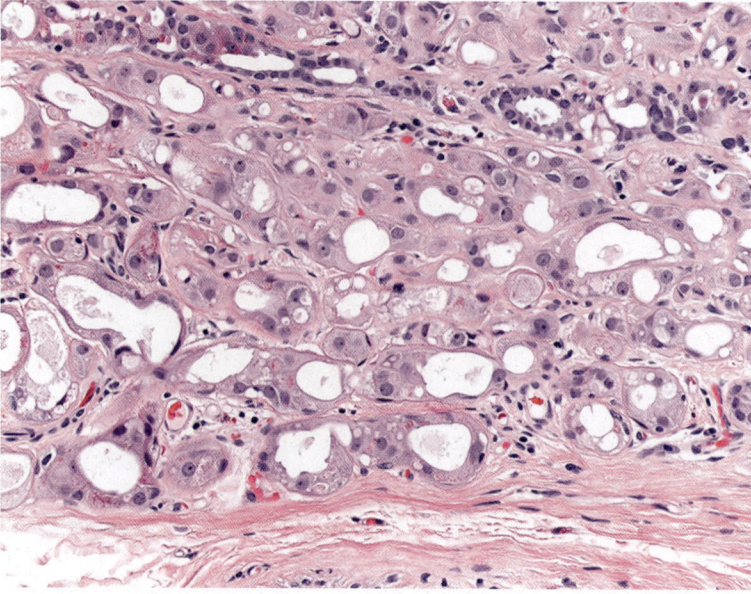

Figure 4-18 A few acini lined by normal cells persist in this atypical apocrine sclerosing lesion. The acini housing the atypical apocrine cells appear larger and have larger lumens than the normal ones. Enlargement of the individual atypical apocrine cells due to the accumulation of cytoplasm rather than to an increase in the number of cells in the acini explains the expansion of the altered glands.

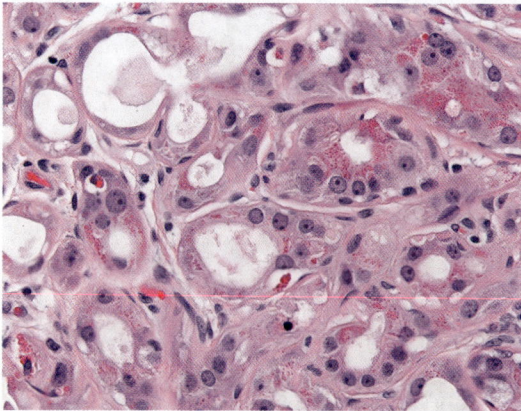

Figure 4-19 The apocrine cells display low-grade cytologic atypia: pallor and vacuolization of the cytoplasm, malposition of the nuclei, and disarray in the location of the granules.

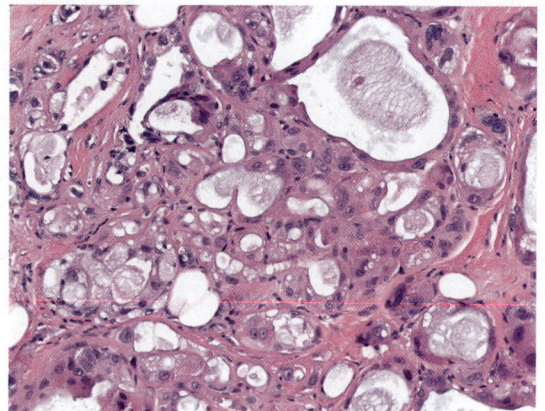

Figure 4-20 The cells lining these acini appear crowded, and a few glands look enlarged.

pathologist searches for other regions of atypia after discovering an atypical apocrine sclerosing lesion. When such a lesion is detected in a core biopsy specimen, excision of the entire lesion would probably serve the patient well.

Atypical apocrine sclerosing lesions can serve as the soil from which apocrine carcinoma germinates. Evidence of cellular proliferation and features of high-grade cytologic atypia would suggest that a malignant proliferation has taken root. Crowding of cells with consequent enlargement of acini and distention of their lumens indicate that the apocrine population has begun to expand (Fig. 4-20). Cellular stratification and the presence of mitotic figures constitute even more compelling evidence

of this sort (Fig. 4-21). Findings such as necrosis, dishesion, and substantial nuclear pleomorphism would clinch the diagnosis of malignancy (Fig. 4-22).

SUMMARY

Proliferations of apocrine cells form a spectrum similar to the one created by conventional ductal cells. Papillary apocrine metaplasia marks one end, and high-grade apocrine ductal carcinoma in situ the other. Pathologists agree on the morphologic characteristics of these extreme members of this family, but no one understands the biologic properties of these lesions sufficiently to partition this collection in a

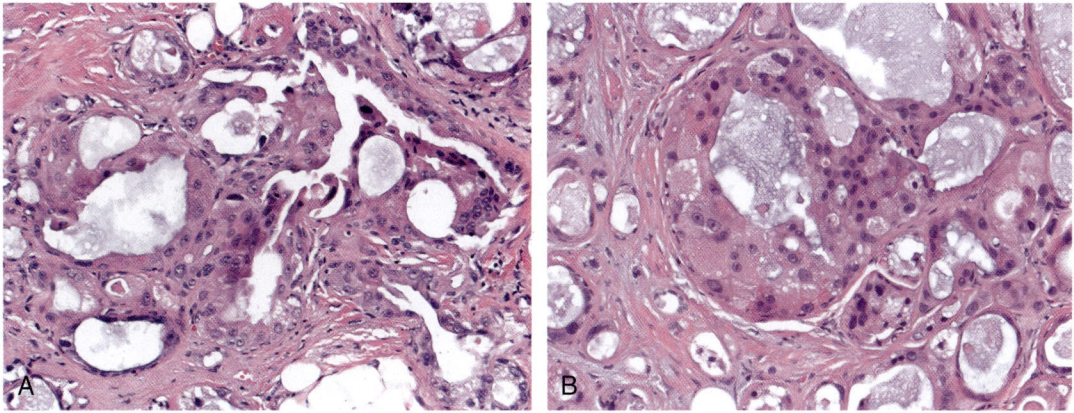

Figure 4-21 **A** and **B,** The atypical apocrine cells pile up in and distend the glands.

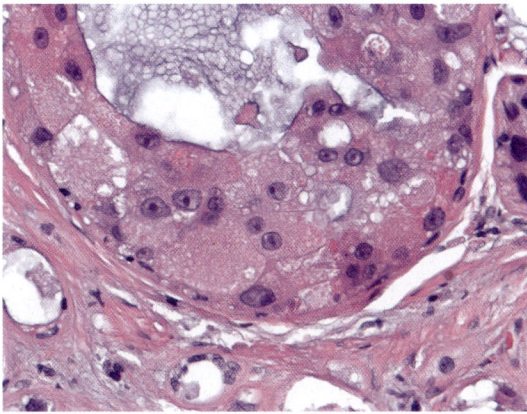

Figure 4-22 The presence of proliferation and marked atypia suggests that apocrine ductal carcinoma in situ has developed in this atypical apocrine sclerosing lesion.

more nuanced way. Heightened awareness of the manifestation of both cytologic and architectural atypia may enhance our understanding of these lesions.

Selected Readings

Carter DJ, Rosen PP: Atypical apocrine metaplasia in sclerosing lesions of the breast: A study of 51 patients. Mod Pathol 1991;4:1-5.

Celis JE, Gromova I, Gromov P, et al: Molecular pathology of breast apocrine carcinomas: A protein expression signature specific for benign apocrine metaplasia. FEBS Lett 2006;580:2935-2944.

Jones C, Damiani S, Wells D, et al: Molecular cytogenetic comparison of apocrine hyperplasia and apocrine carcinoma of the breast. Am J Pathol 2001;158:207-214.

Leal C, Henrique R, Monteiro P, et al: Apocrine ductal carcinoma in situ of the breast: Histologic classification and expression of biologic markers. Hum Pathol 2001;32:487-493.

O'Malley FP, Page DL, Nelson EH, et al: Ductal carcinoma in situ of the breast with apocrine cytology: Definition of a borderline category. Hum Pathol 1994;25:164-168.

O'Malley FP, Bane AL: The spectrum of apocrine lesions of the breast. Adv Anat Pathol 2004;11:1-9.

Pagani A, Sapino A, Eusebi V, et al: PIP/GCDFP-15 gene expression and apocrine differentiation in carcinomas of the breast. Virchows Arch 1994;425:459-465.

Page DL, Dupont WD, Jensen RA: Papillary apocrine change of the breast: Associations with atypical hyperplasia and risk of breast cancer. Cancer Epidemiol Biomarkers Prev 1996;5:29-32.

Raju U, Zarbo RJ, Kubus J, et al: The histologic spectrum of apocrine breast proliferations: A comparative study of morphology and DNA content by image analysis. Hum Pathol 1993;24:173-181.

Seidman JD, Ashton M, Lefkowitz M: Atypical apocrine adenosis of the breast: A clinicopathologic study of 37 patients with 8.7-year follow-up. Cancer 1996;77:2529-2537.

Selim AA, Ryan A, El-Ayat G, et al: Loss of heterozygosity and allelic imbalance in apocrine metaplasia of the breast: Microdissection microsatellite analysis. J Pathol 2002;196:287-291.

Simpson PT, Reis-Filho JS, Gale T, et al: Molecular evolution of breast cancer. J Pathol 2005;205:248-254.

Wells CA, El-Ayat GA: Non-operative breast pathology: Apocrine lesions. J Clin Pathol 2007;60:1313-1320.

Wells CA, McGregor IL, Makunura CN, et al: Apocrine adenosis: A precursor of aggressive breast cancer? J Clin Pathol 1995;48:737-742.

Zagorianakou P, Zagorianakou N, Stefanou D, et al: The enigmatic nature of apocrine breast lesions. Virchows Arch 2006;448:525-531.

5

Mucinous Proliferations

Mammary epithelial cells produce small amounts of mucin on occasion. It ordinarily represents such an inconspicuous component of a lesion that pathologists do not accord its presence any significance, and they may overlook it entirely. Much less commonly, the mucin accumulates in such copious amounts that it dominates the histologic picture. Although such copious quantities of mucin catch one's eye and may even reflect a unique pathogenesis, they do not define the nature of the lesion. Mucin accumulation occurs in several settings and accompanies epithelial proliferations of several types. Apocrine lesions and lobular neoplasia commonly include an element of mucin production, but it usually does not overwhelm the other aspects of the lesions, nor does it complicate the diagnosis. This chapter therefore focuses on lesions of ductal cells characterized by the presence of abundant mucin.

BASIC CONCEPTS

Cellular Properties

The concepts that underlie the analysis of proliferations of conventional ductal cells serve as effectively in the analysis of lesions of mucin-producing ductal cells, but the histologic manifestations of these concepts vary slightly in the latter setting. For example, the accumulation of mucin tends to overshadow the proliferation of cells. They do not pile up very much; instead, they grow in one or just a few layers, which do not fill the ducts and acini. Consequently, cases composed of mucin-producing cells do not usually create the atypical architectural patterns as extensively as their counterparts composed of conventional ductal cells do, and pathologists frequently find that they must base their diagnosis of mucinous proliferations predominantly on cytologic findings. Cytologic atypia takes the same

form in mucin-producing ductal cells as it does in conventional ductal cells; however, atypical mucinous cells often appear small and number only a few, so it takes careful study to detect their cytologic alterations and considerable experience to appreciate the significance of the aberrations. Like commonplace neoplastic ductal cells, neoplastic mucinous cells lack cohesion and display cellular polarization, resulting in the expected basal position of the nucleus and the formation of an apical cytoplasmic compartment.

Mucin Accumulation and Extravasation

Distention of ducts and terminal duct–lobular units by mucin characterizes the family of mucinous ductal lesions. The mucin probably originates from the luminal epithelial cells lining the ducts and acini, but one does not observe mucin droplets in their cytoplasm in conventionally prepared sections. Instead, one finds the mucin in the lumens of the glands (Fig. 5-1). It can stain either faintly blue or pale pink (Fig. 5-2). Besides accumulating in the lumen, the mucin extends beneath the luminal cells, where it separates them from the myoepithelial cells and the basement membrane (Fig. 5-3). The basement membrane confines the mucin for some time, but when this barrier loses its integrity, the mucin escapes into the stroma. This phenomenon can take place in either acini or ducts (Fig. 5-4).

One occasionally observes mucin-filled ducts that seem to have stromal elements or glands within them (Fig. 5-5). Ducts do not have bundles of collagen uncovered by epithelial cells, blood vessels, or acini within their lumens, so this unexpected situation requires an explanation. This pattern can arise only when the ductal epithelium becomes disrupted (Fig. 5-6). Besides allowing for the creation of this unusual configuration, disruption of the ductal

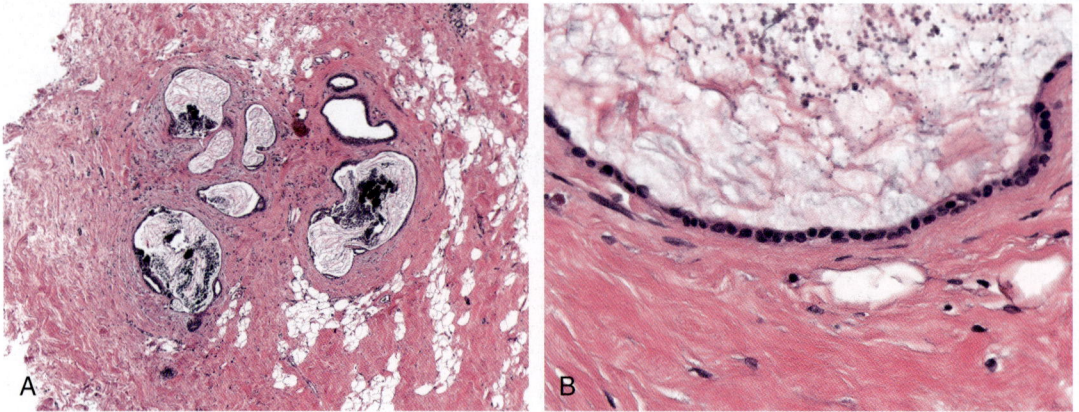

Figure 5-1 A, Mucin and large, chunky calcifications distend terminal ductules and a few acini. **B,** Small bland cells containing just a little cytoplasm line the mucin-filled glands.

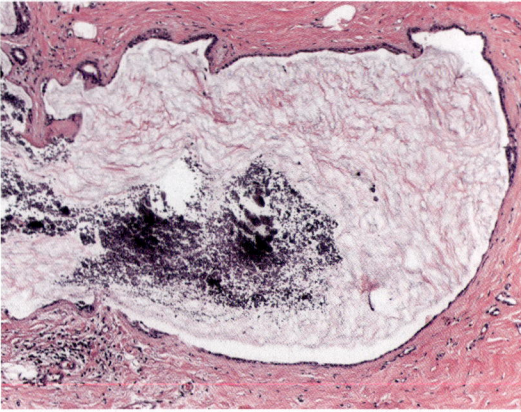

Figure 5-2 The color of the mucin ranges from pink to gray to blue.

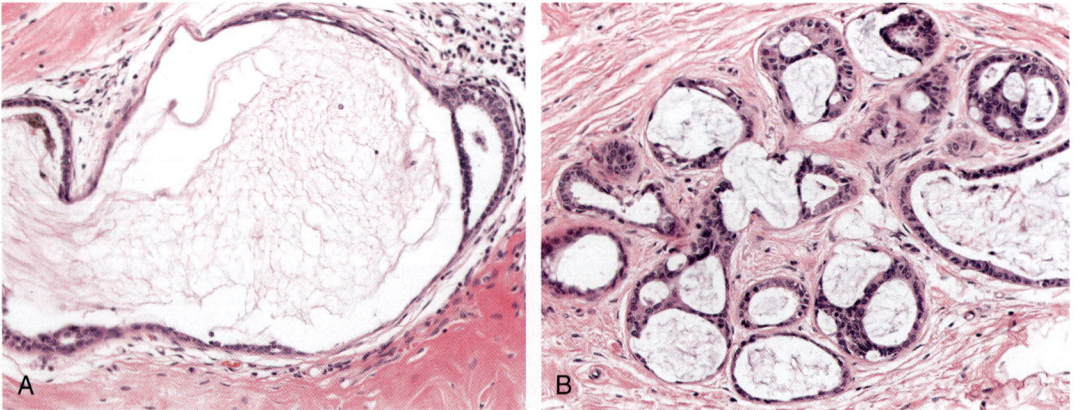

Figure 5-3 Mucin uproots and displaces the epithelium. The process has denuded segments of the wall of the gland in **A;** however, strips of epithelium remain anchored to the basement membrane at several points. One can appreciate the same process involving acini in **B.**

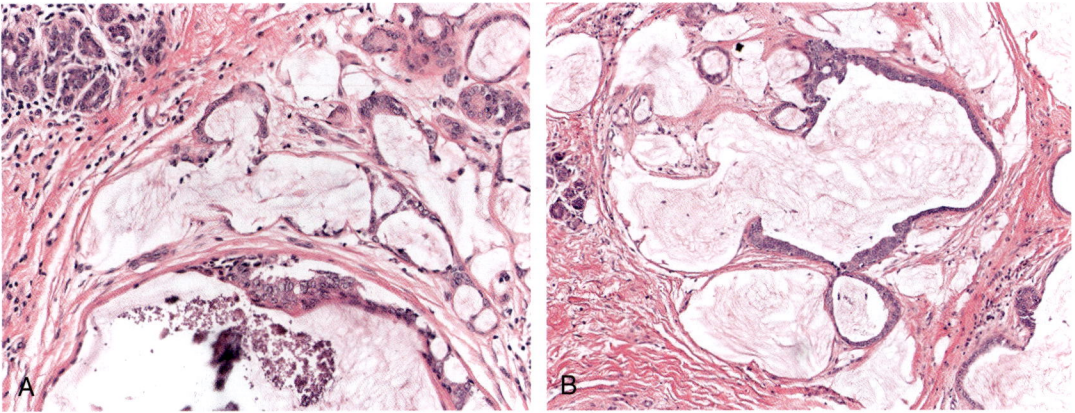

Figure 5-4 Rupture of the basement membrane of acini in **A** or ducts in **B** allows mucin to spill into the stroma.

Figure 5-5 Neither ducts nor acini have naked collagen bundles or stromal cells within their lumens.

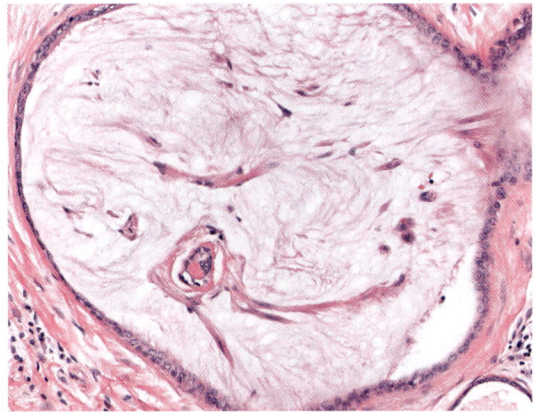

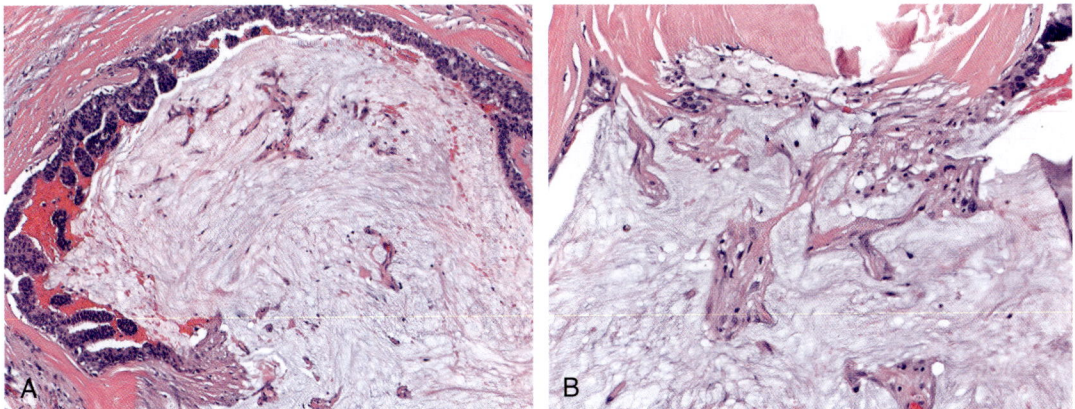

Figure 5-6 The seeming presence of stromal elements within the mucin-filled duct in **A** should prompt a search for other evidence of loss of integrity of the epithelium. The region in **B** illustrates the point of epithelial rupture visible at the bottom of the field in **A**.

epithelium could allow mucin to spread into the stroma; thus, the detection of these structures within a mucin-filled duct should prompt the pathologist to search for the better-recognized evidence of mucin extravasation.

DEFINITIONS AND CLINICOPATHOLOGIC CORRELATIONS

The presence of mucin-filled ducts, ductules, and acini represents the common finding that unites these lesions, but the morphologic characteristics of the epithelial cells lining these structures differ from one type of mucinous proliferation to the next. The epithelium can consist of small, uniform, flattened to low columnar cells growing in a single layer, atypical ductal cells showing only focal stratification and atypical architectural formations, or clearly malignant ductal cells displaying the expected cytologic and architectural characteristics. Many pathologists use the term *mucocele-like lesion* for all cases containing abundant mucin whatever the nature of the epithelial lining, and they go on to qualify the diagnosis with a modifier such as *with atypical ductal hyperplasia* or *with ductal carcinoma in situ* when the epithelial cells display the appropriate features. This approach seems to emphasize the mucin accumulation as the defining characteristic and to relegate the nature of the epithelial cells to the position of an afterthought. Structuring diagnoses in this way recapitulates the pathologist's examination of such a lesion; however, the usage runs the risk of clouding one's understanding of the biologic properties of the entities. The nature of the epithelial proliferation, not the amount of mucin, determines the clinical behavior of the lesion. A potentially more biologically based approach would categorize the abnormalities according to the characteristics of the epithelial cells and designate the presence of abundant mucin as a descriptor. This terminology reserves the diagnosis "mucocele-like lesion" for a lesion composed of benign cells like those cited in the seminal description of this lesion and would use diagnoses such as "atypical ductal proliferation with abundant mucin" and "ductal carcinoma in situ with abundant mucin" for cases containing atypical ductal cells. This usage strikes the author as more biologically focused.

Whatever the terminology, ductal lesions containing abundant mucin seem to form a morphologic continuum and, possibly, a biologic one linking proliferations of bland, mucin-producing ductal cells, at one extreme, with low-grade mucinous ductal carcinomas in situ at the other. One can partition this spectrum into the following three general groups on the basis of the features of the epithelial cells: lesions in which the epithelium consists of normal-appearing ductal cells mostly growing in a single layer (mucocele-like lesion), lesions in which atypical ductal cells grow in a flat or focally complex pattern (atypical ductal proliferation with abundant mucin production), and lesions in which ductal carcinoma in situ lines the mucin-filled structures (ductal carcinoma in situ with abundant mucin production). Conventional ductal hyperplasia showing the usual stratified and fenestrated pattern does not form abundant mucin with any significant frequency, so this type of ductal proliferation does not occupy a place in the spectrum.

Readers will note that the cytologic and architectural patterns of the continuum proposed for mucinous ductal lesions duplicate those seen in the morphologic pathway suggested for conventional ductal proliferations. Normal cells first acquire atypical cytologic characteristics while growing in a flat sheet. At a later stage, the cells stratify to create the atypical type of proliferation. The development of a greater degree of architectural atypia heralds the formation of a carcinoma in situ. Early neoplastic lesions of conventional ductal cells frequently contain a mixture of growth patterns from flat atypia to robust atypical ductal hyperplasia. Lesions composed of mucinous ductal cells also exhibit this variation and, in fact, may vary more than lesions of conventional ductal cells. Consequently, pathologists must examine ductal mucinous lesions thoroughly; the diagnosis should rest on the characteristics of the most abnormal region.

Mucin-containing ductal lesions do not display distinctive clinicopathologic characteristics. The abnormalities arise in adult women of all ages. About half of the lesions consist of palpable nodules; the remainder manifest as mammographic abnormalities. Coarse calcifications sometimes precipitate in the mucin, especially in lesions associated with carcinomas. All lesions in this family can recur if incompletely resected.

The presence of glistening, gelatinous, gray material visible during a macroscopic examination suggests the presence of a mucinous lesion, but one cannot usually detect the accumulation of mucin in small lesions, nor can one differentiate one type of mucinous lesion from the others.

HISTOLOGIC CHARACTERISTICS

Mucocele-Like Lesion

The mucinous ductal proliferation known as the mucocele-like lesion probably represents the rarest member of the family.

Architectural Characteristics

Mucin fills and distends a collection of ducts and lobules (Fig. 5-7). The epithelium lining the structures grows almost entirely as a single layer.

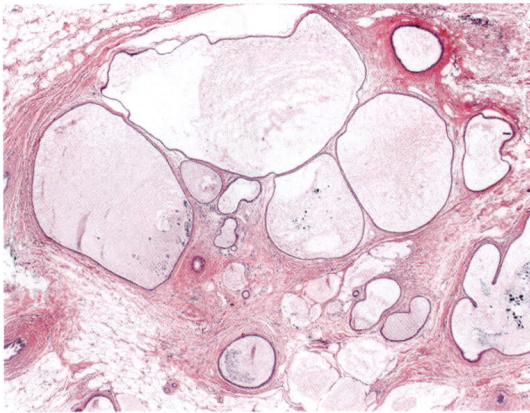

Figure 5-7 Mucin fills a region of the glandular tree in this mucocele-like lesion.

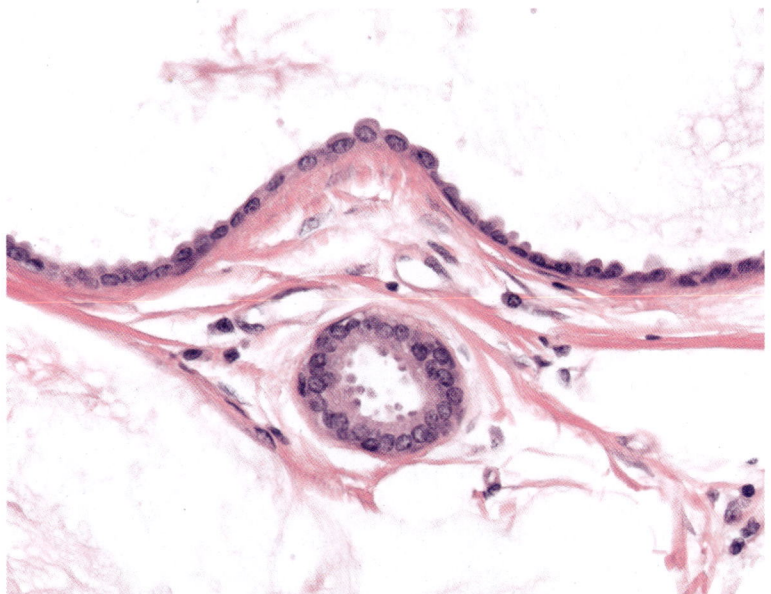

Figure 5-9 The cells vary from cuboidal to flat.

One can observe focal, slight stratification, but the presence of well-developed architectural atypia would preclude this diagnosis.

Cytologic Characteristics

The cells composing the epithelium look like normal ductal cells (Fig. 5-8). They appear small, and they have flat, cuboidal, or low columnar shapes (Fig. 5-9). The nuclei also appear small and exhibit slightly irregular contours, finely granular chromatin, and small nucleoli.

Because of the flat growth pattern, the epithelium of mucocele-like lesions superficially resembles the epithelium of flat epithelial atypia; however, the ductal cells in mucocele-like lesions do not exhibit either the tall columnar shape or the atypical nuclear features characteristic of the cells of flat epithelial atypia. The first descriptions of mucocele-like lesions appeared before

the development of modern ideas about the nature of flat epithelial atypia, so certain early studies of mucocele-like lesions may have included cases containing atypical ductal cells of the flat type. Because flat epithelial atypia probably represents a precursor to ductal carcinoma in situ, it seems safest not to categorize mucinous lesions composed of atypical ductal cells growing in a flat pattern as benign mucocele-like lesions.

Atypical Ductal Proliferation with Abundant Mucin

Most proliferations of mucinous ductal cells are categorized as atypical ductal proliferation with abundant mucin. To qualify for inclusion in this group, the cells must exhibit cytologic atypia, but they can grow in either flat or slightly complex architectural patterns.

Figure 5-8 The cells lining the mucin-filled gland possess less cytoplasm than those lining the nearby ductule; otherwise, the cells in the two locations resemble one another.

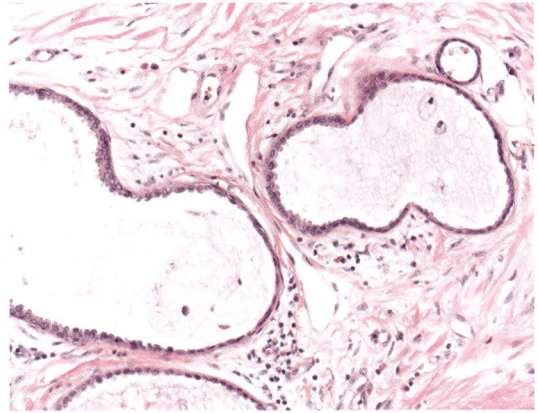

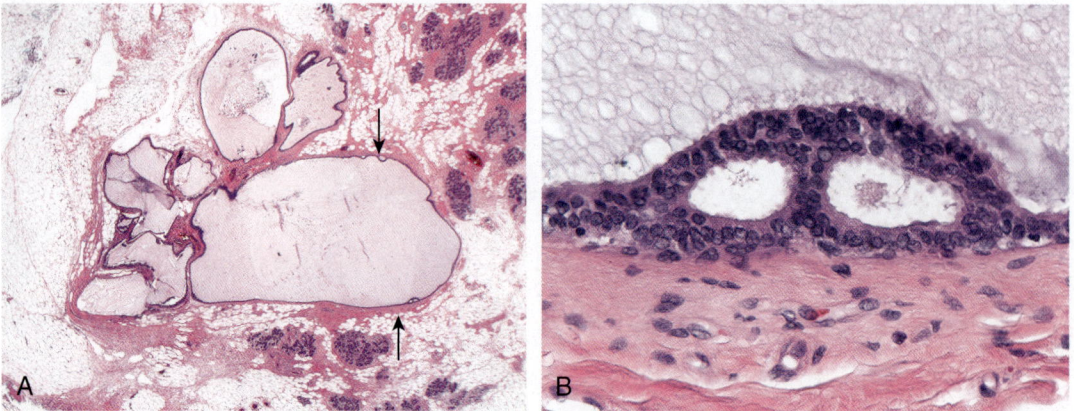

Figure 5-10 Mucin distends a few glandular structures. **A,** Despite the low magnification, one can appreciate that the epithelium looks more complex (*arrows*). **B,** Along a few short stretches of the duct wall, the cells form architecturally complex structures.

Architectural Characteristics

Most of the epithelial proliferation takes the form of a flat sheet. The cells can pile up in a few layers, and they can form a few polarized spaces, bars, or arches (Fig. 5-10). Examples with a flat growth pattern resemble conventional flat epithelial atypia (Fig. 5-11), whereas those forming stratified and architecturally atypical patterns resemble conventional atypical ductal hyperplasia (Fig. 5-12).

Cytologic Characteristics

The level of cytologic atypia ranges from mild to moderate; in most examples, the atypia looks mild. The atypical cells possess smoothly contoured, oval or round nuclei, finely dispersed chromatin, and inconspicuous nucleoli. The cytoplasm usually has an eosinophilic hue (Fig. 5-13).

Ductal Carcinoma In Situ with Abundant Mucin

Atypical mucinous ductal proliferations showing either anaplastic cytologic features or obvious architectural atypia merit the diagnosis of ductal carcinoma in situ with abundant mucin. Pathologists have not agreed on the cytologic criteria that alone would establish the diagnosis of high-grade ductal carcinoma in situ or the extent of architectural atypia needed to substantiate the diagnosis of low-grade ductal carcinoma in situ. Thus, the distinction between an atypical ductal proliferation with abundant mucin and mucinous ductal carcinoma in situ remains ill defined. Pathologists can approach the diagnosis of these mucinous ductal proliferations as they would atypical ductal proliferations composed of conventional ductal cells.

Architectural Characteristics

The polarized cells of atypical mucinous proliferations create the same architectural patterns as the cells of atypical nonmucinous ductal proliferations: cribriform spaces, trabecular bars, and Roman bridges (Fig. 5-14). When created by cells showing low-grade cytologic atypia, these atypical architectural formations substantiate the diagnosis of ductal carcinoma in situ with abundant mucin.

Cytologic Characteristics

The malignant cells display cytologic atypia, which takes the same form as the atypia displayed by the cells of conventional ductal carcinomas in situ (Fig. 5-15). Although the level of atypia can range from mild to severe, most cases fall into the mild category.

Summary

Proliferations of mucin-producing ductal cells form a continuum that nearly duplicates the one created by nonmucinous ductal proliferations. The mucocele-like lesion occupies one end of the spectrum, proliferations of atypical cells with the growth patterns of flat epithelial atypia and atypical ductal hyperplasia the center, and lesions with the architecture of low-grade ductal carcinoma in situ the opposite end. The cells of conventional ductal hyperplasia do not usually produce abundant mucin, so this lesion does not have a place in this family.

PROBLEMS IN THE DIAGNOSIS OF MUCINOUS PROLIFERATIONS

Detection of Invasion

The recognition of invasion is the most common problem posed by mucinous ductal lesions. Although the presence of mucin and malignant

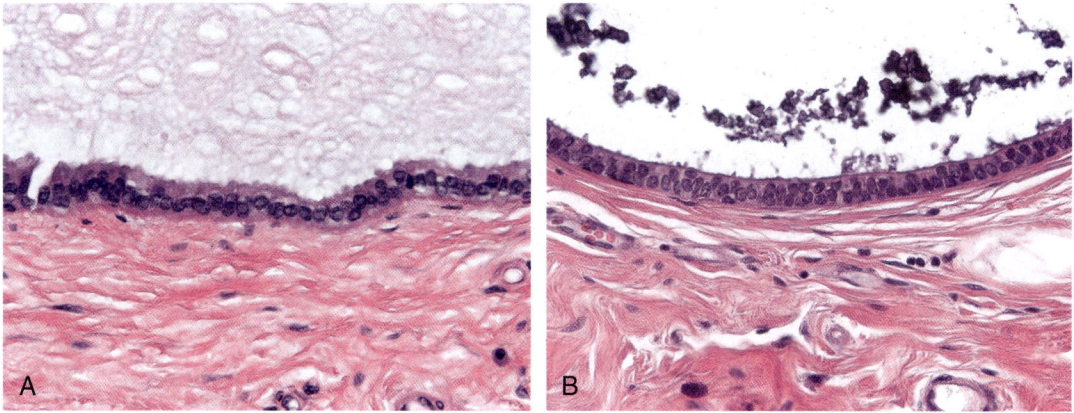

Figure 5-11 The cells composing the atypical ductal proliferation with abundant mucin shown in **A** display the flat pattern of growth, the columnar shape, and the cytologic atypia seen in conventional examples of flat epithelial atypia, shown in **B**.

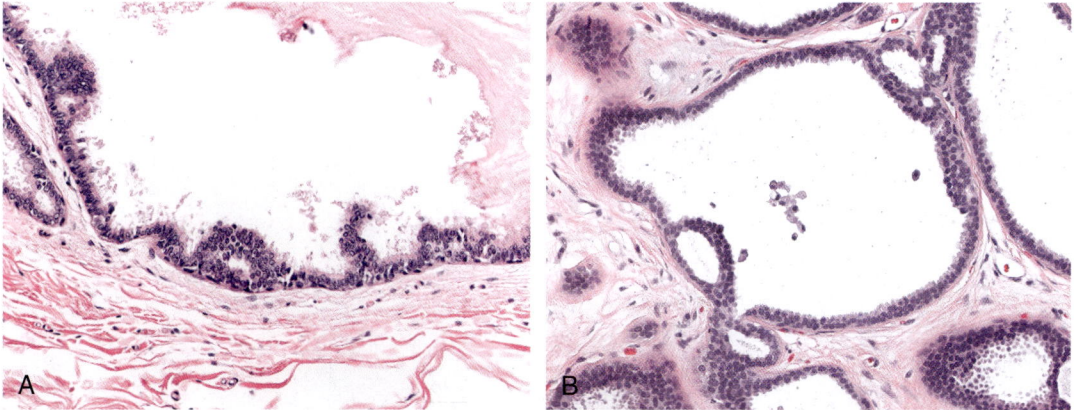

Figure 5-12 The atypical structures of the mucinous lesion in **A** resemble those of conventional atypical ductal hyperplasia, shown in **B**.

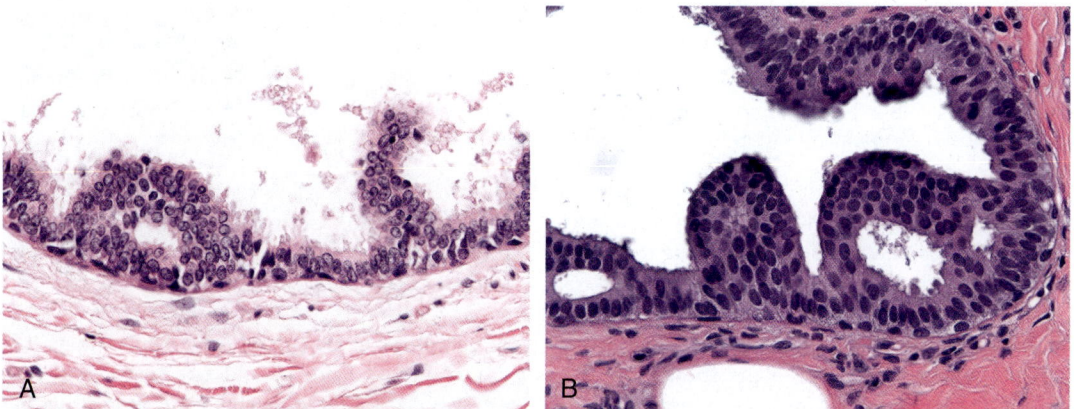

Figure 5-13 The cells in the atypical ductal proliferation with abundant mucin shown in **A** have the same cytologic characteristics as those in conventional atypical ductal hyperplasia, shown in **B**.

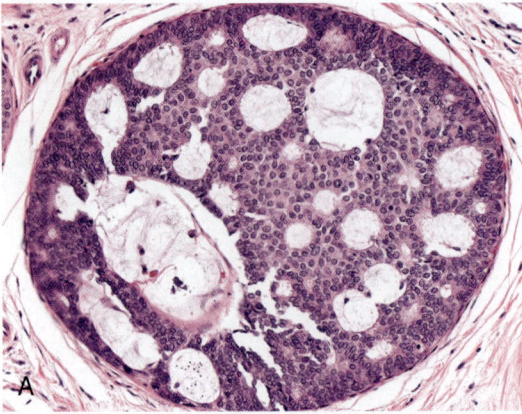

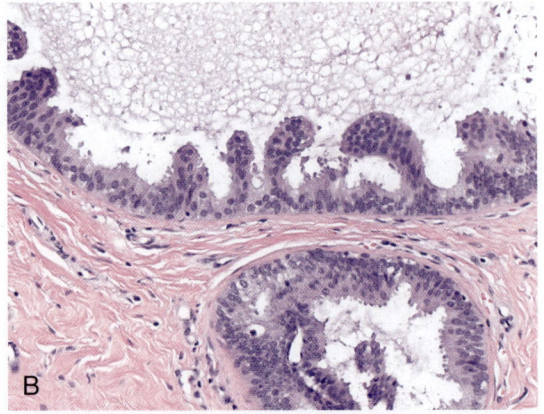

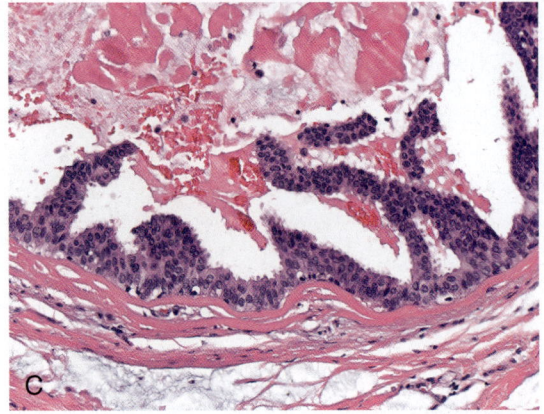

Figure 5-14 Mucin-producing carcinomas give rise to the same cribriform spaces in **A**, micropapillary tufts in **B**, and trabecular bars in **C** that one sees in conventional ductal carcinomas.

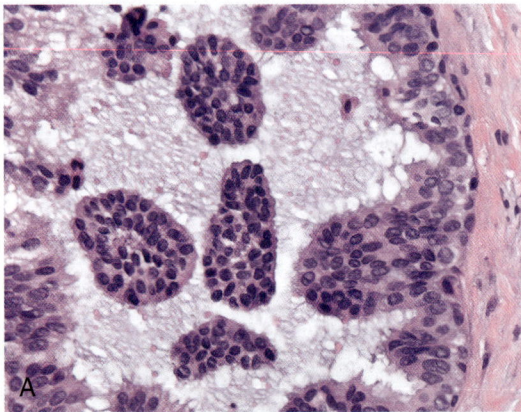

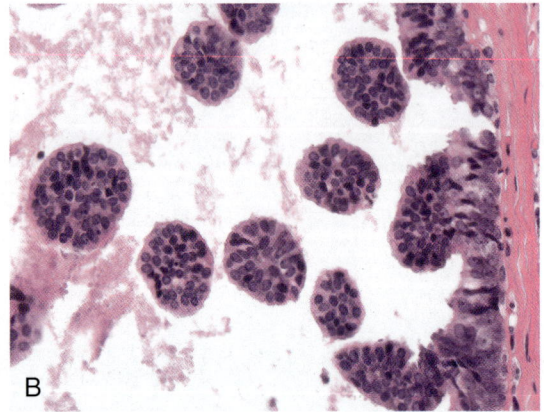

Figure 5-15 The cells in the low-grade mucin-producing ductal carcinoma in **A** look like those of a conventional low-grade ductal carcinoma in situ in **B**.

cells in the stroma ordinarily establishes the diagnosis of invasion, pathologists must keep the following three considerations in mind.

The Origin of the Stromal Mucin Pools

Epithelial mucin can collect in the stroma through different mechanisms. In most examples, it transgresses the wall of the gland on its own accord through undefined mechanisms; less commonly,

the extravasation seems to result from iatrogenic forces. Trauma to the tissue during localization procedures, manipulation of the breast at the time of surgery, and handling of the specimen in the course of pathologic study can all cause mucin to spill into the stroma, and one should not misconstrue mucin extravasated by these mechanisms as invasive mucinous carcinoma. Determining whether the mucin penetrated the stroma for biologic or iatrogenic reasons poses a formidable challenge, and honesty forces one to acknowledge that one cannot identify the mechanism in many instances. Nevertheless, a few points help the observer reach a well-reasoned conclusion (Box 5-1).

First, spontaneous mucin extravasation occurs much more frequently than artifactual extravasation, so pathologists should generally favor the notion that the presence of stromal mucin represents a biologic phenomenon. Second, one should regard stromal mucin as artifactual only when the clinical details

of the case suggest the occurrence of trauma or unusual amounts of manipulation of the tissue. Furthermore, the mechanical forces that lead to artifactual mucin extrusion usually cause other changes. In the setting of a radiologically guided excision, for example, one might observe focal hemorrhage, acute inflammation, or disruption of the integrity of the tissue in the region of the stromal mucin. The presence of marked cautery effect or substantial tissue compression would support the idea that mucin extruded from the ducts during surgery rather than before.

Third, genuine mucin extravasation tends to create space-occupying, round or oval pools, which can displace normal structures. At the edges, bundles of collagen or blood vessels project into the mucin and give the stroma a frayed look (Fig. 5-16). Traumatically extruded mucin, in contrast, often separates collagen bundles and other parenchymal components cleanly. As it flows through the tissue, the mucin sometimes molds around the glandular structures (Figs. 5-17 and 5-18). Fourth, in a minority

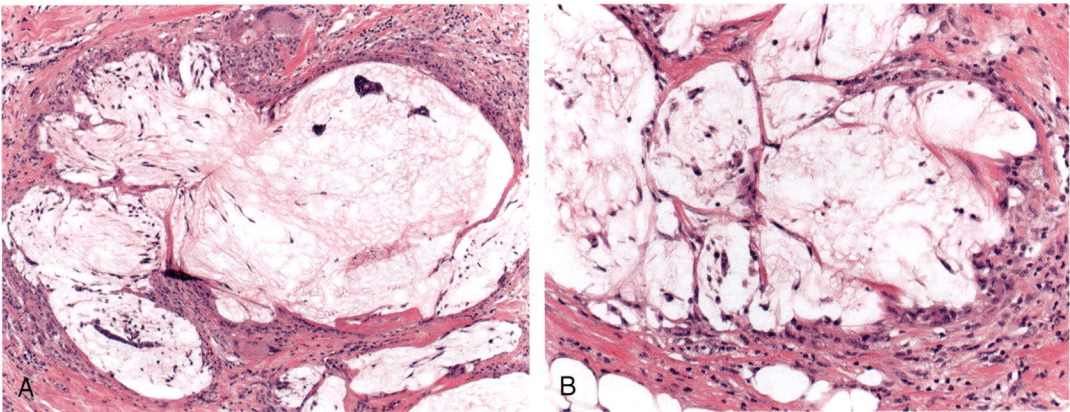

Figure 5-16 A, The pools of stromal mucin produced by invasive mucinous carcinoma have globular shapes and frayed edges. **B,** The mucin at the edge of the pools separates the collagen bundles.

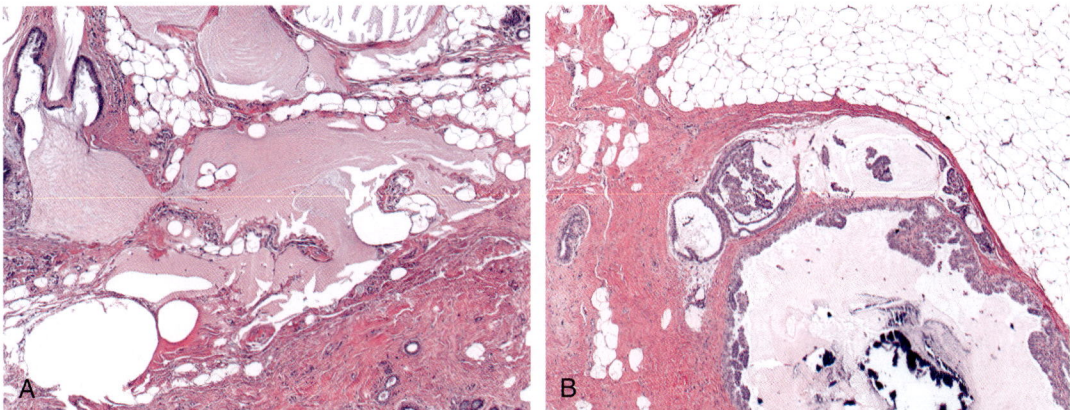

Figure 5-17 A, Trauma during the wire localization of this lesion caused mucin to extrude from the duct and to dissect through the stroma in a linear distribution. **B,** A core biopsy performed prior to this excision pushed mucin into the stroma. It spread along the perimeter of the distended duct.

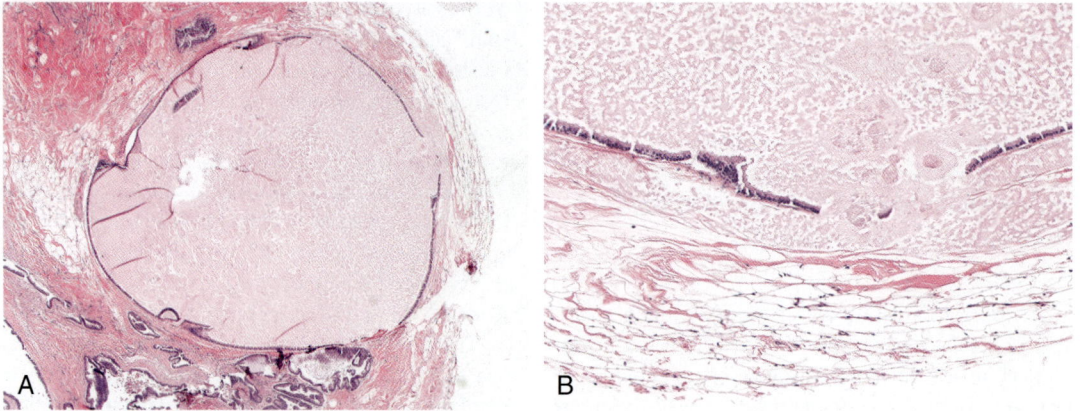

Figure 5-18 A, Manipulation during the excision disrupted this mucin-filled duct. **B,** One can see the tear in the wall and the spread of mucin along the wall of the distended duct.

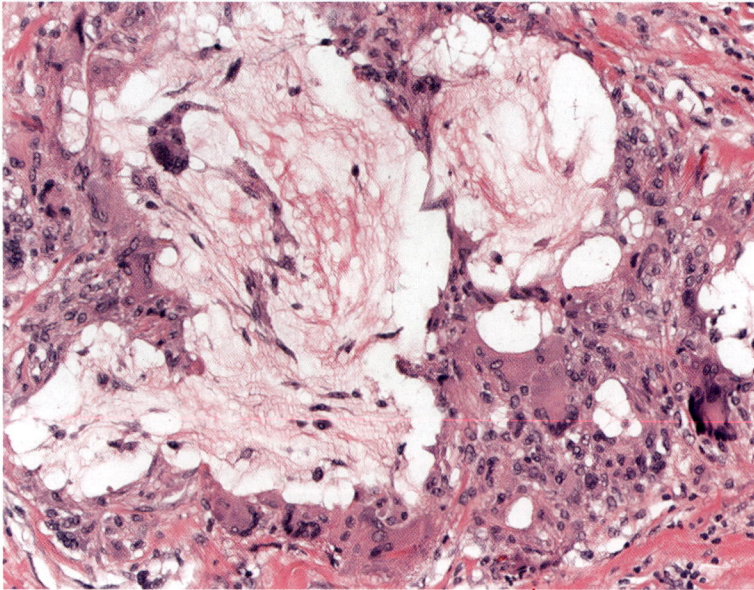

Figure 5-19 The presence of lymphocytes, histiocytes, and giant cells associated with mucin would not fit with the notion of artifactual displacement.

of examples, the mucin incites an inflammatory reaction. If one observes chronic inflammatory cells, especially foreign body giant cells, associated with the mucin or capillaries within it, then one can reasonably conclude that the mucin has occupied the stroma for several days (Fig. 5-19). Fifth, the presence of large calcifications in the mucin would probably argue against the idea of artifactual mucin displacement (Fig. 5-20).

The mere detection of mucin in the stroma does not establish the diagnosis of invasive mucinous carcinoma. To make that interpretation, one must observe malignant cells in the mucin. Certain invasive mucinous carcinomas consist almost entirely of mucin, and it can require an intensive search to discover the rare carcinoma cells in these poorly

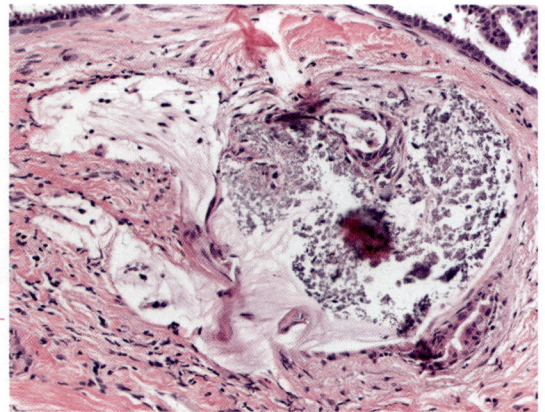

Figure 5-20 The calcifications in this pool of mucin suggest that its presence in the stroma does not represent an artifact.

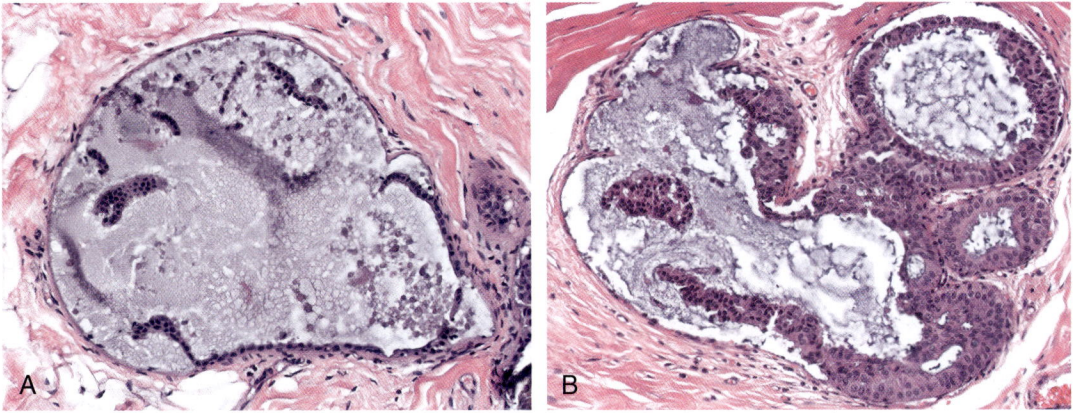

Figure 5-21 A and **B,** Rough handling of the specimen dislodged strips of epithelium from the walls of these ducts.

Box 5-2

Features of displaced epithelium:

- Arrangement of cells in a flat sheet
- Folding or crumpling of the cell clusters
- Presence of crushed cells
- Presence of myoepithelial cells

---

cellular and richly mucinous carcinomas. Because of this phenomenon, the discovery of extravasated mucin should prompt a search for cells within it, especially if atypical cells line the mucin-filled glands. This search sometimes entails submitting many tissue blocks and examining many sections.

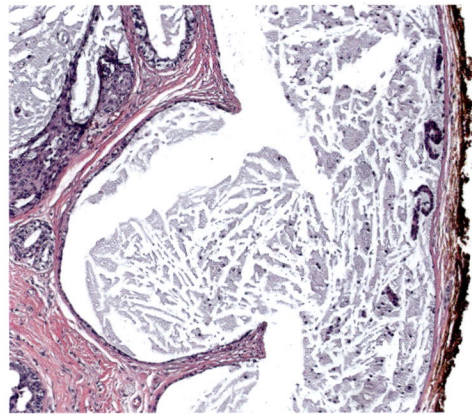

Figure 5-22 Traumatic disruption of the gland led to extravasation of mucin and strips of epithelium.

The Nature of the Cells within the Mucin

Having discovered ductal cells floating in the mucin, one must evaluate both the mechanism by which the cells arrived in the mucin and the nature of the cells. Just as mechanical forces can extrude mucin into the stroma, so, too, can they disrupt the integrity of the epithelium lining the mucin-filled glands. Benign ductal cells, atypical ductal cells, and ductal carcinoma in situ cells can all fall off the basement membrane and collect in the mucin within the glandular lumen. Fragmentation of the epithelium can occur without disrupting the integrity of the gland (Fig. 5-21), and it can accompany the artifactual displacement of mucin into the stroma (Fig. 5-22). If the structure of the gland remains intact, its smooth, rounded shape and sharply defined, smooth border allow one to see that the cells and the mucin occupy a distended duct rather than the stroma. Whether within an intact duct or within mucin displaced into the stroma, the detached epithelial cells usually remain as short, sometimes crumpled, single-layered sheets, poorly preserved small groups, or individual cells (Fig. 5-23). These

formations differ from the three-dimensional clusters and intact small glands formed by invasive mucinous carcinoma (Fig. 5-24). If the intact epithelium grew in a crowded or stratified sheet, the dislodged epithelial strips will appear disorderly, jumbled, and multi-layered (Fig. 5-25). A few myoepithelial cells typically remain attached to the detached luminal cells, and one can highlight their presence using immunohistochemical stains. Pathologists will find this maneuver especially helpful when studying complex epithelial aggregates (Fig. 5-26; Box 5-2).

If one concludes that trauma accounts for the collections of mucin and epithelial cells in the stroma, one can safely overlook them and base the diagnosis of the lesion on the characteristics of the cells within the ducts and lobules. If the cellular groups do not exhibit the characteristics of dislodged epithelium, however, one must consider the diagnosis of invasive mucinous carcinoma. To establish that diagnosis, one must examine the cytologic properties of the suspect cells. They should appear well preserved and intact, and they must exhibit cytologic atypia. The cells of

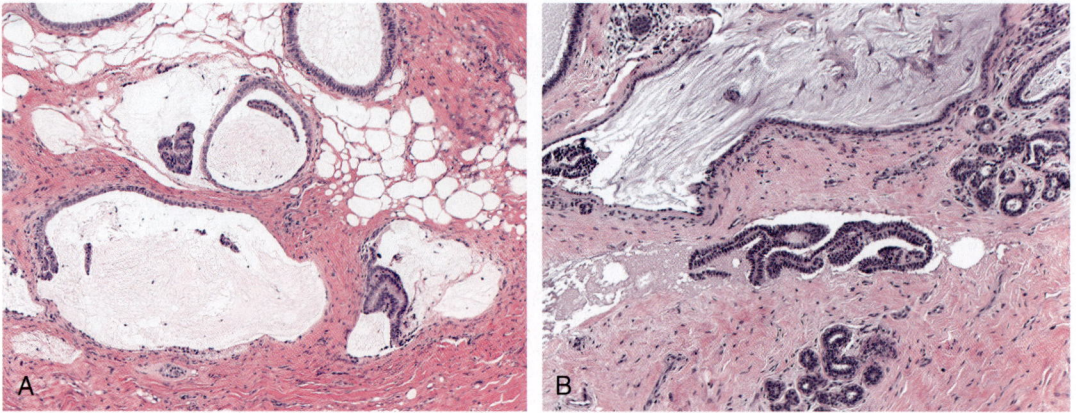

Figure 5-23 A to **C,** Fragments of epithelium dislodged from the walls of the ducts and pushed into the stroma consist of single-layered sheets, crumpled clusters, and a few single cells.

Artifacts

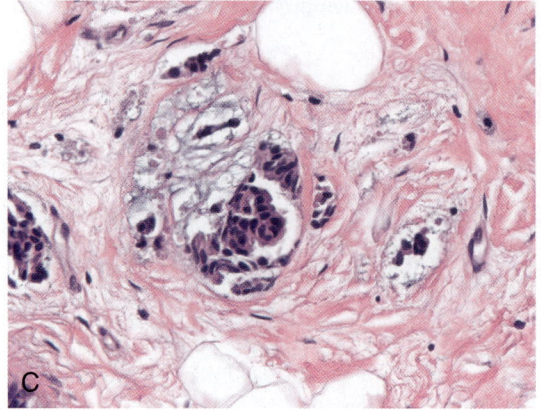

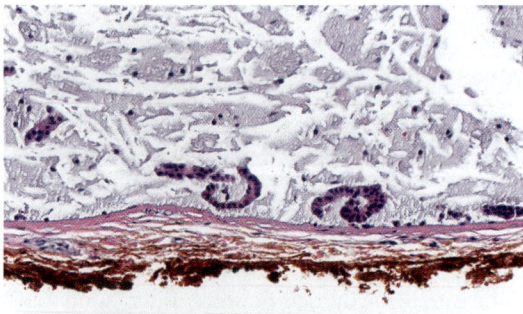

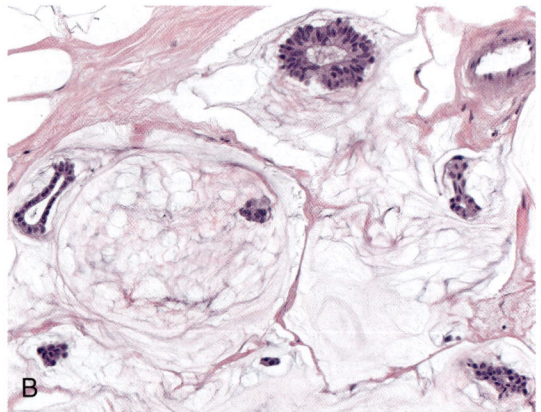

Figure 5-24 The dislodged epithelium shown in **A** does not form the three-dimensional clusters seen in genuine invasive mucinous carcinoma shown in **B.**

invasive mucinous carcinomas usually appear small and possess slightly enlarged nuclei with fine, dark chromatin, and eosinophilic cytoplasm; sometimes, the cytoplasm of a few cells contains small vacuoles. Less common mucinous carcinomas consist of large cells exhibiting marked atypia (Fig. 5-27). The malignant cells can grow in small compact nests, clusters that resemble the papillary formations produced by certain carcinomas growing in body fluids, or loose, dishesive aggregates (Fig. 5-28). The cells display their polarized state by creating glands in the interior of the nests (Fig. 5-29) or forming apical cytoplasmic compartment in the cells at the edges of the groups. Findings such as these favor the diagnosis of invasive

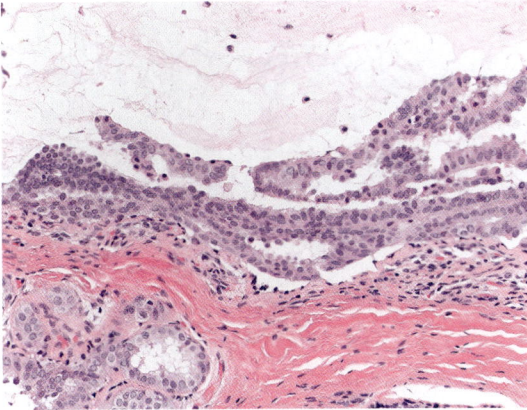

Figure 5-25 Dislodgement of cells growing in complex patterns produces jumbled fragments.

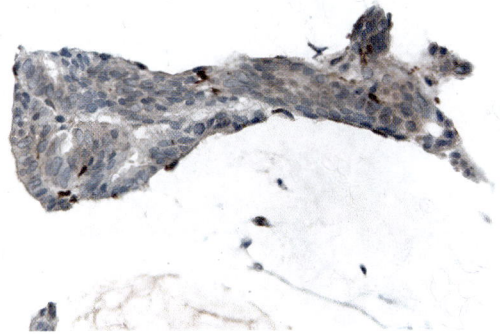

Figure 5-26 Dislodged epithelial fragments usually include a few myoepithelial cells, which one can detect using a stain for p63 protein.

Figure 5-27 A, The cells of invasive mucinous carcinoma typically appear small and possess dark nuclei and eosinophilic cytoplasm. **B,** But occasional examples consist of large cells with marked cytologic atypia.

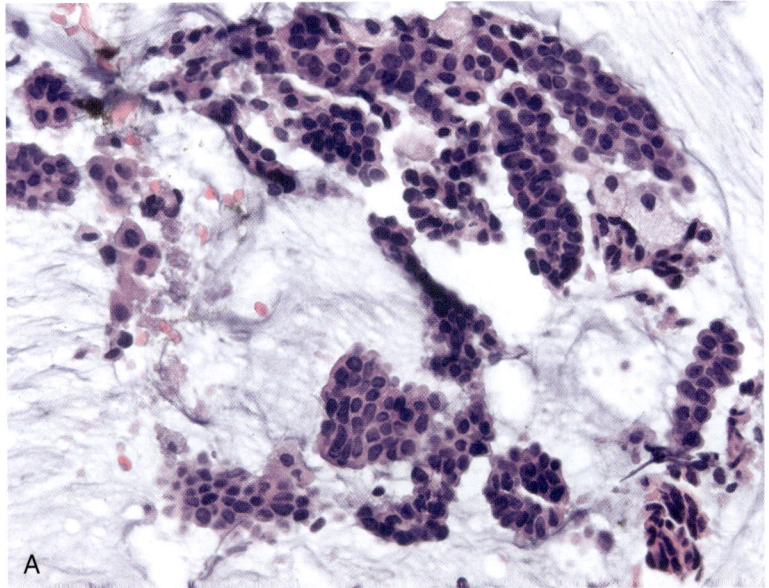

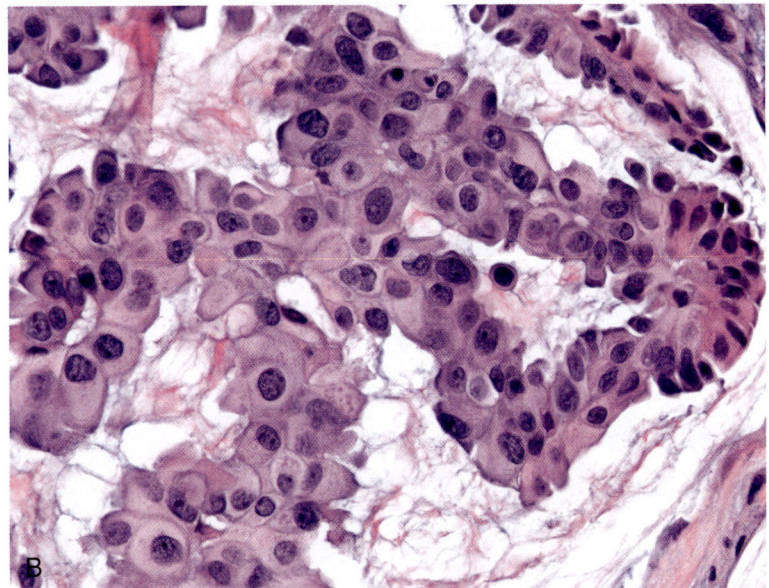

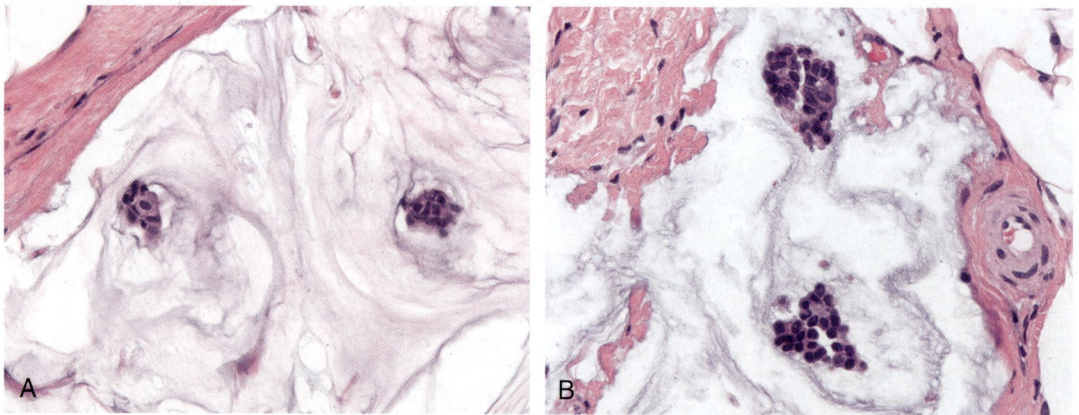

Figure 5-28 A, The clusters of invasive mucinous carcinoma often have a compact, three-dimensional appearance. **B,** But certain groups appear slightly dishesive.

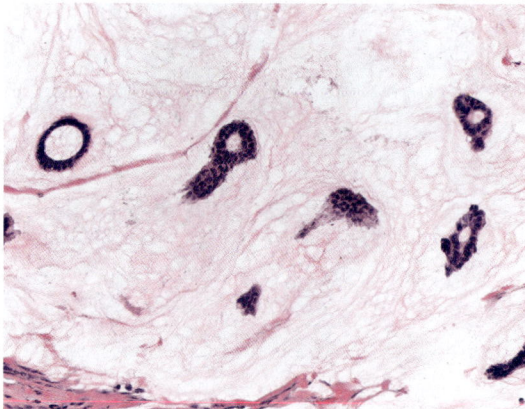

Figure 5-29 The cells in the center of these clusters form cribriform spaces.

mucinous carcinoma rather than dislodged epithelium and mucin, especially in the presence of nearby ductal carcinoma in situ with abundant mucin (Fig. 5-30).

Finally, extruded mucin can surround benign acini and those harboring carcinoma in situ. The smooth contour of the entrapped glands, the presence of a basement membrane and myoepithelial cells, and, in certain cases, the cellular properties distinguish the latter situation from invasive mucinous carcinoma (Fig. 5-31).

The Significance of Malignant Cells and Mucin in the Stroma

One might think that observing pools of mucin and malignant cells in the stroma and mucinous

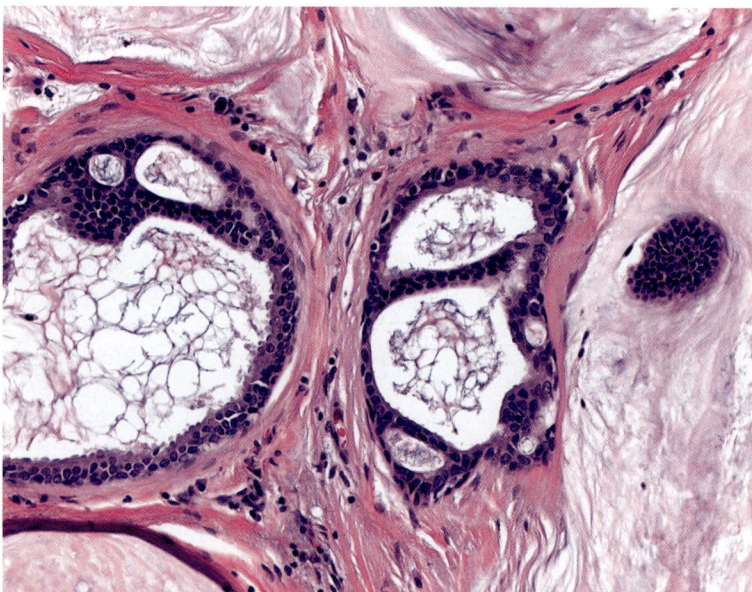

Figure 5-30 The presence of ductal carcinoma in situ with abundant mucin *(left)* should lead one to suspect that the cluster of atypical cells in extravasated mucin *(right)* represents invasive mucinous carcinoma.

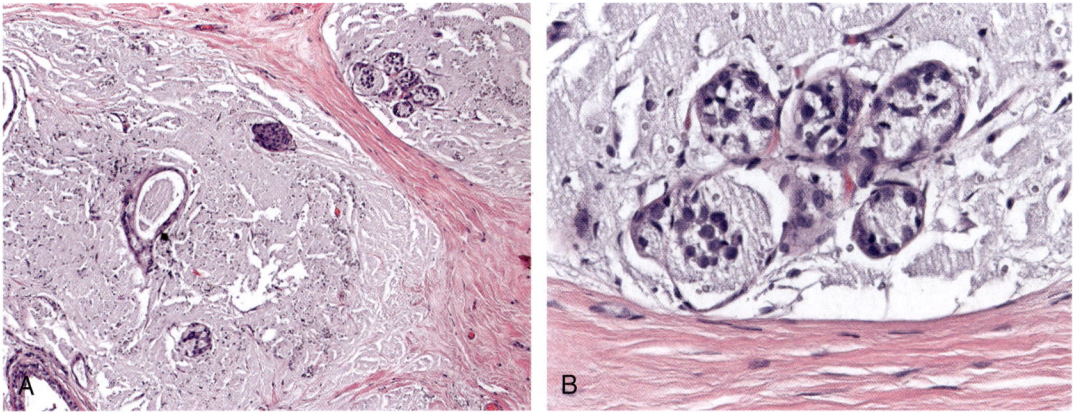

Figure 5-31 A and **B,** Extravasated mucin surrounds a few glands harboring neoplastic lobular cells. **C,** A stain for calponin confirms the noninvasive nature of the cells.

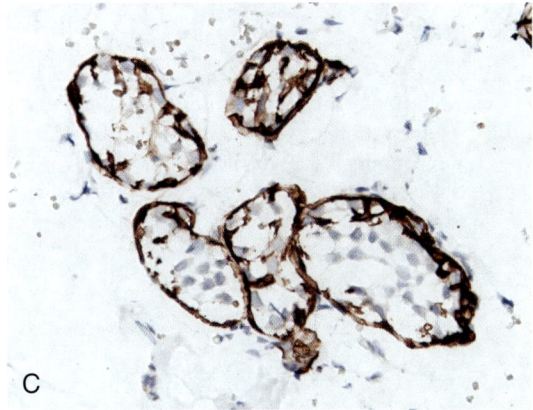

carcinoma in situ in the nearby glands would establish the diagnosis of invasive mucinous carcinoma without controversy, but pathologists disagree about this thinking when the extent of the apparent invasion seems limited (Fig. 5-32). These observers do not object to the diagnosis of invasion because they believe that microinvasive foci do not have clinical relevance. Instead, they believe that these small regions arise from spontaneous rupture of the duct by physical forces rather than from penetration of the duct wall by the tumor cells. According to this line of reasoning, genuine invasion represents an

Figure 5-32 Rupture of the duct allowed mucin and malignant cells to escape into the stroma.

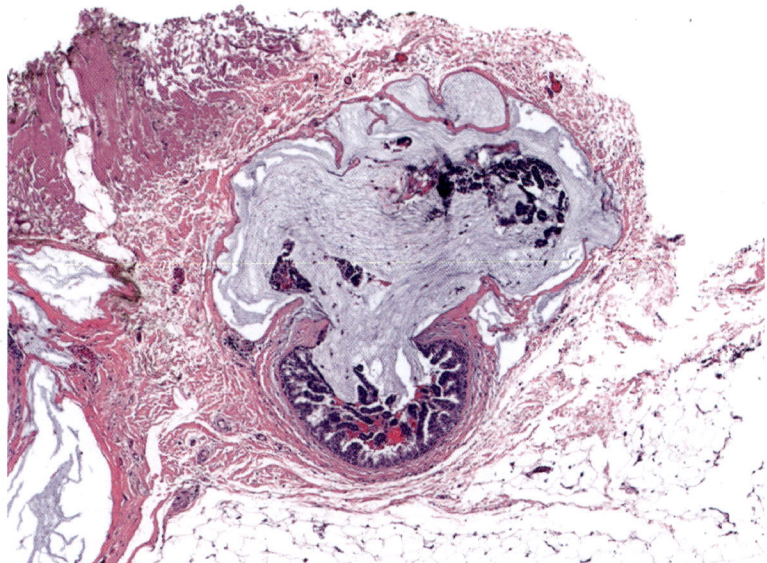

active process carried out, at least in part, by the carcinoma; the passive transport of cells through a tear in the duct wall would not qualify as invasion. Although potentially biologically sound, this reasoning seems hard to apply in practice. After all, on what basis can one determine the mechanism underlying the rupture of a duct harboring ductal carcinoma in situ? Furthermore, once liberated into the stroma by any mechanism, can the carcinoma cells not continue to proliferate? Have they not then become invasive carcinoma, for all practical purposes? Without meaning to diminish the significance of these observers' reservations, the author sets them aside and classifies such foci as invasive.

Selected Readings

Fisher CJ, Millis RR: A mucocele-like tumour of the breast associated with both atypical ductal hyperplasia and mucoid carcinoma. Histopathology 1992;23:69-71.

Fisher ER, Palekar AS, Stoner F, et al: Mucocele-like lesions and mucinous carcinoma of the breast. Int J Surg Pathol 1994;1:213-220.

Hamele-Bena D, Cranor ML, Rosen PP: Mammary mucocele-like lesions (MLL): Benign and malignant. Am J Surg Pathol 1996;20:1081-1085.

Komaki K, Sakamoto G, Sugano H, et al: The morphologic feature of mucinous leakage appearing in low papillary carcinoma of the breast. Hum Pathol 1991; 22:231-236.

Kulka J, Davies JD: Mucocele-like tumours: More associations and possible ductal carcinoma in situ? Histopathology 1993;22:511-512.

Ro JY, Sneige N, Sahin AA, et al: Mucocele-like tumor of the breast associated with atypical ductal hyperplasia or mucinous carcinoma: A clinicopathologic study of seven cases. Arch Pathol Lab Med 1991;115:137-140.

Rosen PP: Mucocele-like tumors of the breast. Am J Surg Pathol 1986;10:464-469.

Weaver MG, Abdul-Karim FW, Al-Kaisi N: Mucinous lesions of the breast: A pathological continuum. Pathol Res Pract 1993;189:873-876.

6

Lobular Proliferations

BASIC CONCEPTS

The morphologic characteristics of lobular neoplasia spring from the same five fundamental cellular properties that give rise to the characteristics of ductal epithelial lesions: cellular proliferation, intercellular cohesion, cellular polarization, cytologic atypia, and architectural atypia. The contributions made by each of these phenomena differ, and this unique mix of properties accounts for the distinctive morphologic attributes of lobular neoplasia. Because the discussion in Chapter 2 has already analyzed many aspects of these basic properties, the following comments highlight only points pertinent to the understanding of lobular proliferations.

Cellular Proliferation

The recognition of the presence of cellular proliferation in lobular neoplasia does not usually pose problems. Accumulation of the cells leads to thickening of the

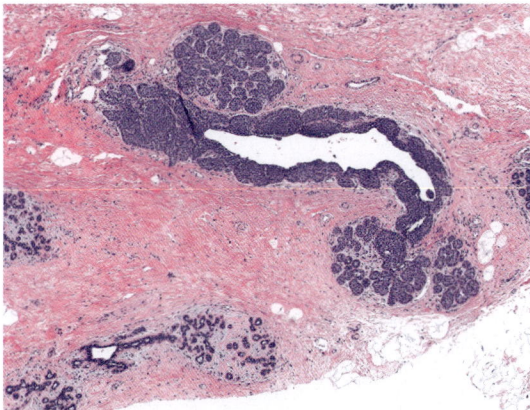

Figure 6-1 Proliferation of the neoplastic lobular cells thickens the epithelium, fills the lumens of acini, and distends small ducts and terminal duct–lobular units.

epithelium, filling of glandular lumens, and, ultimately, distention of ducts and terminal duct–lobular units, findings that stand out at low magnification (Fig. 6-1). One can easily overlook foci of minimal proliferation, of course, and off-center planes of sections can create the appearance of cellular stratification where none exists; however, these difficulties notwithstanding, the recognition of the presence of a proliferative population usually proceeds without difficulty.

Intercellular Cohesion

A lack of intercellular cohesion represents one of the defining characteristics of lobular neoplasia. Writings about this subject often use the term *loosely cohesive* to describe this property of neoplastic lobular cells. Although not, strictly speaking, inaccurate, this usage seems flawed for two reasons. First, it emphasizes the ability of the cells to stick together, when in fact their lack of cohesion represents the definitive attribute. Second, describing the cells of lobular neoplasia as "loosely cohesive" could create the impression that they stick together slightly more than ductal carcinoma cells, which pathologists often describe as dishesive. In reality, the opposite holds true (Fig. 6-2). Neoplastic lobular cells exhibit lower levels of intercellular cohesion, and this property distinguishes them from all other types of proliferative epithelial cells. One recognizes this phenomenon from the presence of gaps between cells (Fig. 6-3). These spaces often appear most obvious in the center of the cellular aggregates. Although the cells of lobular neoplasia always lack cohesion, the extent of cellular separation evident in tissue section varies. Certain examples display only the slightest separation of cells, and uncommon cases do not show any (Fig. 6-4). One must take care to distinguish artifactual disruption of the cells from the genuine lack of cohesion. Rough handling of a tissue specimen, for example,

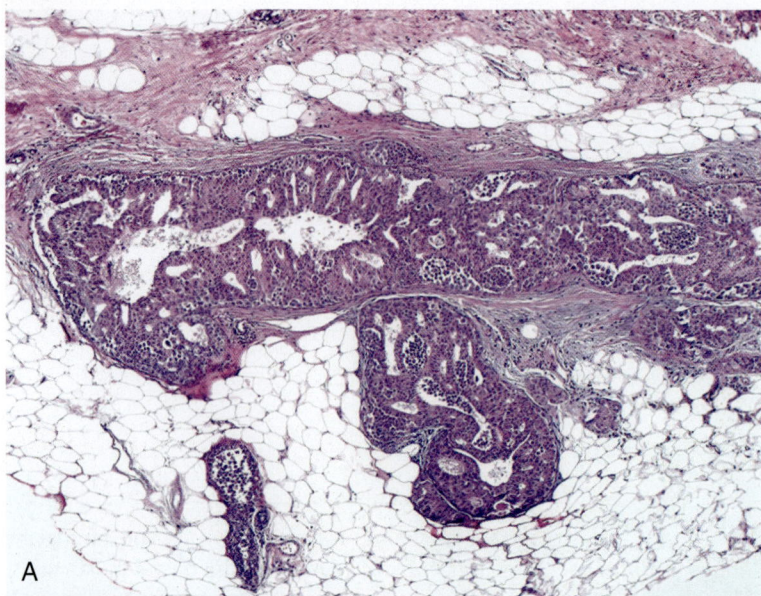

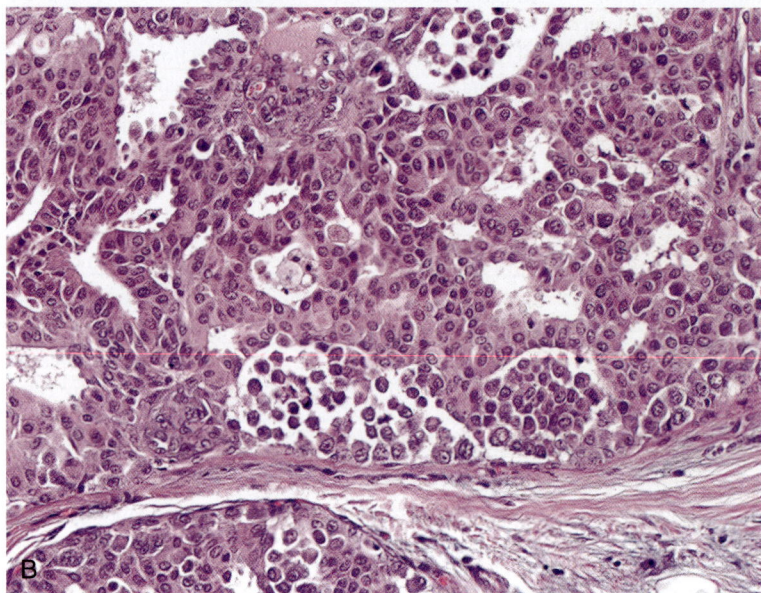

Figure 6-2 A, Lobular carcinoma in situ collides with ductal carcinoma in situ. **B,** The lobular carcinoma cells do not stick together as much as the ductal carcinoma cells do.

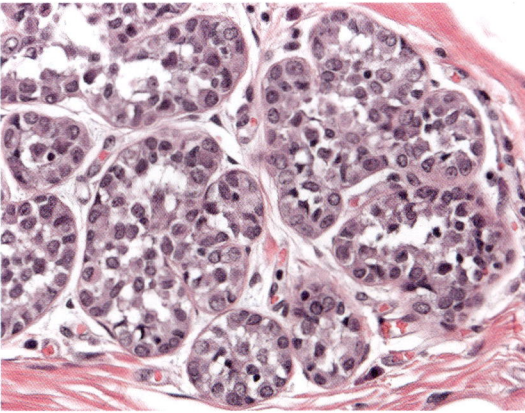

Figure 6-3 The small gaps between the lobular carcinoma cells attest to their dishesive properties.

can make cohesive cells look dishesive, and so can autolysis and cauterization (Fig. 6-5).

Cellular Polarization

The absence of cellular polarity stands as the second fundamental characteristic of lobular neoplasia. In contrast to the columnar shape and eccentric nuclear placement seen in many low-grade ductal carcinoma cells, the cells of lobular neoplasia have round or globular shapes, and the nucleus typically sits near the center of a cell unless displaced by a vacuole or distorted by external forces (Fig. 6-6). The lack of polarization does not differentiate lobular cells from other types of proliferative epithelial cells; hyperplastic ductal cells lack polarity, and so can the cells of high-grade ductal carcinoma.

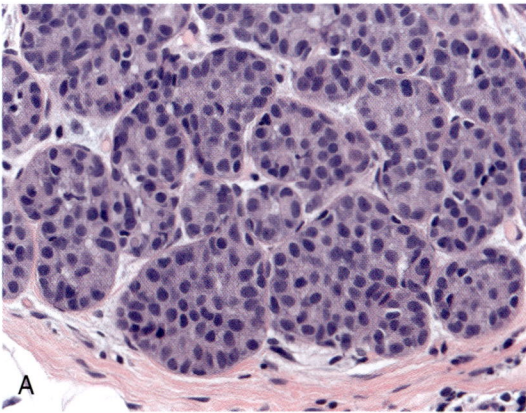

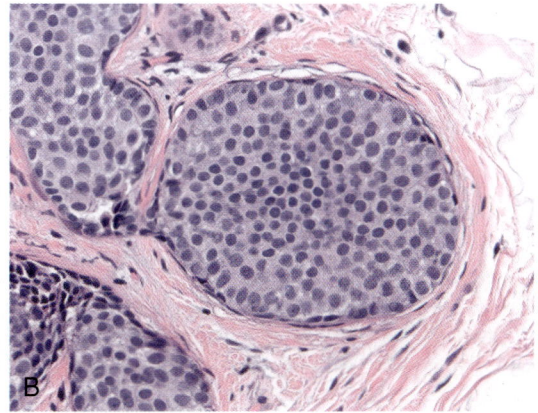

Figure 6-4 The lobular carcinoma cells in **A** show only slight dishesion, and those in **B** virtually none at all.

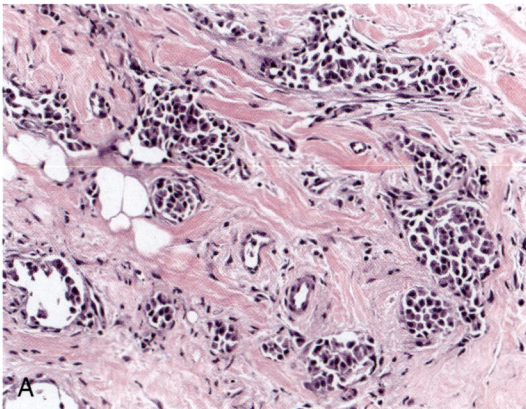

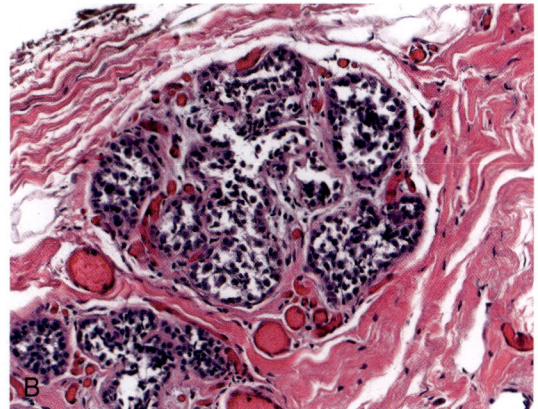

Figure 6-5 Artifacts can make cohesive cells look dishesive. Someone handled the invasive ductal carcinoma in **A** roughly, and someone else compressed the normal lobule at the edge of the specimen in **B.**

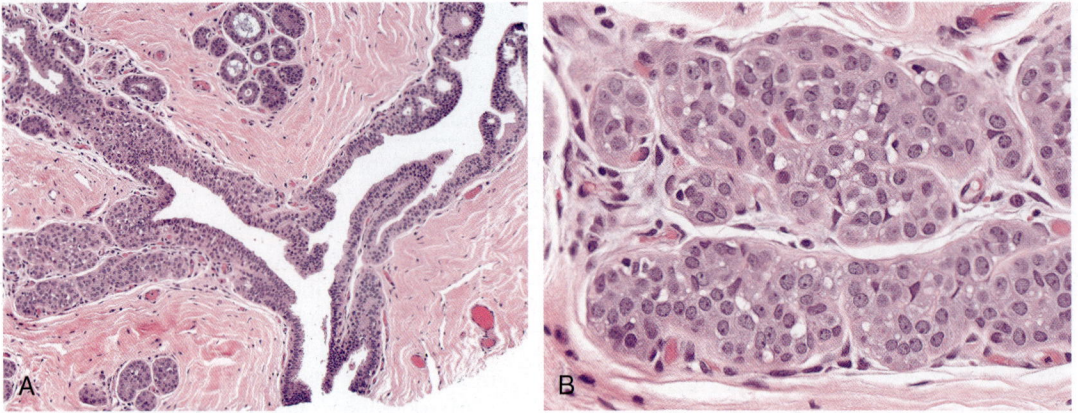

Figure 6-6 A, The juxtaposition of lobular carcinoma in situ and ductal carcinoma in situ in this duct allows one to contrast the nonpolarized lobular carcinoma cells in **B** with their polarized ductal counterparts in **C.**

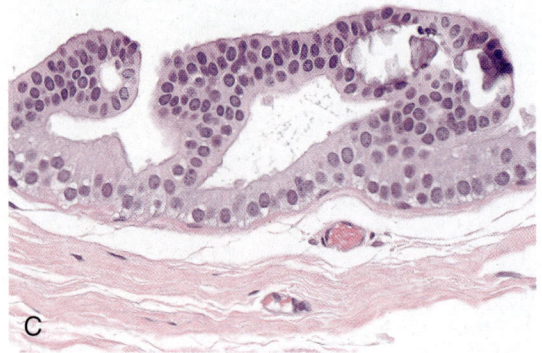

Cytologic Atypia

Cytologic atypia constitutes the third defining feature of lobular neoplasia. As observed with ductal carcinomas, the level of cytologic atypia varies from case to case. Classic cases consist of cells with enlarged nuclei, finely dispersed chromatin, inconspicuous nucleoli, and a slight increase in the amount of cytoplasm, features that one would classify as low-grade atypia; however, the cells in less common examples appear markedly anaplastic (Fig. 6-7).

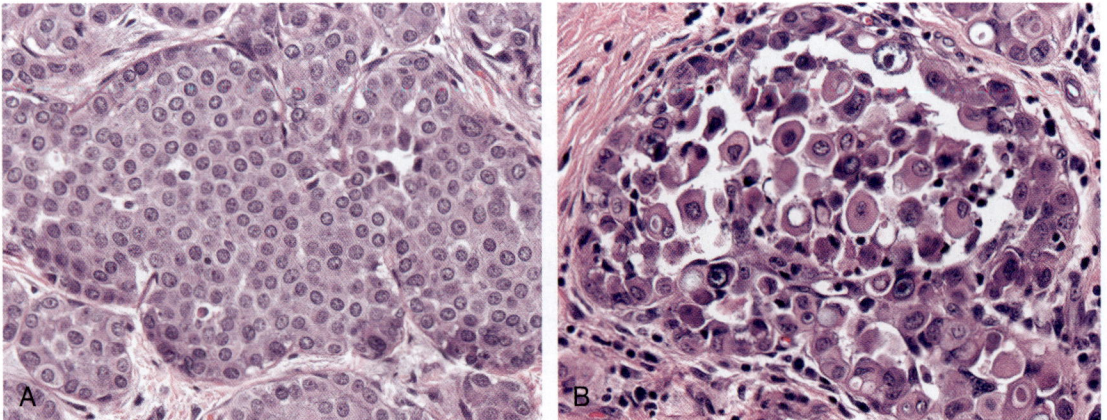

Figure 6-7 The cytologic atypia of neoplastic lobular cells varies from low grade as seen, in **A** to high grade, shown in **B.**

Architectural Atypia

Stratification of cells represents the only manifestation of architectural atypia seen in lobular neoplasia. Because the cells individually lack polarization, they collectively cannot form the architectural patterns that rest on this property: cribriform spaces, trabecular bars, and Roman bridges. Instead, the cells always grow as a dishesive sheet. Uncommon forms of growth can produce patterns that simulate those of architectural atypia, but the presence of genuine cribriform spaces, their variants, or micropapillary structures excludes the diagnosis of lobular neoplasia.

DEFINITIONS AND CLINICOPATHOLOGIC CHARACTERISTICS

Many pathologists separate noninvasive proliferations of neoplastic lobular cells into two categories, *atypical lobular hyperplasia* and *lobular carcinoma in situ*. The cells in the two categories exhibit identical morphologic characteristics; only the quantity of the cells differentiates the two lesions. For this reason and others, certain writers advocate using the all-encompassing term *lobular neoplasia* to refer to both forms of atypical lobular proliferation. This approach seems well suited for discussions of the morphologic characteristics of the two lesions, because descriptions of the cellular characteristics apply equally well to both.

Lobular neoplasia represents a proliferation of atypical, dishesive, and nonpolarized mammary epithelial cells. Pathologists have not pinpointed the cell of origin, but lobular neoplasia would seem to originate from cells basally positioned in the mammary epithelium and distinct from the luminal epithelial cells. Observations of the earliest forms of lobular neoplasia suggest that its precursors reside throughout the mammary glandular tree. Terminal duct–lobular units probably contain many of them, and others probably sit beneath the epithelial cells of ducts. Potential branch points of large ducts seem to represent a favored location for these cells. Wherever they originate, the cells of lobular neoplasia consistently exhibit the following two characteristics: they lack cohesion, and they do not display polarization. These two fundamental properties create the cytologic and architectural attributes that characterize these two lesions.

Most cases of lobular neoplasia occur in women in their later reproductive years. Uncommonly seen in women younger than 40 years, the lesion seems to disappear after menopause. Virtually never does it occur in men.

The typical example does not form a mass, nor do classic cases give rise to calcifications. Thus, lobular neoplasia represents an incidental finding in specimens resected because of an unrelated abnormality.

HISTOLOGIC CHARACTERISTICS

Architectural Characteristics

Box 6-1 summarizes the architectural characteristics of lobular neoplasia.

> **Box 6-1**
>
> Architectural patterns of lobular neoplasia:
>
> - Growth as individual cells and small clusters within benign epithelial cells (*pagetoid involvement*)
> - Growth as structureless sheets

Pattern of Growth

The cells of lobular neoplasia exhibit a consistent and characteristic pattern of growth: the cells in minimal examples proliferate as individuals and small clusters interspersed among preexisting benign cells, and those in well-developed foci form structureless sheets. Typical lobular cells do not give rise to genuine glandular structures. As the cells accumulate, they fill the lumens of the affected acini and ducts, and further expansion of the population leads to distention of the glands. It seems that the acini enlarge to accommodate the expanding mass of neoplastic cells housed within the glands. Therefore, one does not usually observe greatly distended but only partially filled acini or ducts in lobular neoplasia, nor do the cells of lobular neoplasia create lacy festoons, cartwheels, Roman bridges, or micropapillary formations, which occur so commonly in low-grade ductal carcinomas. On the other hand, uncommon ductal carcinomas proliferate solely as sheets of uniform cells, so one cannot regard this solid pattern as a distinctive characteristic of lobular proliferations. Nevertheless, this architectural pattern typifies lobular neoplasia, and deviations from it should make one question the diagnosis.

The appearance of atypical cells as individuals or as groups of two or three along the basement membrane marks the earliest stages of lobular neoplasia (Fig. 6-8). Although certain of the neoplastic cells border the glandular lumen, most sit beneath the luminal cells, sandwiched between them and the basal myoepithelial cells or the basement membrane. This intimate mingling of benign and carcinoma cells

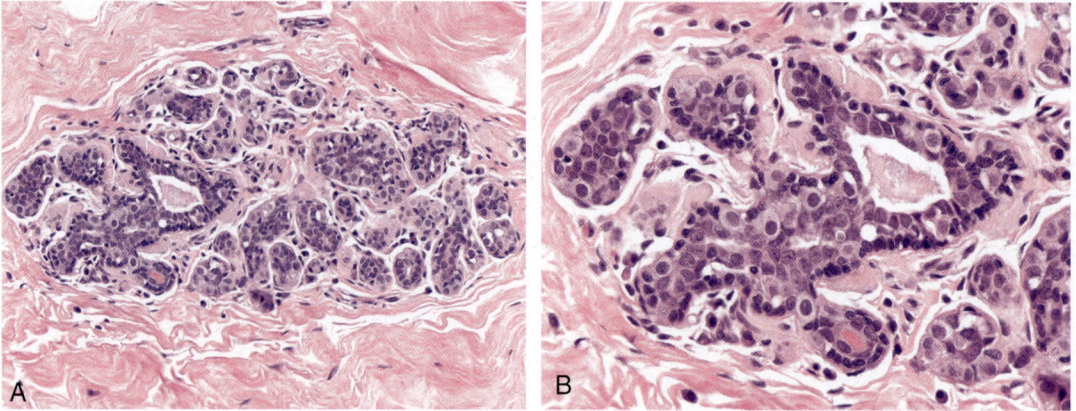

Figure 6-8 A and **B,** In small foci of lobular neoplasia, many of the neoplastic cells sit near the basement membrane. This phenomenon reminded Drs. Foote and Stewart of Paget's disease of the nipple, so they called the pattern *pagetoid.*

does not take place in most carcinomas; malignant cells more commonly grow as a unified mass, which destroys the benign cells rather than coexisting with them. Drs. Foote and Stewart believed that this unusual growth pattern so commonly seen in lobular neoplasia deserves a name. Because it reminded them of the histologic appearance of Paget's disease of the breast, they used the term *pagetoid spread* to refer to it.

The passage of more than half a century has erased the subtlety of histologic study that seems to have underlain the choice of this term. Although terse in their description of the pattern, Drs. Foote and Stewart seemed to use it to describe the growth of scattered individual cells and small clusters within the epithelium. Contemporary pathologists, on the other hand, refer to any pattern in which benign and malignant cells mix as pagetoid spread. Thus, most observers would not hesitate to classify the undermining of luminal cells by a sheet of ductal carcinoma cells, for example, as an example of pagetoid spread. This all-encompassing view of pagetoid spread has robbed the feature of much of its diagnostic significance, for one observes this phenomenon in many examples of ductal carcinomas. In contrast, the pattern of dispersed cells described by Drs. Foote and Stewart, the one most reminiscent of Paget's disease of the breast, occurs in many cases of lobular neoplasia and only rarely in low-grade ductal carcinomas. Thus, the presence of this narrowly defined finding should make one favor the diagnosis of lobular neoplasia. Despite the value of this generalization, pathologists must remember that even when pagetoid spread is defined strictly, its presence does not establish the lobular nature of a malignant population.

In rare cases, the neoplastic lobular cells form spaces of a seemingly glandular nature (Fig. 6-9).

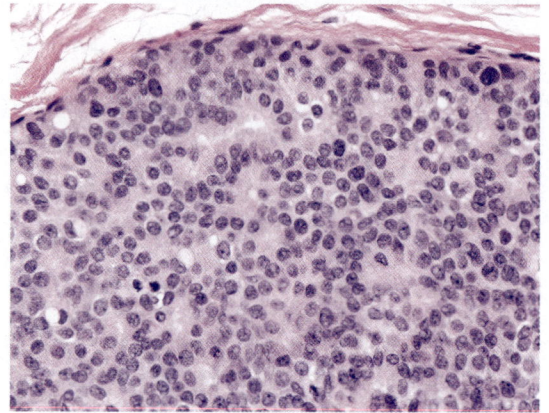

Figure 6-9 The cells in a small region of this case of lobular carcinoma in situ form spaces that look somewhat glandular.

Pathologists disagree about the significance of this finding and the classification of lesions demonstrating these microlumens.

Structural Alterations of Lobules

Growth of lobular neoplasia in terminal duct–lobular units tends to alter the structure of the lobules. These alterations do not spring from fundamental properties of the neoplastic cells, and one can observe the same structural changes in a variety of types of epithelial proliferations. Thus, these structural attributes do not help to determine the nature of the neoplastic population. Recognition of the alterations does further the analysis in a different way, however; it helps buttress one's impression of the presence of an epithelial proliferation. When evaluating lobules that appear only slightly more cellular than expected, one sometimes has trouble deciding whether they harbor an excessive number of epithelial cells.

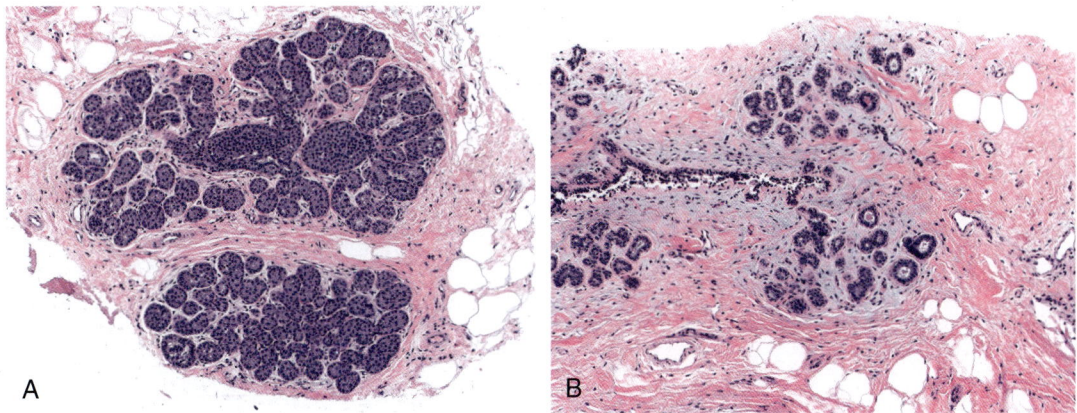

Figure 6-10 Lobular carcinoma in situ has enlarged the terminal ductules and lobules in **A**. Compare them with adjacent, uninvolved cells in **B**.

Recognizing the presence of an expansion of the epithelial population represents the first step in making a confident diagnosis. Attention to the following four generalizations about the structure of lobules involved by lobular neoplasia often enables one to form a secure opinion regarding the presence of an epithelial proliferation:

1. The lobules appear enlarged (Fig. 6-10). The recognition of lobular enlargement proves trickier than one might first assume, because geometric and physiologic variations complicate the analysis. Geometric considerations arise because lobules have dimensions greater than the 4 or 5 μm that encompass the usual histologic sections, which consequently include only a portion of each lobule. If the plane of section does not traverse the center of the lobule, it will appear smaller than its greatest dimension. Furthermore, the likelihood of underestimating the size of a lobule rises as the size of the lobule increases. Physiologic variations also confound the estimation of lobular size, for lobules change in size and complexity as women age. Lobules enlarge and develop more acini during the reproductive years, and most lobules atrophy following menopause; therefore, a lobule of normal size for a woman in her fourth decade might look pathologically enlarged if encountered in a specimen from a postmenopausal woman.

   Neither source of variation prevents the recognition of extreme lobular enlargement, but pathologists find it difficult to detect minor degrees of expansion without reference to a standard. The literature does not contain such a point of reference, so one must turn to the uninvolved lobules in the specimen under study. They exist in the same physiologic state as the suspect lobules, thereby eliminating one source of variation. By scanning 10 or 20 normal lobules, one can estimate the range of their sizes. If the average size of the pathologic lobules exceeds the average size of the uninvolved ones, then one can safely regard the altered lobules as enlarged. This conclusion rests on particularly solid ground if the smallest of the pathologic lobules appears larger than the largest of the uninvolved ones.

2. The acini appear enlarged and vary in size to a greater extent than expected. The estimation of acinar dimension entails the same difficulties as the evaluation of lobular size; once again, coexisting, uninvolved counterparts provide a reliable point of reference. The acini of normal lobules exhibit a narrow range in their dimensions, whereas the diameters of those involved by lobular neoplasia differ by as much as tenfold. The majority of the involved acini appear larger than normal.

3. The number of the acini appears increased and certain of them display unusual shapes. In the most fully developed cases of lobular neoplasia, the involved lobules seem to contain more acini than the uninvolved lobules (Fig. 6-10). Moreover, the altered acini lose their round profiles; they may exhibit irregular or teardrop shapes or configurations that suggest the process of budding (Fig. 6-11).

4. The specialized stroma does not seem to respond to the presence of the neoplastic cells. The enlarging acini seem to crowd out the stromal cells and make them difficult to discern (Fig. 6-12). In occasional examples, the intralobular stroma exhibits reactive, myxoid changes (Fig. 6-13); however, involvement of the lobules by processes other than the lobular neoplasia most often accounts for changes in the specialized stroma.

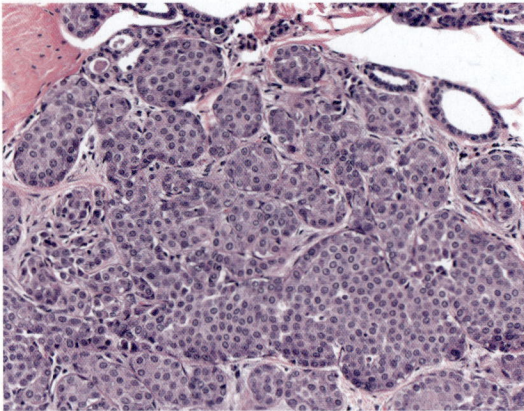

Figure 6-11 Certain of the acini filled and distended by lobular carcinoma cells have irregular shapes.

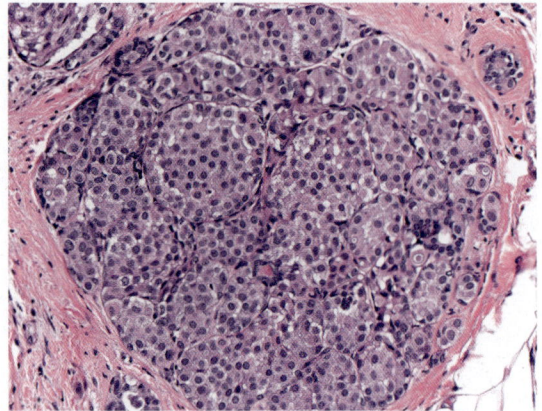

Figure 6-12 The few delicate strands of collagen coursing between distended acini represent the remnants of the specialized stroma.

Structural Alterations of Ducts

Besides altering the structure of terminal duct–lobular units, lobular neoplasia subtly changes the configuration of ducts. Most commonly, the proliferative cells accumulate among the preexisting ones and thicken the epithelium (Fig. 6-14). One can usually appreciate this alteration at even low magnification (Fig. 6-15). The neoplastic cells also accumulate at points of potential branching in ducts of a certain size. These ductal buds consist of evenly spaced, tiny pockets of cells that cause the basement membrane to bulge outward. The simplest of these aggregates consists of just one or two myoepithelial cells, a few basal cells, and an occasional luminal cell, whereas more complex examples contain ductules and acini (Fig. 6-16). The clusters seem to represent sites from which side branches or lobules sprout. When lobular neoplasia involves ducts, the neoplastic cells first become apparent in these clusters (Fig. 6-17). Accumulation from the lobular cells fills and distends the outpouchings, eventually leading to formation of the "cloverleaf" configuration (Fig. 6-18). The least common of these alterations of ductal structure arises when the lobular cells replace the indigenous epithelial cells, fill the lumen, and distend the duct (Fig. 6-19).

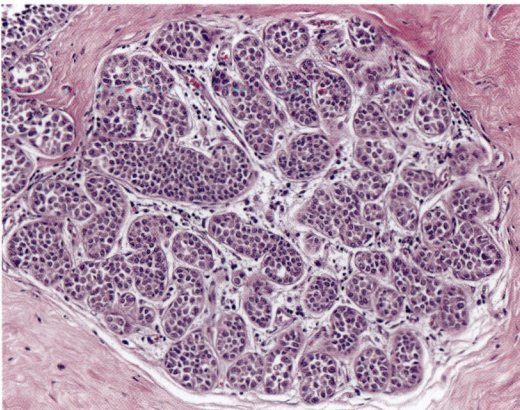

Figure 6-13 The specialized stroma in this lobule involved by lobular neoplasia exhibits a slight myxoid quality.

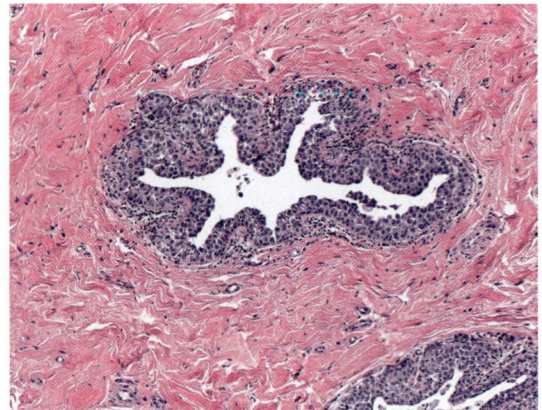

Figure 6-14 Accumulation of neoplastic lobular cells has thickened the epithelium of this large duct.

Figure 6-15 A, Even at scanning magnification, one can appreciate the thickening of the epithelium in the duct to the left of the center, especially when contrasted with the epithelium in the duct to the right of center. **B,** Examination of the involved duct at higher magnification (*left*) and comparison with the uninvolved one (*right*) validates one's initial impression.

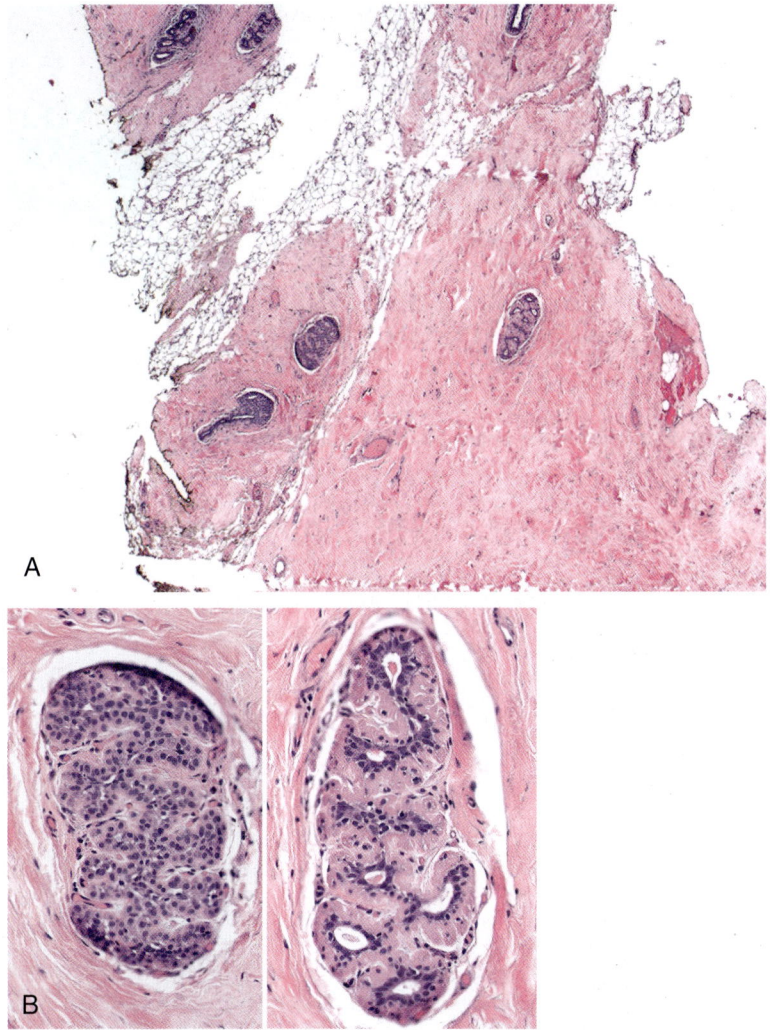

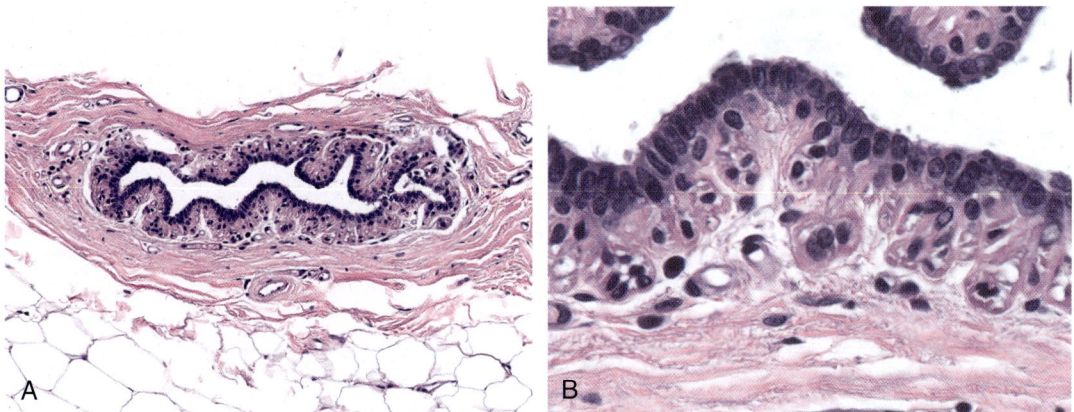

Figure 6-16 A, The epithelium of certain large ducts forms periodically spaced clusters of cells, which probably represent sites of potential branching. **B,** The clusters consist of a few basal epithelial cells enveloped by myoepithelial cells.

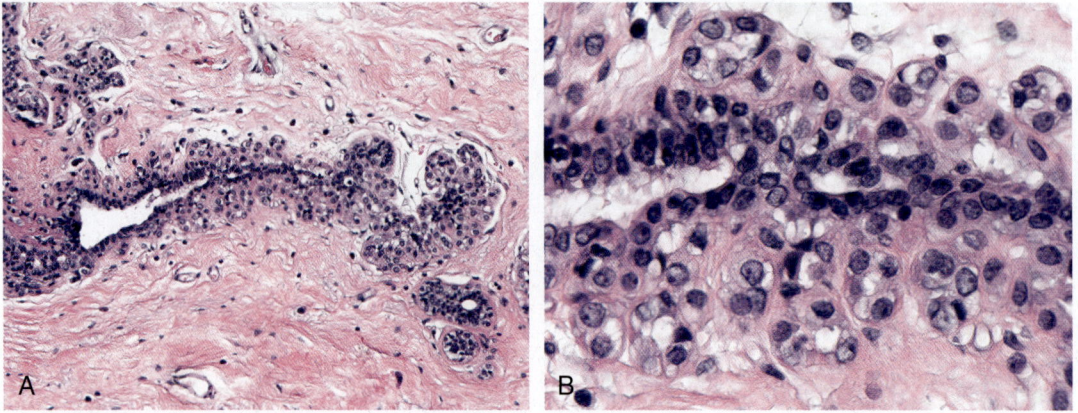

Figure 6-17 When lobular neoplasia involves large ducts in **A**, it seems to begin in the epithelial buds as in **B**.

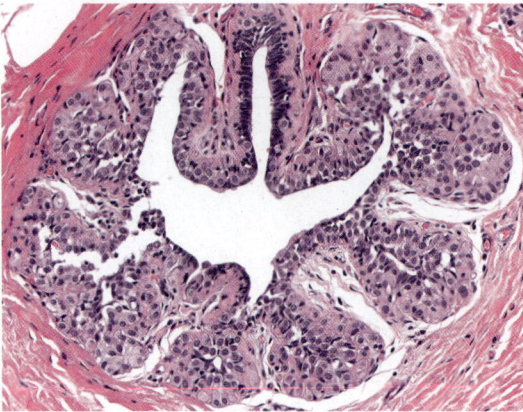

Figure 6-18 Accumulation of neoplastic lobular cells in the walls of large ducts creates the "cloverleaf" pattern.

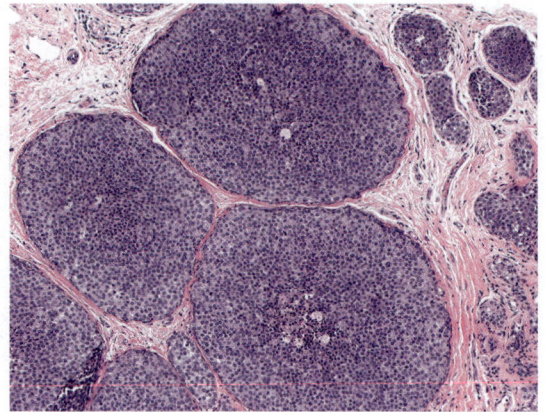

Figure 6-19 Lobular neoplasia can displace the epithelium of large ducts and entirely fill the structures with neoplastic cells.

Cytologic Characteristics

Box 6-2, on page 127, summarizes the cytologic characteristics of lobular neoplasia.

Cellular Properties

With certain exceptions, the cytologic details of lobular neoplasia do not vary much from case to case. Like the cells of most other types of mammary carcinoma, those of lobular neoplasia appear larger than normal epithelial cells. The difference in size stands out clearly in regions of early pagetoid growth, where the benign and malignant cells sit side-by-side (Fig. 6-20). The neoplastic cells enlarge because they contain more cytoplasm and larger nuclei than normal cells. The carcinoma cells have round or oval shapes (Fig. 6-21). The cells along the perimeter of a

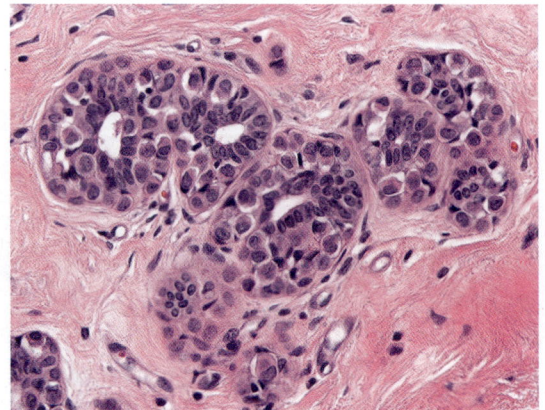

Figure 6-20 Apposition of the neoplastic cells with the normal ones allows one to appreciate the relatively larger size of the former.

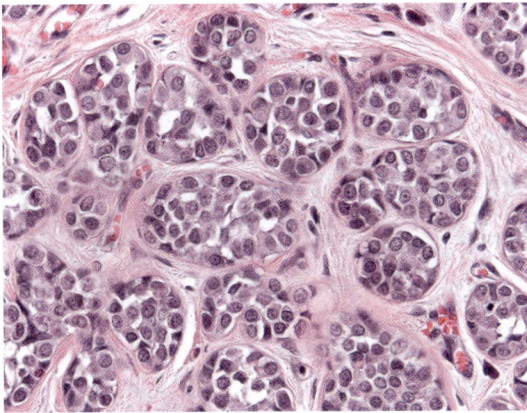

Figure 6-21 Neoplastic lobular cells usually have round or oval shapes.

distended gland occasionally look slightly cuboidal, and their nuclei sit at the bases of the cells (Fig. 6-22). Certain observers claim that this feature should lead one to favor a diagnosis of ductal carcinoma rather than lobular neoplasia, but this author does not hold that view. The occasional formation of cuboidal cells with eccentric nuclei aside, never does one observe well-developed columnar cells with substantial apical cytoplasmic compartments in lobular neoplasia. Because of the dishesive nature of the cells, they often look frayed or slightly disrupted and somewhat disheveled. One has difficulty appreciating the cell membranes, although they sometimes stand out clearly when the cells grow in a closely packed sheet (Fig. 6-23).

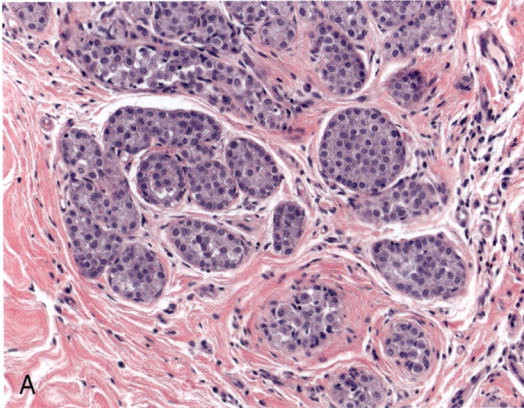

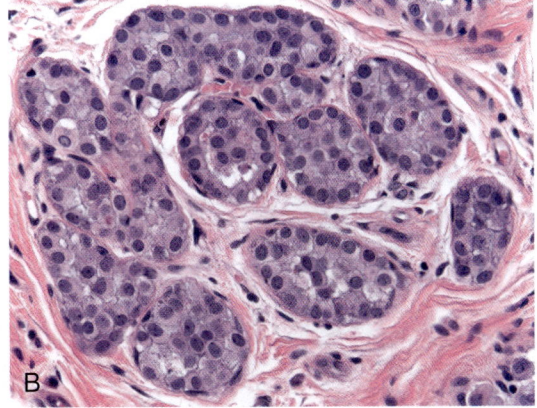

Figure 6-22 A and **B,** The neoplastic lobular cells along the basement membrane sometimes look cuboidal or slightly columnar, and their nuclei have eccentric positions closer to the basement membrane than the lumen.

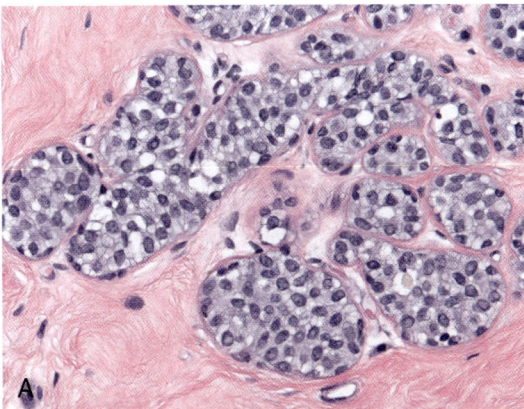

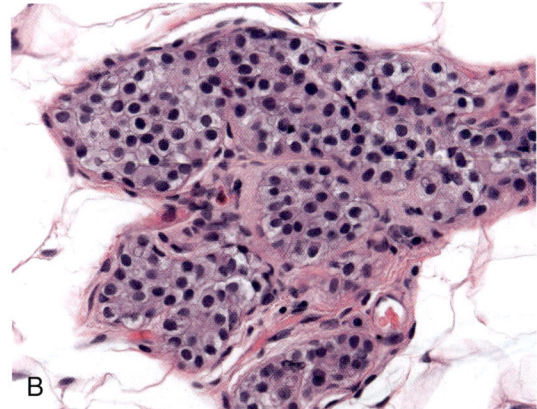

Figure 6-23 A, The cell membranes of neoplastic lobular cells do not usually appear well-defined. **B,** They can stand out clearly when the cells grow closely packed.

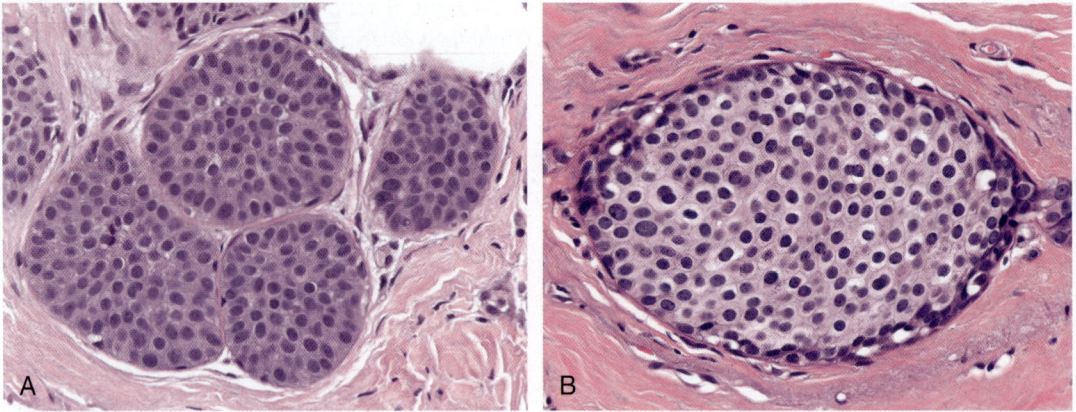

Figure 6-24 The nuclei of lobular carcinoma in situ, shown in **A** can appear identical to those of ductal carcinoma in situ, as seen in **B**.

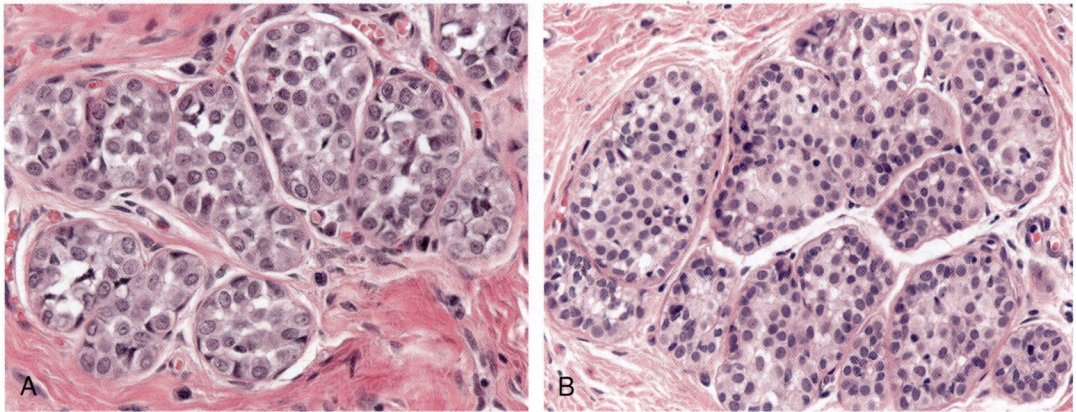

Figure 6-25 A and **B,** The nuclei of lobular neoplasia can vary from one case to the next. The chromatin appears pale and granular in many examples, but others have homogeneous, dark nuclear material.

The nucleus tends to occupy the center of the cell. Both the polygonal shape of the cells and the central location of their nuclei arise because of the lack of cellular polarization. The shapes of the nuclei vary from one case to the next and even from one cell to the next in individual cases. Those of typical cases appear nearly round, whereas less common examples consist of cells with variably shaped nuclei. The nuclei often have slightly irregular contours and exhibit subtle notches and small folds, features that bring to mind the nuclei of hyperplastic ductal cells. In other cases of lobular neoplasia, the nuclei have smooth contours, like the nuclei of low-grade ductal carcinoma (Fig. 6-24). Thus, nuclear characteristics alone cannot differentiate lobular neoplasia from certain other types of epithelial proliferation. The characteristics of the chromatin vary somewhat among cases. The nuclear material usually has a finely granular texture, which imparts a pale appearance to the nuclei, and one can often discern a

tiny nucleolus. In other examples, the chromatin appears homogeneous, finely dispersed, and hyperchromatic, making it impossible to detect nucleoli (Fig. 6-25).

The cytoplasm of neoplastic lobular cells typically appears homogeneous and stains faintly with eosin. Almost all cases contain at least a few cells with mucin in their cytoplasm, and such cells sometimes constitute the dominant population. The mucin forms miniscule droplets, which gives the cytoplasm a frothy quality (Fig. 6-26). Coalescence of these droplets forms large collections of mucin and the creation of signet ring cells (Fig. 6-27).

A few decades ago, a strongly voiced debate concerning the use of *signet ring cell* in lobular neoplasia briefly enlivened the literature. The purists involved in this minor tempest pointed out that many of the cytoplasmic structures that look like large mucin vacuoles instead constitute intracytoplasmic lumens, and these

Figure 6-26 The cytoplasm of neoplastic lobular cells usually appears pale or slightly eosinophilic, and the presence of mucin droplets often creates a slightly frothy quality.

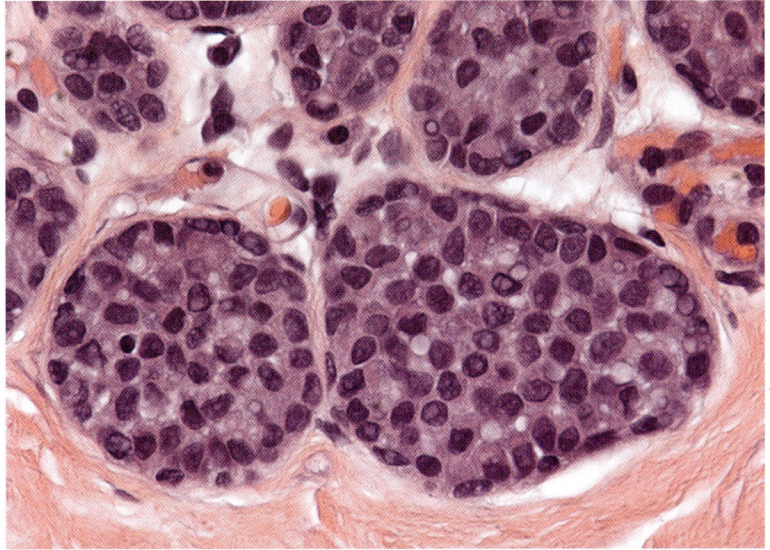

writers insisted that microscopists should reserve the term signet ring cell for those cells containing mucin-filled vacuoles. Because one often cannot distinguish intracytoplasmic lumens from mucin-filled vacuoles without the use of electron microscopy, this distinction seems impractical for everyday use; furthermore, common parlance does usually take its cue from linguistic precision. For better or worse, pathologists have come to regard any cell containing a large cytoplasmic space, and most precisely, a cell in which the space distorts the shape of the nucleus, as a signet ring cell.

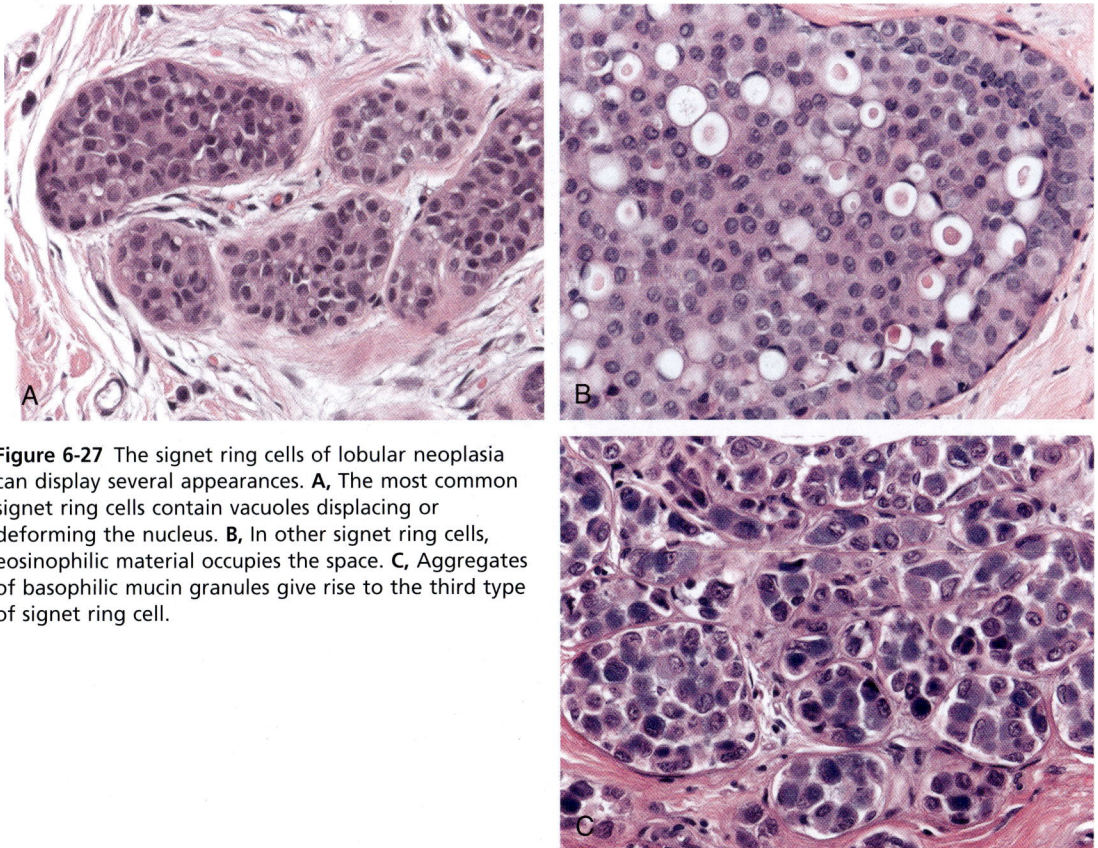

Figure 6-27 The signet ring cells of lobular neoplasia can display several appearances. **A,** The most common signet ring cells contain vacuoles displacing or deforming the nucleus. **B,** In other signet ring cells, eosinophilic material occupies the space. **C,** Aggregates of basophilic mucin granules give rise to the third type of signet ring cell.

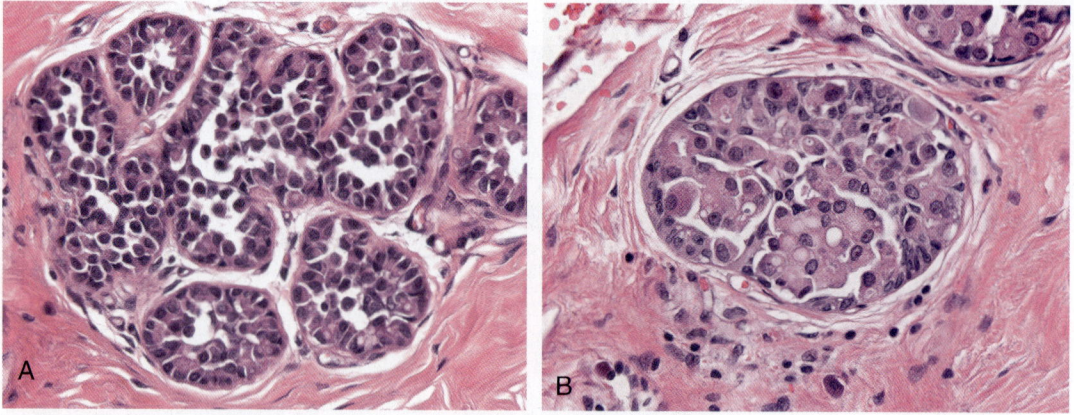

Figure 6-28 A, The dense, eosinophilic color of the cytoplasm and the dark staining of the nuclei give these neoplastic lobular cells a myoid quality. **B,** The abundance of the cytoplasm in these cells suggests apocrine differentiation.

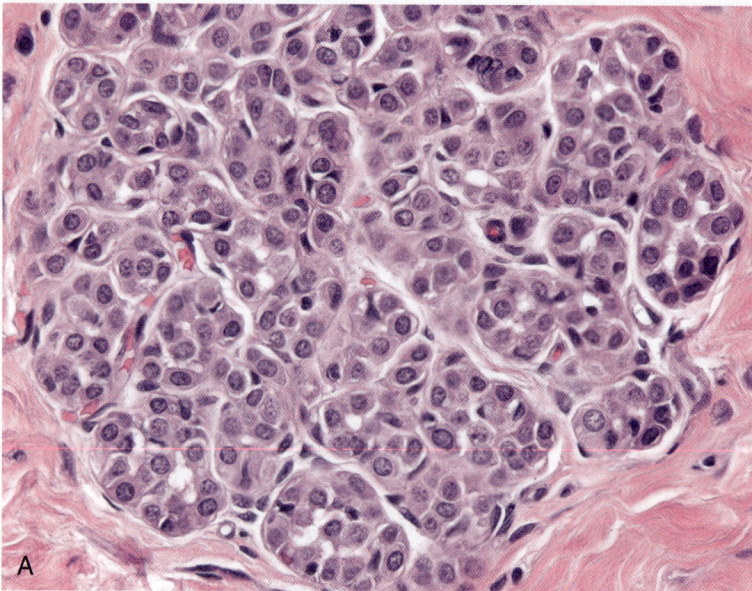

Figure 6-29 A, The type B neoplastic lobular cells appear slightly larger than classic, type A cells, and the former have slightly larger nuclei, more cytoplasm, and more easily seen nucleoli than in the latter.
B, The lobule contains a mixture of type A (*left*) and type B (*right*) carcinoma cells.

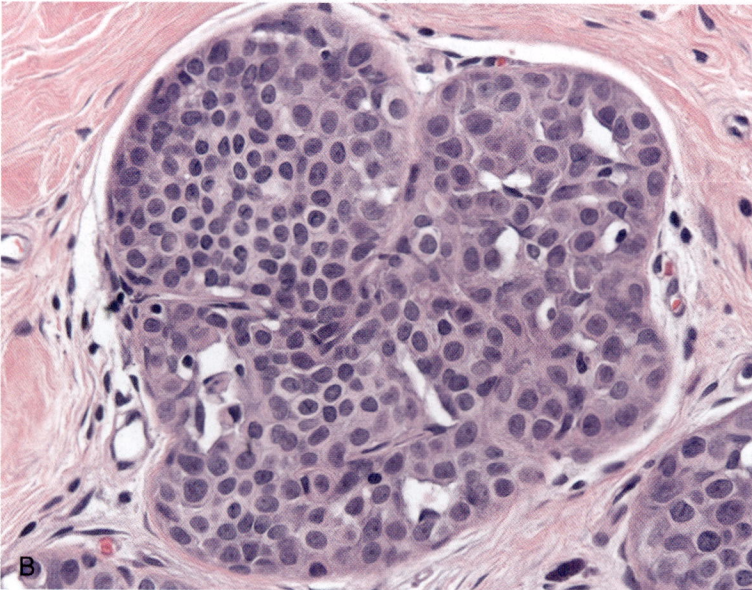

The signet ring cells in lobular neoplasia sometimes contain a blob of eosinophilic material within the vacuole. This *targetoid* pattern occurs much less commonly in ductal carcinomas, so the presence of cells like these should lead one to favor classifying the neoplastic cells as lobular. For the purpose of completeness, one must point out that breast carcinomas can create signet ring cells through yet another mechanism: uniform, minute, basophilic granules of mucin fill the cytoplasm without forming a vacuole (see Fig. 6-27), and they often displace the nucleus to one side of the cell. Signet ring cells of this type do not arise commonly in any type of breast cancer, so one should not regard their presence as a reliable way of subclassifying carcinoma cells.

The cytoplasm can assume other appearances, although it does so only rarely. It can condense and become deeply eosinophilic. If the nuclei also stain darkly, the cells resemble rhabdomyoblasts, so pathologists sometimes refer to this appearance as *myoid* (Fig. 6-28A). The cytoplasm can also become voluminous and eosinophilic, so that the cells resemble apocrine cells (Fig. 6-28B). Finally, unusual cases of lobular neoplasia consist of cells with clear cytoplasm.

When Drs. Foote and Stewart first described lobular carcinoma in situ, they characterized the cells as "surprisingly uniform in size." Later, Dr. Haagensen noted that certain cases of lobular neoplasia include cells slightly larger than the typical ones and that these enlarged cells possess abundant cytoplasm, large and slightly pleomorphic nuclei, granular chromatin, and easily seen nucleoli (Fig. 6-29). He referred to such cells as *type B* to distinguish them from the typical, smaller, and more uniform *type A* cells. One can find at least a few type B cells in many cases of lobular neoplasia, and in certain examples, they form the dominant population. Their presence does not seem to have diagnostic or clinical significance, although one can find it difficult to distinguish type B cells from cells of pleomorphic lobular carcinoma.

Box 6-2

Cytologic characteristics of lobular neoplasia:

- Absence of cellular polarization
- Absence of cellular cohesion

Ancillary Characteristics

Although the following three findings do not represent cytologic characteristics in the strict sense, they can provide diagnostic information. One must use this information judiciously, because each of the three generalizations has important exceptions.

Mitotic Activity

One has difficulty finding division figures in most cases of conventional lobular neoplasia, but uncommon examples do contain easily observed dividing cells. Such cells tend to show slightly larger nuclei than usual (the Haagensen type B pattern). The presence of mitotic figures need not argue against the diagnosis of lobular neoplasia if other characteristics of the proliferation support that interpretation.

Necrosis

Although most examples of conventional lobular neoplasia contain scattered apoptotic cells, typical lesions do not show abundant luminal necrotic debris (Fig. 6-30). A problem of classification therefore arises in those rare instances in which cells of a lobular nature exhibit central coagulative necrosis (*comedonecrosis*), a phenomenon that seems to occur mostly in ducts distended by the neoplastic proliferation. Pathologists of the past regarded such a marked degree of cellular death as incompatible with the diagnosis of lobular neoplasia, and they classified these forms of carcinoma in situ either as ductal or as carcinomas with mixed ductal and lobular features. Later observations have reversed this thinking. Mostly on the basis of the results of immunohistochemical staining for E-cadherin, pathologists have come to believe that foci of lobular neoplasia can undergo extensive necrosis. The phenomenon takes place most commonly in ducts distended by cells showing cellular and nuclear enlargement and variability (Fig. 6-31). Thus, the presence of abundant necrosis does not argue against the diagnosis of lobular neoplasia according to current thought.

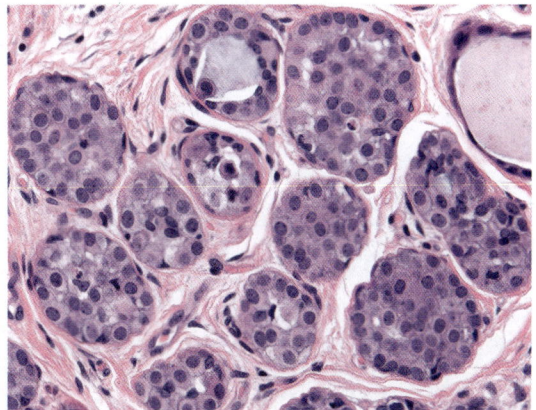

Figure 6-30 Most cases of lobular neoplasia do not display abundant necrosis, but many examples contain a few apoptotic cells.

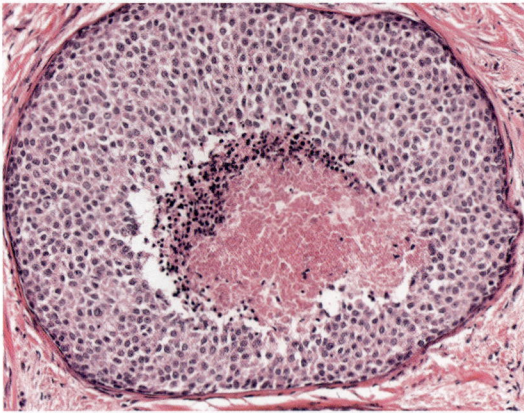

Figure 6-31 When neoplastic lobular cells appear larger and more variable than usual, one can observe abundant necrosis, especially of cells growing in ducts.

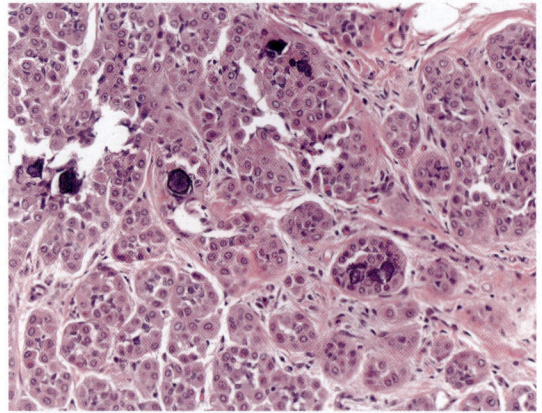

Figure 6-32 This example of lobular carcinoma in situ contains calcifications.

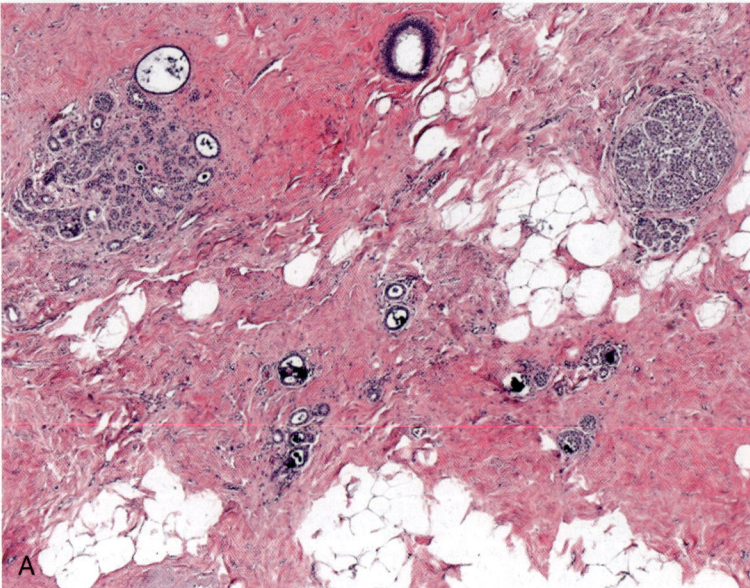

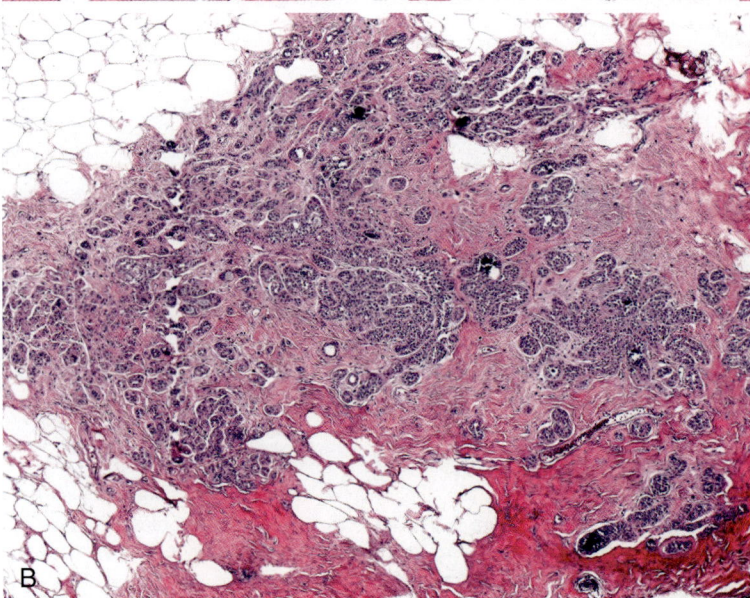

Figure 6-33 A, Lobular neoplasia involves glands in the upper right, and fibrocystic changes have produced calcifications in microcysts in the center. **B,** Lobular neoplasia occupies lobules distorted by sclerosing adenosis and containing preexisting calcifications.

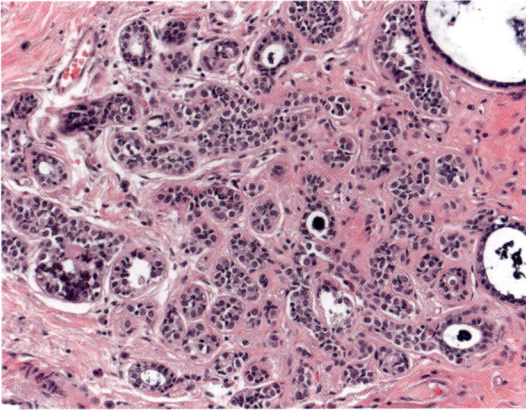

Figure 6-34 When lobular neoplasia involves lobules already altered by fibrocystic changes or sclerosing adenosis, the neoplastic cells can engulf the preexisting benign calcifications.

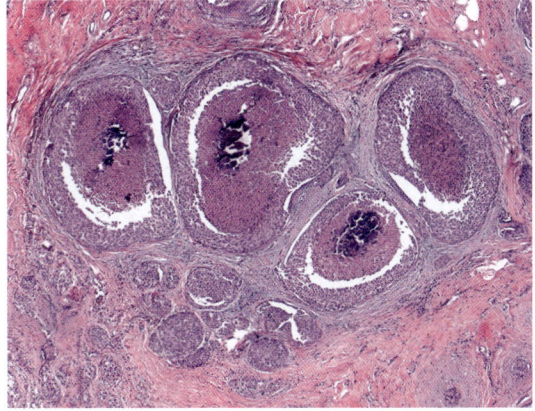

Figure 6-35 If the cells of lobular neoplasia undergo extensive necrosis, the debris can serve as a nidus for calcification.

Lobular neoplasia refers to in situ lesion

Calcification

The conventional teaching holds that the cells of lobular neoplasia do not produce calcifications; however, one can observe calcium deposits within aggregates of neoplastic lobular cells in a minority of cases (Fig. 6-32). This situation can arise through two mechanisms. First, the proliferation of the neoplastic cells can surround preexisting, benign calcifications. Lobular neoplasia most often arises in tissue that also displays fibrocystic changes or sclerosing adenosis. Calcium phosphate regularly precipitates in the dilated acini of microcysts and the compressed acini of sclerosing adenosis (Fig. 6-33). Frequently, lobular neoplasia comes to involve the lobules altered by these benign conditions, and sometimes the cells of lobular neoplasia actually enclose the calcium crystals (Fig. 6-34). Thus, the lobules first undergo microcyst formation or sclerosing adenosis, which leads to microcalcification; later, the malignant cells colonized the lobule. This theory can explain most instances in which conventional lobular neoplasia and calcifications occupy the same terminal duct–lobular unit. The second mechanism of calcification in lobular neoplasia occurs in examples showing abundant central necrosis. Just as in cases of high-grade ductal carcinoma in situ with comedonecrosis, the cellular debris resulting from the death of the neoplastic lobular cells serves as a nidus for the precipitation of calcium crystals, and calcifications identical to the casting calcifications of comedocarcinoma result (Fig. 6-35). Keeping in mind these exceptions, one should avoid making a diagnosis of lobular neoplasia in cases in which the neoplastic cells seem to give rise to calcifications.

IMMUNOHISTOCHEMICAL CHARACTERISTICS OF LOBULAR NEOPLASIA

A large body of literature documents the absence of E-cadherin in almost all forms of lobular neoplasia (Fig. 6-36). With beta-catenin and other molecules, E-cadherin forms intercellular junctions, and its absence from the neoplastic cells might explain their dishesive properties. Both benign and malignant ductal cells, in contrast, express E-cadherin. This generalization holds true for even the smallest foci of atypical lobular hyperplasia. The development of robust, specific antibodies to this protein has given pathologists a powerful tool for the diagnosis of lobular neoplasia; however, the interpretation of immunohistochemical staining for E-cadherin requires experience and careful correlation with findings present in conventionally stained sections.

The cells of lobular neoplasia show consistent patterns of expression of other molecules, also. For example, classic examples of lobular neoplasia stain for estrogen receptor protein and stain only weakly or not at all for cytokeratin 5/6. Although these properties might contribute diagnostic information in certain uncommon and narrowly defined situations, the characteristics do not help to solve the usual problem of distinguishing lobular neoplasia from ductal carcinoma in situ, because cells in both lesions stain in the same way with respect to these two proteins.

Summary

Neoplastic lobular cells show remarkably consistent characteristics. They always lack well-developed polarity, and they usually lack cohesion. As a result, the cells grow in loosely aggregated, structureless

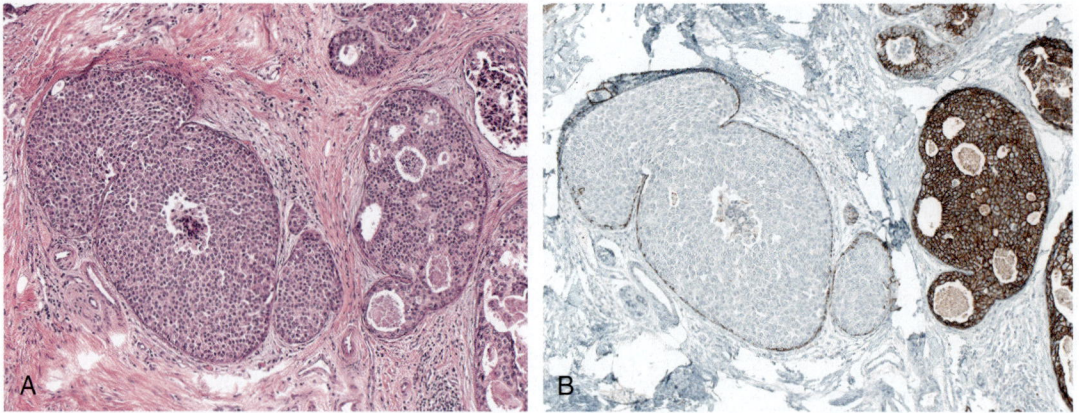

Figure 6-36 A, and **B,** The lobular carcinoma in situ shown on the *left* does not stain for E-cadherin, but the ductal carcinoma in situ on the right does.

sheets, and they mingle with benign epithelial cells in an intimate way. The accumulation of these cells fills and expands acini and ducts and renders the specialized stroma inconspicuous. The cells of the typical case possess uniform nuclei and scant, often foamy, cytoplasm, but both the nuclei and the cytoplasm vary in appearance. Enlargement and pleomorphism of the nucleus represent the most problematic variations. One does not observe significant mitotic activity in the usual example, the neoplastic lobular cells do not produce calcifications, and noticeable necrosis does not occur except in uncommon cases. Neoplastic lobular cells do not express E-cadherin or cytokeratin 5/6.

PROBLEMS IN THE DIAGNOSIS OF LOBULAR NEOPLASIA

The dishesive and nonpolarized nature of neoplastic lobular cells create such distinctive patterns that pathologists do not have difficulty recognizing typical cases of lobular neoplasia. Exceptional lobular proliferations appear more cohesive than the usual, and pathologists struggle to differentiate this variety of lobular neoplasia from the solid type of ductal carcinoma in situ. Certain forms of myoepithelial hyperplasia can also closely resemble a lobular proliferation. The mingling of the lobular cells with indigenous epithelial cells or proliferative ductal cells produces complex patterns, which demand close study to understand. Involvement of lobules altered by pathologic processes and physiologic changes alters the architectural configurations created by lobular proliferations in ways that mimic the appearances of other lesions.

Immunohistochemical staining for E-cadherin provides a tool for distinguishing neoplastic lobular cells from most other cells of the breast and for unraveling the complexities of these situations, but it requires experience and careful correlation with conventional sections to interpret the patterns of staining accurately. The recognition that neoplastic lobular cells can display pleomorphism has introduced a new entity, *pleomorphic lobular carcinoma*. Pathologists have not clearly defined its characteristics, nor have they established criteria to separate this lesion from high-grade ductal carcinoma that lacks E-cadherin. Pathologists traditionally divide lobular proliferations into two subgroups on the basis of the quantity of neoplastic cells; one could debate the rationale for this subdivision. Finally, the small size of neoplastic lobular cells and their insidious manner of stromal infiltration create problems in detecting small foci of invasion. The following paragraphs address certain aspects of these problems.

Distinction of Solid Ductal Carcinoma In situ from Lobular Carcinoma In Situ

The differentiation from solid ductal carcinoma in situ represents the most difficult problem in the differential diagnosis of lobular neoplasia. Classic examples of lobular neoplasia do not pose this problem, of course, because their loosely cohesive cells and disheveled appearance distinguish these populations from ductal carcinomas in situ, which typically consist of cells with slightly cohesive properties and an orderly arrangement. The cells of lobular neoplasia do not always exhibit their dishesive properties clearly, and in certain cases, the cells remain closely apposed. The differentiation of this pattern of lobular neoplasia from solid ductal carcinoma in situ always poses difficulties.

Pathologists of the past have used the presence of marked nuclear pleomorphism and abundant

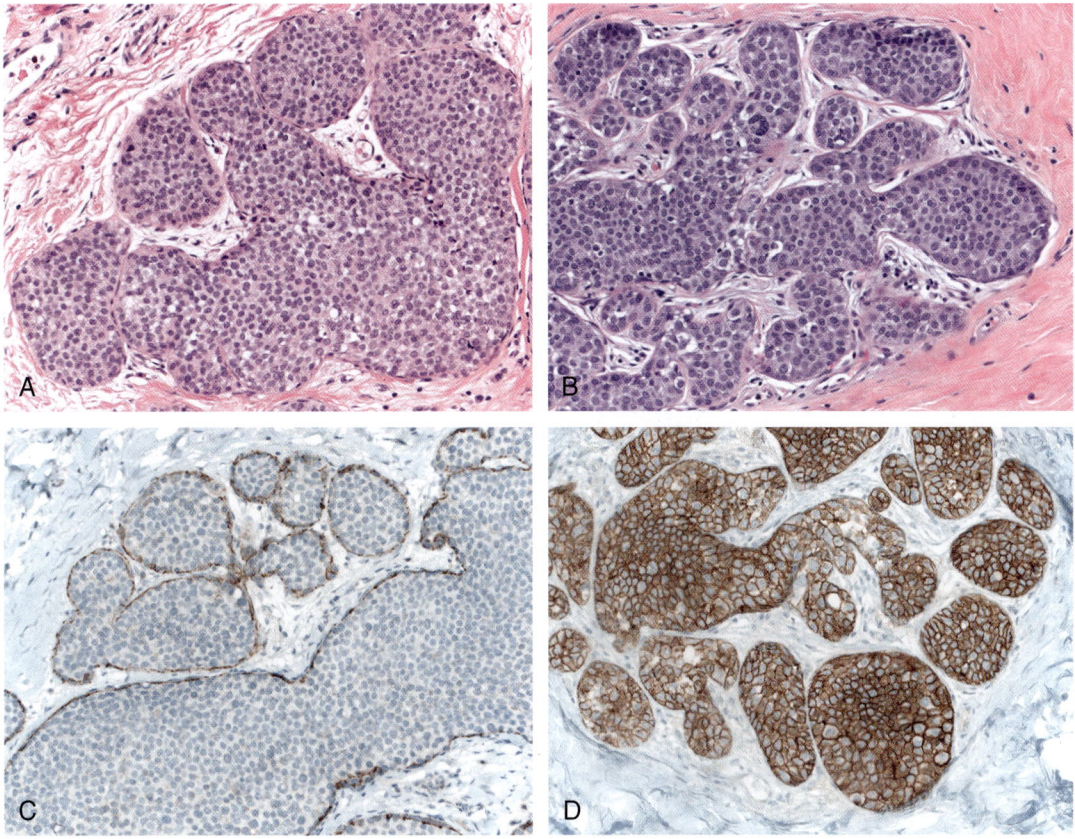

Figure 6-37 The lobular carcinoma in situ in **A** does not appear as dishesive as many examples and it resembles the solid ductal carcinoma in situ in **B**. Immunohistochemical stain for E-cadherin fails to demonstrate the protein in the lobular carcinoma cells as seen in **C**, whereas the cells of the ductal carcinoma stain strongly in **D**.

necrotic debris to classify ambiguous solid carcinomas in situ as ductal, but the realization that both findings can occur in lobular neoplasia renders these criteria useless. Other observers have suggested that the formation of a pavement pattern, which consists of evenly spaced cells showing distinct cell membranes, and the creation of microacini favor the diagnosis of solid ductal carcinoma in situ. Neither criterion bears up under careful scrutiny. It seems that staining for E-cadherin provides the most reliable way to distinguish between lobular neoplasia and solid ductal carcinoma in situ (Fig. 6-37). Most cases of carcinoma in situ that look ambiguous in conventional sections yield unambiguous results when stained for E-cadherin. Rare examples exhibit variable staining results; however, we do not know the significance of such findings, nor do we know how to classify such cases. Finally, rare low-grade carcinomas that form convincing cribriform spaces and therefore look like conventional ductal carcinoma in situ can fail to stain for E-cadherin. In such cases, the author has not allowed this immunohistochemical staining result to override the diagnosis based on conventionally stained sections. A carcinoma showing the typical architectural patterns of ductal carcinoma but lacking E-cadherin probably represents ductal carcinoma that has lost E-cadherin expression rather than an unusual type of lobular carcinoma in situ.

Distinction from Myoepithelial Proliferations

Proliferations of myoepithelial cells can take three forms; two occur within lobules, and the third in ducts. Each form can simulate lobular neoplasia to a greater or lesser degree. Within lobules, myoepithelial cells most commonly proliferate within the stroma. In doing so, they cause the lobules to look unusually cellular (Fig. 6-38). Although such foci resemble the hypercellular lobules of lobular neoplasia at low magnification, close inspection shows that the extra cells sit within collagenous stroma between acini rather than within them. Furthermore, the myoepithelial cells do not appear atypical, nor do they display the other cellular characteristics of atypical lobular cells (Fig. 6-39). In a much more unusual lesion, myoepithelial cells of the lobule proliferate

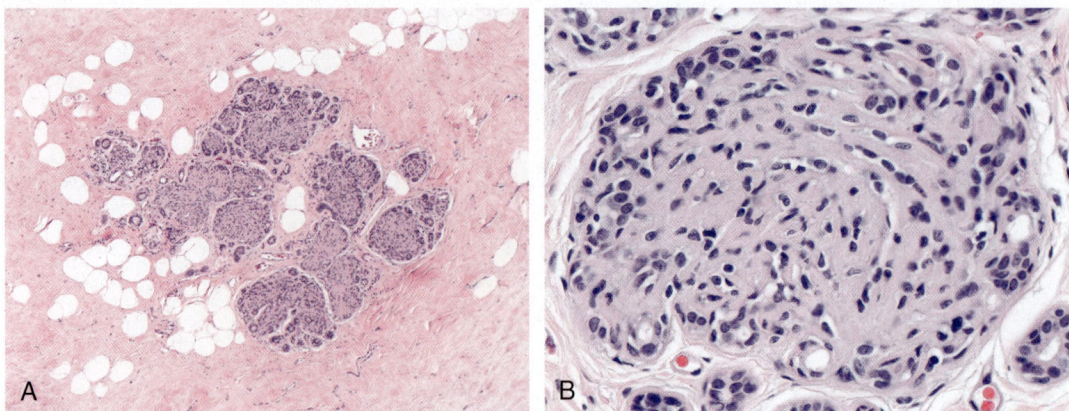

Figure 6-38 A, When viewed at low magnification, the cellularity and lobular shape of this focus of intralobular myoepithelial hyperplasia suggest the diagnosis of lobular neoplasia. **B,** Examination at high magnification reveals that myoepithelial cells and collagen occupy most of the lobule and that only a few acini persist at its periphery.

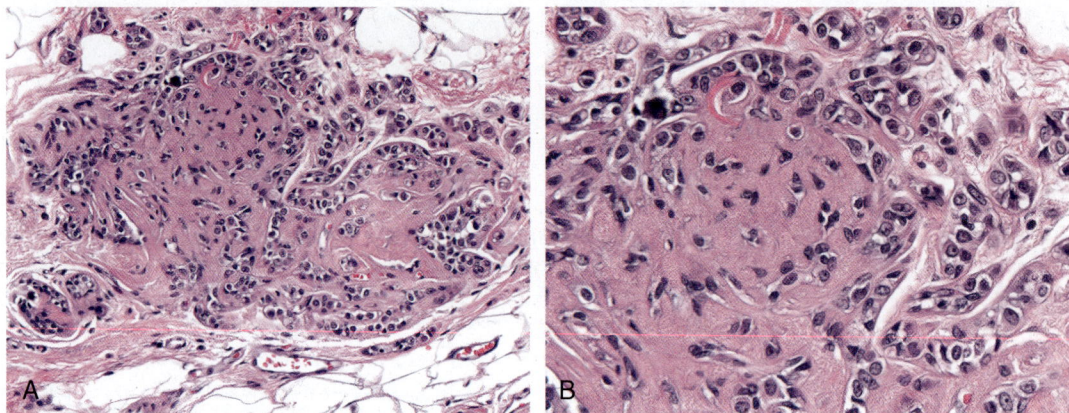

Figure 6-39 A, Lobular neoplasia has colonized this region of intralobular myoepithelial hyperplasia. **B,** High magnification allows one to appreciate that the neoplastic cells appear larger than the myoepithelial cells and that the former possess larger nuclei than the latter. Furthermore, the neoplastic lobular cells display dishesion not demonstrated by the myoepithelial cells.

as a single layer sandwiched between the luminal cells and the basement membrane (Fig. 6-40). This situation creates a pattern that brings to mind the pagetoid pattern of lobular neoplasia; however, hyperplastic myoepithelial cells have more cytoplasm than neoplastic lobular cells, and the former do not display the loose cohesion exhibited by the latter. A stain for a myoepithelial marker distinguishes between a myoepithelial proliferation and lobular neoplasia.

Besides growing within lobules, myoepithelial cells can proliferate as single cells or a multicellular layer within the epithelium of ducts. This process creates a picture that virtually duplicates the appearance of the pagetoid growth of lobular neoplasia (Fig. 6-41). It requires careful attention to cellular characteristics, the results of ancillary studies, and considerable experience to distinguish these two lesions. Hyperplastic myoepithelial cells tend to display subtle variation in spacing and a hint of clustering (Fig. 6-42). Thin slips of collagen often encase individual cells or small groups. Although certain of these characteristics overlap with those of neoplastic lobular cells, attention to a few features helps distinguish the two lesions. First, hyperplastic myoepithelial cells have more cytoplasm and a lower nucleus-to-cytoplasm ratio than neoplastic lobular cells. Second, the nuclei of hyperplastic myoepithelial cells show more pronounced variation in shape than lobular cells do. Third, the nuclei of hyperplastic myoepithelial cells often contain obvious nucleoli, whereas conventional lobular carcinoma cells do

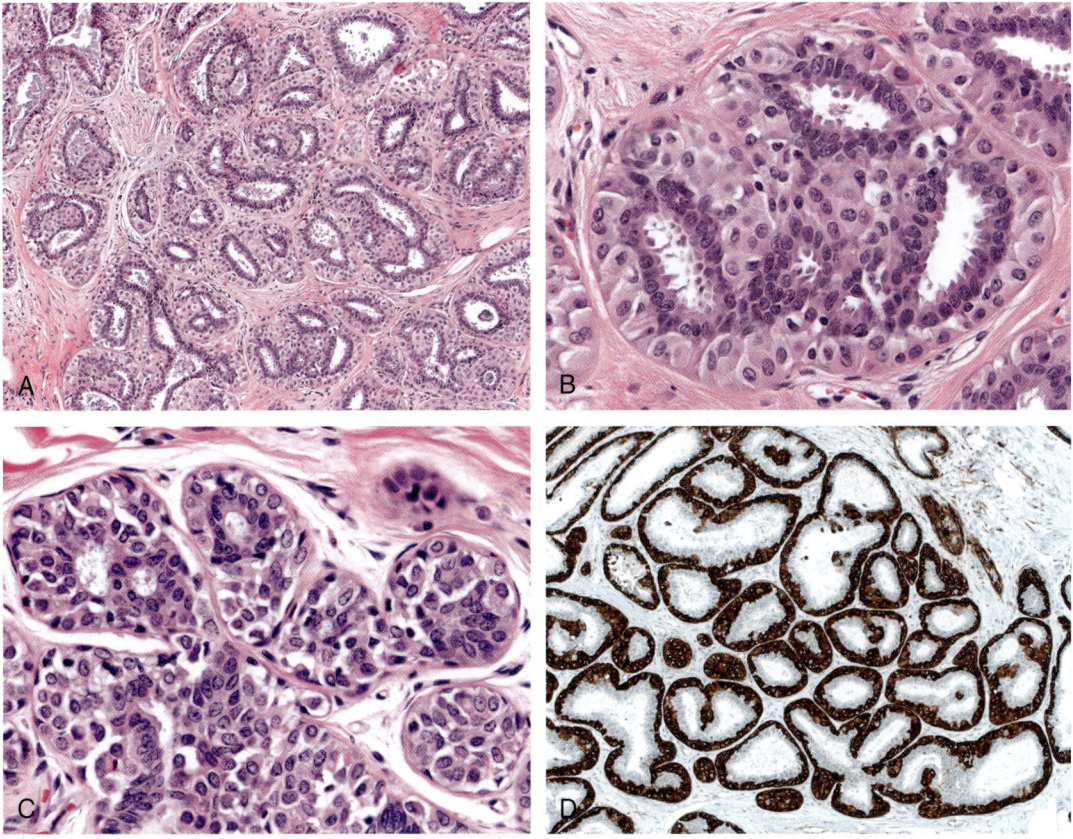

Figure 6-40 A and **B,** Myoepithelial cells can proliferate within the lobule as a single layer. The pattern suggests the phenomenon of intralobular pagetoid spread, but the abundance of the cytoplasm and the lack of cytologic atypia distinguish this form of myoepithelial proliferation from lobular neoplasia growing in a pagetoid pattern in a lobule, seen in **C. D,** A stain for myosin heavy chain confirms the myoepithelial nature of the proliferative cells.

Figure 6-41 Lobular carcinoma in situ occupies the lobule at the *left* and myoepithelial hyperplasia thickens the epithelium of the duct at the *right.*

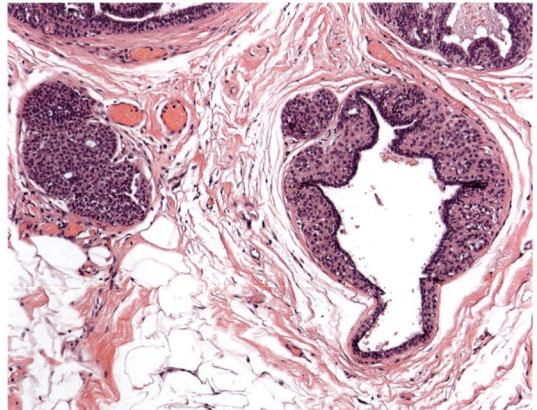

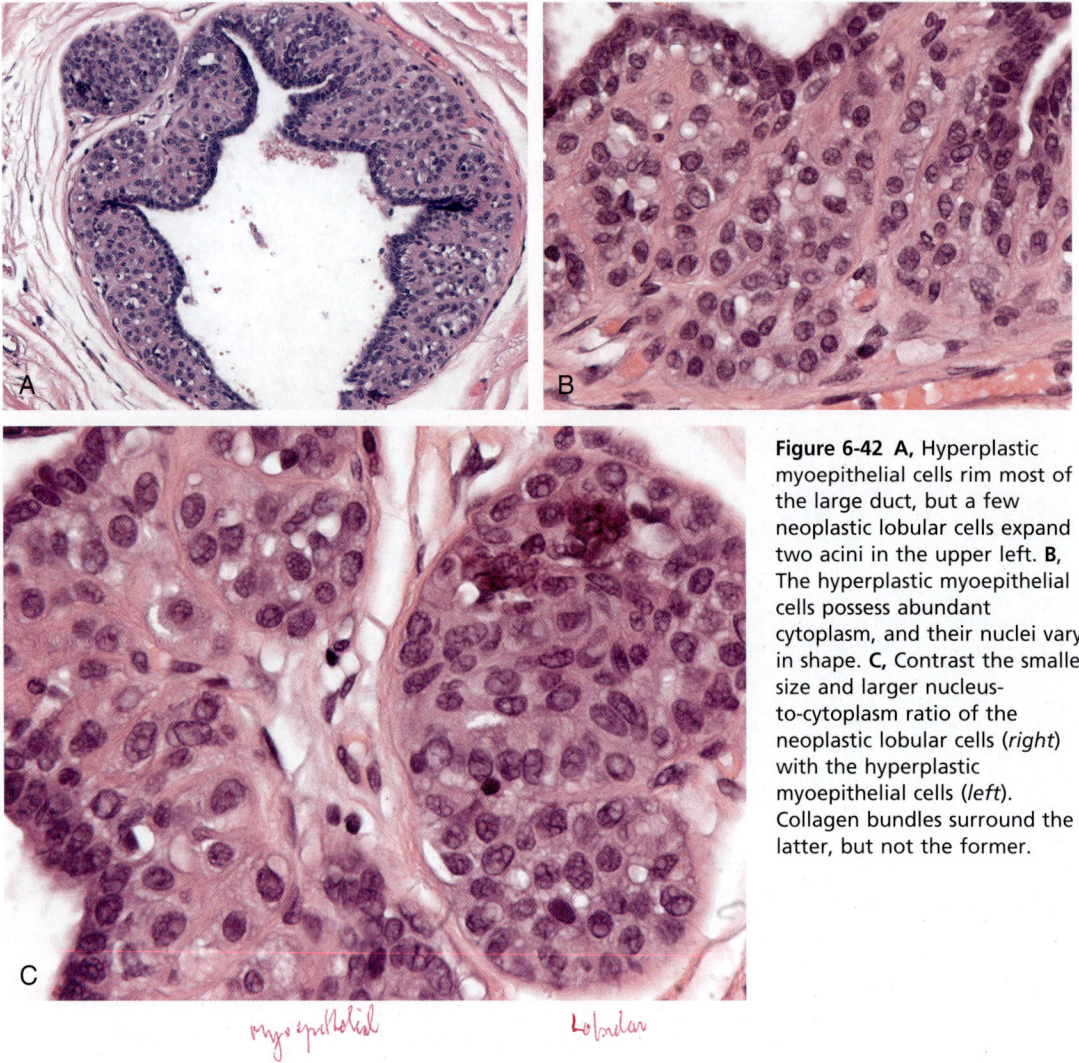

Figure 6-42 A, Hyperplastic myoepithelial cells rim most of the large duct, but a few neoplastic lobular cells expand two acini in the upper left. **B,** The hyperplastic myoepithelial cells possess abundant cytoplasm, and their nuclei vary in shape. **C,** Contrast the smaller size and larger nucleus-to-cytoplasm ratio of the neoplastic lobular cells (*right*) with the hyperplastic myoepithelial cells (*left*). Collagen bundles surround the latter, but not the former.

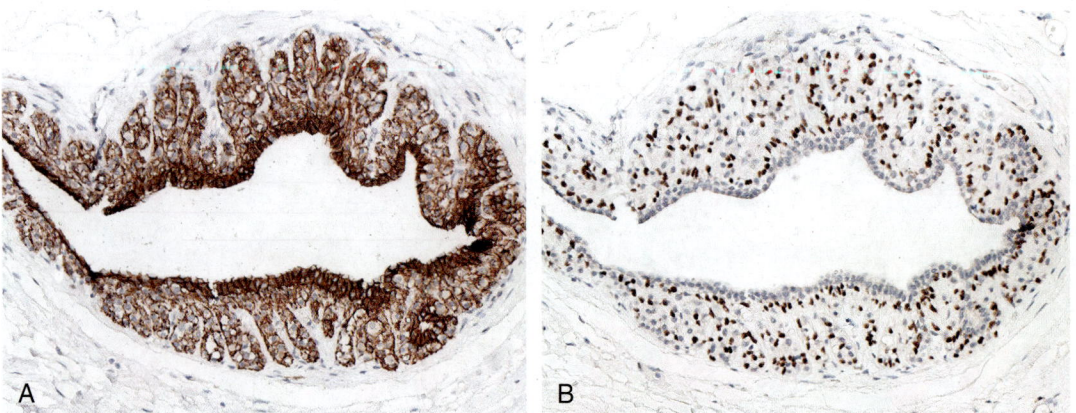

Figure 6-43 The positive reaction of stains for myosin heavy chain in **A** and p63 protein in **B** confirm the myoepithelial nature of the cells in the ductal wall.

not. Fourth, myoepithelial cells do not display the dishesion exhibited by neoplastic lobular cells. Finally, bands of collagen do not surround neoplastic lobular cells to the extent seen in many cases of ductal myoepithelial hyperplasia.

Reading this list of morphologic differences, one could conclude that differentiating myoepithelial hyperplasia from lobular neoplasia would amount to little more than a trivial exercise. Experience proves the contrary, because the cells of lobular neoplasia can possess more than the usual amount of cytoplasm, their nuclei can vary in size and shape, and they can contain clearly evident nucleoli. Moreover, neoplastic lobular cells usually entrap preexisting benign cells, which can make the cell clusters look slightly pleomorphic and somewhat jumbled, and the dishesion of lobular cells does not always appear obvious. Pathologists often find it helpful to use immunohistochemical staining to evaluate the impression based on the study of conventionally stained sections (Fig. 6-43). Staining for E-cadherin and a myoepithelial marker such as p63 protein often leads to an unambiguous conclusion.

Infrequently Emphasized Patterns of Pagetoid Growth

Instead of eradicating preexisting benign cells, as most carcinoma cells do, neoplastic lobular cells seem willing to mingle with the indigenous population. This intermingling of cell types gives rise to the pattern loosely regarded as pagetoid spread. Although pathologists most often think of the phenomenon as a process affecting ducts, this manner of growth can occur in structures throughout the mammary glandular tree, including structures already home to other pathologic processes. By doing so, the cells create confusing patterns that can lead the pathologist to make an erroneous diagnosis.

Intralobular Growth

The pagetoid growth of lobular neoplasia within terminal duct–lobular units produces a picture that resembles the appearance of cribriform ductal carcinoma in situ. The process begins as individual neoplastic cells collect along the basement membrane of the terminal ductules and acini (Fig. 6-44). Accumulation of the cells uproots the luminal cells from the basement membrane, and at times, these preexisting benign cells persist as intact acini entrapped within the neoplastic population (Fig. 6-45). Because the acini consist of polarized cells forming well-defined glands, the structures bring to mind the appearance of cribriform spaces. Minimal examples of this phenomenon might go unnoticed or provoke only passing curiosity (Fig. 6-46), but large regions of intralobular pagetoid spread could lead to an erroneous diagnosis of atypical ductal hyperplasia, ductal carcinoma in situ, or carcinoma in situ with mixed ductal and lobular features (Figs. 6-47 and 6-48).

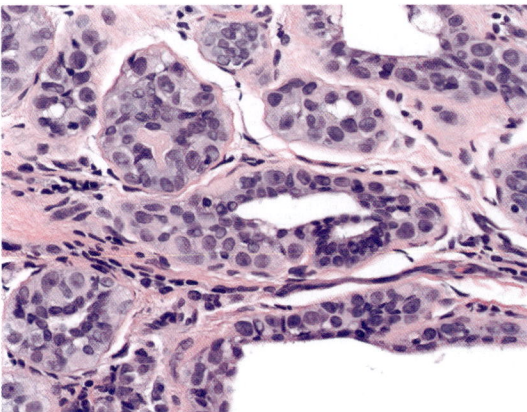

Figure 6-44 The neoplastic lobular cells have lifted the luminal cells from the basement membrane. The latter remain in a flattened sheet or intact acini.

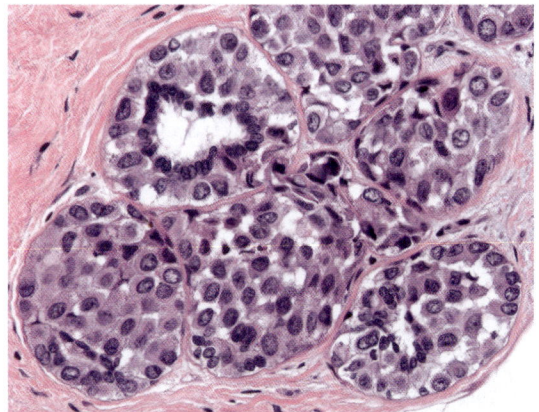

Figure 6-45 Preexisting luminal cells persist in the form of intact glands surrounded by the neoplastic population.

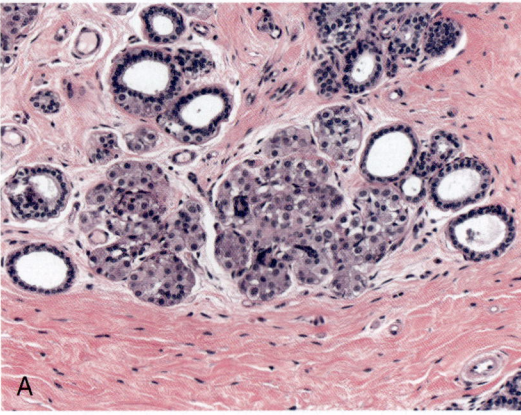

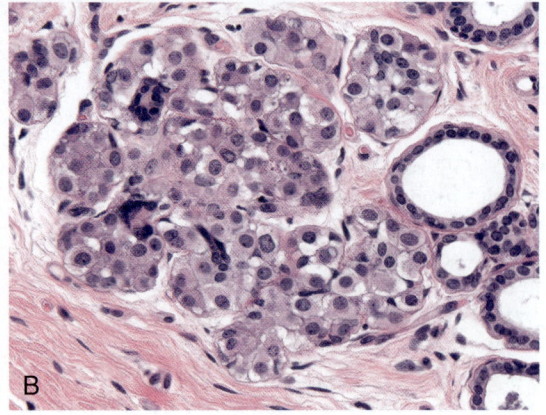

Figure 6-46 A and **B,** This small region of intralobular pagetoid growth would probably not attract much attention or interest.

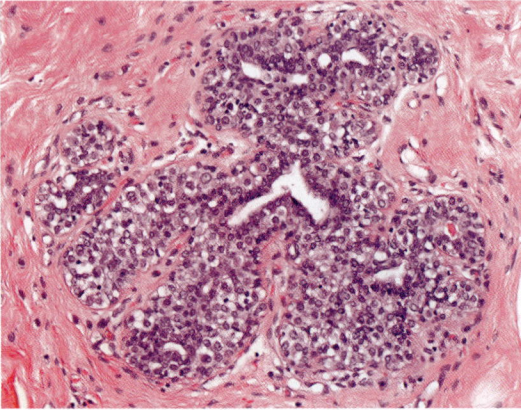

Figure 6-47 Intralobular pagetoid growth of lobular neoplasia suggests diagnoses such as atypical ductal hyperplasia, ductal carcinoma in situ, or carcinoma in situ with mixed ductal and lobular features.

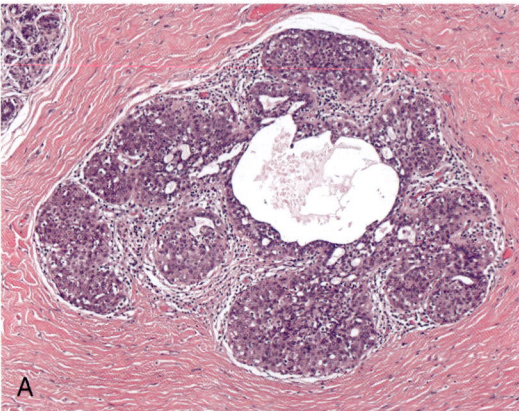

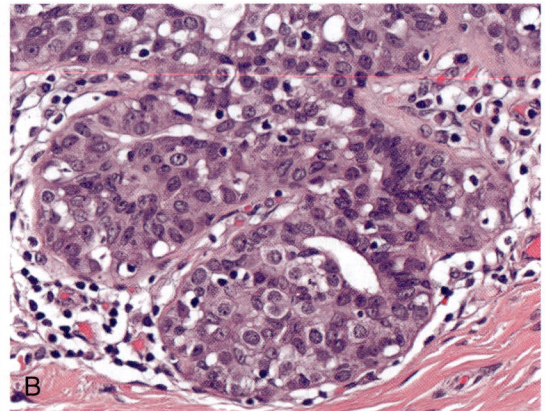

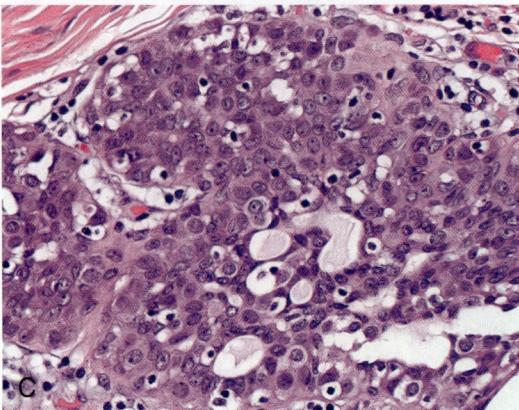

Figure 6-48 A to **C,** One could misinterpret the neoplastic lobular cells growing in a pagetoid way in these primitive lobules as a population of atypical ductal cells.

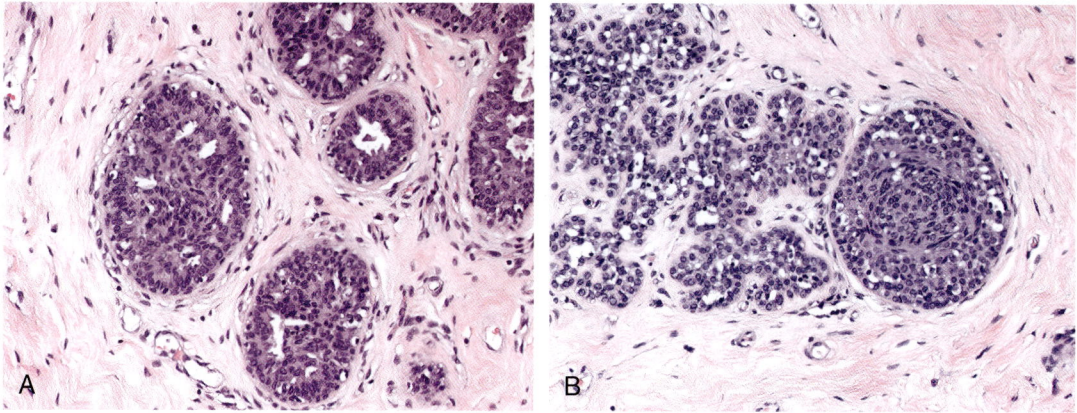

Figure 6-49 A, Hyperplastic ductal cells populate small ducts and acini. **B,** Neoplastic lobular cells occupying glands in the left have infiltrated the periphery of the focus of conventional ductal hyperplasia in the right, which is also shown in **C.**

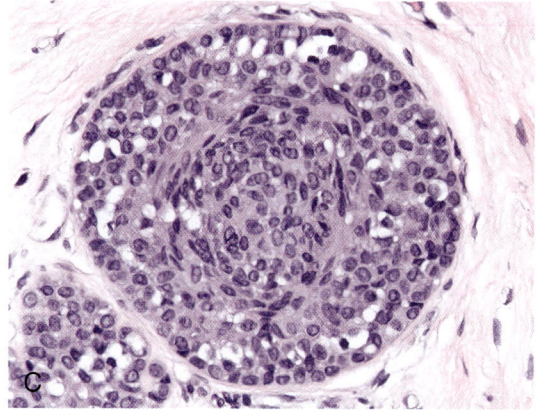

Involvement of Conventional Ductal Hyperplasia

Besides populating pristine ducts and lobules, lobular neoplasia can grow in ducts and acini already involved by ductal hyperplasia. As they do in other anatomic locations, the cells of lobular neoplasia involving ductal hyperplasia make their appearance along the basement membrane (Fig. 6-49). As they increase in number, the neoplastic cells usually encase the hyperplastic population, which remains in the center of the gland; less often, the lobular cells displace the hyperplastic ones to the edge of the acinus (Fig. 6-50). This peripheral location of the atypical cells and their encircling of the benign cells represent the first clues

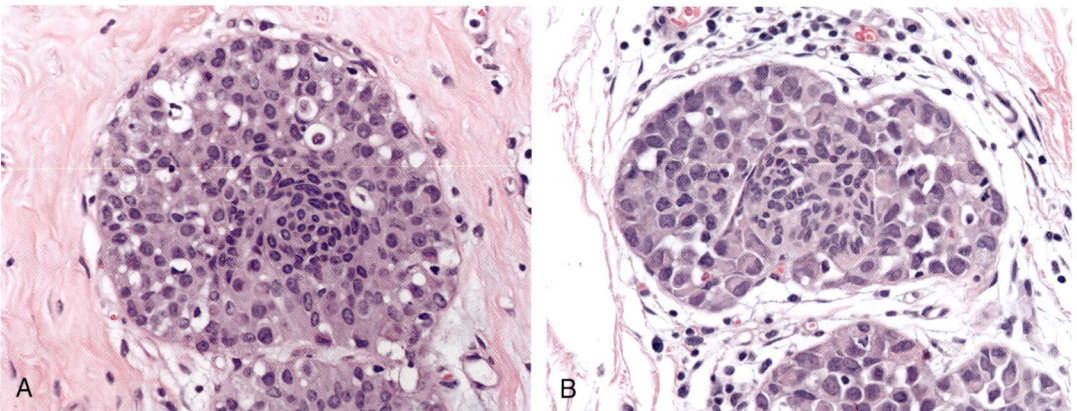

Figure 6-50 Neoplastic lobular cells usually displace hyperplastic ductal cells towards the center of the gland in **A,** but the benign cells sometimes remain in an eccentric position in **B.**

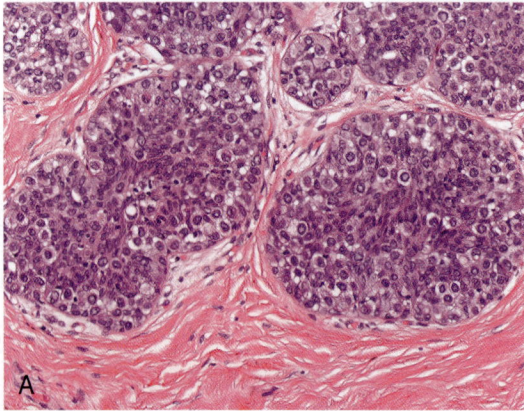

Figure 6-51 A, Neoplastic lobular cells can percolate among hyperplastic ductal cells. **B,** The side-by-side position of the two types of cells allows one to appreciate the differences in their cellular properties.

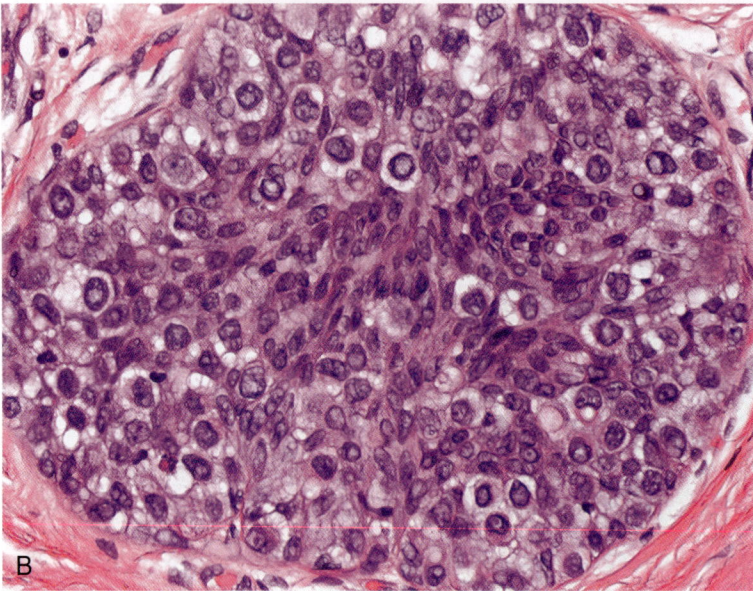

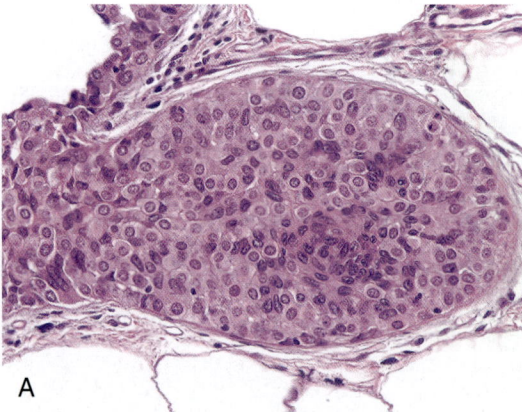

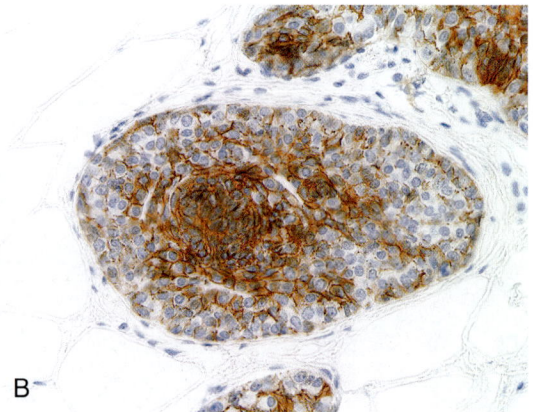

Figure 6-52 A, The focus of ductal hyperplasia mixed with lobular neoplasia presents a confusing picture but staining for E-cadherin reveals its true nature. **B,** The hyperplastic ductal cells stain for the protein, whereas the neoplastic lobular cells do not.

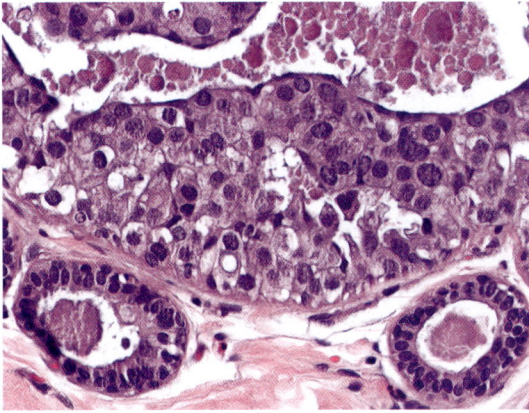

Figure 6-53 One could confuse this focus of immature ductal hyperplasia with lobular neoplasia growing in a pagetoid pattern, but the immature ductal cells look more cohesive than neoplastic lobular cells usually appear.

that two types of epithelial cells coexist in such a focus. With further proliferation, the neoplastic lobular cells percolate among the hyperplastic ductal cells (Fig. 6-51). The intimate mixing of the two types of cells makes the differences in their fundamental cellular properties obvious: the neoplastic lobular cells appear larger than the hyperplastic ductal cells, and the former lack the marked cohesion of the latter. Once one appreciates these differences, the proper classification of the cells does not usually pose a problem. Staining for E-cadherin should resolve cases of an uncertain nature; lobular carcinoma cells fail to stain, whereas hyperplastic ductal cells express the protein (Fig. 6-52).

Distinguishing immature ductal hyperplasia from the pagetoid involvement of conventional ductal hyperplasia by lobular neoplasia probably represents the most challenging aspect of this situation, because one finds large cells along the basement membrane in both lesions. Attention to the cohesive properties of the cells usually allows one to differentiate the two types of proliferation. Immature hyperplastic ductal cells appear cohesive, whereas neoplastic lobular cells display their characteristic dishesive qualities (Fig. 6-53).

Involvement of Ductal Carcinoma In Situ

When lobular neoplasia colonizes ducts harboring ductal carcinoma in situ, the neoplastic lobular cells do so in their characteristic fashion: they accumulate along the basement membrane and displace the ductal carcinoma cells from their peripheral position (Fig. 6-54). The close apposition of the cells allows one to appreciate differences in properties of the two populations. The ductal cells appear polarized and slightly cohesive, whereas the lobular cells lack both qualities.

Involvement of Altered Lobules

Just as lobular neoplasia can grow in a pagetoid way in ducts and lobules harboring preexisting epithelial proliferations, so, too, can the neoplastic cells populate lobules altered by preexisting benign processes. Growth in such terminal duct–lobular units produces patterns that mimic other lesions, so the pathologist must pay special attention to avoid erroneous diagnoses.

Figure 6-54 The cells of lobular carcinoma in situ have undermined the malignant ductal cells. One can appreciate that the former lack the polarization and cohesion of the latter.

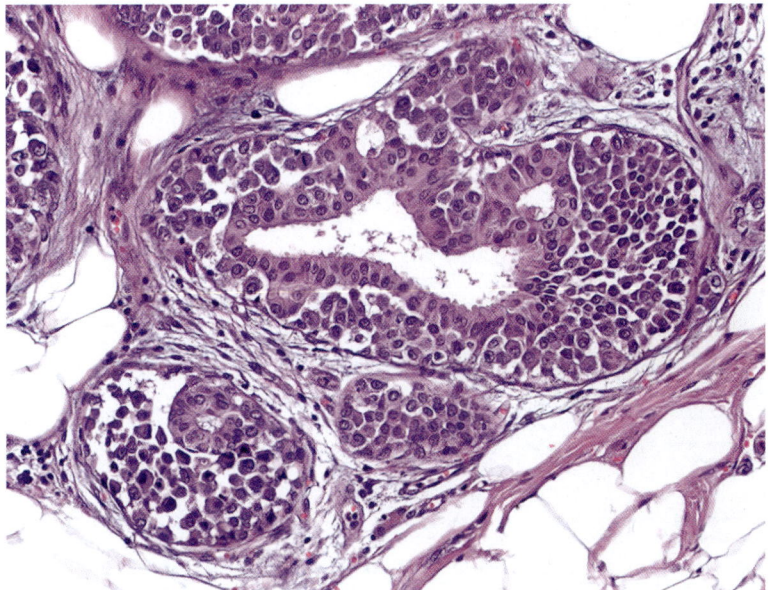

Collagenous Spherulosis

Collagenous spherulosis represents a benign sclerosing process in which nodules of basement membrane proteins enclosed by myoepithelial cells compress the acini and ductules (Fig. 6-55). Although the lesion looks like a form of intraductal epithelial proliferation, study of the early phases demonstrates that the process usually affects lobules. It often coexists with radial scars and papillomas. Because of the round shape of the spherules and the seemingly intraductal location of the process, the lesion superficially resembles cribriform ductal carcinoma in situ, and the collision of lobular neoplasia with collagenous spherulosis heightens this resemblance. When lobular neoplasia extends into a focus of collagenous spherulosis, the neoplastic cells displace the indigenous luminal cells but leave the myoepithelial cells and the enclosed spherules in place. Thus, the neoplastic cells surround round, neatly punched-out spaces, thereby recalling the appearance of low-grade, cribriform ductal carcinoma in situ (Fig. 6-56).

Table 6-1 lists three features that distinguish lobular neoplasia involving collagenous spherulosis from cribriform ductal carcinoma in situ: the contents of the spaces, the nature of the cells surrounding the spaces, and the extent of cohesion of the atypical cells. First, in cases of spherulosis, the spaces contain either the densely eosinophilic spherules or radiating, bluish ground substances (Fig. 6-57). Cribriform spaces usually appear empty or contain detached carcinoma cells or cellular debris. Although the spaces in ductal carcinomas occasionally contain eosinophilic material or mucin, the secretory material does not resemble collagenous spherules, nor does the flocculent mucin look like the stellate aggregates of ground substances seen in spherulosis. Second, myoepithelial cells create most of the spaces in spherulosis. These cells appear long and flattened and they

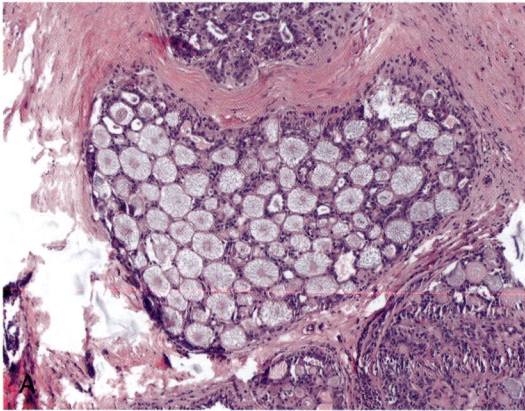

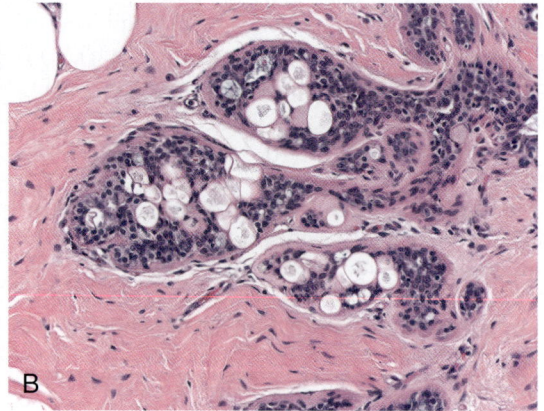

Figure 6-55 A and **B,** Collagenous spherulosis represents a sclerosing process characterized by the deposition of spherules of basement membrane proteins.

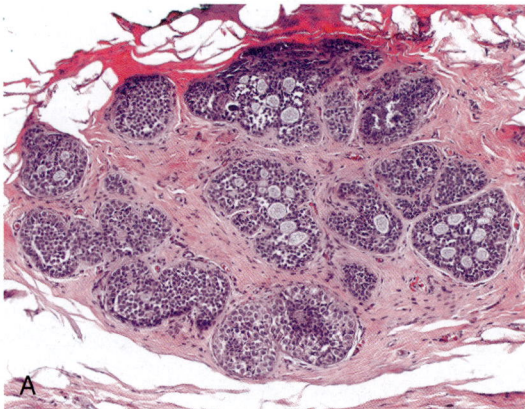

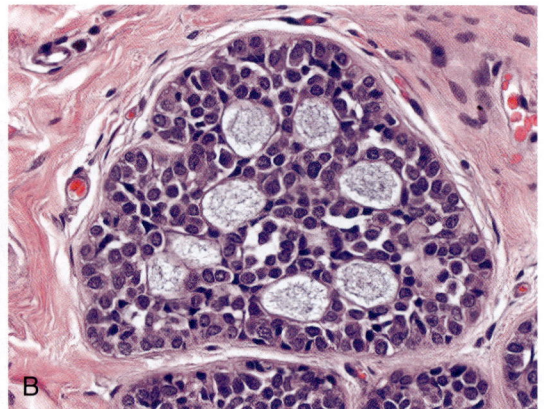

Figure 6-56 A, Lobular neoplasia has colonized a region of collagenous spherulosis. **B,** The coexistence of atypical epithelial cells and round spaces brings to mind the appearance of cribriform ductal carcinoma in situ.

Table 6-1   Histological Attributes of Lobular Neoplasia Involving Collagenous Spherulosis and Cribriform Ductal Carcinoma in Situ

	Lobular Neoplasia Involving Collagenous Spherulosis	Cribriform Ductal Carcinoma In Situ
Contents of spaces	Pink or blue basement membrane proteins	Usually empty Occasionally detached cells, debris, protein, or mucin
Nature of cells surrounding spaces	Flattened myoepithelial cells, normal luminal cells	Polarized atypical ductal cells
Extent of cohesion of atypical cells	Dishesive	Slightly cohesive

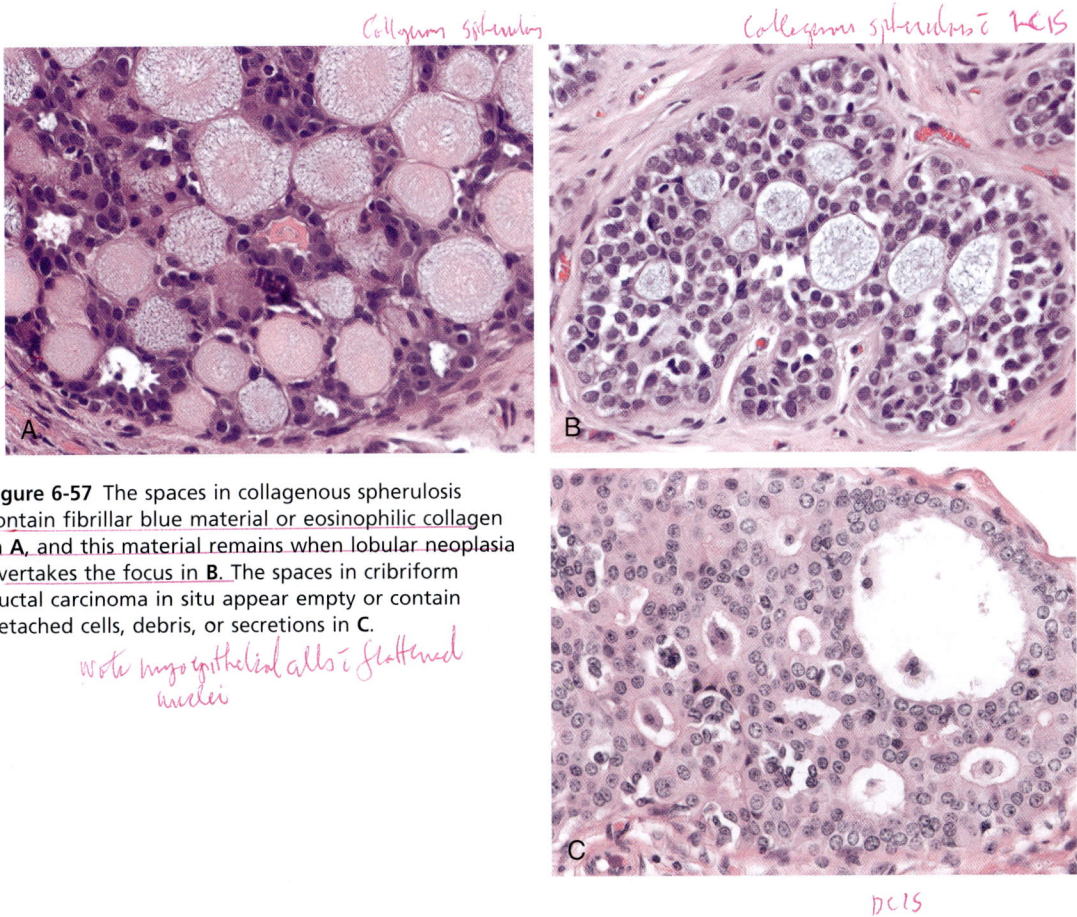

Collagenous spherulosis   *Collagenous spherulosis c̄ LCIS*

Figure 6-57 The spaces in collagenous spherulosis contain fibrillar blue material or eosinophilic collagen in **A**, and this material remains when lobular neoplasia overtakes the focus in **B**. The spaces in cribriform ductal carcinoma in situ appear empty or contain detached cells, debris, or secretions in **C**.

Note myoepithelial cells c̄ flattened nuclei

DCIS

possess thin, hyperchromatic nuclei and densely eosinophilic cytoplasm (Fig. 6-58). When this lesion becomes colonized by lobular neoplasia, the myoepithelial cells remain as a layer between the neoplastic cells and the spherules. In carcinomas, on the other hand, malignant epithelial cells abut the spaces. Furthermore, the carcinoma cells surrounding cribriform spaces look polarized; the nuclei sit near the basal aspect of the cell, and apical cytoplasm accumulates next to the lumen. Third, the cells of lobular neoplasia do not display intercellular cohesion, so they tend to detach from their neighbors even when growing in a focus of collagenous spherulosis (Fig. 6-59). The cells of cribriform ductal carcinoma in situ, in contrast, do not tend to separate. In difficult cases, immunohistochemical stains reveal the myoepithelial nature of the cells surrounding the spherules (Fig. 6-60). If one pays attention to these three points, however, one usually does not need special studies.

Rem of material ~ CS

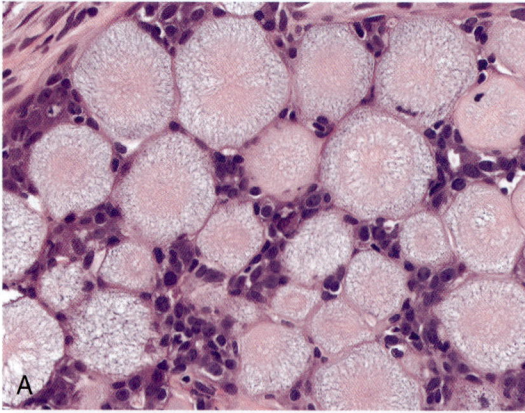

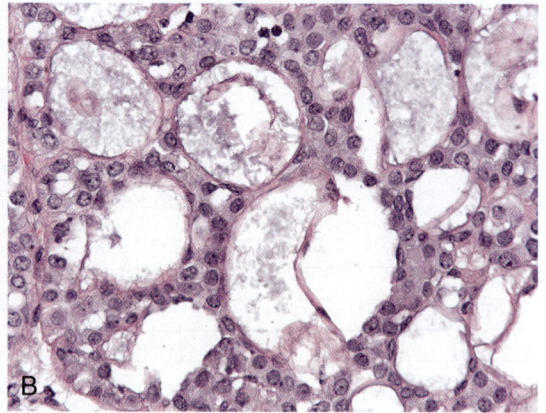

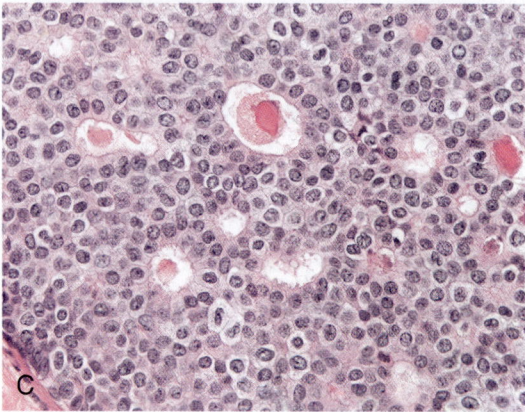

Figure 6-58 Myoepithelial cells surround the spherules in collagenous spherulosis in **A** even when the lesion contains neoplastic lobular cells, as seen in **B**. One does not observe myoepithelial cells in foci of ductal carcinoma in situ in **C**.

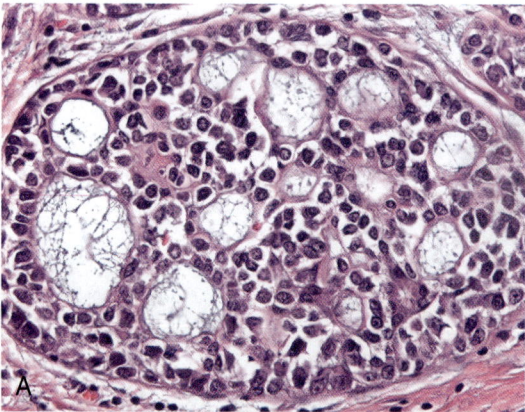

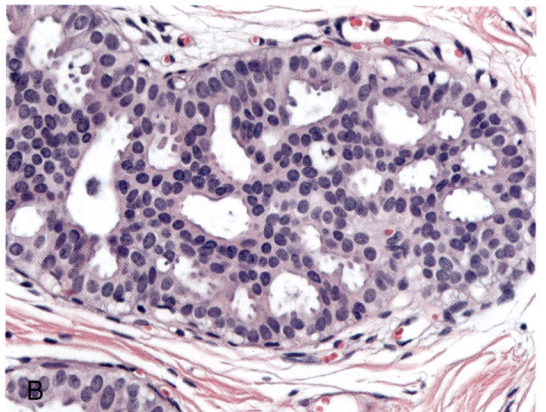

Figure 6-59 The cells of lobular neoplasia involving collagenous spherulosis appear dishesive in **A**, whereas those of ductal carcinoma in situ do not, as shown in **B**.

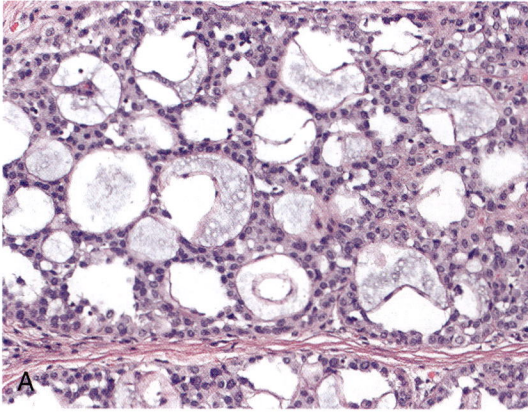

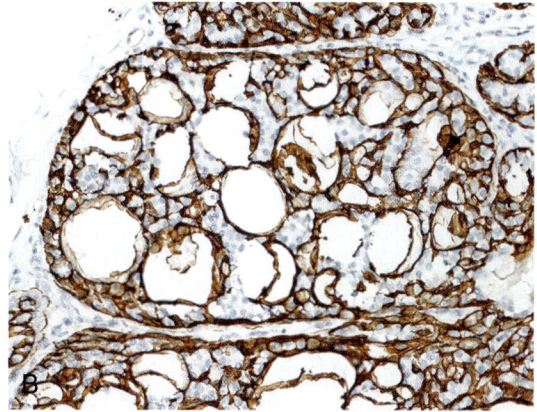

Figure 6-60 A, Immunohistochemical staining can help to resolve problematic cases like the one shown here. Staining for myosin heavy chain in **B** and keratin in **C** reveals the underlying structure of collagenous spherulosis.

Have to use SMM Heavy chain to see myoepithelial cells

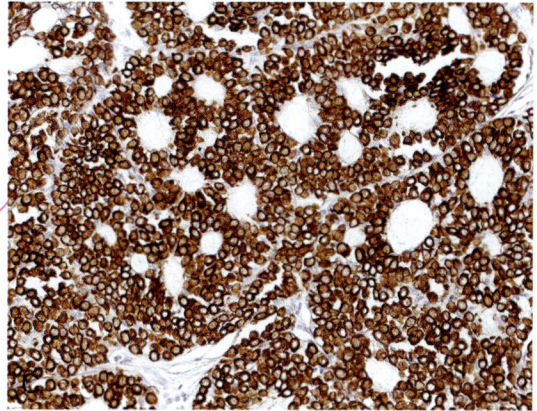

Sclerosing Adenosis

The growth of lobular neoplasia in lobules deformed by sclerosing adenosis produces an appearance that superficially resembles that of invasive carcinoma (Fig. 6-61). Examination of such foci at high magnification does little to aid in this distinction; in fact, this approach only makes the problem more difficult. Using low magnification, one can appreciate that regions of sclerosing adenosis harboring lobular neoplasia retain their lobulated contour, swirling character, and orderly relationship between the stroma and acini even when involved by the neoplastic cells (Fig. 6-62). By comparing problematic areas with foci of uninvolved sclerosing adenosis, one can often appreciate the underlying similarities in structure. Special stains for markers of myoepithelial cells

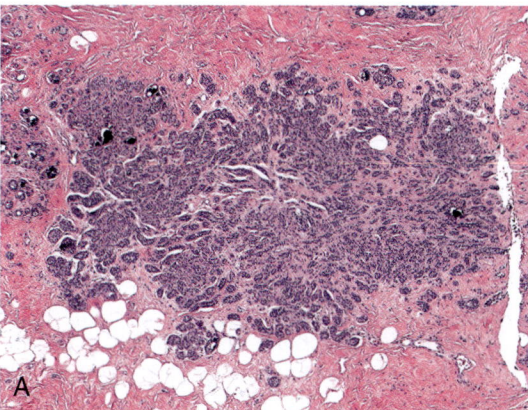

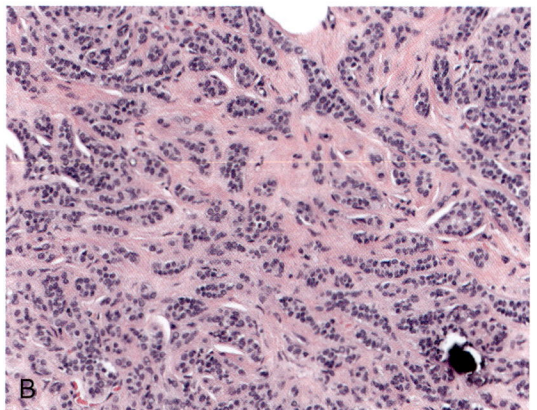

Figure 6-61 A, Lobular neoplasia has colonized this nodule of sclerosing adenosis. **B,** High magnification makes the lesion look like invasive carcinoma.

Need myoepithelial stain to see myoepithelial cells

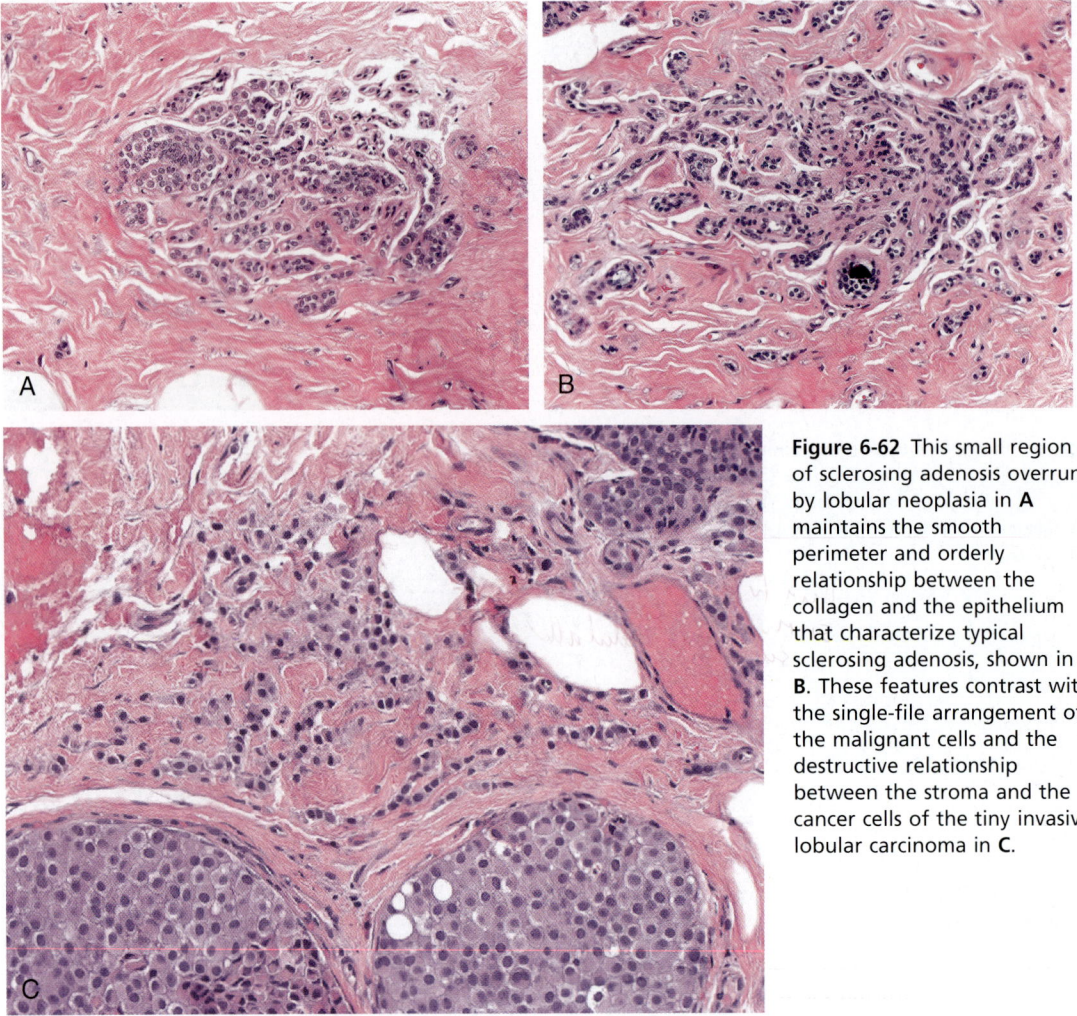

Figure 6-62 This small region of sclerosing adenosis overrun by lobular neoplasia in **A** maintains the smooth perimeter and orderly relationship between the collagen and the epithelium that characterize typical sclerosing adenosis, shown in **B**. These features contrast with the single-file arrangement of the malignant cells and the destructive relationship between the stroma and the cancer cells of the tiny invasive lobular carcinoma in **C**.

may also help to highlight the noninvasive aspects of this lesion.

Atrophy

Lobular neoplasia typically affects women late in their reproductive years, a time of life when terminal duct–lobular units appear complex. During the perimenopausal period, the lobules atrophy and so, too, it seems, do the cells of lobular neoplasia. If they persist, they usually number only a few and they sit in diminutive acini and slender ducts (Fig. 6-63). The small size of the affected structures makes it difficult to detect the neoplastic cells at low magnification; furthermore, the paucity of the cells makes it hard to discern their fundamental properties. This author cannot suggest a fail-safe way of recognizing lobular neoplasia in atrophic tissue; however, paying particular attention to subtle increases in the size of the glandular structures often allows one to spot the presence of a few extraneous epithelial cells (Fig. 6-64). Having detected a suspicious focus, one can then compare the suspect glands with uninvolved ones. Such comparisons usually enable one to establish or exclude the presence of an epithelial proliferation (Fig. 6-65). The mere presence of proliferative epithelial cells does not cement the diagnosis of lobular neoplasia. One must also evaluate the morphologic characteristics and, sometimes, the immunohistochemical characteristics of the cells. Lobular neoplasia growing in atrophic tissue exhibits the expected cytologic atypia, lack of cellular polarization, and lack of cellular cohesion, and the cells do not stain for E-cadherin.

Subclassifying lobular neoplasia becomes imprecise when the proliferation involves atrophic tissue. Most pathologists require filling and distention of at least half the acini in a lobule to make a diagnosis of lobular carcinoma in situ; lesser degrees of

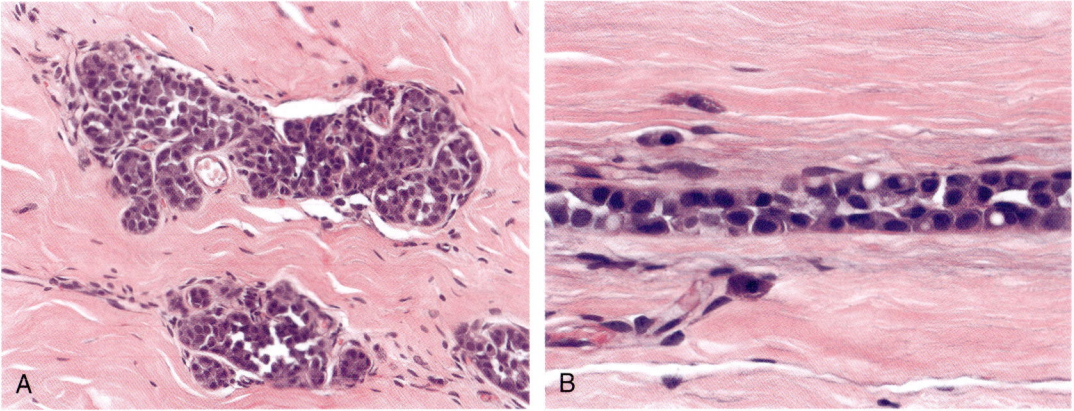

Figure 6-63 When lobular neoplasia involves atrophic breast tissue, the abnormal lobules may appear small in **A** and the ducts slender in **B**.

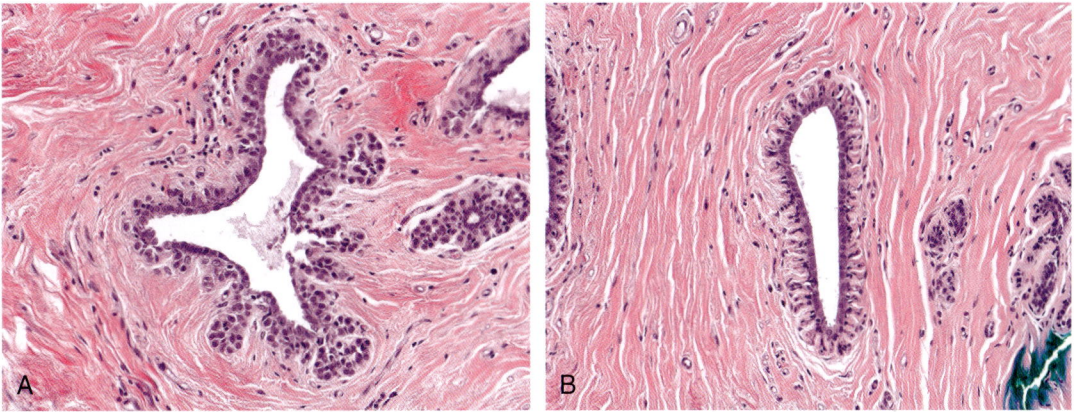

Figure 6-64 The duct in the center of **A** and the lobule to its right might not seem noteworthy until one contrasts them with normal structures in **B**.

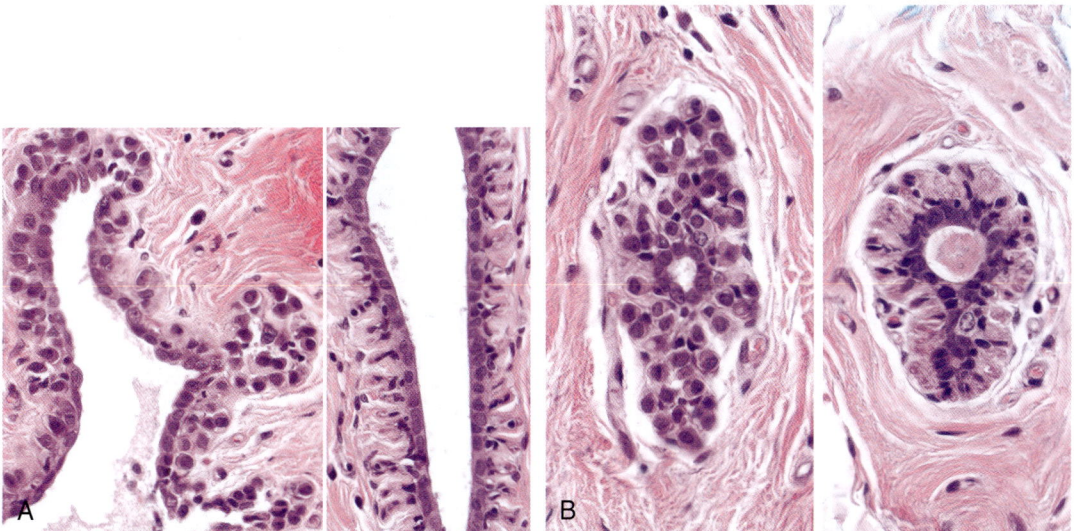

Figure 6-65 High magnification of the ducts in **A** and lobules in **B** from Figure 6-64 makes the presence of neoplastic lobular cells obvious.

proliferation merit the diagnosis of atypical lobular hyperplasia. As the lobules atrophy, the acini become so small that it takes just a few neoplastic cells to produce filling and distention of the glands. If one follows a strict interpretation of the usual criteria, foci such as the one pictured in Figure 6-63 would qualify for the diagnosis of lobular carcinoma in situ if encountered in atrophic breast tissue; however, many pathologists would make the diagnosis of atypical lobular hyperplasia for the same focus if seen in tissue from a woman in her reproductive years. Researchers have not determined whether pathologists must modify the criteria for distinguishing atypical lobular hyperplasia from lobular carcinoma in situ in the setting of atrophy. Because treatment of the patient does not usually depend on this distinction, it seems prudent to adopt a conservative approach to this situation and to require the presence of substantial distention of glands before making a diagnosis of lobular carcinoma in situ in the atrophic breast.

Atrophy takes place for other reasons than the postmenopausal loss of estrogen. Therapeutic irradiation of the breast causes massive atrophy of lobules, and administration of certain cytotoxic agents can cause subtle shrinkage in the size of the acini. Recognizing lobular neoplasia in these settings poses the same problems as those encountered in postmenopausal atrophy, and one tackles the difficulties in the same way.

Interpretation of Immunohistochemical Stains for E-cadherin

The discovery that the cells of lobular neoplasia lack E-cadherin and the development of reliable immunohistochemical staining protocols to detect the protein have given pathologists a robust technique to aid in the recognition of lobular neoplasia. The secure interpretation of the results of such staining requires knowledge of the staining properties of both normal cells and carcinomas and an understanding of the growth patterns of lobular neoplasia.

Normal mammary epithelial cells show consistent staining reactions for E-cadherin. Luminal cells throughout the gland exhibit uniform and intense staining of their cell membranes and therefore appear completely enclosed by a thick, dense, E-cadherin–positive rim. Myoepithelial cells and other cells of the basal layer, on the other hand, usually display discontinuous staining of their cell membranes, which creates a granular appearance (Fig. 6-66). The cells of lobular neoplasia fail to stain for E-cadherin, whereas ductal carcinoma cells usually show strong and continuous linear membrane staining.

Despite these straightforward and consistent characteristics, complicated staining patterns can develop when E-cadherin–negative lobular cells mingle with the variably staining benign cells or ductal carcinoma cells (Fig. 6-67). An increase in the number of myoepithelial cells, the close proximity between these cells and the neoplastic lobular cells, and structural alterations of the affected lobules complicate the interpretation of the results of E-cadherin staining, and off-center planes of section add to the confusion. In certain cases of lobular neoplasia, especially those comprising only a few neoplastic cells, the basal cells seem especially numerous. The granular staining of the basal cell membranes for E-cadherin makes it difficult to appreciate the lack of staining of the neoplastic lobular cells when the two types of cells sit in close proximity (Fig. 6-68). The author finds it useful to search for clusters, or even pairs, of suspicious cells

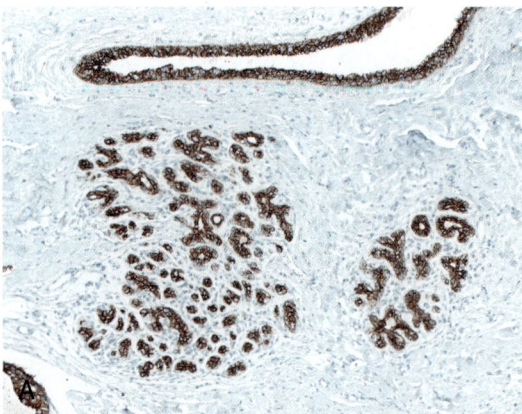

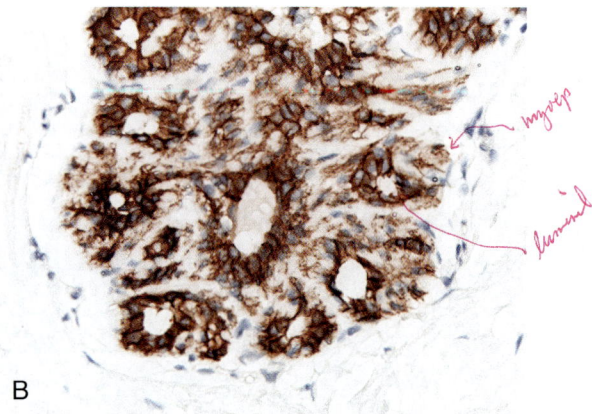

Figure 6-66 A, Luminal cells in ducts and lobules stain for E-cadherin. **B,** An off-center plane of section highlights the myoepithelial cells in this slightly developed lobule. They exhibit granular staining for E-cadherin, whereas the luminal cells display strong linear staining of their membranes.

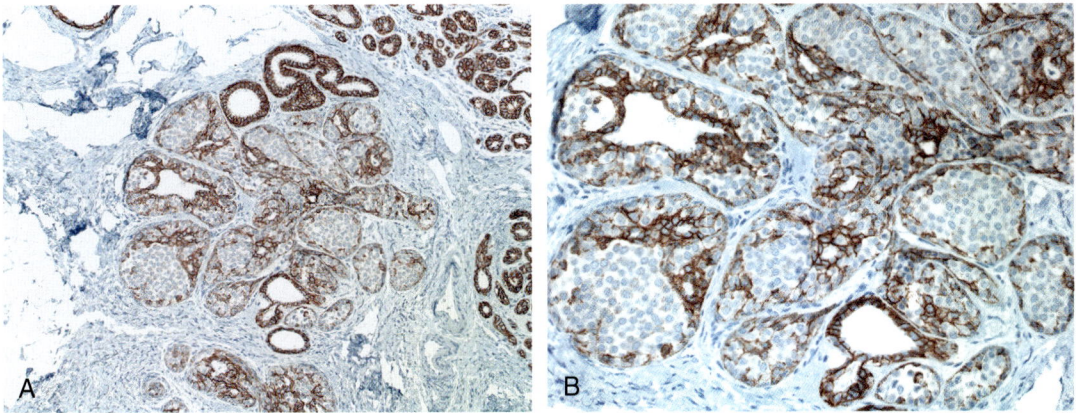

Figure 6-67 A, The intermingling of the lobular carcinoma cells and benign cells creates a complicated and confusing picture. **B,** Cells showing intense, circumferential reactivity are residual luminal cells, and those with faint, punctate staining are myoepithelial cells. The lobular carcinoma cells do not stain at all.

and to pay particular attention to the segments of the cell membranes where the atypical cells touch each other. Failure of these regions of the membranes to stain for E-cadherin provides strong evidence for the absence of the protein; in certain cases, it provides the only secure evidence of this finding. The difficulty

detecting the lack of staining of the lobular cells is not limited to cases with numerous myoepithelial cells. The same problem arises whenever the lobular cells grow as single cells or pairs dispersed within the indigenous epithelial cells. One can usually resolve these difficulties in the same way.

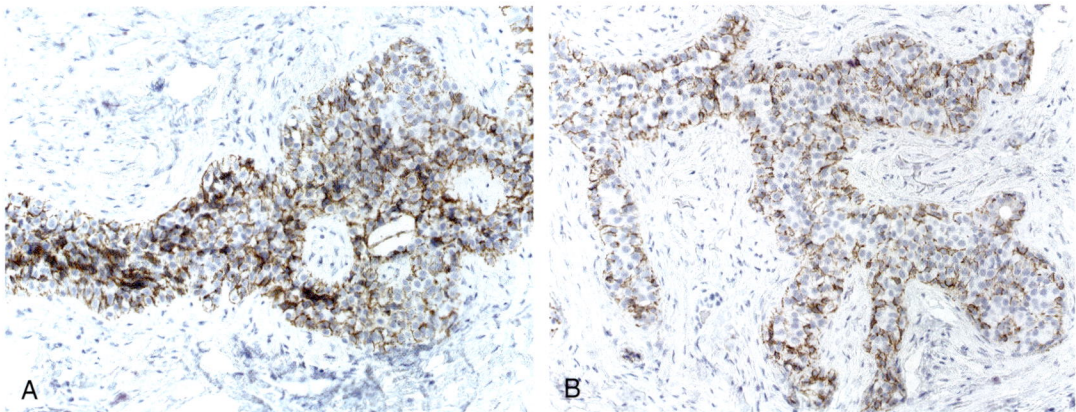

Figure 6-68 A, The large number of myoepithelial cells and the off-center plane of section make it hard to appreciate the lack of E-cadherin in the few neoplastic cells in the small duct. **B,** This more nearly central plane of section of the duct facilitates the recognition of the carcinoma cells. **C,** Attention to the apposed membranes allows one to appreciate the lack of E-cadherin staining of the neoplastic cells.

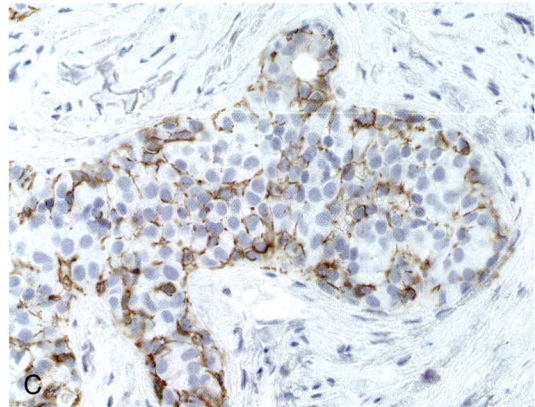

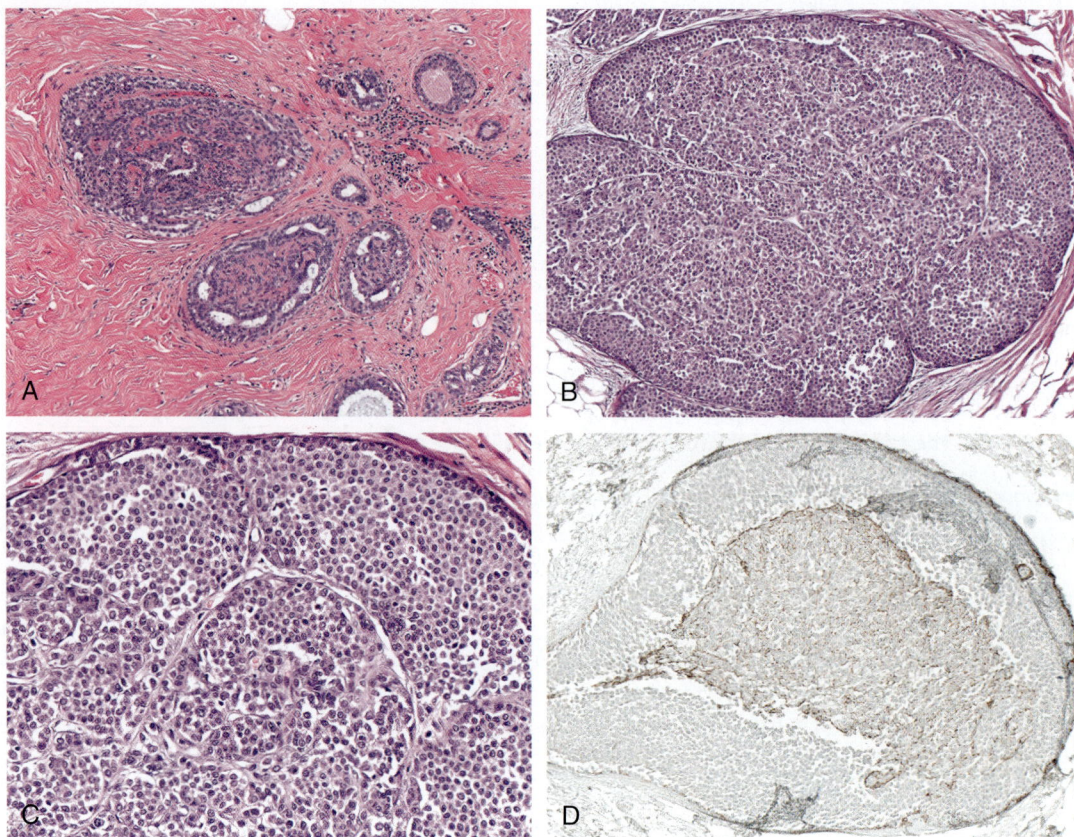

Figure 6-69 A, These two lobules show stromal and myoepithelial proliferation in their centers. When lobular neoplasia affects a lobule distorted in this way, the myoepithelial and stromal cells become engulfed by the neoplastic population in **B** and **C**, and a confusing pattern of E-cadherin staining ensues in **D.**

Distortion of lobules by unnamed benign processes can alter their structure in ways that create confusing examples of E-cadherin staining. For example, in one type of lobular alteration, proliferation of stromal cells in the center of the lobule traps the central acini in a mass of myoepithelial cells and fibroblasts. The nodule of stromal cells compresses the peripheral acini against surrounding stroma, so that they come to form a discontinuous ring of flattened tubules encircling the lobule (Fig. 6-69). When lobular neoplasia involves such a structure, the intermixed myoepithelial and stromal cells create a perplexing picture, especially in sections stained for E-cadherin. The presence of both stained and unstained cells could lead one to conclude that the carcinoma in situ exhibits both ductal and lobular features; however, careful study and correlation of the immunohistochemical results with those of the conventionally stained sections reveal the truth. The neoplastic cells fail to stain for E-cadherin, but the entrapped myoepithelial cells show their characteristic, granular staining pattern.

Pleomorphic Lobular Carcinoma In Situ

Dr. Haagensen's observation that neoplastic lobular cells sometimes appear slightly pleomorphic did not seem to disconcert pathologists, but these same observers apparently refused to believe that cells of lobular neoplasia could display marked pleomorphism. Consequently, throughout the second half of the twentieth century, pathologists dutifully classified all pleomorphic mammary carcinomas as ductal even though the other cellular attributes of certain cases seemed more in keeping with cells of a lobular nature. The belief that all pleomorphic mammary carcinomas have a ductal nature has finally disappeared, first for invasive carcinomas, then for noninvasive ones, and pathologists now accept the notion that the cells of lobular carcinoma in situ can exhibit marked pleomorphism. Despite the acceptance of this belief, microscopists have yet to define criteria to distinguish pleomorphic lobular carcinoma in situ from the Haagensen type B variety of conventional lobular carcinoma in situ (Fig. 6-70).

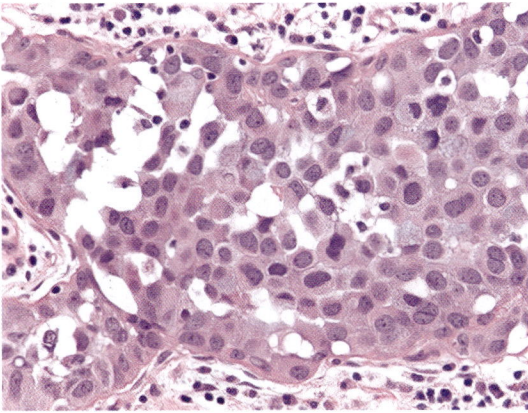

Figure 6-70 Do these neoplastic lobular cells display sufficient pleomorphism to merit the diagnosis of pleomorphic lobular carcinoma?

This author cannot fill this void, although the presence of central necrosis, calcified cellular debris, or frequent mitotic figures in a lobular carcinoma showing only modest pleomorphism would probably lead

him to classify the proliferation as pleomorphic lobular carcinoma in situ rather than Haagensen type B lobular carcinoma in situ.

E-cadherin–Negative High-Grade Carcinoma In Situ

Distinguishing pleomorphic lobular carcinoma in situ from high-grade ductal carcinoma in situ can pose a difficult problem. In the proper context, failure of the cells to express E-cadherin probably serves as reliable evidence of a lobular nature; however, the current thinking may have taken this idea to an extreme. Many pathologists classify all high-grade carcinomas lacking E-cadherin as lobular despite the observation that ductal carcinomas can lose expression of E-cadherin. A more nuanced position might allow that E-cadherin–negative high-grade carcinomas in situ can have either a lobular or a ductal nature. For examples, certain E-cadherin–negative high-grade carcinomas in situ coexist with a conventional lobular carcinoma (Fig. 6-71).

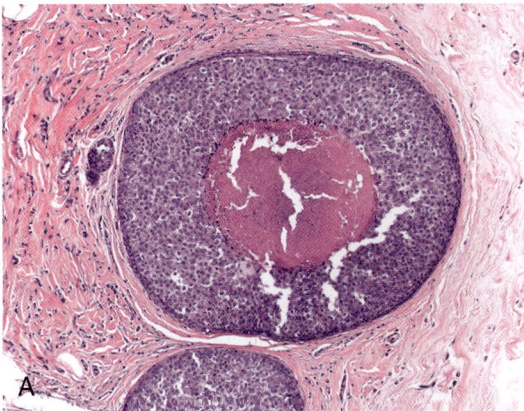

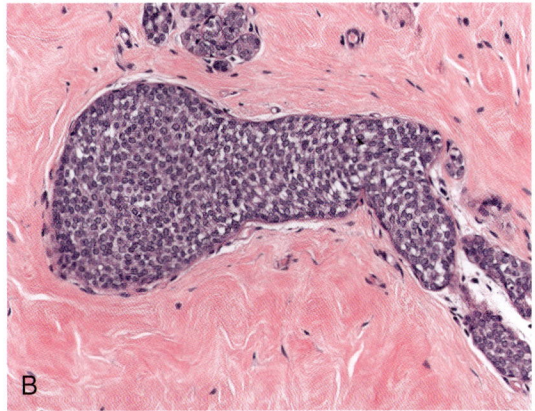

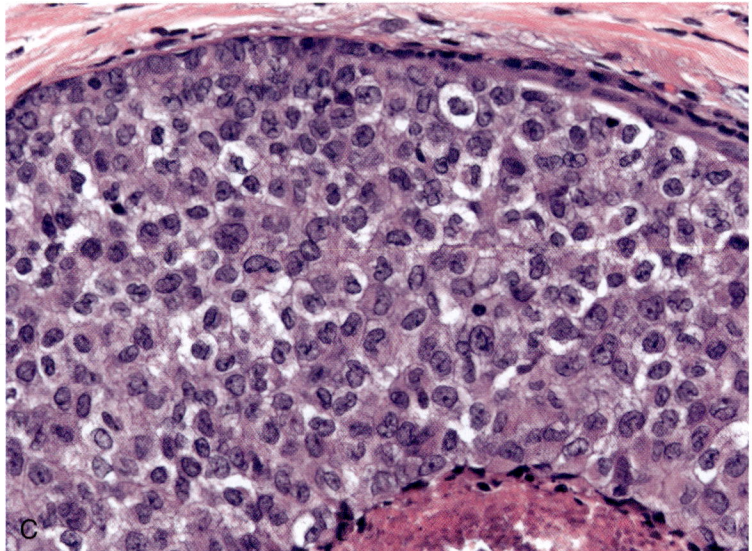

Figure 6-71 A, This E-cadherin–negative high-grade carcinoma coexists with conventional invasive lobular carcinoma and lobular carcinoma in situ in **B. C,** The neoplastic cells appear larger than conventional neoplastic lobular cells and their nuclei vary in shape; they contain finely dispersed chromatin, nucleoli of a noticeable size, and fragile foamy cytoplasm.

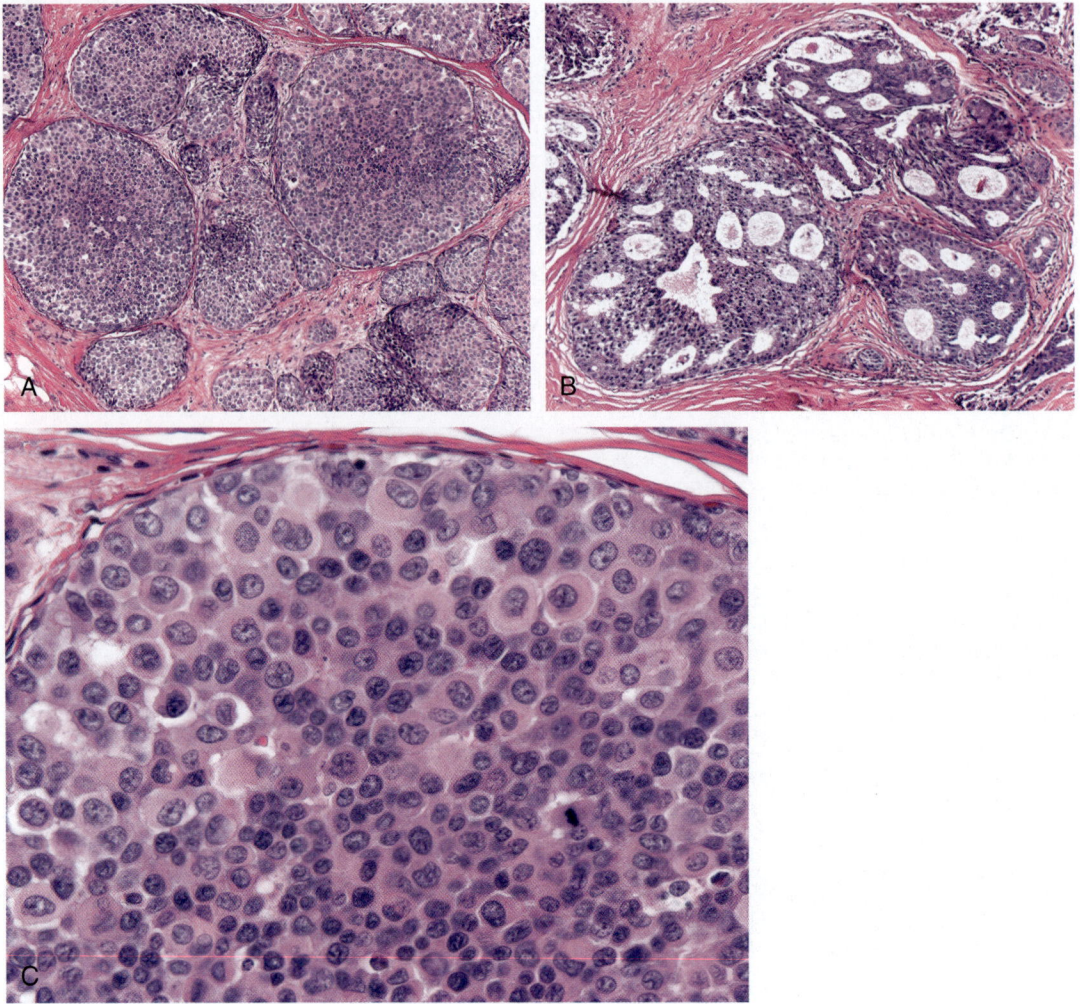

Figure 6-72 A, This E-cadherin—negative high-grade carcinoma coexists with conventional ductal carcinoma in situ, as shown in **B. C,** The cells growing in a solid pattern possess dense, eosinophilic cytoplasm, clearly defined cell borders, nuclei of varying size and shape, clumpy chromatin, and large nucleoli.

These occurrences probably represent genuine lobular neoplasia displaying a spectrum of atypia. Other E-cadherin—negative high-grade carcinomas merge with clear-cut ductal carcinomas, which stain for E-cadherin (Fig. 6-72). These E-cadherin—negative carcinomas probably represent ductal carcinomas that have abandoned expression of the protein. Cases such as the one pictured in Figure 6-73 may illustrate an intermediate stage in this phenomenon. Pathologists may wish to consider the possibility that E-cadherin—negative high-grade carcinomas in situ can have either a lobular or a ductal nature. Experience recounted in the literature and clinical practice indicate that invasive carcinomas do exist with E-cadherin—negative high-grade carcinomas in situ more frequently than with corresponding low-grade carcinomas in situ. Pathologists would do well to keep this observation in mind when examining E-cadherin—negative high-grade carcinomas, because the foci of invasion sometimes consist of just a few cells, which can escape detection easily.

Distinction from Atypical Lobular Hyperplasia

Pathologists tend to think of atypical hyperplasia as a type of neoplastic proliferation composed of cells

Figure 6-73 A, This carcinoma forms cribriform spaces and dishesive sheets. The cells with glandular features express E-cadherin at low levels in **B,** and the dishesive cells show only focal, weak staining for the molecule in **C.**

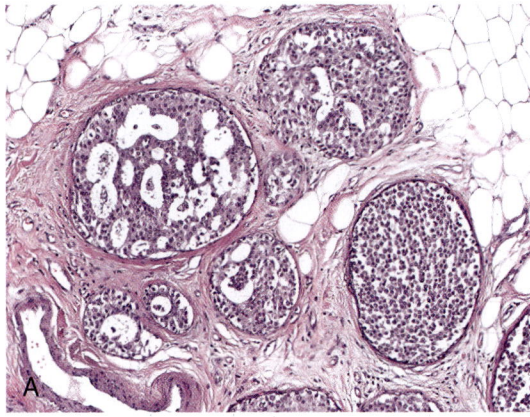

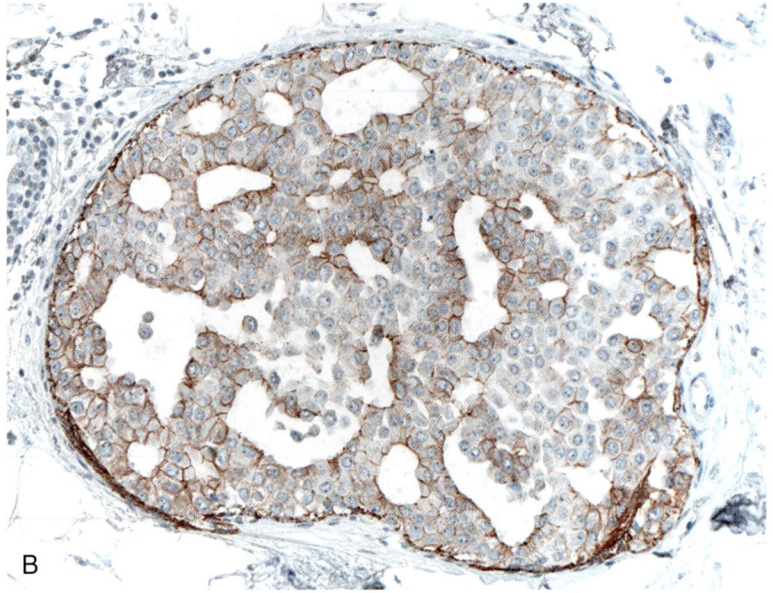

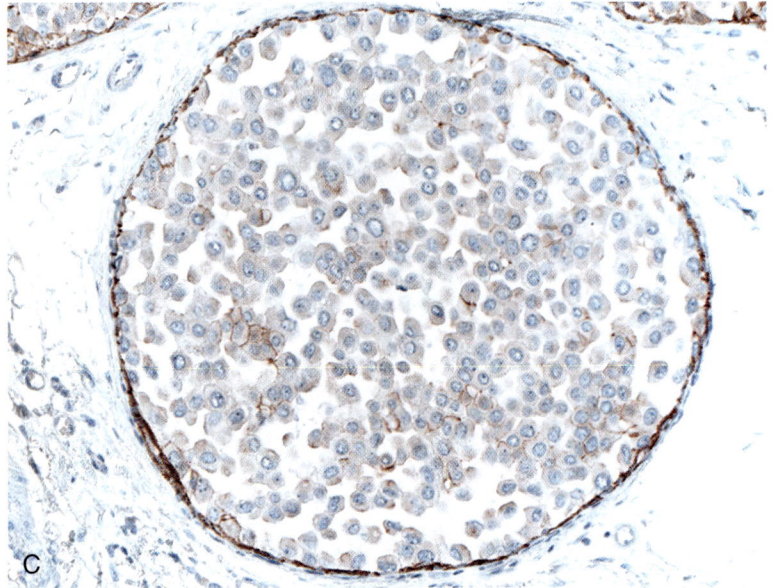

lacking fully malignant characteristics. According to this concept, atypical hyperplasia occupies an intermediate position in the morphologic continuum linking normal cells with malignant ones, and the cells of atypical hyperplasia differ in certain, still undefined, properties from both their normal and their malignant counterparts. The current classification of lobular neoplasia takes a different approach, one based on the quantity of the neoplastic cells. The commonly used definition of lobular carcinoma in situ requires that the characteristic cells constitute the entire epithelial population in a terminal duct–lobular unit, fill all the acini in the lobule, and expand or distort at least half of them. Less extensive involvement merits the diagnosis of atypical lobular hyperplasia. According to this formulation, the cells appear identical in both lesions; only their numbers differ, and atypical lobular hyperplasia represents a miniature form of lobular carcinoma in situ.

Perhaps one should take a more fluid approach to this distinction. Pathologists may wish to take into account factors such as the clinical practice of the treating physicians, the nature of the specimen, and the extent of involvement in relation to the size of the specimen when evaluating ambiguous examples. For instance, one might prefer the diagnosis of lobular carcinoma in situ for a borderline lesion detected in a core biopsy specimen if such a diagnosis would provoke an excision and the diagnosis of atypical lobular hyperplasia would not. On the other hand, one might favor the diagnosis of atypical lobular hyperplasia for an identical borderline lesion if it represents the only collection of neoplastic cells in an excision specimen of substantial size. Such an approach would conflict with the philosophy of certain procrustean physicians; thus, one cannot advocate its general use. For certain pathologists, it offers a nuanced way of dealing with the currently inescapable uncertainties in the evaluation of lobular neoplasia. Molecular studies hint at genetic differences between atypical lobular hyperplasia and lobular carcinoma in situ. Confirmation of these results and determination of their clinical implications might lead to a clinically meaningful way of stratifying forms of lobular neoplasia.

Detection of Invasion

All practicing pathologists have firsthand experience with the difficulties in detecting small foci of invasive lobular carcinoma. The author can offer just a few, seemingly self-evident, tips to help with this problem. First, having established a diagnosis of lobular neoplasia, a wise pathologist will look at all the sections again, paying close attention to the stroma. When examining breast tissue, most pathologists instinctively focus on the glandular tissue, and the presence of a diagnostically difficult epithelial proliferation only encourages this instinct. As a result, the stroma can remain only superficially examined, and foci of invasive carcinoma can go undetected. To avoid this error, a seasoned pathologist consciously and conscientiously inspects the stroma in all cases showing lobular neoplasia.

Second, when searching for foci of invasion, one should pay particular attention to even subtle increases in stromal cellularity (Fig. 6-74). Viewed at

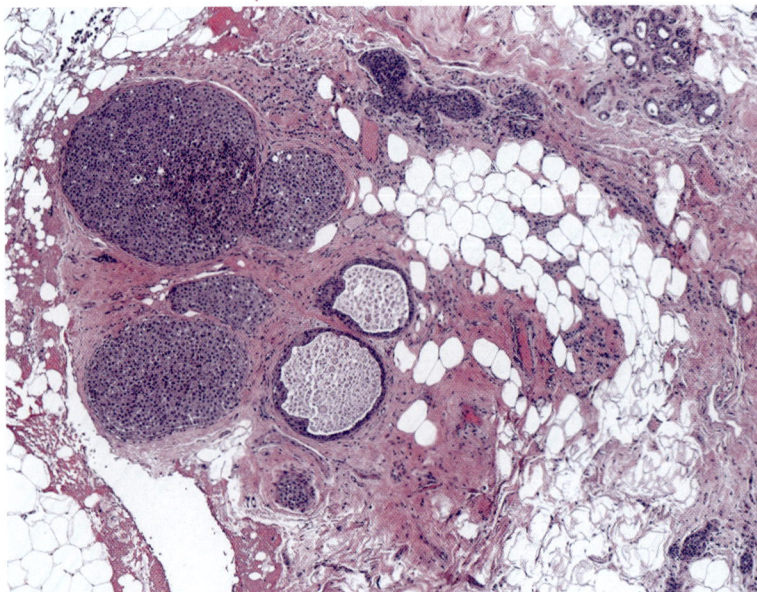

Figure 6-74 Attention to the noninvasive carcinoma could distract one from the presence of the few invasive cells in the neighboring stroma.

low magnifications tiny regions of invasive lobular carcinoma can resemble pseudoangiomatous stromal hyperplasia, fat necrosis, nonspecific chronic inflammation, and the healing reaction to an earlier procedure. It seems unwise to assume that a benign process such as these accounts for the presence of extra cells in the stroma in tissue harboring lobular neoplasia. Many times, benign changes such as these explain the cellularity of the foci, but inspection at high magnification and the liberal use of immunohistochemical staining for keratin ensure that one will not overlook a miniscule focus of invasive lobular carcinoma.

Third, when studying tissue resected from the region of a recent procedure, one should look with special suspicion upon foci separated from the site of the procedure in which the stroma looks hypercellular. The inflammatory reaction and granulation tissue formation resulting from the prior procedure usually form a continuous zone surrounding the operative site. Regions of cellular stroma distant from the reactive tissue and separated from it by unaltered breast tissue should always provoke careful study. Finally, pleomorphic lobular carcinomas in situ frequently invade the stroma, so one must remain especially alert when examining these high-grade carcinomas.

Besides failing to detect small nests of invasive lobular cells, pathologists can overlook invasive lobular carcinoma when the cells grow in round nests. This growth pattern, termed *alveolar*, simulates the appearance of lobular carcinoma in situ (Fig. 6-75). Although the round nests of carcinoma cells do look like acini distended by neoplastic cells, the arrangement of the clusters does not duplicate the structure of a lobule. Thus, the low-magnification appearance provides the best tool for avoiding this mistake and one can evaluate one's impression by carrying out immunohistochemical staining for myoepithelial cells.

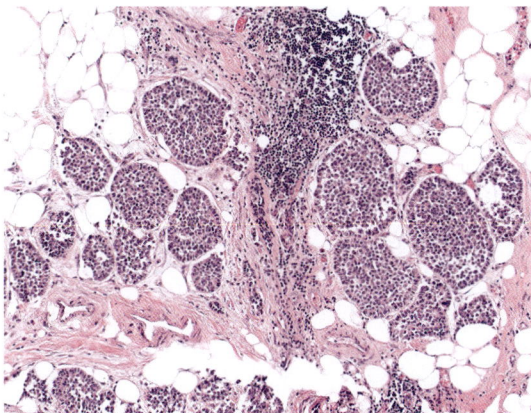

Figure 6-75 These well-defined, globular nests of invasive lobular carcinoma could pass for lobular carcinoma in situ, but the lack of a lobular arrangement announces their invasive nature.

Selected Readings

Abdel-Fatah TM, Powe DG, Hodi A, et al: High frequency coexistence of columnar cell lesion, lobular neoplasia, and low-grade ductal carcinoma in situ with invasive tubular carcinoma and invasive lobular carcinoma. Am J Surg Pathol 2007;31:417-426.

Acs G, Lawton TJ, Rebbeck TR, et al: Differential expression of E-cadherin in lobular and ductal neoplasms of the breast and its biologic and diagnostic implications. Am J Clin Pathol 2001;115:85-98.

Bànkfalvi À, Terpe H-J, Breukelmann D, et al: Immunophenotypic and prognostic analysis of E-cadherin and β-catenin expression during breast carcinogenesis and tumour progression: A comparative study with CD44. Histopathology 1999;34:25-34.

Bentz JS, Yassa N, Clayton F: Pleomorphic lobular carcinoma of the breast: Clinicopathologic features of 12 cases. Mod Pathol 1998;11:814-822.

Bratthauer GL, Tavassoli FA: Lobular intraepithelial neoplasia: Previously unexplored aspects assessed in 775 cases and their clinical implications. Virchows Arch 2002;440:134-138.

De Leeuw WJ, Berx G, Vos CB, et al: Simultaneous loss of E-cadherin and catenins in invasive lobular breast cancer and lobular carcinoma in situ. J Pathol 1997;183:404-411.

Fadare O, Dadmanesh F, Alvarado-Cabrero I, et al: Lobular intraepithelial neoplasia [lobular carcinoma in situ] with comedo-type necrosis: A clinicopathologic study of 18 cases. Am J Surg Pathol 2006;30:1445-1453.

Fechner RE: Lobular carcinoma in situ in sclerosing adenosis: A potential source of confusion with invasive carcinoma. Am J Surg Pathol 1981;5:233-239.

Foote FW, Stewart FW: Lobular carcinoma in situ: A rare form of mammary cancer. Am J Pathol 1941;17:491-495.

Goldstein NS, Bassi D, Watts JC, et al: E-cadherin reactivity of 95 noninvasive ductal and lobular lesions of the breast: Implications for the interpretation of problematic lesions. Am J Clin Pathol 2001;115:534-542.

Haagensen CD, Lane N, Lattes R, et al: Lobular neoplasia (so-called lobular carcinoma in situ) of the breast. Cancer 1978;42:737-769.

Jacobs TW, Pliss N, Kouria G, et al: Carcinoma in situ of the breast with indeterminate features: Role of E-cadherin staining in categorization. Am J Surg Pathol 2001;25:229-236.

Lerwill MF: The evolution of lobular neoplasia. Adv Anat Pathol 2006;13:157-165.

Lu YJ, Osin P, Lakhani SR, et al: Comparative genomic hybridization analysis of lobular carcinoma in situ and atypical lobular hyperplasia and potential roles for gains and losses of genetic material in breast neoplasia. Cancer Res 1998;58:4721-4727.

Mastracci TL, Shadeo A, Colby SM, et al: Genomic alteration in lobular neoplasia: A microarray comparative genomic hybridization signature for early neoplastic proliferation in the breast. Genes Chromosomes Cancer 2006;45:1007-1017.

Mastracci TL, Tjan S, Bane A, et al: E-cadherin alterations in atypical lobular hyperplasia and lobular carcinoma in situ of the breast. Mod Pathol 2005;18:741-751.

Morandi L, Marucci G, Foschini MP, et al: Genetic similarities and differences between lobular in situ neoplasia (LN) and invasive lobular carcinoma of the breast. Virchows Arch 2006;449:14-23.

Page DL, Kidd TE Jr, Dupont WD, et al: Lobular neoplasia of the breast: Higher risk for subsequent invasive cancer predicted by more extensive disease. Hum Pathol 1991;22:1232-1239.

Reis-Filho JS, Simpson PT, Jones C, et al: Pleomorphic lobular carcinoma in situ: Role of comprehensive molecular pathology in characterization of an entity. J Pathol 2005;207:1-13.

Resetkova E, Albarracin C, Sneige N: Collagenous spherulosis of breast: Morphologic study of 59 cases and review of the literature. Am J Surg Pathol 2006;30:20-27.

Rosen PP, Lieberman PH, Braun DW Jr, et al: Lobular carcinoma in situ of the breast: Detailed analysis of 99 patients with average follow-up of 24 years. Am J Surg Pathol 1978;2:225-251.

Sgroi D, Koerner FC: Involvement of collagenous spherulosis by lobular carcinoma in situ: Potential confusion with cribriform ductal carcinoma in situ. Am J Surg Pathol 1995;19:1366-1370.

Vos CB, Cleton-Jansen AM, Berx G, et al: E-cadherin inactivation in lobular carcinoma in situ of the breast: An early event in tumorigenesis. Br J Cancer 1997;76:1131-1133.

Part
II

PAPILLARY PROLIFERATIONS

7

Concepts Basic to the Analysis of Papillary Proliferations

Papillary lesions form two distinct groups distinguished, in part, by their size: large papillary neoplasms and ductal epithelial proliferations growing as microscopic papillary tufts. The distinction between these two categories seems obvious to most, but a few observations help illustrate the differences. Large, or macropapillary, tumors (Fig. 7-1) manifest as discrete, individual structures, evident on macroscopic examination and usually numbering no more than a few in a specimen. They grow as warty masses, often attached to only one portion of the duct wall, and they consist of epithelium, stroma, and blood vessels. The small, or micropapillary, proliferations (Fig. 7-2) consist of hundreds or thousands of minuscule papillary tufts that are invisible to the naked eye, each cluster containing a relatively small number of cells. These micropapillae usually consist only of epithelial cells, although uncommon examples do have stromal cores. Micropapillary proliferations usually merge with other, more common forms of ductal epithelial proliferation. Micropapillary hyperplasia blends with usual ductal hyperplasia, and micropapillary ductal carcinoma in situ coexists with cribriform ductal carcinoma in situ.

The separation of papillary lesions into macropapillary and micropapillary categories, by itself, does not establish a diagnosis, because both groups contain both benign and malignant members. One makes this distinction mainly because the two groups of papillary lesions display different clinicopathologic characteristics, and the approaches to diagnosis of the two groups differ.

PROPERTIES OF MACROPAPILLARY TUMORS

The diagnosis of macropapillary tumors begins with an assessment of three features: the geometric characteristics of the fronds, the amount of the

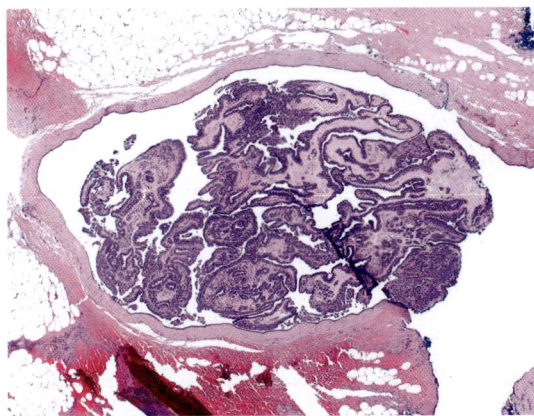

Figure 7-1 One could detect this macropapillary tumor with the naked eye. The single nodule consists of many types of cells.

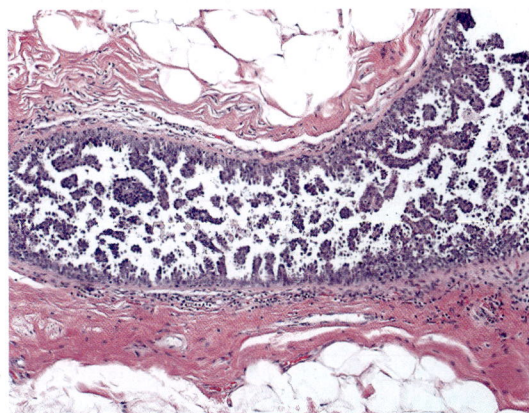

Figure 7-2 One would not detect this micropapillary proliferation during a macroscopic examination. It consists of innumerable papillary tufts composed almost exclusively of epithelial cells.

stroma, and the cellular characteristics of the epithelium (Box 7-1). By evaluating these three aspects of a lesion and integrating the information elucidated by the evaluation, pathologists can readily classify the majority of large papillary tumors. Additional pathologic processes, such as scarring and epithelial proliferation, alter the appearance of these fundamental features and thereby complicate the analysis; nevertheless, consideration of these three attributes forms the backbone of the diagnosis of macropapillary tumors.

Fundamental Characteristics

Geometric Characteristics of the Fronds

Pathologists have not established a precise definition of the term *frond*; nevertheless, most observers intuitively understand the meaning of this designation for the subunits of papillary neoplasms. Because the formation of fronds represents a defining characteristic of these lesions, the structural attributes of the fronds reflect the nature of the neoplasm; thus, studying the structural attributes of these structures gives the pathologist valuable diagnostic information. One should estimate the number of fronds, study their size and shape, determine the extent of variation of these two properties, and evaluate the arrangement of the fronds. Papillomas consist of just a few fronds, generally similar in size and shape, that fit together neatly; in contrast, most papillary carcinomas contain many fronds of greatly varying configuration, which form a shaggy, disorderly mass. Only rarely do papillary tumors deviate from this generalization, so an assessment of these geometric characteristics, evident at even low magnification, gives the pathologist a solid start in establishing the diagnosis of a papillary neoplasm.

Amount of Stroma

Papillary tumors vary in the quantity of stroma that they contain; papillomas contain copious collagen, whereas carcinomas do not contain as much. One would find it impractical to measure the amount of stroma, but estimating the ratio of stroma to epithelium offers an easily performed and reliable surrogate marker. The typical papilloma contains at least as much stroma as epithelium and often much more. In the commonplace papillary carcinoma, the epithelium overwhelms the stroma, creating the impression that the collagen exists only to support the neoplastic epithelial cells. One can appreciate this difference in the ratio of stroma to epithelium in most uncomplicated cases; however, epithelial proliferations of several types overrun papillomas, and the superimposition of these processes makes it impossible to determine the proportions of stroma and epithelium

> **Box 7-1**
>
> Features of primary importance in the analysis of papillary tumors:
>
> - Geometric characteristics of the fronds
> - Amount of the stroma
> - Cellular characteristics of the epithelium

present before the epithelial cells are multiplied. Thus, one must remain alert to the presence of superimposed epithelial proliferation when evaluating the amount of stroma in a papillary tumor.

Characteristics of the Epithelium

The characteristics of the neoplastic epithelial cells establish the nature of a papillary tumor. When examining the epithelial cells, pathologists must take note of two aspects of the population: the number of layers of cells, and the cytologic features of the epithelial cells. A normally structured, two-layered ductular epithelium composed of benign luminal and myoepithelial cells covers the fronds of the usual papilloma. Proliferation of either the epithelial or myoepithelial cells alters the structure of the epithelium; however, in the absence of a superimposed proliferation, the epithelium of a papilloma consists of two layers of cells and two types of cells, and neither type of cell appears atypical. The neoplastic epithelium of a papillary carcinoma, on the other hand, consists entirely of malignant ductal cells, which can grow in any number of layers. Like the malignant cells in other forms of ductal carcinoma, those that compose papillary carcinomas exhibit cytologic features of malignancy. Most often this atypia appears low to intermediate grade, but occasional papillary carcinomas exhibit a higher level of anaplasia.

Ancillary Characteristics

When confronted with papillary tumors exhibiting unusual patterns or combinations of processes or when seeking evidence to buttress a diagnosis based on the fundamental findings, pathologists find that consideration of three ancillary aspects of the tumor and examination of the epithelium apart from the lesion usually provide the needed diagnostic evidence (Box 7-2). The three ancillary features are the level of mitotic activity, the presence of dishesion, and the pattern of calcification. Although both papillomas and papillary carcinomas can show mitotic activity, papillary carcinomas contain division figures more frequently and in greater numbers than papillomas. The epithelial cells of papillomas stick together

Papillomas - Stroma

tightly, whereas those of carcinomas do not. Calcium precipitates in the stroma of papillomas and in the glandular lumens of carcinomas.

Examination of the epithelium apart from the lesion often helps because the epithelial cells of papillary tumors frequently cover the walls of the ducts harboring the papillary tumor and sometimes extend into the adjoining ducts and lobules. Because cellular proliferations in these locations lack the architectural complexities introduced by the underlying papillary architecture, their diagnosis can proceed according to the criteria and approach set forth for conventional ductal epithelial proliferations. One must restrict the examination to epithelial cells in ducts within a few millimeters of the papillary tumor, of course; the farther away one ventures, the less likely it becomes that a coexisting epithelial proliferation represents the same process as the papillary tumor.

PROPERTIES OF MICROPAPILLARY PROLIFERATIONS

Micropapillary proliferations do not constitute distinct entities. As members of the family of ductal proliferations, they represent either conventional ductal hyperplasia or ductal carcinoma in situ growing in a flat and filiform architecture. When ductal cells multiply in the usual, fenestrated pattern, they pile on top of one another, fill the lumen, and distend the gland. In micropapillary lesions, the cells do not stratify extensively; rather than piling up, they grow in just a few layers. To accommodate this expanding sheet of cells without impinging on the lumen of the gland, the diameter of the structure must increase. Modest increases in the numbers of cells lead to only a modest increase in the diameter of the duct, whereas substantial cellular proliferation enlarges the duct to a much greater extent.

The cells do not grow only as a flat sheet. In independent, scattered foci, the epithelial cells pile up, and these heaps of cells constitute the micropapillae. If the expansion of the proliferative population takes place in an orderly and regulated fashion, the micropapillae appear uniform in both distribution and structure features, but poorly regulated and uncoordinated cellular proliferation gives rise to variability in the placement and architecture of the papillary tufts. In addition to determining the extent of glandular enlargement and the structure of the micropapillae, the fundamental nature of the cells determines their cytologic characteristics. Hyperplastic ductal cells demonstrate marked cohesion, lack nuclear atypia, and undergo maturation. Malignant ductal cells demonstrate the opposite characteristics; they lack cohesion, exhibit atypia, and fail to mature.

Fundamental Characteristics

Building on the preceding ideas, one can formulate the following five properties that allow one to classify micropapillary proliferations: the extent of glandular distention, the size and configuration of the micropapillae, the contents of the gland lumen, the cytologic characteristics of the proliferative cells, and the presence of maturation (Box 7-3).

Extent of Glandular Distention

Micropapillary lesions distend the glands in which they grow without filling them with cells. Pathologists often fail to consider this finding, in part because slight amounts of distention do not attract their attention. Many observers find it helpful to turn to nearby uninvolved structures as a reference point. By contrasting the diameters of normal-appearing glands with those of glands harboring a micropapillary proliferation, one can easily gauge the extent of glandular enlargement. Micropapillary hyperplasia causes only modest distention of the glands, whereas micropapillary carcinoma usually enlarges them greatly.

Size and Configuration of the Micropapillae

Size and configuration of the micropapillae refer to the variability in the structural characteristics of the micropapillae. The orderly and regulated growth of hyperplastic ductal cells imparts uniformity to the papillary tufts, whereas the disorganized proliferation of carcinoma cells results in obvious variation in the size and configuration of the papillary structures.

Contents of the Gland Lumen

The contents of glands harboring micropapillary growths offer a window on the cohesive properties of the proliferative cells. Firmly bound to one another, cohesive hyperplastic cells do not slough into the lumen. Dishesive carcinoma cells, on the other hand, separate from their neighbors and fall into the duct, where they degenerate. In doing so, they create the "dirty background" familiar to cytopathologists. Thus, dying cells and cellular debris collect in the lumens of glands overtaken by micropapillary carcinoma.

Cytologic Characteristics of the Proliferative Cells

The cytologic characteristics of micropapillary proliferations identify the nature of the cells, and this property represents the most persuasive of the five properties used to evaluate micropapillary lesions. Benign ductal cells growing in a micropapillary architecture display the cellular characteristics of conventional ductal hyperplasia, whereas those of micropapillary ductal carcinoma in situ look like the malignant cells in other types of ductal carcinoma. No matter what other findings a micropapillary lesion might show, one cannot consider it malignant if the cells display cellular characteristics of benign cells. In most cases of micropapillary ductal carcinoma in situ, the cells demonstrate only low-grade atypia, so one must evaluate the remaining properties of the population to substantiate or to exclude a diagnosis of malignancy. Rare micropapillary proliferations consist of such obviously anaplastic cells that one can make the diagnosis of carcinoma without regard to other diagnostic elements.

Presence of Maturation

Micropapillary proliferations provide pathologists with some of the best opportunities to master the morphologic manifestations of the phenomenon of maturation, one of the fundamental concepts in the analysis of ductal proliferations discussed in Chapter 2. The formation of slender micropapillary structures makes it easy to evaluate the cytologic properties of the cells at different positions with the papillae. Pathologists will find it

Box 7-3

Criteria for the analysis of micropapillary proliferations:

- Extent of glandular distention
- Size and configuration of the micropapillae
- Contents of the duct lumen
- Cytologic characteristics of the proliferative cells
- Presence of maturation

especially illustrative to compare the features of the cells at the tips of the micropapillae with those of the cells near the basement membranes. When present in a micropapillary lesion, the phenomenon of maturation usually stands out clearly. Most benign micropapillary lesions demonstrate this pattern, but malignant lesions do not.

Selected Readings

Azzopardi JG: Problems in Breast Pathology. (Major Problems in Pathology, vol 11.) London, WB Saunders, 1979.

Kraus FT, Neubecker RD: The differential diagnosis of papillary tumors of the breast. Cancer 1962;15:444-455.

Murad TM, Contesso G, Mourisesse H: Papillary tumors of large lactiferous ducts. Cancer 1981;48:122-133.

Ohuchi N, Abe R, Kasai M: Possible cancerous change of intraductal papillomas of the breast: A 3-D reconstruction study of 25 cases. Cancer 1984;54:605-611.

Oyama T, Koerner FC: Noninvasive papillary proliferations. Semin Diagn Pathol 2004;21:32-41.

Sapino A, Botta G, Cassoni P, et al: Multiple papillomas of the breast: Morphologic findings and clinical evolution. Anat Pathol 1996;1:205-218.

8

Papilloma

DEFINITIONS AND CLINICOPATHOLOGIC CHARACTERISTICS

Papillomas are neoplasms formed from mammary glandular tissue and stroma. We do not know whether the cellular alterations that give rise to papillomas affect the glandular cells, the stromal cells, or both; however, one can easily see that both types of tissue proliferate during the formation of the lesion. Papillomas arise in the walls of ducts, and the resulting tumor usually protrudes into the lumen. If the growing mass does not impinge on the lumen or if the neoplasm originates outside the wall of the duct, the nodule develops the features of a variant of a papilloma.

Papillomas can arise at any point in the ductal system, but they show a predilection for its extremes, the lactiferous sinuses and the terminal ductules. Central papillomas usually arise singly, whereas the small duct (peripheral) papillomas typically occur in clusters (Fig. 8-1). Tumors involving the large ducts look like genuine neoplastic masses, but careful study of small duct papillomas shows that certain of them might arise through a process of lobular sclerosis and distortion rather than growth of a tumor within a small duct. About three-quarters of patients with central papillomas complain of a nipple discharge, whereas women with small duct papillomas usually either describe a mass or do not report any symptoms. Tumors in both locations display identical histologic characteristics.

If one wishes to preserve the clinical and pathologic purity of lesions classified as papillomas, one must maintain a strict definition of the entity. One should restrict the diagnosis to neoplasms composed of glands and stroma arising from the wall of a duct. Artifacts of tissue sectioning and perturbations in the relationships between the glands and the stroma can result in foci that superficially resemble papillomas. For example, when sectioned in certain planes, small lobules can seem to protrude into ducts, especially if the latter have become dilated. One should not classify such foci as papillomas. Enlargement of acini sometimes brings them into a back-to-back arrangement, and the delicate bands of entrapped stroma seem to form a papillary skeleton. Lobules altered in this way do not represent papillomas, either. In a phenomenon known as *unfolding of the lobule*, distention and coalescence of the outermost acini of a lobule form a space that resembles a small duct, and entrapment of strands of intralobular stroma creates a branching stromal structure that looks like the framework of a papilloma. This process, which probably represents a variation of the acinar distention seen in flat epithelial atypia, accounts for the formation of many small duct papillomas.

The frequent coexistence of papillomas and ductal carcinoma in situ raises the question of a causal link between the two. Many of the most eminent physicians of the 19th century, for example, believed that breast cancers typically arise from papillomas. By the middle of the 20th century, the common thinking

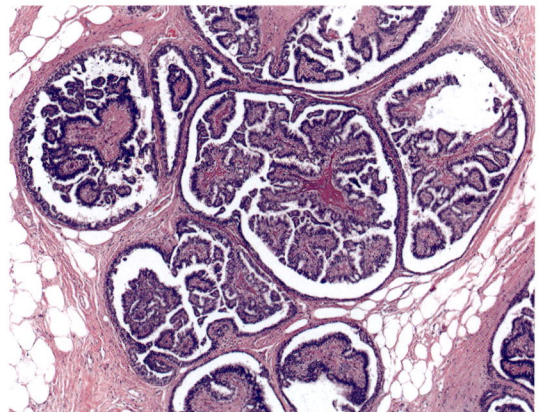

Figure 8-1 A cluster of small papillomas occupies a region of the terminal ductal tree.

had swung to the opposite point of view, so most contemporary physicians regard papillomas as completely innocuous. Early studies of the relationship between papillomas and carcinoma suffer from many problems that limit the interpretation of the results, but modern investigations have consistently shown that women with papillomas face a slightly higher risk for the development of invasive carcinoma than women without papilloma. Evidence of several types suggests that the higher risk applies mostly to patients with multiple papillomas. For example, one finds microscopic foci of ductal carcinoma in situ in about a quarter of breast specimens containing papillomas, most commonly cases of multiple, peripheral papillomas, and women with multiple papillomas develop carcinomas more frequently than women with single papillomas. The notion that the unfolding of the lobule that gives rise to small duct papillomas represents a form of atypical ductal proliferations offers a rationale for the association between multiple small duct papillomas and ductal carcinoma in situ.

At the macroscopic level, a papilloma looks like a verrucous mass protruding from a portion of the wall of a duct. The mass distends the duct and usually fills it, and accumulation of serous fluid can enlarge the duct further to create a partly cystic lesion. Infarction, hemorrhage, and scarring commonly occur and alter the usual macroscopic characteristics in obvious ways.

HISTOLOGIC CHARACTERISTICS

Fundamental Characteristics

Geometric Properties of the Fronds

Low magnification shows that the fronds of a papilloma are few in number and display polygonal shapes with broad and blunt configurations (Fig. 8-2). The term *broad* refers to the observation that the two dimensions of an individual frond do not vary by more than a factor of four or five, and the designation *blunt* describes the smooth overall contour of the frond. Furthermore, the facing sides of adjacent fronds usually run parallel to each other. Because of this molding of the fronds to their neighbors, they seem to fit together like pieces of a simple jigsaw puzzle and thereby to form a compact mass.

Amount of Stroma

Each frond contains abundant stroma composed of collagen, fibroblasts, and blood vessels (Fig. 8-3). The proportions of stroma and glands can vary from one region of a papilloma to the next (Fig. 8-4), and so can the character of the stroma. In older papillomas,

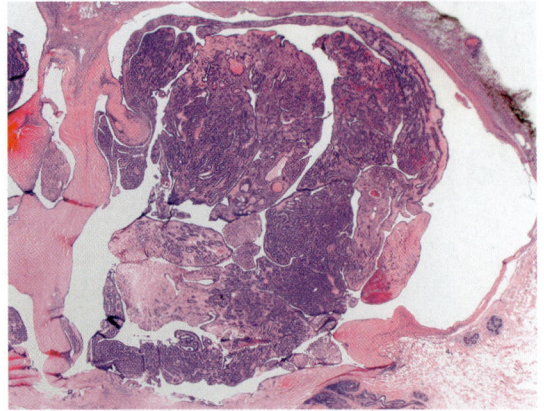

Figure 8-2 A typical papilloma consists of just a few fronds, which display broad, blunt, polygonal shapes and smooth arching contours. The dimensions of the fronds do not vary markedly, and the fronds fit together neatly.

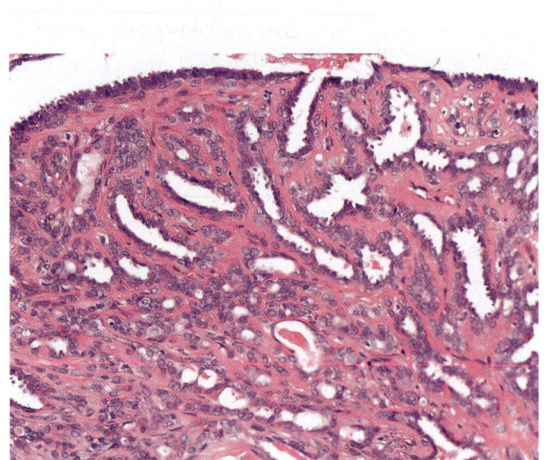

Figure 8-3 The stroma of this papilloma composes about half of the tumor's mass. The stroma consists of collagen, fibroblasts, and blood vessels.

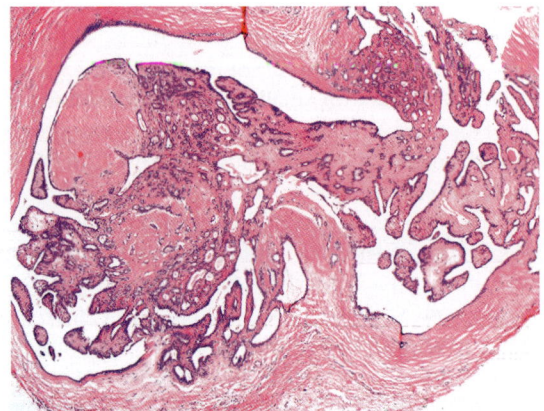

Figure 8-4 The proportion of stroma and glands in this papilloma varies from one region to the next.

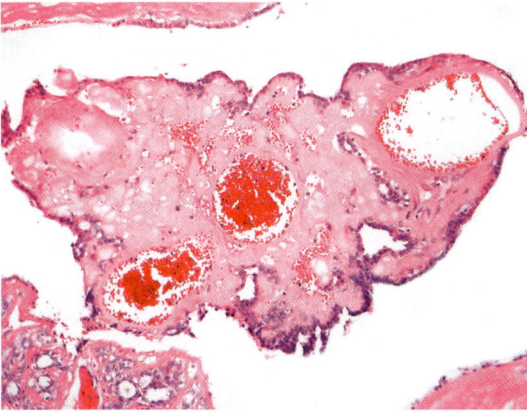

Figure 8-5 The stroma demonstrates hyalinization, loss of stromal cells, and dilatation of capillaries.

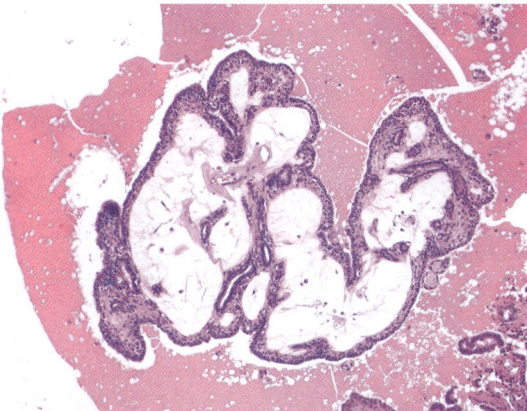

Figure 8-6 The fronds of this papilloma display marked edema.

the stroma undergoes hyalinization, the fibroblasts disappear, and the capillaries can become dilated (Fig. 8-5). In other situations, the stroma becomes edematous (Fig. 8-6). Although the amount of the stroma can help distinguish papillomas from papillary carcinomas, the composition of the stroma does not provide diagnostic information. Both benign and malignant papillary tumors can have either cellular or hyalinized stroma, and the stroma of these lesions can either contain blood vessels or lack them.

Characteristics of the Epithelium

The epithelium of a papilloma varies in its morphology. It can appear flat and inconspicuous or tall and cellular (Fig. 8-7). Whatever its appearance, it consists of a complex, yet organized, mixture of cells (Fig. 8-8). The basement membrane often appears distinct, and above it sits the myoepithelium. The myoepithelial cells sometimes look inconspicuous, but more often they stand out clearly or even prominently. Such cells appear large and they possess abundant clear cytoplasm and a large, irregular, convoluted, pale, oval nucleus containing a nucleolus of modest size. Less conspicuous myoepithelial cells have flattened, elongate shapes and contain dark, spindly nuclei and dense, eosinophilic cytoplasm. A layer of luminal cells covers the myoepithelium. They most often look like conventional ductal cells and frequently show apocrine change. Eosinophilic secretory material or a few histiocytes sometimes occupy the duct in which the papilloma grows; only extremely rarely does it contain sloughed cells or cellular debris. In most cases, the duct contains only the papilloma (Box 8.1).

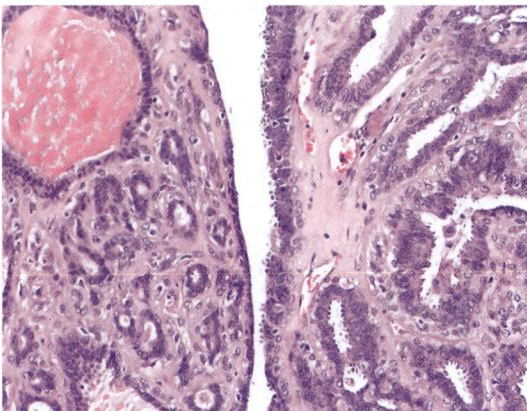

Figure 8-7 The epithelium varies from flat to columnar.

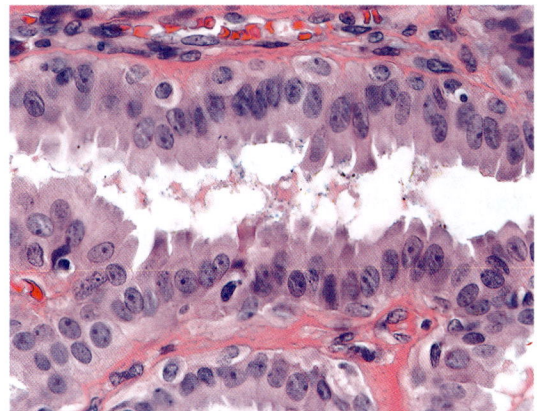

Figure 8-8 The epithelium of a papilloma comprises two layers of cells and two types of cell. The luminal cells have columnar shapes, oval nuclei, and eosinophilic cytoplasm. The myoepithelial cells appear polygonal and possess folded nuclei and pale cytoplasm.

Ancillary Characteristics

One has difficulty detecting mitotic figures in most papillomas. It usually requires an unreasonably long search to find even one or two. A rare papilloma possesses easily detected division figures, which might reflect the hormonal stimulation of the luteal phase. One can probably ignore their presence if all other features of such a case fit with the diagnosis of papilloma. The epithelial cells of a papilloma adhere to one another tightly, so the lumen does not usually contain detached cells or cellular debris. In cases of florid conventional ductal hyperplasia involving a papilloma, a few superficial cells can wither, flake off the mass, and fall into the lumen, and after infarction, the epithelium can fragment and degenerate. Besides these circumstances, the epithelial cells of a papilloma do not exhibit dishesion.

The majority of papillomas do not harbor calcifications. When they do develop, the calcifications usually crystallize in stromal locations, such as the dense collagen laid down by sclerosing papillomas, the fibrotic reaction that can surround conventional papillomas, and the hyalinized stromal cores of an ancient papilloma. The presence of other patterns of calcification would make one reconsider the diagnosis of papilloma. Finally, papillomas often involve only a portion of the wall of the duct, and the epithelium covering the remainder of the wall appears flattened, normal, or slightly hyperplastic. The presence of these benign cells usually bolsters the diagnosis of papilloma for the papillary tumor (Box 8-2).

Summary

Papillomas consist of a few orderly fronds composed of abundant stroma and a normally structured epithelium containing benign luminal and myoepithelial cells. Most examples do not show significant mitotic activity, cellular dishesion, or calcification.

PROBLEMS IN THE DIAGNOSIS OF PAPILLOMAS

Commonplace papillomas like those already illustrated do not cause diagnostic problems for experienced pathologists; however, the superimposition of secondary processes on a papilloma creates confusing patterns, which can lead to an erroneous diagnosis of malignancy. The most common of these complicating processes are alteration of the cytologic features, scarring and entrapment of benign glands, and proliferation of epithelial cells. Papillomas occassionlly give rise to secondary changes in lobules, which can confuse pathologists unfamiliar with this phenomenon. The morphologic attributes of papillomas overlap with those of adenomyoepithelioma and ductal adenomas. These shared features blur the distinction between the entities, making it difficult to clarify certain cases. Sampling a papilloma with a core biopsy can displace fragments of the papilloma, and the presence of epithelial cells or bits of papilloma in unexpected locations can confuse observers. The following paragraphs examine these problem areas.

Unexpected Cytologic Findings

The cells of benign papillomas sometimes display unexpected cytologic characteristics. Because these changes occur so uncommonly, pathologists may not know of their existence, and this lack of awareness creates uncertainty about the nature of these alterations. Changes of this type affect both luminal cells and myoepithelial cells. Active luminal cells, for example, can appear slightly enlarged and can contain slightly enlarged

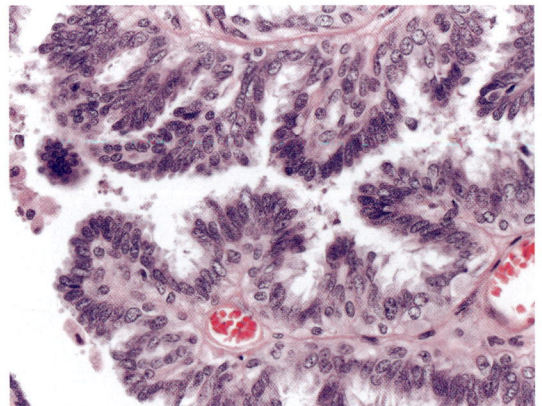

Figure 8-9 The luminal cells have slightly enlarged nuclei and frayed apical cytoplasm. The orderly epithelium composed of a single layer of luminal cells and distinct myoepithelial cells reflects the lesion's benign nature.

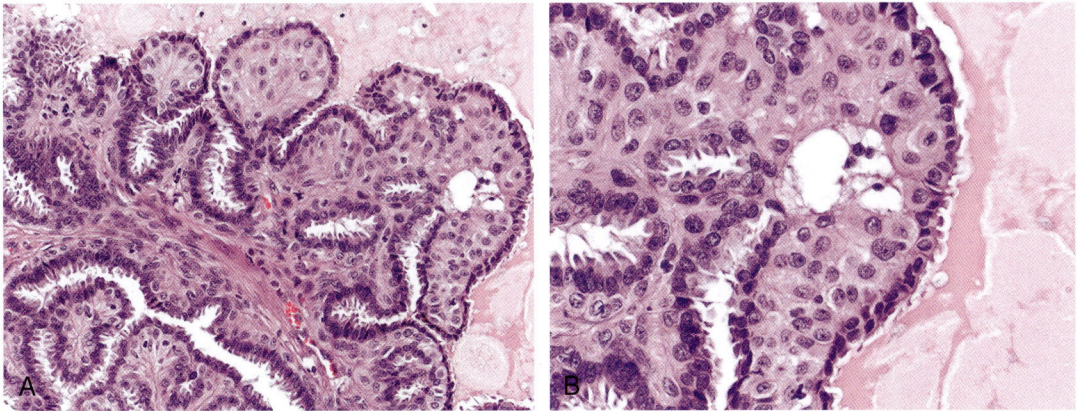

Figure 8-10 A, The myoepithelial cells in the lower left appear prominent, and in the upper right, they show proliferation and stratification. **B,** High magnification allows one to appreciate the bland characteristics of the myoepithelial cells.

nuclei and modest amounts of apical cytoplasm, which sometimes forms blebs (Fig. 8-9). As long as these prominent luminal cells form only a single layer and overlie a row of myoepithelial cells, one can ignore such cells.

Myoepithelial cells, too, sometimes look out-of-the-ordinary. They can enlarge so that they form a prominent layer or even aggregate to produce cell clusters (Fig. 8-10). These active myoepithelial cells have abundant, clear cytoplasm, centrally placed nuclei, and a distinct nucleolus. Their presence beneath the luminal cells reminds one of the appearances of pagetoid involvement by carcinoma in situ; however, the cytologic characteristics of active myoepithelial

cells differ from those of carcinoma cells (Fig. 8-11). Myoepithelial cells have lower nucleus-to-cytoplasm ratios than carcinoma cells and usually have slightly irregular, indented nuclei and small nucleoli. Myoepithelial cells also undergo a degenerative phenomenon in which the cells and their nuclei swell to enormous sizes (Fig. 8-12). The chromatin becomes widely dispersed and clumped, and large regions of the nucleus become clear. The bizarre appearance of such cells does not seem to have any clinical significance. Once pathologists become familiar with the ranges of appearance of both luminal and myoepithelial cells, the presence of these cytologic characteristics should not cause diagnostic confusion.

Figure 8-11 *Left,* The prominent myoepithelial cells might suggest the appearance of lobular carcinoma growing in a pagetoid pattern, but cytologic features distinguish the two lesions. *Right,* The cells of lobular carcinoma involving a papilloma have less cytoplasm than the myoepithelial cells and demonstrate dishesion not seen in the myoepithelial cells.

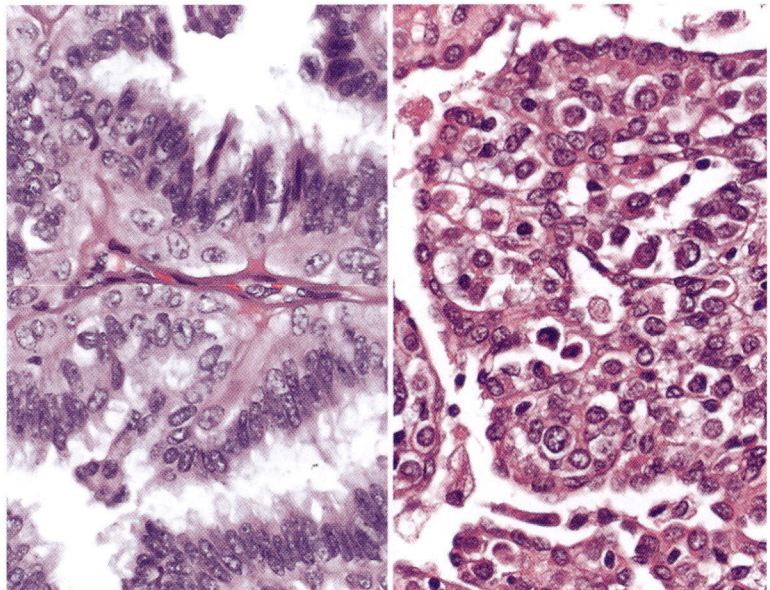

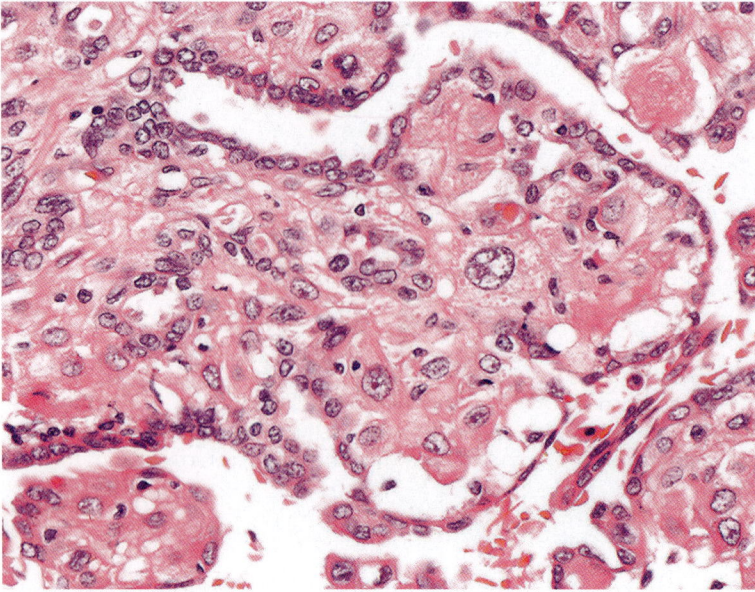

Figure 8-12 Several myoepithelial cells show degenerative changes; their nuclei appear huge and their chromatin pale and washed-out.

Sclerosing papilloma

Scarring and Entrapment of Benign Glands

Papillomas commonly undergo fibrosis, which sometimes results from spontaneous infarction. When the sclerosis becomes extreme, one can make the diagnosis of *sclerosing papilloma* (Fig. 8-13). Whether minimal or marked, the fibrosis can entrap and distort glands in the region of the papilloma. Early observers misinterpreted this entrapment as invasion and thereby misdiagnosed papillomas as papillary carcinomas. One might wonder how this error became so commonplace, because pathologists of the 19th and early 20th centuries made especially detailed observations and gave them considerable thought.

The literature does not provide an explicit answer to this question, but it would seem that these investigators made two mistakes. First, they mistook the irregular glands trapped in the sclerosing reaction as invasive carcinoma. Then, on the basis of the presence of these "invasive" glands, these pathologists erroneously concluded that the papillary tumor must represent papillary carcinoma. Drs. Kraus and Neubecker emphasized the frequency of this error, and Dr. Azzopardi places scarring and distortion on the top of his list of the causes of the misdiagnosis of papillomas as papillary carcinomas. To refrain from misinterpreting a papilloma as a papillary carcinoma, pathologists must avoid this error. One must not base the diagnosis of malignancy on the presence of epithelial nests that seem to represent invasive carcinoma. Instead, the diagnosis of carcinoma must rest on the cytologic and architectural characteristics of the papillary tumor itself.

Only after determining that a papillary tumor displays criteria of malignancy should one consider the

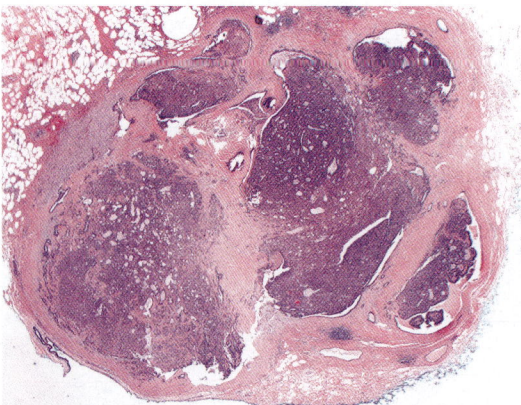

Figure 8-13 This papilloma has evoked an intense scarring reaction.

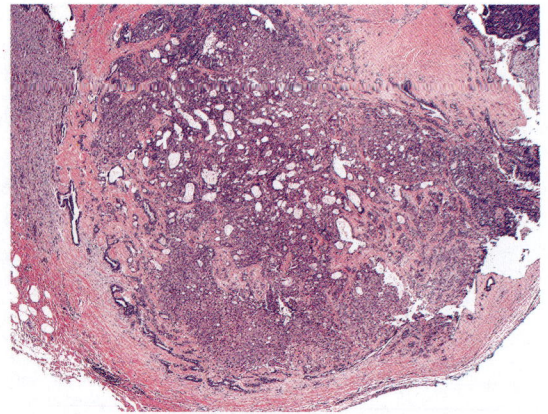

Figure 8-14 The glands entrapped within the scarring reaction flow around the periphery of the involved duct.

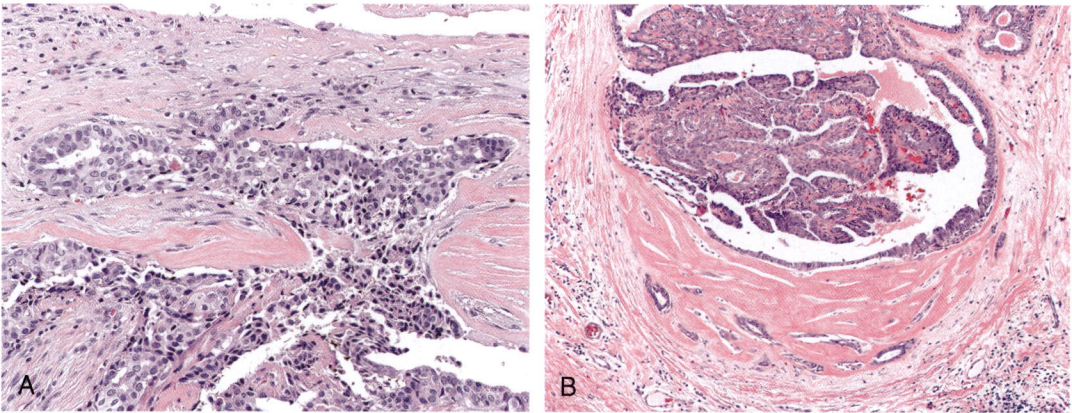

Figure 8-15 A, A desmoplastic and fibrotic reaction has entrapped an aggregate of benign cells, which run in the direction of the fibroblasts and collagen bundles. **B,** The benign glands trapped in the fibrous reaction to this papilloma flow in a circular direction around the wall of the duct.

Pseudoinvasion associated with altered stroma.

question whether irregular epithelial clusters reflect entrapment or invasion. Several features help differentiate these two phenomena. Entrapped epithelium consists of benign cells arranged in irregular but smoothly contoured clusters, which tend to flow in the direction of the fibroblasts and bundles of collagen as they sweep around the periphery of the involved duct (Fig. 8-14). The stroma can appear either desmoplastic or collagenous (Fig. 8-15). Whatever the composition of the stroma, the glands maintain an orderly relationship with the stromal components. The nests typically exhibit a polygonal shape, but they can become compressed into long, slender cords, which closely resemble the single-file pattern of invasive carcinoma (Fig. 8-16). In cases of pronounced fibrosis, the nests may not exhibit circular, flowing distribution (Fig. 8-17). Nevertheless, one must not forget that the glands assume their

unusual shapes and pseudoinvasive pattern because of the scarring process. Consequently, the suspect clusters always reside in altered stroma; never do they permeate normal tissue.

Besides studying the shape and pattern of the entrapped glands, one should examine the cytologic characteristics of the cells composing the nests. Entrapped benign glands consist of both luminal cells and myoepithelial cells, both of which look small and bland. The detection of myoepithelial cells provides especially important evidence to establish the benign nature of glandular clusters. One can usually recognize myoepithelial cells in conventionally stained sections, but immunohistochemical stains facilitate their recognition.

Nests of invasive carcinoma also grow in the scarred stroma, of course, but they exhibit a destructive and permeative relationship with the fibroblasts and

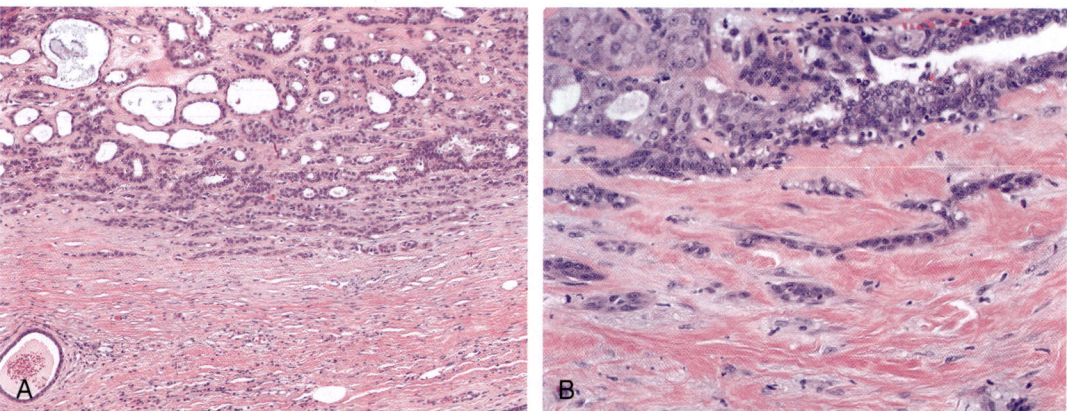

Figure 8-16 A, Scarring has compressed glands into long, thin cords. **B,** This arrangement simulates the pattern of invasion, but the nests flow in the direction of the fibroblasts and collagen.

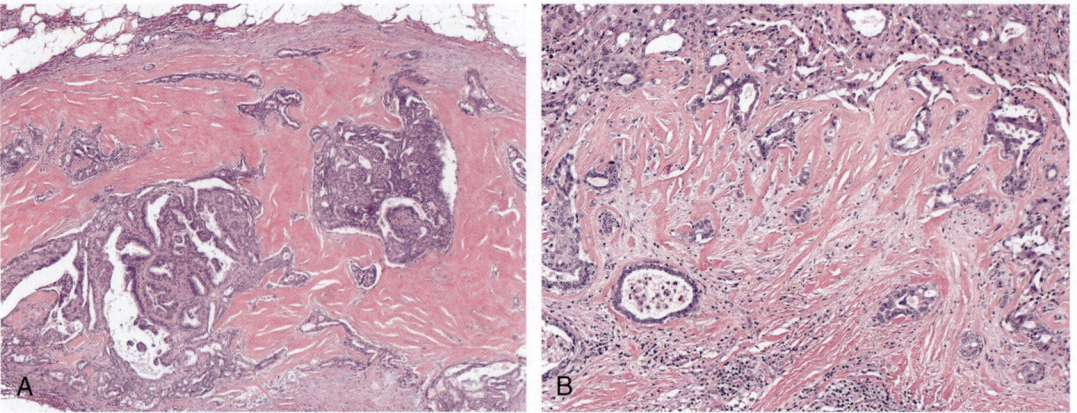

Figure 8-17 A and **B,** Pronounced, dense scarring has entrapped haphazardly disposed, irregular clusters of benign cells. These entrapped glands do not show the typical circular, flowing arrangement seen in many scarred papillomas.

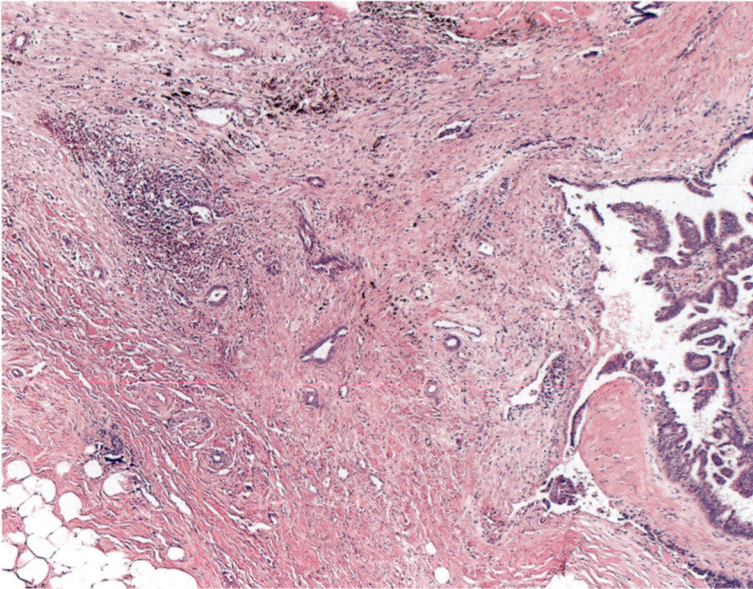

Figure 8-18 The invasive glands adjacent to this carcinoma do not flow with the stroma.

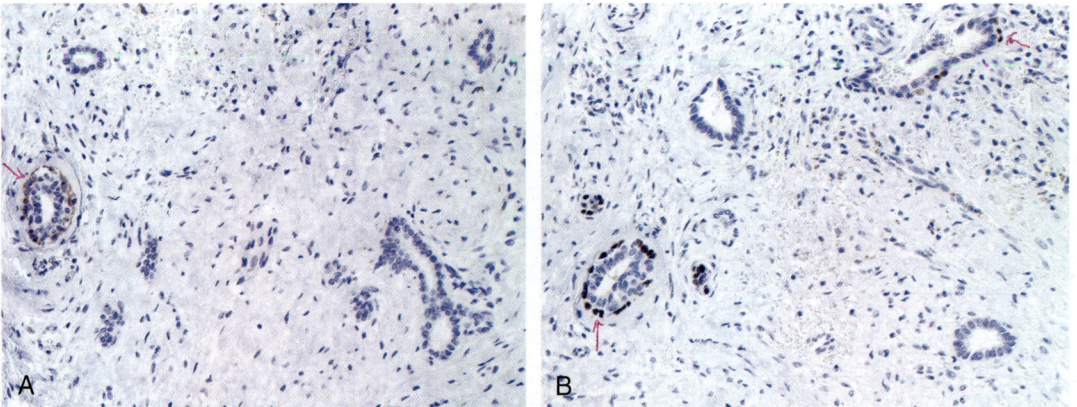

Figure 8-19 Immunohistochemical stains for myosin heavy chain in **A** and p63 protein in **B** reveal that the invasive glands lack myoepithelial cells but that the entrapped, benign glands possess them.

collagen (Fig. 8-18); the cells lining them look malignant, and the glands lack myoepithelial cells (Fig. 8-19). Furthermore, the glands frequently invade normal tissues.

Superimposed Epithelial Proliferations

Like normal ducts and terminal duct–lobular units, papillomas can serve as the seat of both benign and malignant epithelial proliferations. This phenomenon occurs commonly, and the superimposition of epithelial proliferations on preexisting papillomas gives rise to some of the most common problems in the diagnosis of papillary tumors. Solving these problems requires careful observation and clear, stepwise thinking. Pathologists must first recognize the presence of an underlying benign papilloma by observing regions displaying the expected characteristics of that lesion: broad, blunt fronds and two-layer epithelium composed of two types of cells showing benign cytologic features. Then, observers must determine the location and the pattern of the proliferative cells.

Epithelial proliferations superimposed on papillomas can assume two different patterns. The first, a *superficial stratified pattern* (Fig. 8-20A), arises when the cells accumulate in several layers on the surface of the fronds. Conventional ductal hyperplasia, atypical ductal hyperplasia, and ductal carcinoma in situ all can grow in this way. The second, the *inverted adenosis pattern* (Fig. 8-20B), develops when the cells form small glands or clusters within the stalk of the papilloma. When this glandular proliferation becomes florid, a lesion that closely mimics the appearance of cribriform ductal carcinoma in situ results. These two forms of proliferation require different approaches to their diagnosis.

Epithelial Proliferations on the Surface (Superficial Stratified Pattern)

When cells in this location proliferate, they pile on top of one another in several layers and often bridge the surface of the papilloma and the wall of the duct. One can analyze these superficial proliferations using the standard cytologic and architectural criteria for epithelial proliferations within ducts presented in Chapter 3. The approach suggested for proliferations within ducts works just as well for proliferations superimposed on a papilloma.

Although concepts derived for proliferations within ducts apply to those occupying the surfaces of papillomas, one must make allowances for artifacts produced by the extreme three-dimensional complexity of papillomas when evaluating certain criteria. The evaluation of the extent of cellular proliferation, for example, does not pose any problem when one is examining a cross section of a duct, but with the curving surfaces of a papilloma, it is especially easy to produce tangential planes of section and thereby to create the impression of proliferation where none exists (Fig. 8-21A). One should require the presence of several layers of cells that fill the space between individual fronds or between the fronds and the duct wall before concluding that proliferation has taken place. Distortion of the orderly, geometric structure of the underlying mass also helps bolster the impression of genuine stratification. Off-center sectioning of the folded, curving structure of a papilloma can also make polarized luminal cells growing in a single layer look like an aggregate of cells forming cribriform spaces (Fig. 8-21B). Finally, sectioning the tips of papillae can give rise to an appearance that suggests cellular dishesion (Fig. 8-21C). Partial separation of the cells from their neighbors along the perimeter of a cell cluster, fraying of the cytoplasmic

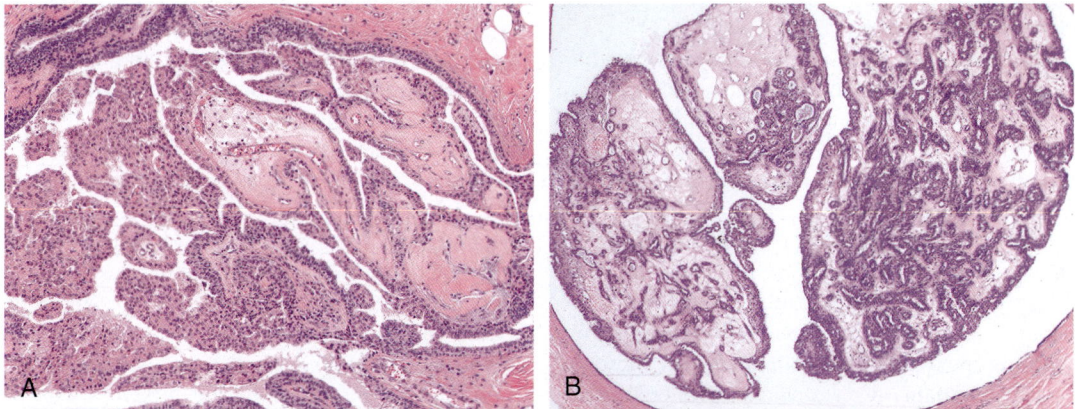

Figure 8-20 A, The epithelial proliferation in this papilloma has formed several layers on the surface of the papillary skeleton. This appearance represents the superficial stratified pattern of epithelial proliferation. **B,** The glands within the largest frond of the papilloma show modest proliferation, which creates the inverted adenosis pattern.

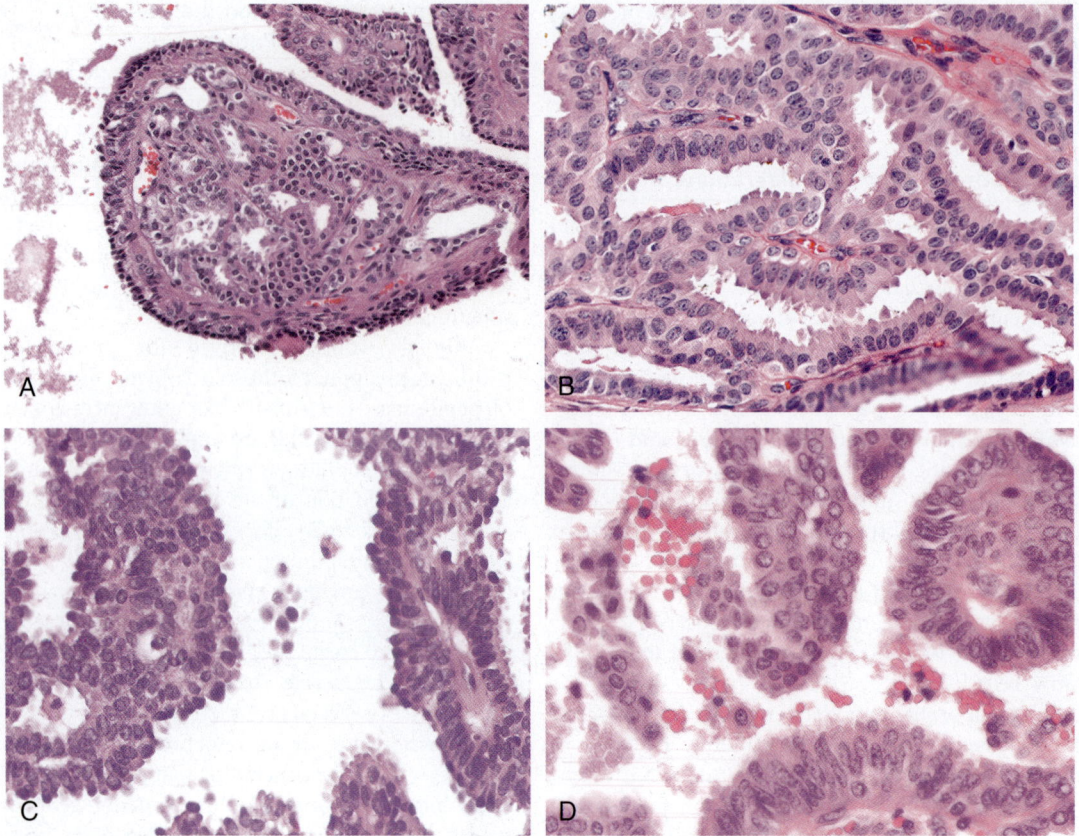

Figure 8-21 A, An off-center plane of section creates the impression of cellular proliferation where none exists. **B,** The same phenomenon makes these curving tubules lined by a single layer of columnar cells look like cribriform spaces. **C,** The group of about ten cells in the center probably represents the tip of a papillary structure cut in an off-center plane rather than sloughed epithelial cells. **D,** The separation of cells from their neighbors, the fraying of cytoplasm, and the degeneration of the apparently detached cells all serve as more reliable indications of the lack of intercellular cohesion.

borders, and degeneration of seemingly detached cells all serve as more reliable indications of the lack of cellular cohesion (Fig. 8-21D).

Applying the standard criteria with these modifications, one would make the diagnosis of conventional ductal hyperplasia involving a papilloma for a proliferation of cohesive cells lacking cytologic atypicality. As Figure 8-22 illustrates, the proliferative cells in such a lesion display the characteristic features of hyperplastic ductal cells, and the cells growing on the papilloma look like those growing in ducts uninvolved by the papilloma. Of the forms of epithelial proliferation superimposed on a papilloma, this one occurs most commonly. The presence of cells with anaplastic cytologic features establishes the diagnosis of intermediate- or high-grade ductal carcinoma involving a papilloma (Fig. 8-23). When the proliferative cells exhibit both low-grade cytologic atypism and architectural atypism, one would

make the diagnosis of low-grade ductal carcinoma in situ involving a papilloma (Fig. 8-24). One would classify proliferations characterized by low-grade cytologic atypicality but lacking architectural atypicality as atypical ductal hyperplasia or flat epithelial atypia (Fig. 8-25).

When evaluating epithelial proliferations on the surface of a papilloma, one should keep in mind that certain examples of florid conventional ductal hyperplasia sometimes exhibit two types of changes not usually seen in routine situations. First, the uppermost cells can become especially small, their nuclei shrunken and pyknotic, and their cytoplasm especially eosinophilic, and a few can detach from one another and fall into the lumen, where they degenerate (Fig. 8-26). This phenomenon, which seems to represent an exaggerated form of commonplace maturation, accounts for certain rare papillomas that display epithelial necrosis.

Figure 8-22 A, Conventional ductal hyperplasia grows on the surface of the fronds of this papilloma. **B,** High magnification demonstrates cellular features identical to those of hyperplastic cells distant from the papilloma, shown in **C.**

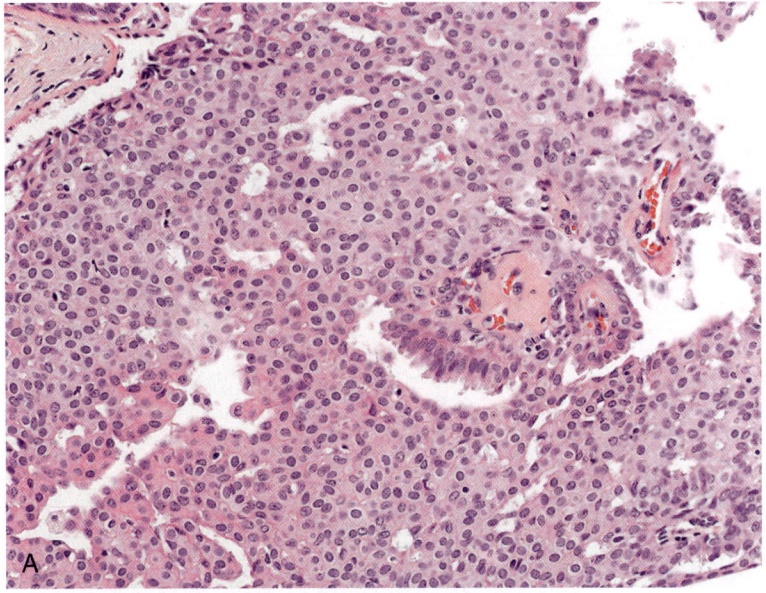

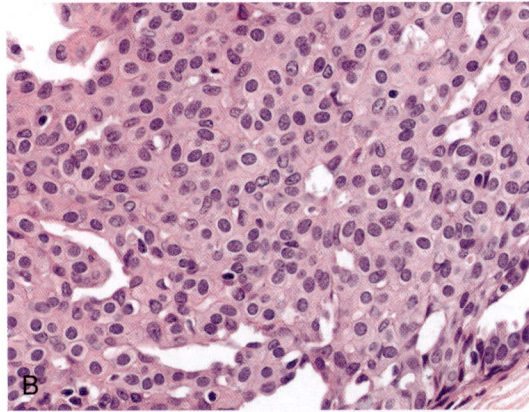

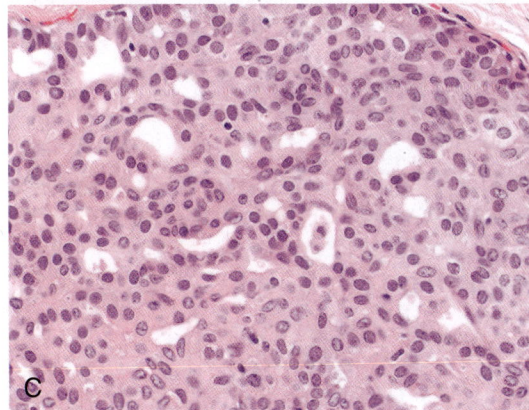

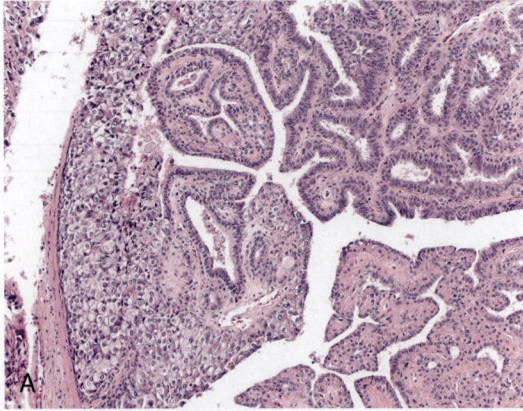

Figure 8-23 A, Intermediate-grade ductal carcinoma occupies the surface of this papilloma. **B,** High magnification discloses the anaplastic cellular features.

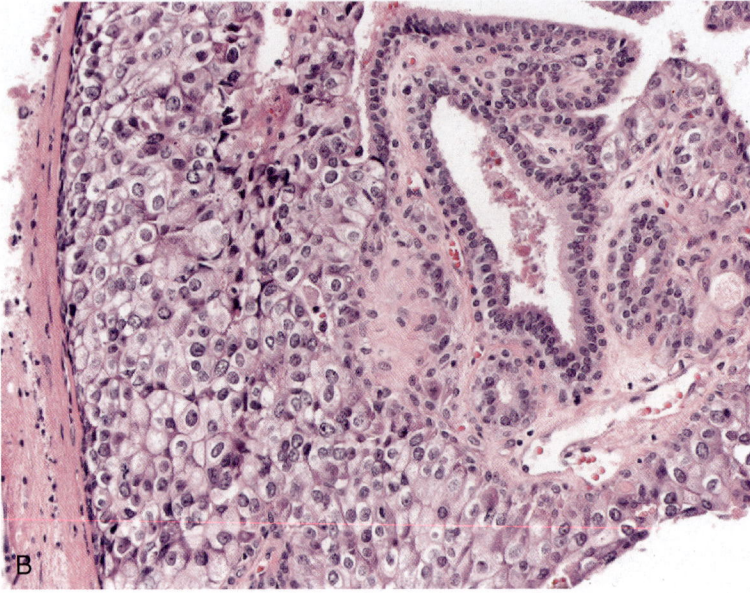

Intermediate grade DCIS

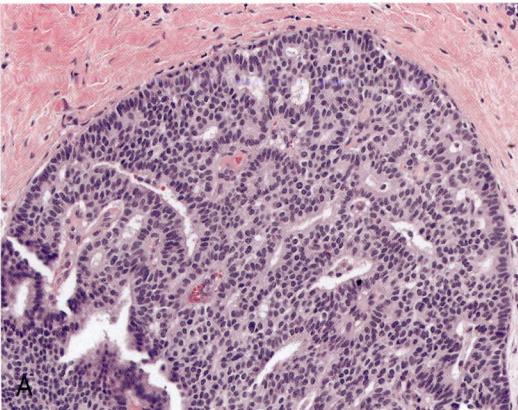

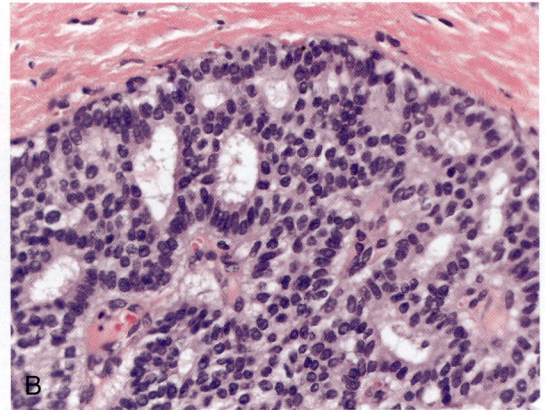

Figure 8-24 A, The proliferation on the surface of the fronds of the papilloma displays features of low-grade ductal carcinoma in situ. **B,** High magnification illustrates the cytologic atypia and formation of cribriform spaces that establish the diagnosis.

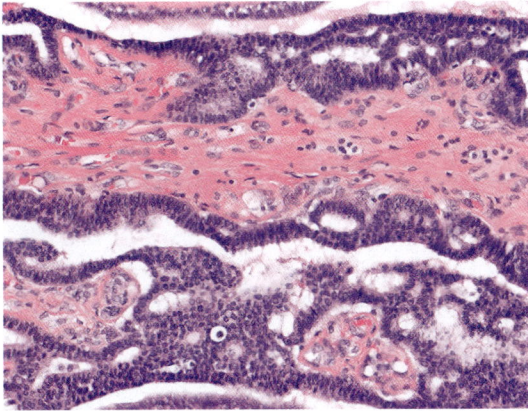

Figure 8-25 The epithelial proliferation growing on the surface of these fronds displays cytologic atypia but lacks convincing architectural atypia.

ADH   or   Flat ep atypia

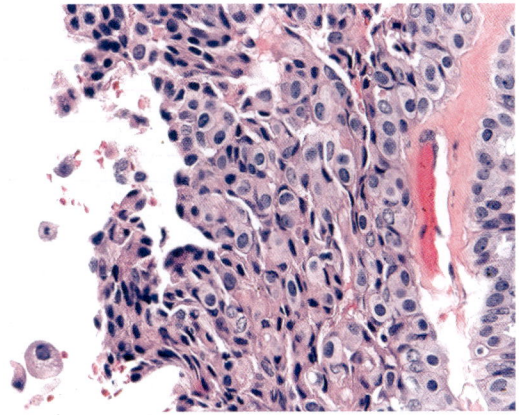

Figure 8-26 Usual ductal hyperplasia grows on the surface of this papilloma. The most superficial cells appear especially small, and their nuclei especially dark. The cells fall away from their neighbors to degenerate in the lumen of the duct.

p.170 text

In the second type of change, the ductal cells accumulate abundant, eosinophilic cytoplasm that often contains vacuoles and sometimes pigment. The nuclei vary from dark to pale. Most commonly, they look pale and display irregular contours, irregular nuclear membranes, and prominent nucleoli. The cells frequently contain two nuclei (Fig. 8-27). These changes probably represent a degenerative process affecting apocrine cells. Cells of this type become dishesive and fall into the lumen of the duct, and they often appear in a discharge from the patient's nipple, where they can alarm the inexperienced observer.

nipple discharge

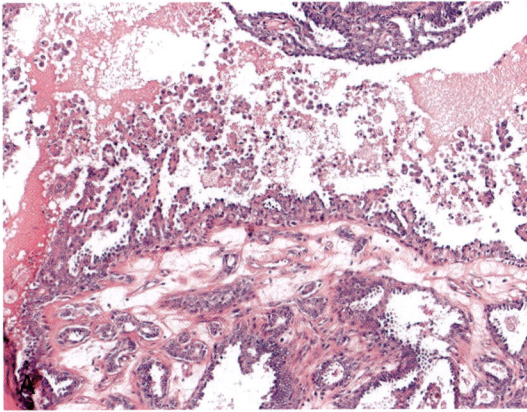

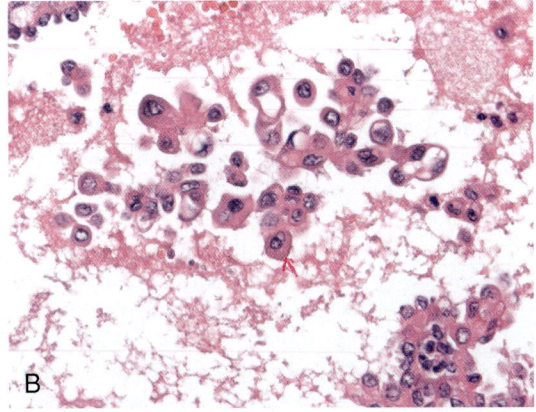

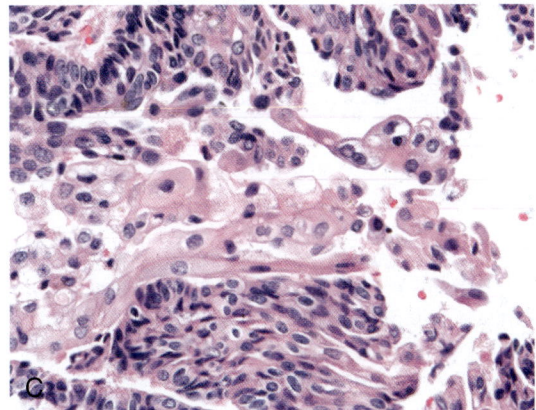

Figure 8-27 A, The hyperplastic cells on the surface of this papilloma show degenerative changes. **B,** The cells possess dense, eosinophilic, vacuolated cytoplasm, and their nuclei have irregular contours, irregular nuclear membranes, and prominent nucleoli. Several cells contain two nuclei. **C,** A minority of cells contain dark, smudgy chromatin.

Lack of cellular cohesion is dyshesion

Although this phenomenon reflects a lack of cellular cohesion, one must not mistake it for the dishesion inherent in carcinoma cells. Attention to cytologic features, such as the degenerative qualities of the nuclei and the low ratio of nucleus to cytoplasm identifies the cells as benign and the features as degenerative rather than neoplastic.

Epithelial Proliferations within the Stalk (Inverted Adenosis Pattern)

Virtually all papillomas harbor glands within their stalks; in fact, the presence of such glands led certain pathologists of the 19th century to use the term *intraductal sclerosing adenosis* instead of *papilloma*. In the presence of the typical number of glands growing in the usual pattern, pathologists need not pay much attention to these glands; however, they can multiply to form closely packed acini and cell clusters (Fig. 8-28). This phenomenon creates a pattern quite different from the pattern produced by surface proliferations and one that requires a different and especially cautious diagnostic approach. The actively growing cells within the stalk of a papilloma often appear a bit larger than one would expect, and they often possess slightly enlarged nuclei, findings that ordinarily suggest the presence of atypia. Furthermore, the architectural complexity of a papilloma makes it easy for tangential sectioning of the proliferative glands to produce a cribriform-like appearance. Thus, this pattern of epithelial proliferation simulates both cytologic and architectural atypicality and can mislead pathologists into making an erroneous diagnosis of malignancy (Fig. 8-29). One cannot exaggerate the potential for the inappropriate diagnosis of carcinoma in the evaluation of glandular proliferations within the body of a papilloma.

To guard against mistaking the complex glandular pattern for low-grade cribriform ductal carcinoma in situ, one should look for delicate strands of collagen and capillaries surrounding each cell cluster (Fig. 8-30). The presence of this attenuated stroma identifies the glands as closely packed acini growing in an adenosis pattern, and careful inspection shows that each acinus consists of a single layer of luminal cells overlying a row of myoepithelial cells. In contrast, foci of ductal carcinoma in situ lack internal collagen bands. One does not observe stroma surrounding the individual cribriform spaces of a cribriform carcinoma, nor does one observe myoepithelial cells.

Because of the possibility of confusing the complex glandular pattern of a papilloma with low-grade cribriform ductal carcinoma in situ, one must hesitate before making the latter diagnosis for an epithelial proliferation involving only the stalk of a papilloma. To consider this diagnosis, one must first observe a large mass of epithelial cells completely

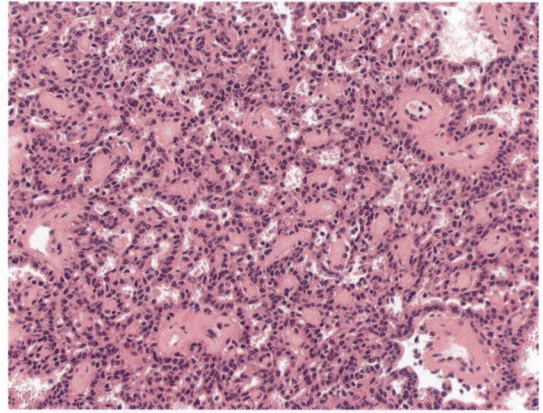

Figure 8-28 The glands within the stalk of this papilloma have multiplied and become confluent.

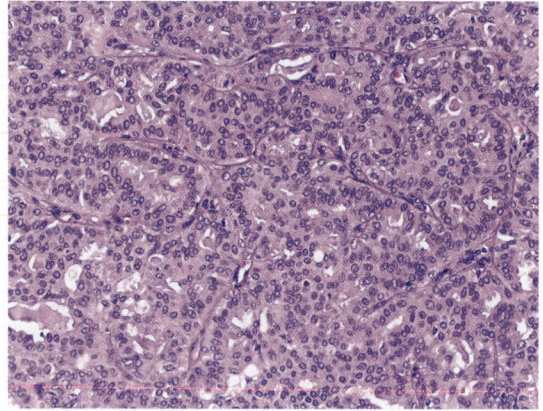

Figure 8-29 Proliferation of ductal cells, off-center planes of section, and confluence of the glands within the stalk of this papilloma create an appearance similar to that of ductal carcinoma in situ.

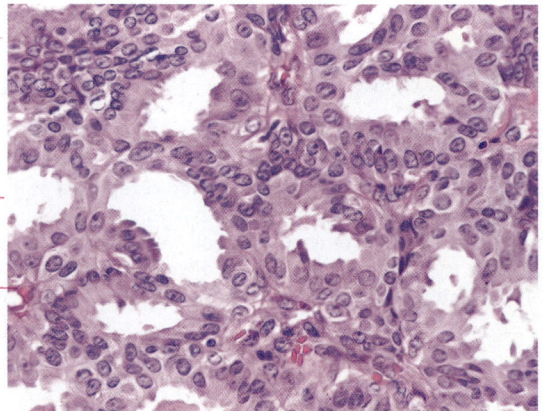

Figure 8-30 The presence of delicate strands of collagen and capillaries between the glands indicates that this region represents the complex glandular pattern rather than ductal carcinoma in situ.

Delicate strands of collagen + capillaries.

Figure 8-31 A, A collection of epithelial cells lacking intervening stroma deforms the structure of this papilloma. **B,** The cells display cytologic and architectural atypia.

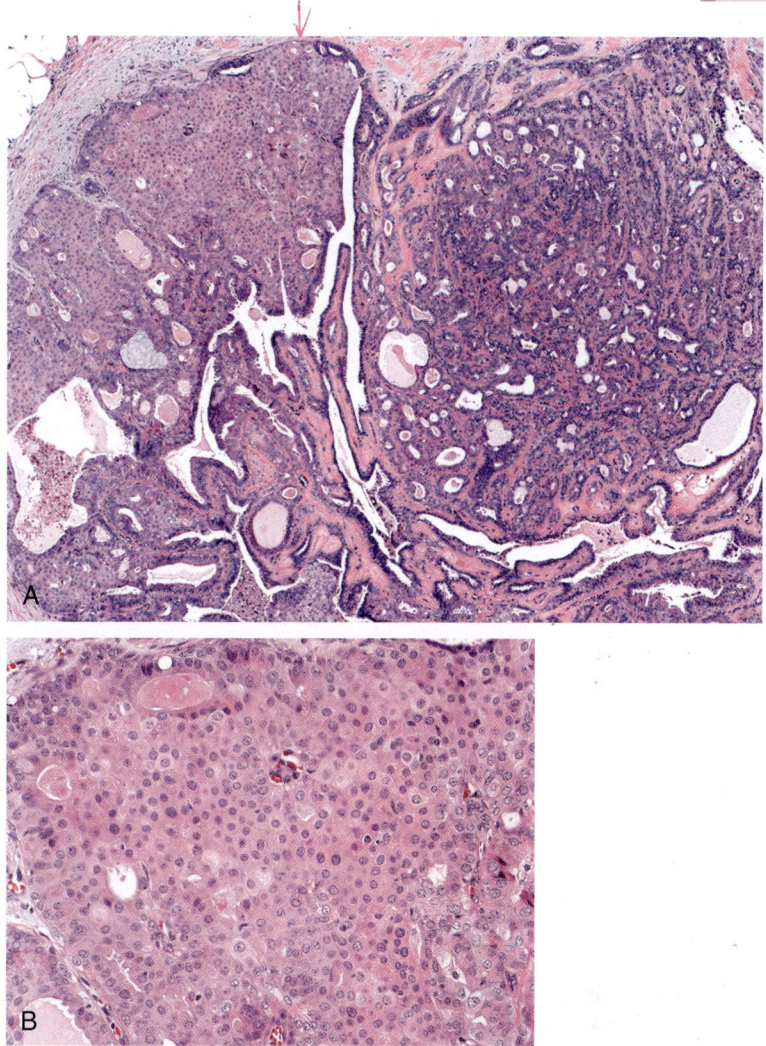

devoid of internal stroma. Such a mass usually forms a bulging nodule that displaces and distorts the neighboring portions of the papilloma. Having identified a proliferative focus, one must then evaluate the cytologic and architectural characteristics of the proliferative cells, searching for convincing evidence of both cytologic and architectural atypism (Fig. 8-31). Only in the presence of all three features (proliferation, cytologic atypia, and architectural atypia) should one consider the diagnosis of low-grade ductal carcinoma in situ involving the stalk of a papilloma, and even in the presence of these findings, certain pathologists would refrain from making the diagnosis of malignancy as a matter of principle. No less a pathologist than Dr. Arthur Purdy Stout, for example, advocated this conservative line of thought.

The practice of avoiding the diagnosis of low-grade ductal carcinoma in situ involving the stalk of a papilloma has much to recommend it, for it simplifies the task of the pathologist while satisfying the clinical needs of the patient and the surgeon. Despite its appeal, this line of reasoning has two limitations. First, it applies to only those cases in which the suspicious cells reside exclusively in the body of the papilloma and do not spread onto the wall of the involved duct or into nearby ducts. Pathologists should take a more aggressive approach to the diagnosis when they see the neoplastic cells straying in this manner, because the excision of the papillary tumor in this situation can no longer guarantee the complete excision of the neoplastic population. Second, this pragmatic approach may not satisfy the curiosity of those observers who wish to understand the pathologic processes in the specimens under study. The more detailed analysis and classification of these proliferative nodules, on the other hand, reveal their

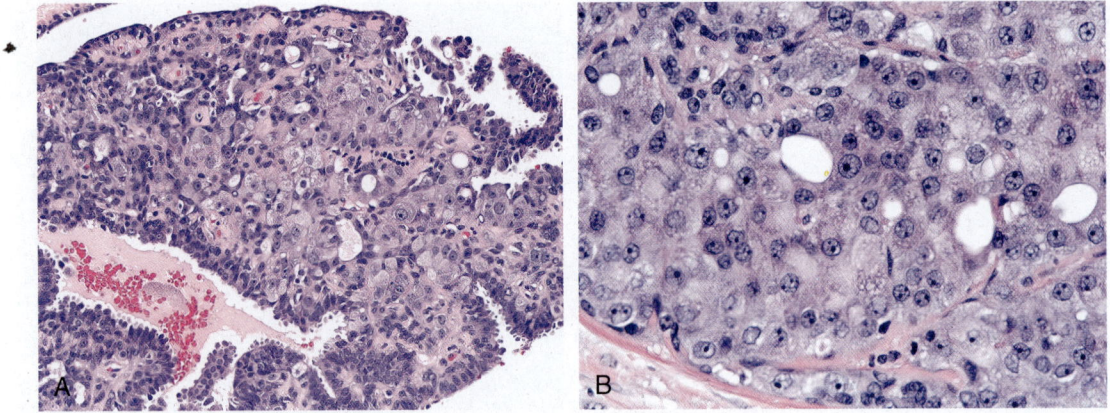

Figure 8-32 A, This papilloma contains a population of atypical cells. **B,** High magnification reveals the large size and atypical nuclei of the malignant cells.

nature, and a full understanding of the pathologic changes allows pathologists to recognize the origin of a ductal carcinoma within a papilloma and to distinguish this lesion from a genuine papillary carcinoma.

Unlike the recognition of low-grade ductal carcinoma in situ involving the stalk of a papilloma, which frequently challenges the pathologist, the detection of high-grade ductal carcinoma in situ within a papilloma usually proceeds without much difficulty. When the cells exhibit sufficiently anaplastic cytologic characteristics, one can make the diagnosis of carcinoma without regard to the architectural properties or even the limitations created by the complexity of the papillary architecture (Fig. 8-32).

Proliferation of Cells with Granular and Eosinophilic Cytoplasm

Many pathologists regard all cells with eosinophilic, granular cytoplasm within papillomas as innocuous apocrine cells. One can understand this bias, because many papillomas do contain conventional apocrine cells (Fig. 8-33). Nevertheless, the practice of dismissing all apocrine-like cells as inconsequential can lead to a failure to recognize neoplastic or preneoplastic populations within a papilloma. Such processes arise in two situations, one common and one rare. First, pathologists must remember that carcinomas arising in large duct papillomas commonly consist of cells with finely granular and somewhat eosinophilic cytoplasm and nuclei containing granular and pale chromatin. Because the chromatin does not display the finely dispersed texture and hyperchromasia seen in commonplace low-grade ductal carcinoma cells, one can understand pathologists' failure to appreciate the cytologic atypia of this neoplastic population.

The overlap of the cytoplasmic properties between the atypical cells and conventional apocrine cells makes it especially easy to overlook the presence of this atypical population. Two properties distinguish these atypical cells from everyday apocrine cells, the nucleus-to-cytoplasm ratio and the characteristics of the nuclei (Fig. 8-34). Although both types of cells possess abundant cytoplasm, the amount present in apocrine cells noticeably exceeds the quantity seen in the atypical cells, and the former have much lower nucleus-to-cytoplasm ratios than the latter. One can appreciate the difference in the nucleus-to-cytoplasm ratios by noting that the nuclei of the atypical cells look more densely packed. The nuclear characteristics of the two types of cells differ, also. The chromatin of the atypical cells appears uniform and finely granular and the nucleoli look inconspicuous. Conventional apocrine cells, in contrast, usually possess pale nuclei, clumped chromatin, and prominent nucleoli. Attention to these cytologic features and an appreciation of their significance help to keep pathologists

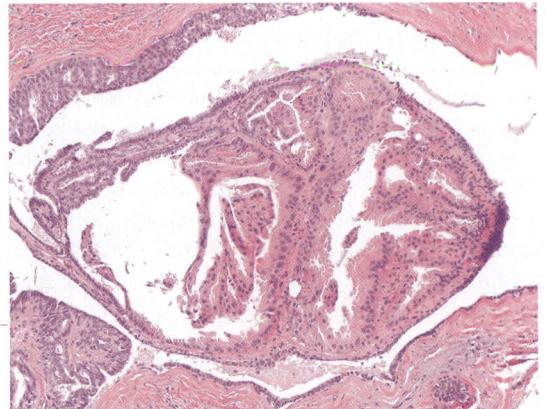

Figure 8-33 This small papilloma contains especially numerous apocrine cells.

Figure 8-34 The atypical cells in **A** appear more closely packed than the apocrine cells in **B.** The nuclei in **A** have finely dispersed, slightly hyperchromatic chromatin and inconspicuous nucleoli, which contrast with the paler chromatin and more prominent nucleoli of the nuclei in **B.**

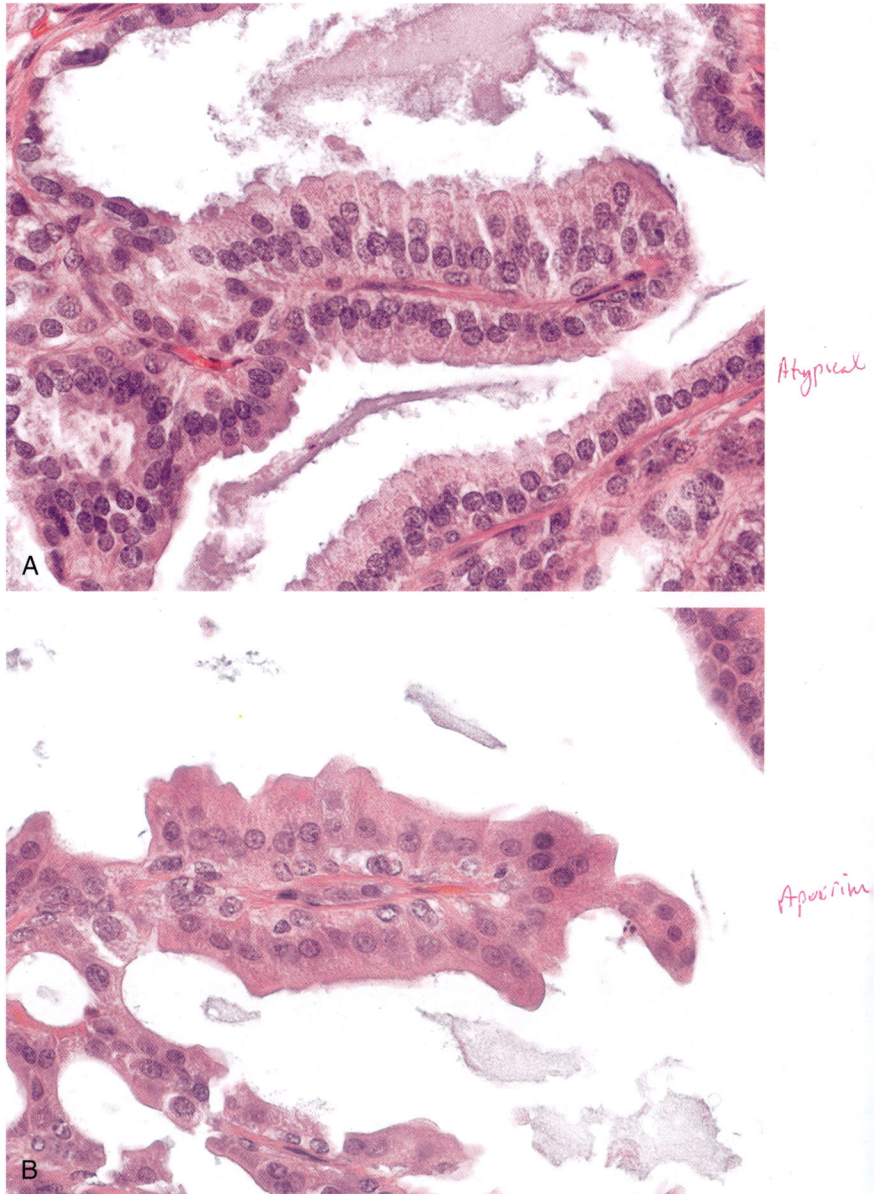

from failing to recognize the presence of a neoplastic proliferation within a preexisting papilloma.

Although these cellular alterations indicate the presence of low-grade atypia, they do not identify the cells as malignant. The diagnosis of ductal carcinoma in situ in this setting requires the presence of significant proliferation and both cytologic and architectural atypia just as it does in other proliferations of a low-grade nature. To evaluate these phenomena, one should use the approach and the criteria set forth in the previous discussions. Foci showing minimal proliferation and only suggestive cribriform spaces (Fig. 8-35) merit the diagnosis of atypical ductal hyperplasia. The diagnosis of ductal carcinoma in situ would seem appropriate for larger nodules that lack internal strands of collagen, deform the structure of the papilloma, and contain several convincing cribriform spaces (Fig. 8-36).

Rare proliferations composed of cells with abundant granular cytoplasm represent examples of apocrine neoplasia (Fig. 8-37); therefore, the correct categorization of cells as apocrine does not mean that one can eliminate the possibility of malignancy from consideration. Pathologists must conduct a careful search for evidence of cytologic atypia in the apocrine cells. The criteria used for assessing the presence and extent of atypia of apocrine cells in other settings apply to apocrine proliferations occurring in papillomas.

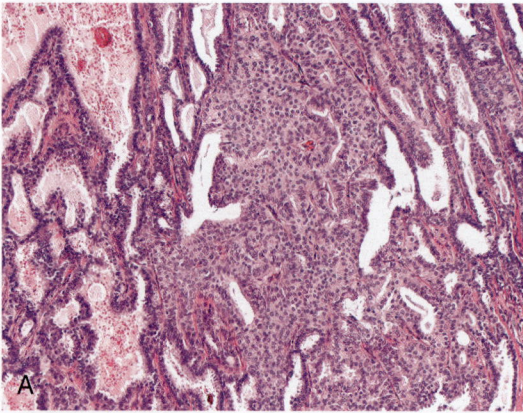

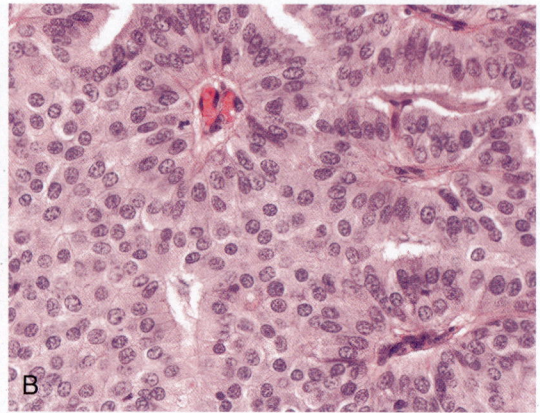

Figure 8-35 A, Atypical cells occupy a portion of this papilloma. Most of the cells grow in a single layer, but those in the center form a small nodule, which distorts the arrangement of the adjacent glands. **B,** The cells display low-grade cytologic atypicality and they might pile up. One space suggests the appearance of a cribriform space, but it could just as well reflect an off-center plane of section.

ADH (text p 177)

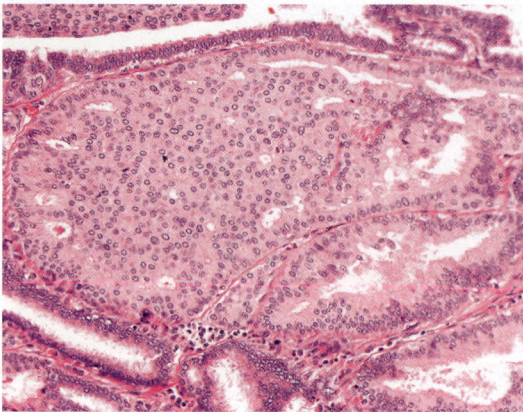

Figure 8-36 The cells in this nodule have eosinophilic cytoplasm reminiscent of that seen in benign apocrine cells; however, those in this focus are malignant. The epithelial cells form a small nodule lacking internal stroma, deforming the structure of the underlying papilloma, and containing several cribriform spaces.

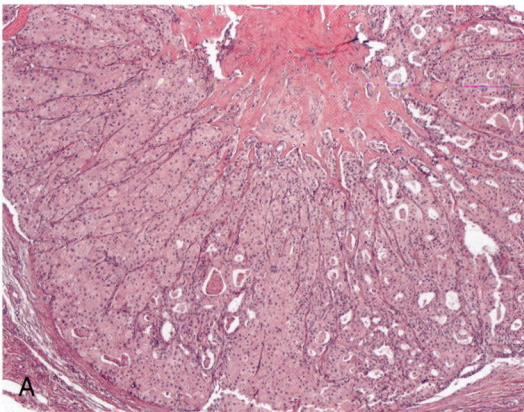

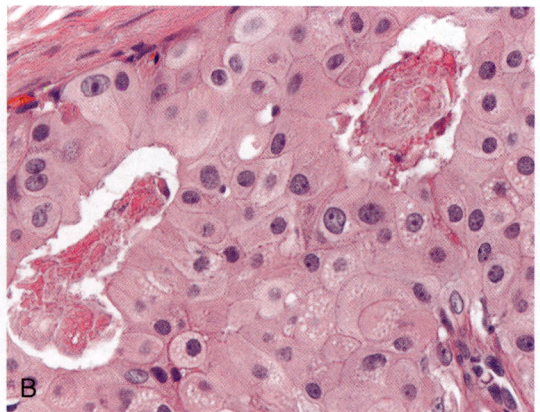

Neoplasia

Figure 8-37 A, A population of atypical apocrine cells has overrun this papilloma. **B,** The atypical apocrine cells show stratification, loss of the basal position of their nucleus, vacuolization of their cytoplasm, and mild pleomorphism of their nuclei and nucleoli.

The Nature of "Atypical Papilloma"

Certain pathologists advocate the use of the term *atypical papilloma* for lesions in which low-grade ductal carcinoma occupies less than a third of a papilloma or for papillomas displaying cytologic atypicality of a low-grade nature. This approach does eliminate certain problems classifying borderline cases, but the practice may create more problems than it solves. By applying a single diagnosis to slightly different patterns of proliferation, this usage blurs the nuances of pathogenesis that pathologists can appreciate. Furthermore, investigators have yet to establish the clinical implications of lesions classified as atypical papillomas. Do these tumors have a behavior different from that of papillomas harboring small foci of low-grade ductal carcinoma in situ? Considering these difficulties, certain pathologists may find it preferable to use existing diagnostic terms to describe the pathologic processes evident in a papillary tumor. This approach would favor diagnoses such as "ductal carcinoma in situ involving a papilloma" and "atypical ductal hyperplasia involving a papilloma," for example, rather than "atypical papilloma."

Secondary Lobular Changes

Terminal duct–lobular units in the tissue in the vicinity of a papilloma can undergo reactive changes that cause the acinar epithelial cells to appear unusual. One type of lobular change resembles an inflammatory reaction centered on lobules. The affected lobules appear slightly enlarged. The presence of abundant myxoid ground substance, extra stromal cells, and inflammatory cells makes the intralobular stroma appear prominent, and dilatation of the acini enlarges the glandular tissue (Fig. 8-38). The distended glands contain eosinophilic material, which probably represent products of secretion because the luminal cells lining the acini often contain eosinophilic droplets in their cytoplasm (Fig. 8-39). These glandular cells vary in cytologic features. Some appear flat and vaguely squamous, whereas others have abundant, foamy cytoplasm that sometimes contains yellow-brown pigment (Fig. 8-40). The latter cells possess large nuclei, coarsely granular chromatin, and prominent nucleoli (Fig. 8-41).

Researchers have not identified the nature of this lobular alteration; however, it seems to depend on the presence of a papilloma, because one does not encounter these changes in other settings. The inflammatory quality of the stroma suggests that irritating substances such as blood or mammary secretions have found their way into the glandular lumen, and one occasionally observes rupture of the glands with leakage of their contents into the stroma (Fig. 8-42). The offending papilloma often shows infarction and hemorrhage, so blood seems an especially likely culprit. Because the densely eosinophilic intracellular droplets resemble those of conventional apocrine cells, secretion of a damaging compound could also incite the inflammation. Whatever the pathogenesis of this abnormality, pathologists should not interpret it as a neoplastic phenomenon.

The second type of lobular alteration occurs in the setting of papillomas with sclerosis. The stromal reaction to the tumor engulfs neighboring lobules. Besides causing the scarring and distortion of acini

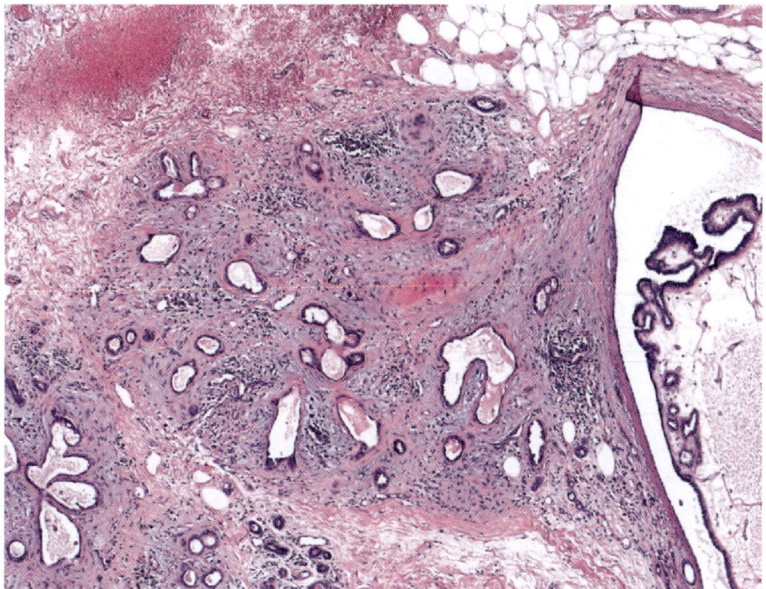

Figure 8-38 The lobule adjacent to this papilloma appears enlarged because of edema and inflammation of the intralobular stroma and dilatation of the acini.

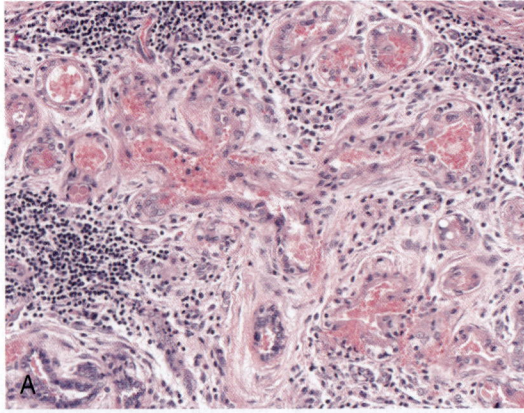

Figure 8-39 A, The lumens of the acini contain pink secretions and eosinophilic droplets. **B,** The cytoplasm of the acinar cells contains identical droplets.

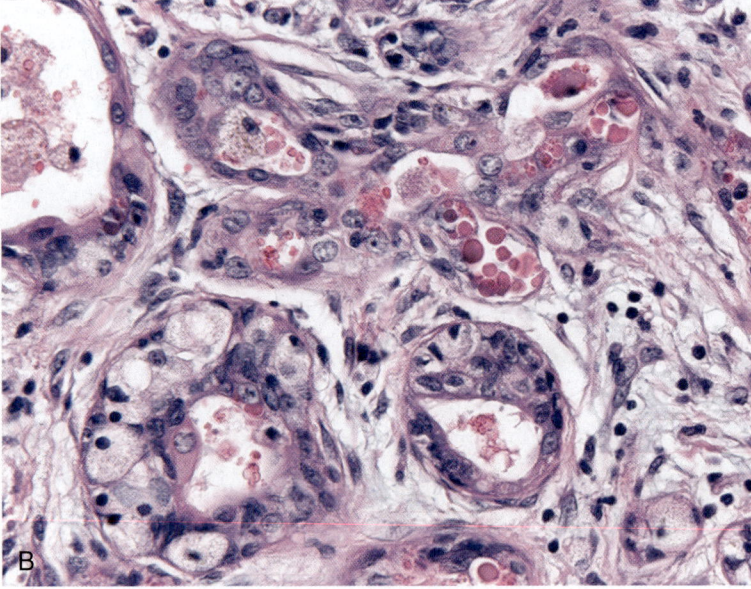

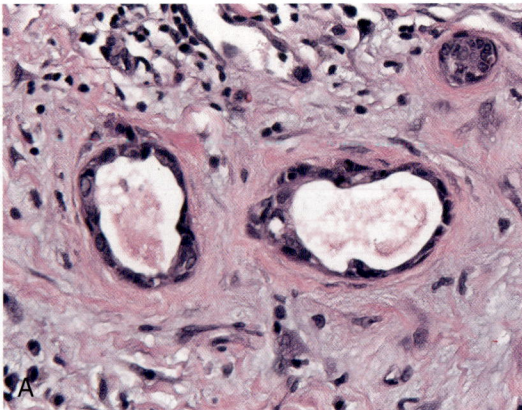

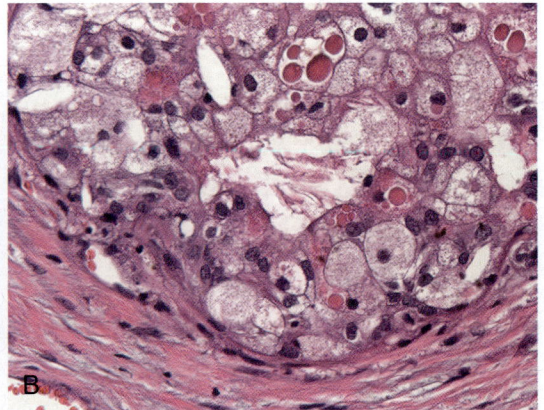

Figure 8-40 A, When the cells lining the acini contain only modest amounts of cytoplasm, they have a low cuboidal or flat shape. **B,** In other examples, the cell contains abundant foamy cytoplasm.

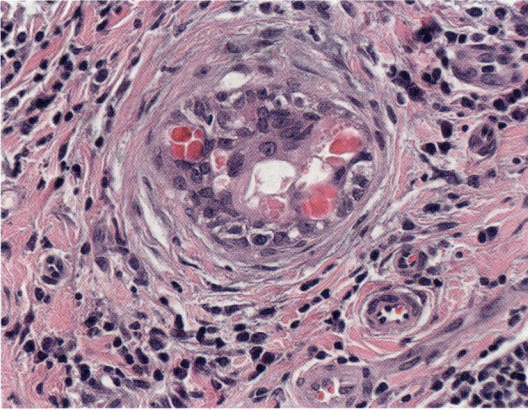

Figure 8-41 The nuclei can appear large, the chromatin pale, and the nucleoli prominent.

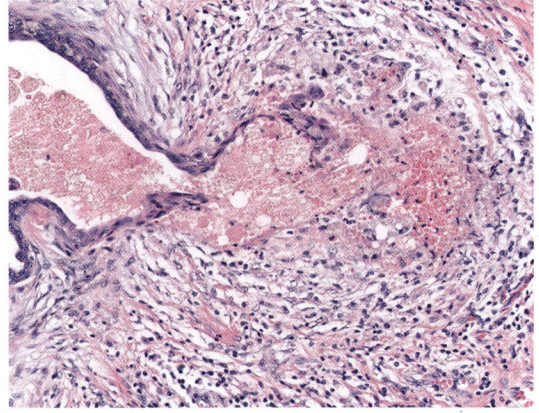

Figure 8-42 Rupture of this duct has spilled material into the stroma.

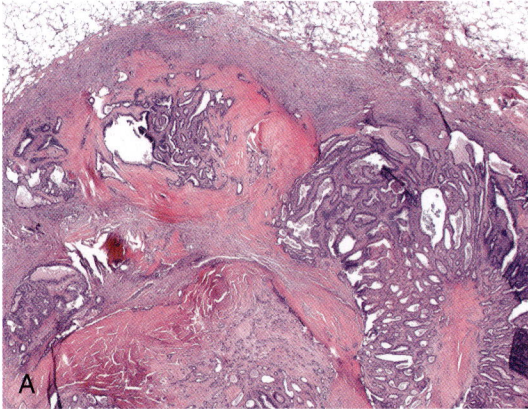

Figure 8-43 A, The desmoplastic reaction of this sclerosing papilloma has surrounded a lobule shown in **B. C,** The densely eosinophilic cytoplasm gives the cells a squamous appearance, and the cells possess barely detectable intercellular bridges.

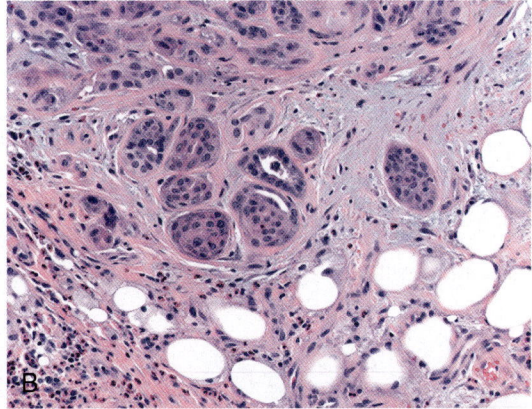

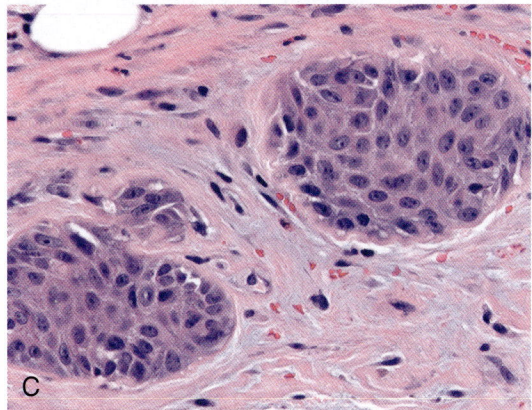

already illustrated, the sclerosing reaction can cause the acinar cells to assume squamous characteristics (Fig. 8-43). The cells possess dense, eosinophilic cytoplasm and nuclei that vary from small to plump. The chromatin can stain darkly or less so, and the larger nuclei usually contain easily detected nucleoli. These changes do not have any clinical significance, but they do complicate the detection and diagnosis of low-grade adenosquamous carcinoma. This complication represents a significant concern, because this variety of invasive carcinoma frequently emerges in the bed of a sclerosing papilloma (Fig. 8-44).

Several findings allow one to distinguish reactive squamous metaplasia of acini from low-grade adenosquamous carcinoma. First, reactive lobules maintain

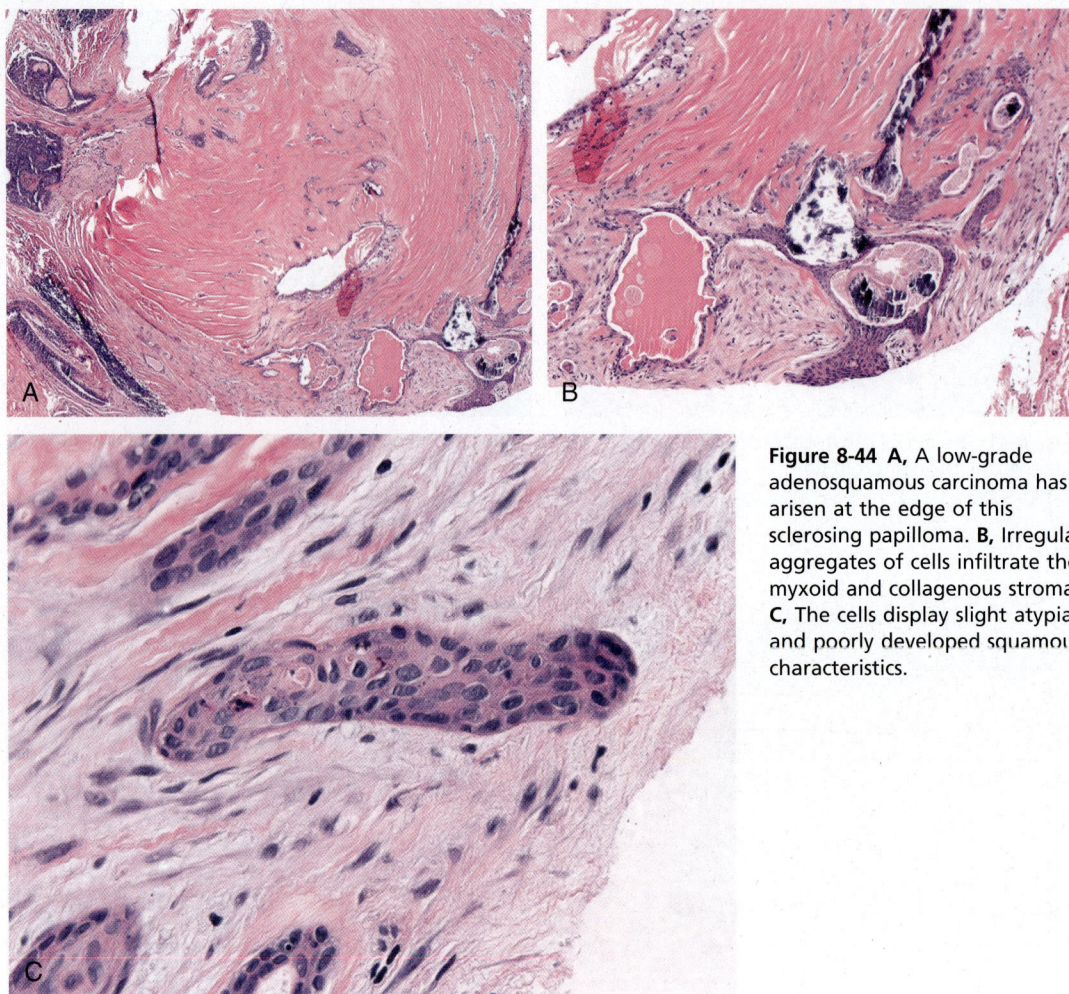

Figure 8-44 A, A low-grade adenosquamous carcinoma has arisen at the edge of this sclerosing papilloma. **B,** Irregular aggregates of cells infiltrate the myxoid and collagenous stroma. **C,** The cells display slight atypia and poorly developed squamous characteristics.

their underlying structural organization, and the distribution of their acini recalls that of a normally formed terminal duct–lobular unit. The glands of low-grade adenosquamous carcinoma grow haphazardly without recreating a lobular structure. Second, the nuclei in reactive squamous cells appear bland, whereas those of carcinomas display subtle enlargement, pleomorphism, and atypia. Finally, immunohistochemical staining of reactive acini for myoepithelial proteins reveals the usual patterns. When applied to low-grade adenosquamous carcinomas, these stains usually produce unexpected results, which vary from gland to gland. Attention to these findings helps pathologists avoid overlooking this subtle type of carcinoma.

Variants of Papillomas

When pathologic processes that give rise to papillomas unfold in slightly different ways or in slightly different locations, lesions representing variations of

papillomas develop. The three lesions in this family are adenomyoepithelioma, ductal adenoma, and pleomorphic adenoma. These lesions grow as well-defined, space-occupying masses within the mammary parenchyma, and they compress the adjacent uninvolved tissue. Each consists of newly formed stroma and glandular structures lined by normally positioned luminal and myoepithelial cells. Many examples of these lesions coexist with conventional papillomas. Descriptions of these three entities record many common features, and individual cases often exhibit a mixture of findings; consequently, pathologists need not fret about the choice of diagnosis in a given case. Once one establishes the benign nature of such a tumor, personal preference can guide further classification of the nodule.

Displaced Epithelium and Fragments

Growing as most do within cavities, papillomas seem more easily fragmented than many other lesions. The

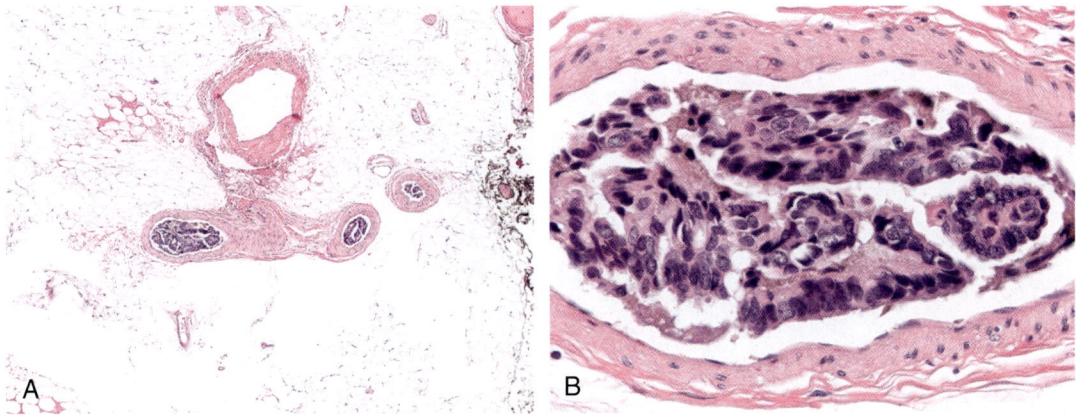

Figure 8-45 A, Mechanical forces created during either this biopsy or the prior one probably account for the presence of these crumpled strips of epithelium and a fragment of a papilloma inside a small vein. **B,** One can identify a few myoepithelial cells and a bit of stroma in the tissue fragments.

mechanical trauma generated during a core needle biopsy or an aspiration procedure can dislodge clusters of hyperplastic cells from the surface of papillomas harboring florid conventional ductal hyperplasia, and the groups often become implanted in the granulation tissue of the needle track. Chapter 13, devoted to radial scars, discusses the histologic characteristics of this phenomenon in detail. The same forces that dislodge clusters of hyperplastic cells can push fragments of the papilloma into lymphatic vessels and blood vessels (Fig. 8-45), and the pieces can even migrate to lymph nodes. Once the pathologist becomes familiar with these phenomena, they need not cause confusion.

Selected Readings

Azzopardi JG: Problems in Breast Pathology. (Major Problems in Pathology, vol 11.), London, WB Saunders, 1979.

Ciatto S, Andreoli C, Cirillo A, et al: The risk of breast cancer subsequent to histologic diagnosis of benign intraductal papilloma: Follow-up study of 339 cases. Tumori 1991;77:41-43.

Haagensen CD, Stout AP, Phillips JS: The papillary neoplasms of the breast. I: Benign intraductal papilloma. Ann Surg 1951;133:18-36.

Kraus FT, Neubecker RD: The differential diagnosis of papillary tumors of the breast. Cancer 1962;15: 444-455.

Krieger N, Hiatt RA: Risk of breast cancer after benign breast diseases: Variation by histologic type, degree of atypia, age at biopsy, and length of follow-up. Am J Epidemiol 1992;135:619-631.

Murad TM, Contesso G, Mourisesse H: Papillary tumors of large lactiferous ducts. Cancer 1981;48:122-133.

Nagi C, Bleiweiss I, Jaffer S: Epithelial displacement in breast lesions: A papillary phenomenon. Arch Pathol Lab Med 2005;129:1465-1469.

Ohuchi N, Abe R, Kasai M: Possible cancerous change of intraductal papillomas of the breast: A 3-D reconstruction study of 25 cases. Cancer 1984;54:605-611.

Page DL, Salhany KE, Jensen RA, et al: Subsequent breast carcinoma risk after biopsy with atypia in a breast papilloma. Cancer 1996;78:258-266.

Raju UB, Lee MW, Zarbo RJ, et al: Papillary neoplasia of the breast: Immunohistochemically defined myoepithelial cells in the diagnosis of benign and malignant papillary breast neoplasms. Mod Pathol 1989;2: 569-576.

Sapino A, Botta G, Cassoni P, et al: Multiple papillomas of the breast: Morphologic findings and clinical evolution. Anat Pathol 1996;1:205-218.

Youngson BJ, Cranor M, Rosen PP: Epithelial displacement in surgical breast specimens following needling procedures. Am J Surg Pathol 1994;18:896-903.

9

Papillary Carcinoma

DEFINITIONS AND CLINICOPATHOLOGIC CHARACTERISTICS

Papillary carcinomas are malignant neoplasms in which neoplastic ductal cells grow on an arborizing stromal framework. Despite the superficial similarities between papillomas and papillary carcinomas, the two lesions do not share fundamental properties, and the former do not give rise to the latter. Both the stroma and the glandular tissue of a papilloma have a neoplastic origin, whereas only the glandular cells constitute the neoplastic component of a papillary carcinoma. The stroma represents preexisting mammary stroma overrun by the malignant cells and remodeled by them to create the characteristic branching skeleton.

Like papillomas, papillary carcinomas can affect any region of the ductal tree. Tumors growing in large ducts commonly provoke a bloody discharge from the nipple. Those situated more peripherally might create a mass or a mammographic abnormality, but they also may not produce clinical symptoms or signs. Papillary carcinomas tend to affect women somewhat older than those with either commonplace breast cancers or papillomas. Thus, papillary tumors in women older than 70 years most often represent carcinomas. Papillary carcinomas account for a higher proportion of breast cancers in men.

On macroscopic examination, one cannot reliably distinguish a conventional papillary carcinoma from a papilloma, but the former often appears pink-tan and exceptionally fragile. Certain special types of papillary carcinoma—solid papillary carcinoma and intracystic papillary carcinoma—frequently exhibit the distinctive macroscopic features described later.

HISTOLOGIC CHARACTERISTICS

Fundamental Characteristics

Geometric Properties of the Fronds

At low magnification, the typical papillary carcinoma displays a disorderly architecture composed of a large number of fronds (Fig. 9-1). The fronds vary greatly in size and shape, and many have filiform or ribbon-like configurations (Fig. 9-2). The two dimensions of these long, slender structures differ greatly; one dimension of one of these filiform fronds often measures much more than the other dimension. The fronds of a papillary carcinoma do not fit together neatly in the way that those of a papilloma do; consequently, papillary carcinomas have a disorderly and shaggy appearance, which contrasts with the compact look of a papilloma (Fig. 9-3). When the carcinoma cells proliferate exuberantly, they can obscure the underlying papillary architecture and thereby make

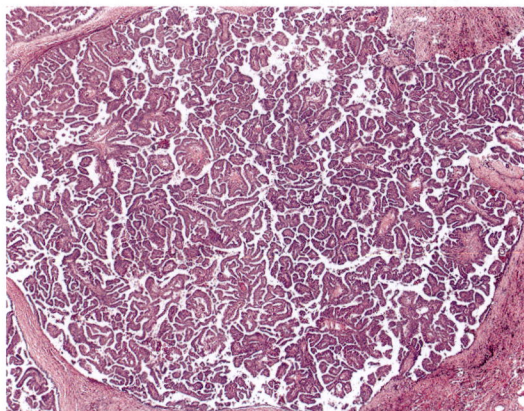

Figure 9-1 This papillary carcinoma consists of many fronds that vary dramatically in size and shape.

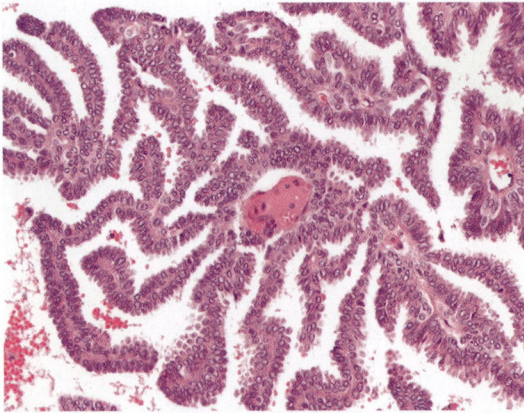

Figure 9-2 The lengths of the filiform papillae of this papillary carcinoma measure much more than their widths.

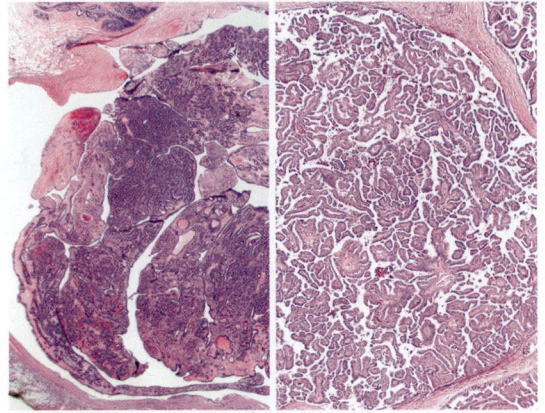

Figure 9-3 The papilloma (*left*) consists of just a few, broad and blunt fronds that fit together smoothly, whereas the papillary carcinoma (*right*) forms a shaggy mass composed of innumerable, irregular fronds.

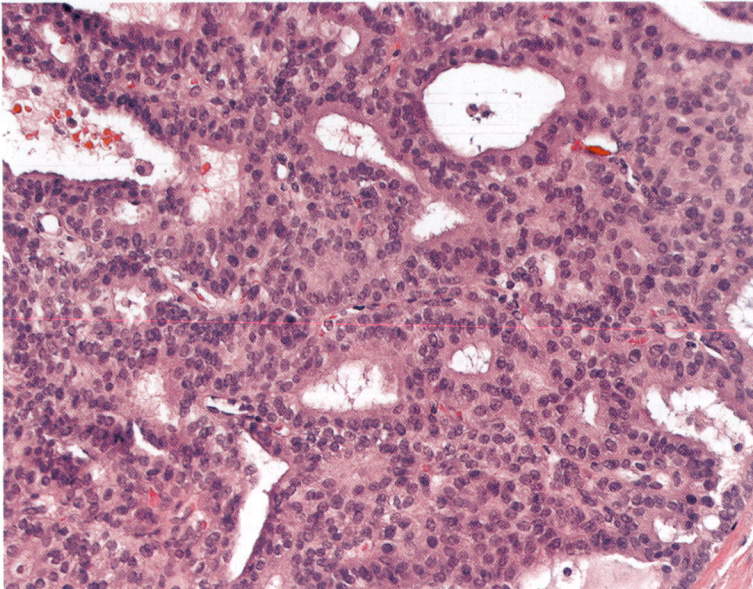

Figure 9-4 The florid proliferation of the carcinoma cells obscures the papillary architecture of this papillary carcinoma, but the engorged capillaries reveal the branching configuration of the supporting fibrovascular skeleton.

a papillary carcinoma look somewhat solid; however, close inspection reveals the papillary architecture of the supporting fibrovascular skeleton (Fig. 9-4).

Amount of Stroma

A few fronds contain only epithelial cells, but most have a fibrous connective tissue core. The fibrous connective tissue typically accounts for only a minimal portion of the frond, and the skimpiness of the stroma gives the impression that it participates in the growth of the tumor only to support the epithelium (Fig. 9-5). Figure 9-6 shows the difference in typical

amount of stroma between a papillary carcinoma and a papilloma.

Characteristics of the Epithelium

Atypical ductal cells constitute the epithelium of a papillary carcinoma; myoepithelial cells do not participate in the formation of this lesion. Furthermore, the malignant ductal cells always display cytologic atypicality and usually show stratification. The cytologic features of most papillary carcinomas resemble those of low-grade ductal carcinoma in situ. The cells appear enlarged, look cuboidal or polygonal,

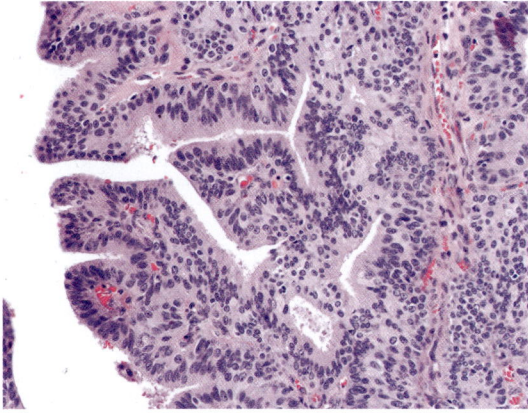

Figure 9-5 Epithelial cells constitute most of this papillary carcinoma, whereas the stroma accounts for only a little of the lesion's bulk.

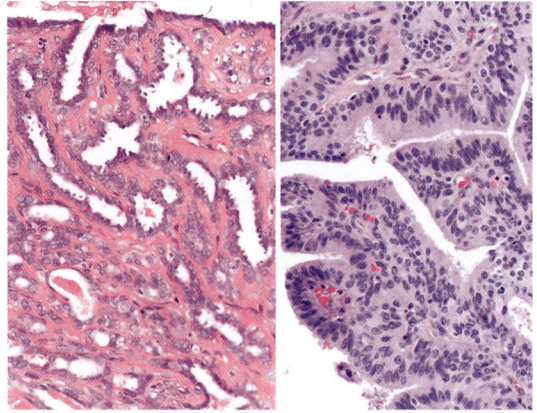

Figure 9-6 Contrast the abundant stroma in the papilloma (*left*) with the scant amount of stroma in the papillary carcinoma depicted (*right*).

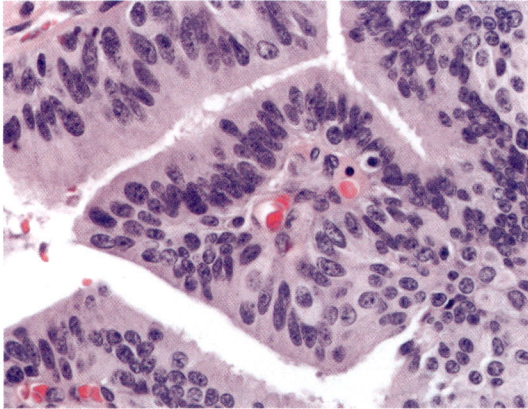

Figure 9-7 The epithelium of this papillary carcinoma consists of just one type of cell, which displays low-grade cytologic atypicality. The tumor cells possess slightly enlarged, oval nuclei, homogeneous and dark chromatin, inconspicuous nucleoli, and abundant apical cytoplasm.

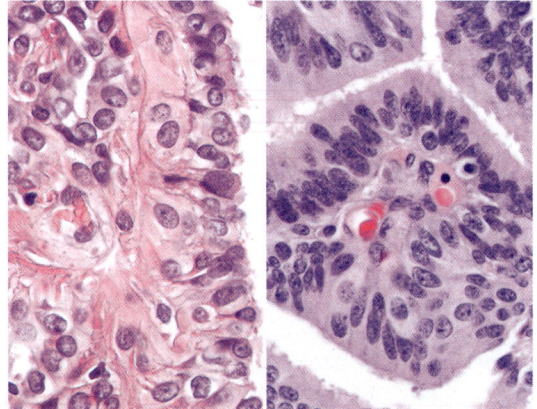

Figure 9-8 Contrast the two-layered epithelium composed of two types of benign cells in the papilloma (*left*) with the multilayered epithelium consisting of only malignant luminal epithelial cells in the papillary carcinoma (*right*).

and contain slightly enlarged, smoothly contoured oval or round nuclei, homogeneous dark chromatin, inconspicuous nucleoli, and ample cytoplasm (Fig. 9-7). The cells usually grow in several layers and form cribriform spaces and trabecular bars. Thus, the characteristics of the epithelium of a papillary carcinoma contrast with those of papilloma in three ways. In the former, the epithelium consists of one type of cell that appears cytologically atypical and demonstrates architectural atypicality, whereas the epithelium of a papilloma consists of two types of cells, both benign, which grow in an orderly, two-layered arrangement (Fig. 9-8) (Box 9-1).

Box 9-1

Fundamental characteristics of papillary carcinoma:

- Numerous fronds that vary greatly in size and shape
- Preponderance of the epithelium over the stroma
- A proliferative population composed solely of neoplastic epithelial cells

Table 9-1 Histologic Characteristics of Papilloma and Conventional Papillary Carcinoma

	Papilloma	Conventional Papillary Carcinoma
Fundamental Characteristics		
Fronds	Few, broad, blunt	Many, variable in size and shape
Stroma	Abundant	Minimal
Epithelium	Two layers; two types of benign cells	Atypical luminal cells only
Associated epithelial proliferation	Conventional ductal hyperplasia	Ductal carcinoma in situ
Ancillary Characteristics		
Mitotic rate	Rare	Occasional
Dishesion	None	Present
Calcification	Stromal	Luminal

Ancillary Characteristics

One can usually find mitotic figures easily in a papillary carcinoma, in contrast to papillomas, which rarely exhibit division figures. The malignant cells of a papillary carcinoma tend to separate from one another and to slough into the duct lumen as single cells or small clusters. When the cells degenerate, nuclear debris and degenerating cytoplasm collect within the duct lumen. The dishesion of papillary carcinomas contrasts with the marked cohesion of the epithelial cells of papillomas. If calcifications form in a papillary carcinoma, they typically precipitate in the luminal debris, in cribriform spaces, or in the nearby stroma. Calcium deposits do not commonly form within the fibrovascular skeleton of a carcinoma, as they sometimes do in papillomas. In many papillary carcinomas, the malignant cells completely coat the wall of the affected duct, and the carcinoma cells may extend into neighboring ducts. Malignant cells growing in these locations most often display the characteristic cytologic and architectural features of low-grade ductal carcinoma in situ (Box 9-2).

Summary

Papillary carcinomas develop when malignant ductal cells grow in a manner that remodels the existing mammary fibrous connective tissue to form a branching skeleton. They usually consist of innumerable, irregular, filiform fronds forming a shaggy mass. Carcinoma cells supported by scant fibrous tissue compose the fronds. One can usually detect evidence of cell division and dishesion, and calcifications often form within the carcinoma. Conventional ductal carcinoma in situ often involves the duct harboring a

Box 9-2

Ancillary characteristics of papillary carcinomas:

- Numerous mitotic figures
- Cellular dishesion
- Luminal calcifications
- Coexisting ductal carcinoma in situ

papillary carcinoma and the ducts adjacent to it. Table 9-1 contrasts the fundamental characteristics and the ancillary findings of papillomas and papillary carcinomas.

PROBLEMS IN THE DIAGNOSIS OF PAPILLARY CARCINOMA

Although pathologists find that application of the basic criteria for the diagnosis of papillary tumors identifies many papillary carcinomas without ambiguity, three problematic areas remain. First, two uncommon patterns of conventional papillary carcinomas display histologic features that can lead one to confuse these carcinomas with benign or atypical lesions. Second, the recognition of invasion poses problems in many papillary carcinomas. Finally, two special types of papillary carcinoma raise problems of their own.

Uncommon Histologic Features of Conventional Papillary Carcinoma

Two variations in cellular morphology seen in conventional papillary carcinomas give rise to patterns

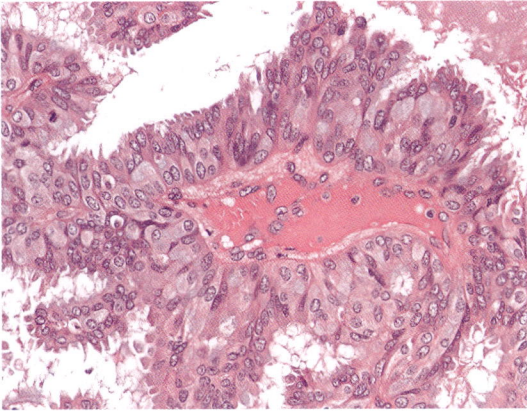

Figure 9-9 The cells growing along the stalk of this papillary carcinoma possess pale, bluish gray cytoplasm. Pathologists sometimes refer to such cells as *dimorphic cells* and tumors containing many of them as *dimorphic papillary carcinomas.*

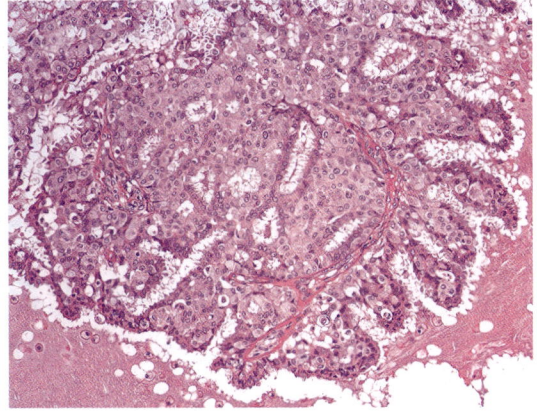

Figure 9-10 The dimorphic cells in this papillary carcinoma constitute the dominant population.

that cause diagnostic confusion. The first variation consists of clearing of the cytoplasm, a process that seems to favor cells growing along the basement membrane. Growth of the carcinoma as a single layer of tall, columnar cells is the second variation.

Carcinomas Containing Cells with Clear Cytoplasm (Dimorphic Cells)

As many as a third of papillary carcinomas contain a distinct population of cells growing adjacent to the basement membrane and possessing abundant clear cytoplasm similar to that seen in myoepithelial cells (Fig. 9-9). These cells usually form a layer just one or two cells thick, but they can accumulate in such

numbers that they become the dominant population (Fig. 9-10). Lefkowitz and colleagues[1] referred to these cells as *dimorphic tumor cells*, and pathologists occasionally refer to a tumor containing many of these cells as a *dimorphic papillary carcinoma*. Because the cytologic features of these basally situated malignant cells differ from those of the overlying epithelial cells, one could easily misinterpret them as either myoepithelial cells or as lobular carcinoma cells growing in a pagetoid pattern (Fig. 9-11) and thereby misclassify a papillary carcinoma as a papilloma harboring myoepithelial hyperplasia or lobular carcinoma in situ.

To prevent these errors, one has only to appreciate that the cells represent a single population rather than

Figure 9-11 Λ, The myoepithelial cells in this papilloma have proliferated to form a small nodule.

(Continued)

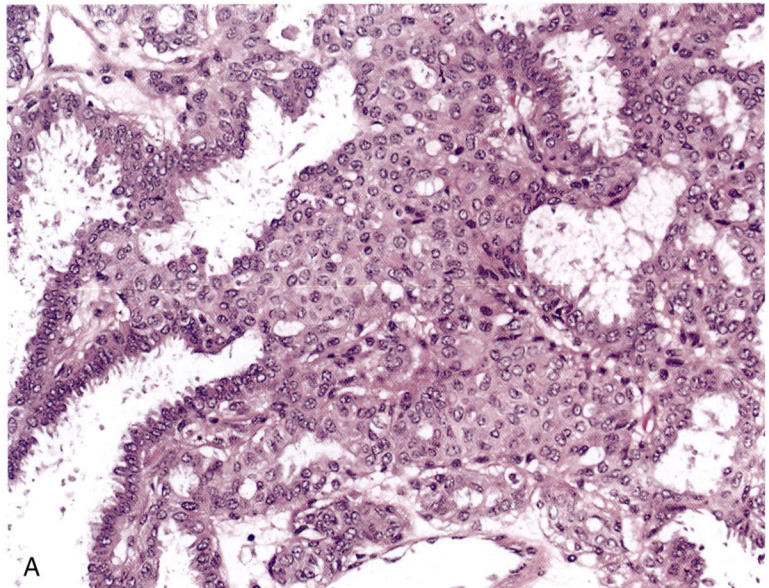

A

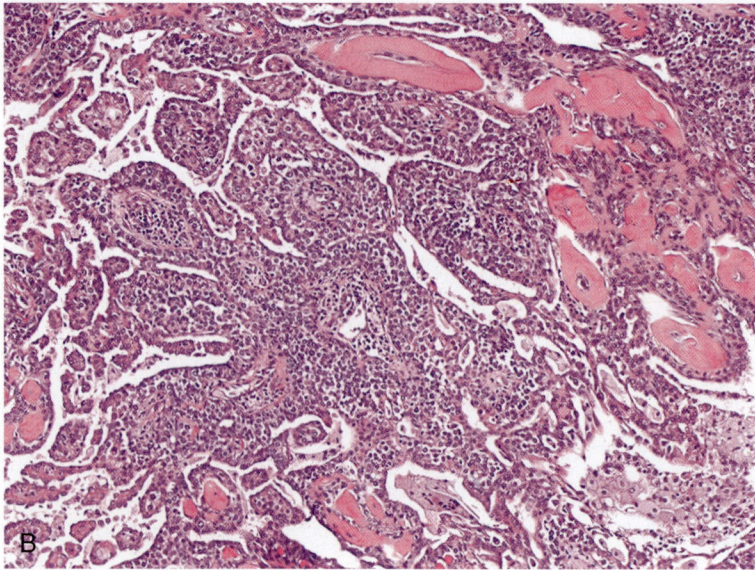

Figure 9-11–cont'd B, Lobular carcinoma in situ extensively involves this papilloma.

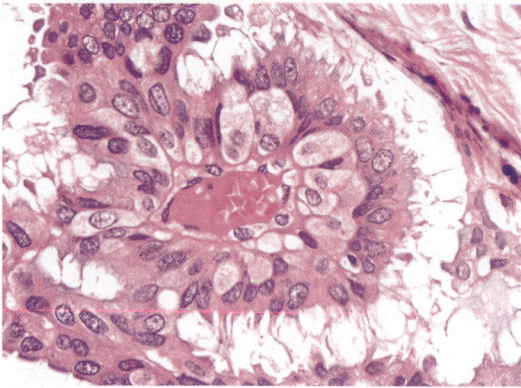

Figure 9-12 The nuclei of the basal cells with pale cytoplasm (the dimorphic cells) appear identical to those of the more superficial carcinoma cells, which possess eosinophilic cytoplasm.

two distinct clans; attention to the nuclear characteristics of the two types of cells allows one to recognize their common heritage. Dimorphic tumor cells possess nuclei identical to those of the more superficial carcinoma cells (Fig. 9-12), whereas myoepithelial cell nuclei differ from those of the overlying epithelial cells (Fig. 9-13A), and so do the nuclei of lobular carcinoma cells (Fig. 9-13B). Furthermore, the cells of lobular neoplasia usually display the lack of cohesion characteristic of this lesion, whereas dimorphic cells look somewhat more cohesive. One could also use the results of immunohistochemical staining for keratin, myosin heavy chain, calponin, and p63 protein to differentiate dimorphic cells from myoepithelial cells. Carcinoma cells would stain for keratin but not for the other three proteins, whereas myoepithelial cells would show the opposite reaction pattern.

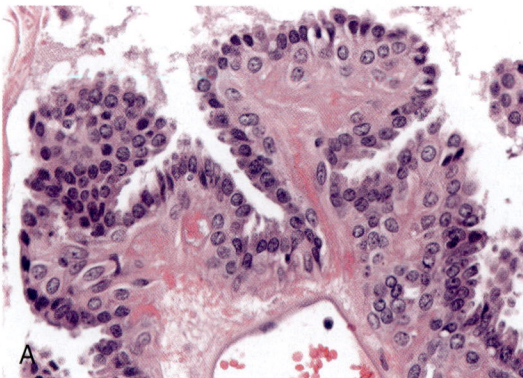

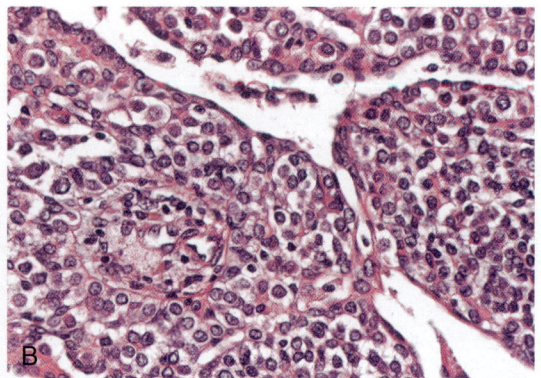

Figure 9-13 A, The myoepithelial cells in this papilloma have larger nuclei and paler chromatin than the overlying luminal cells. **B,** Lobular carcinoma grows within the epithelium of this papilloma. The polygonal carcinoma cells have larger nuclei and paler cytoplasm than the overlying, flattened benign cells. The former appear dishesive, whereas the latter look cohesive.

A positive staining reaction for E-cadherin would distinguish dimorphic carcinoma cells from lobular carcinoma.

Carcinomas Composed of Tall, Columnar Cells

The neoplastic cells of certain papillary carcinomas do not form multiple layers; instead, they grow as a single layer of columnar cells (Fig. 9-14). They appear unusually tall, and their nuclei occupy the basal region of the cell, creating a well-developed apical cytoplasmic compartment. In cases of minimal cellular proliferation, the nuclei sit at the same position in each cell, producing a parallel array and a deceptively orderly appearance. With more advanced proliferation, the nuclei become crowded and either very long and thin or pseudostratified. Whatever their shape, the nuclei have smooth contours, homogeneous chromatin, and inconspicuous nucleoli.

One can observe a few cells with these characteristics in many otherwise conventional papillary carcinomas (Fig. 9-15), and occasional papillary carcinomas with complex branching and scant stroma consist almost entirely of such cells; however, papillary carcinomas composed primarily of tall, columnar cells often differ from typical papillary carcinoma. This type of papillary carcinoma tends to form short, stubby fronds that show a simple branching pattern. The fronds usually contain abundant stroma and capillaries, and the epithelium grows predominantly in a single layer (Fig. 9-16). The simplicity of the papillary architecture, the abundance of the collagen, the minimal level of epithelial proliferation, the orderliness of the epithelium, and the minimal nature of the cytologic atypicality together create an appearance that superficially mimics that of a papilloma, and one can understand why pathologists often find the diagnosis of such cases difficult.

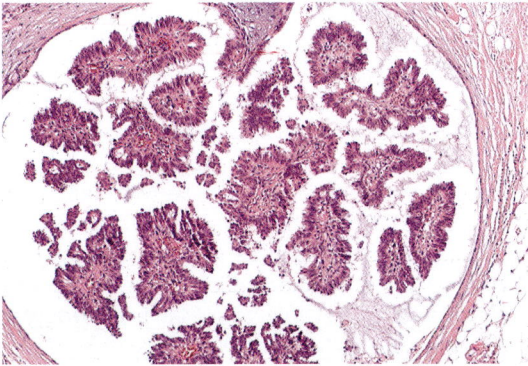

Figure 9-14 This papillary carcinoma consists of just a few short, stubby fronds containing abundant stroma and covered by a single layer of epithelial cells.

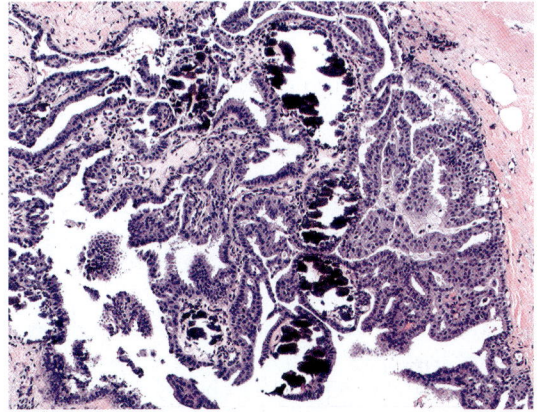

Figure 9-15 In a few areas, the malignant cells in this papillary carcinoma grow as a single layer of columnar cells, but most regions show piling up of cuboidal or polygonal cells.

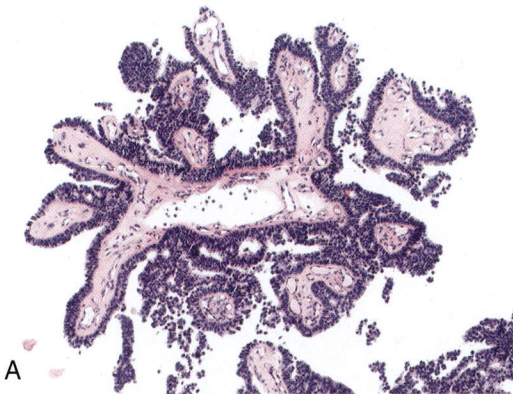

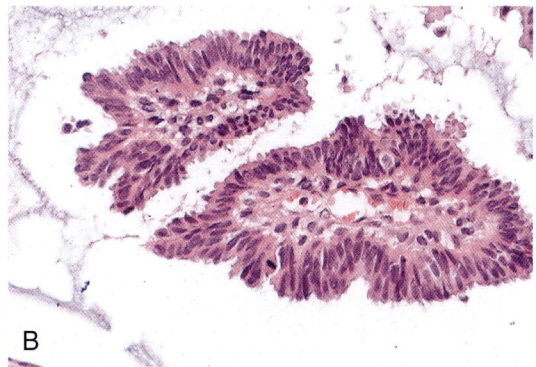

Figure 9-16 A, The fronds of this form of papillary carcinoma consist of abundant stroma covered by a single layer of epithelial cells. **B,** The epithelial cells have columnar shapes, oval nuclei, and homogeneous and dark chromatin, and they grow in a crowded, pseudostratified layer.

Attention to the following four characteristics helps minimize this difficulty: the shape of the cell, the shape of the nucleus, the properties of the chromatin, and the arrangement of the cells. Normal columnar ductal epithelial cells have a height only a few times their width, whereas malignant columnar cells appear much taller than their width. Mirroring these cellular proportions, benign nuclei appear relatively short and plump, whereas malignant nuclei look long and slender. Benign ductal cells have slightly granular chromatin, which can show clearing, but malignant columnar cells usually possess homogeneous and finely granular chromatin. Finally, normal ductal cells do not show the crowding or the nuclear pseudostratification seen in these papillary carcinomas.

Distinction between Papilloma Involved by Ductal Carcinoma In Situ and Papillary Carcinoma

Papilloma harboring ductal carcinoma in situ and papillary carcinoma seem to represent different lesions arising through different pathogenetic pathways. The former begins its life as a benign papilloma, which either gives rise to ductal carcinoma in situ or becomes colonized by ductal carcinoma cells originating in ducts beyond the one housing the papilloma. The latter, on the other hand, grows as a papillary carcinoma from its inception. Despite this conceptual difference, neither oncologists nor pathologists maintain a sharp distinction between the two entities. Distinguishing these two lesions does not have clinical importance, of course, because physicians recommend the same treatment for both.

Nevertheless, the pathologist may wish to differentiate the two lesions as often as the cases permit, because this careful approach allows the pathologist to develop expertise with the application of the diagnostic criteria for macropapillary tumors and to appreciate the pathogenesis of the lesions more fully.

To distinguish a papilloma colonized by ductal carcinoma in situ from a papillary carcinoma, one must discover evidence of the preexisting papilloma. Such evidence consists of two elements: the broad, blunt fronds composed of abundant collagen characteristic of a papilloma, and benign epithelial cells of either luminal or myoepithelial type (Fig. 9-17). The presence of broad fronds strongly suggests the existence of an underlying papilloma; however, this finding alone does not establish this point, because certain varieties of papillary carcinoma characteristically have fronds with these characteristics. Recognition of either benign luminal cells or myoepithelial cells within the papillary structures, however, is persuasive evidence of an underlying papilloma, because conventional papillary carcinomas do not contain significant numbers of benign cells. Careful, detailed study of conventional hematoxylin and eosin—stained sections often discloses these benign cells, and immunohistochemical staining for markers of myoepithelial cells highlights their presence (Fig. 9-18). One should probably observe both the broad fronds and the benign cells to identify an underlying papilloma with confidence. The absence of these findings does not exclude the possibility of a preexisting papilloma, but one would find it difficult to substantiate this impression without them.

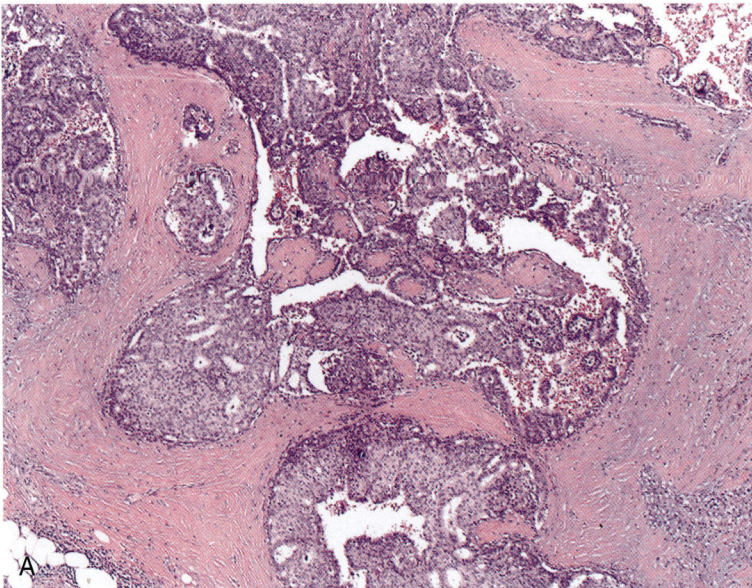

Figure 9-17 A, This malignant papillary tumor has the thick, collagenous stromal cores characteristic of a papilloma.

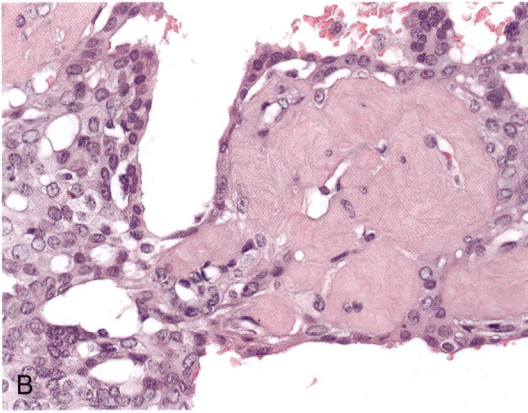

Figure 9-17–cont'd B, High magnification reveals a few residual benign luminal cells and myoepithelial cells.

If one consistently maintains a distinction between papillomas involved by ductal carcinoma in situ and papillary carcinomas, one will note several clinicopathologic differences between the two entities. First, patients with genuine papillary carcinoma tend to be a few years older on average than those with ductal carcinoma in situ involving a papilloma.

Second, a papilloma involved by ductal carcinoma in situ may lack a coexisting invasive carcinoma, whereas a papillary carcinoma typically exhibits at least minimal invasion. Finally, when invasive carcinoma develops in the setting of a papilloma harboring ductal carcinoma in situ, the invasive cancer usually takes the form of a conventional ductal carcinoma of no special type. Papillary carcinomas, on the other hand, invade mostly in a papillary architecture, although one sometimes sees a few small clusters or single cells.

Recognition of Blunt Invasion

When evaluating conventional types of carcinoma in situ for the presence of invasion, many pathologists rightfully adopt a conservative stance to prevent misinterpreting scarred or distorted glands occupied by malignant cells as invasive carcinoma. The assessment of invasion of papillary carcinoma requires the opposite approach. Pathologists must remain ever vigilant, because invasive papillary carcinoma often takes the form of well-defined, smoothly contoured nests that simulate the appearance of ducts overrun by noninvasive papillary carcinoma. Moreover, the desmoplastic response evoked by the

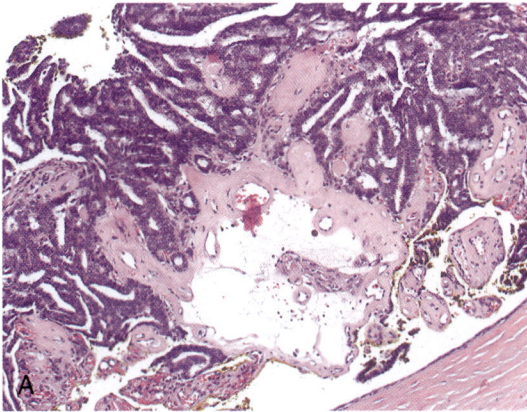

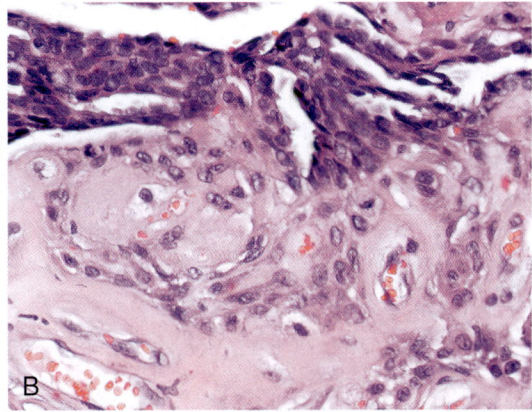

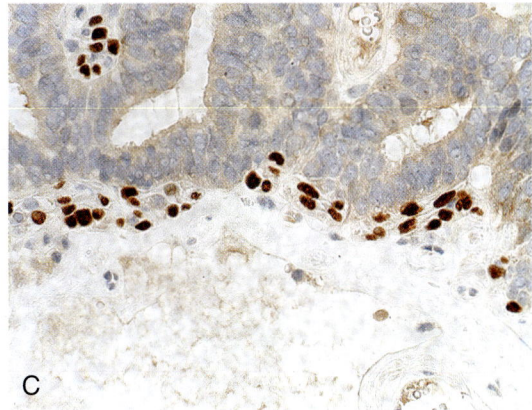

Figure 9-18 A, This papillary tumor has the broad, collagenous fronds commonly seen in papillomas. **B,** The pale cells growing in strands within the collagen of the stalk represent preexisting, benign myoepithelial cells. **C,** A stain for p63 protein discloses the myoepithelial cells.

(not with tumor cells)
Evidence of pre-existing papilloma.

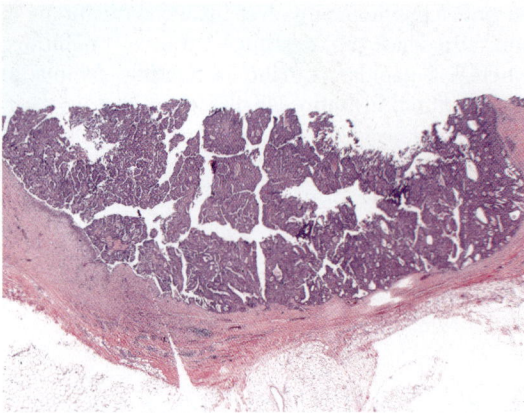

Figure 9-19 This large mass of papillary carcinoma invades in a blunt manner.

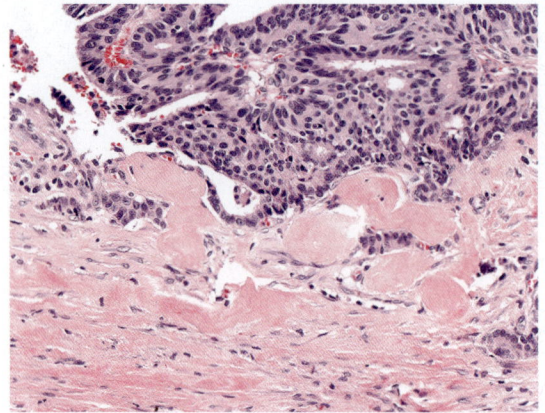

Figure 9-20 Irregular small clusters of carcinoma cells extend between bundles of collagen.

invasive carcinoma looks like the reactive fibrosis that often surrounds ducts involved by ductal carcinoma in situ. To recognize this pattern of blunt invasion, pathologists must study the lesion at both low and high magnification.

Using low magnification, one should determine whether the nests of tumor cells display sizes compatible with those of distended glands and whether the arrangement of the nests resembles the architecture of the mammary glandular tree. The presence of extremely large masses of cells or aggregates displaying shapes inconsistent with dichotomously branching ducts or lobulated terminal duct–lobular units should raise the possibility of invasion. The mass shown in Figure 9-19, for example, has a smooth contour, but its enormous size alone makes a diagnosis of noninvasive carcinoma unlikely. With high magnification, one must carefully inspect the

interface between the masses of carcinoma cells and the stroma. One should suspect the presence of invasion if even small regions of the papillary mass have irregular or angulated contours. Furthermore, one must look for subtle extension of the carcinoma cells between fibroblasts or collagen bundles abutting the tumor (Fig. 9-20). Such invasive cells may not wander far from the main mass (Fig. 9-21), so the intrusion of even a few small nests or columns of malignant cells between fibroblasts or near distended blood vessels or the entrapment of just a few collagen bundles within the mass (Fig. 9-22) should suggest the diagnosis of invasion. The use of immunohistochemical stains for myoepithelial proteins facilitates the recognition of the phenomenon, and with experience, one can develop confidence in the interpretation of the subtle changes evident in conventionally stained sections.

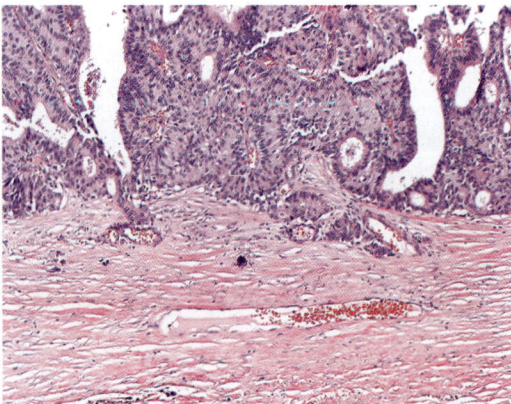

Figure 9-21 Irregular and oddly shaped glands extend a short distance into the stroma and penetrate very close to small blood vessels. The entire mass represents invasive carcinoma.

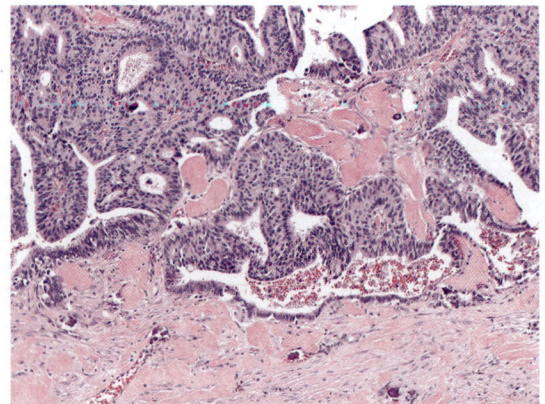

Figure 9-22 Blunt invasion has incorporated collagen bundles into this invasive papillary carcinoma.

Figure 9-23 This small focus of papillary carcinoma spans only a few millimeters, yet the entire mass represents invasive carcinoma.

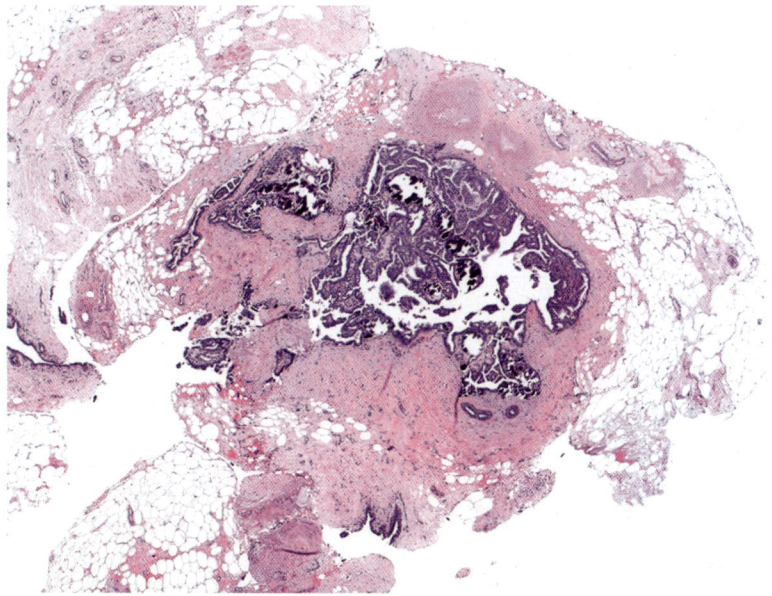

The phenomenon of blunt invasion is not restricted to large masses of carcinoma cells. The early stages of invasion, too, can display this pattern, and so can small tumors (Fig. 9-23). The existence of small papillary carcinomas growing in this fashion suggests that the process of blunt invasion represents an intrinsic property of this type of carcinoma, present in even tiny cancers. It also seems that most genuine, conventional papillary carcinomas demonstrate this pattern of invasion, at least in part, and that one should think carefully before making the diagnosis of papillary ductal carcinoma in situ of conventional type.

Uncommon Varieties of Papillary Carcinoma

Most carcinomas displaying a papillary architecture represent either conventional papillary carcinomas or papillomas overrun by ductal carcinoma in situ; however, the category of papillary carcinoma also encompasses two less common varieties, solid papillary carcinoma and intracystic papillary carcinoma. Both entities raise problems in diagnosis.

Solid Papillary Carcinoma

Solid papillary carcinoma, a form of ductal carcinoma with endocrine differentiation, usually presents in women older than 60 years and often causes a bloody discharge from the nipple. To the unaided eye, the color of these carcinomas often borders on shades of red or pink, and the nodules usually feel a bit softer than conventional breast cancers. Microscopic examination shows that hyalinized cores of stroma and delicate strands of collagen form a branching, papillary skeleton supporting a compact and densely cellular, multilayered epithelial population. Although the collagenous stromal fronds appear obvious immediately, it requires close inspection to appreciate the delicate strands of collagen and the capillaries coursing through the solid, cellular nests (Fig. 9-24). The inconspicuous nature of the papillary architecture in these cellular areas explains the choice of the term *solid* for this variety of papillary carcinoma.

The carcinoma cells appear generally uniform and bland. Their shapes vary from polygonal to fusiform (Fig. 9-25). The nuclei vary in size; most appear only minimally enlarged, but rare ones look gigantic compared with their neighbors. The nuclear shapes vary from nearly round to long and spindly (Fig. 9-26). Many nuclei have irregular contours, the chromatin of most appears pale and granular, and the nuclei usually contain small nucleoli (Fig. 9-27). One can find mitotic figures without a diligent search. The cytoplasm typically has a gray or amphophilic hue; dense core granules sometimes collect in such numbers that the cytoplasm takes on an eosinophilic and finely granular appearance (Fig. 9-28). The cells abutting the stromal cores frequently line up so that their nuclei create a palisade arrangement (Fig. 9-29). The stroma adjacent to the cell nests often contains hemosiderin.

Most examples of solid papillary carcinoma produce mucin, which can accumulate in three locations. Intracellular mucin usually appears as tiny droplets in the cytoplasm; it can also aggregate to form vacuoles (Fig. 9-30A) or even to create signet ring cells. Extracellular mucin forms pools either within epithelial-lined spaces or within the stroma (Fig. 9-30B and C). A mucicarmine stain often reveals

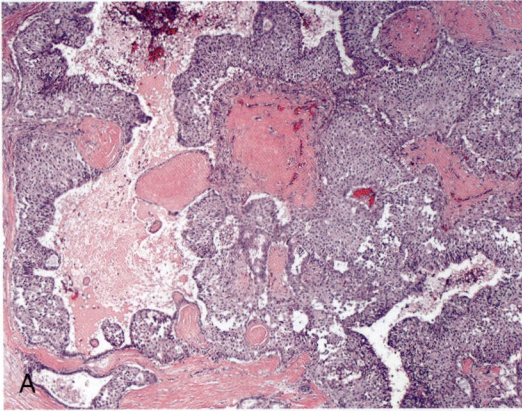

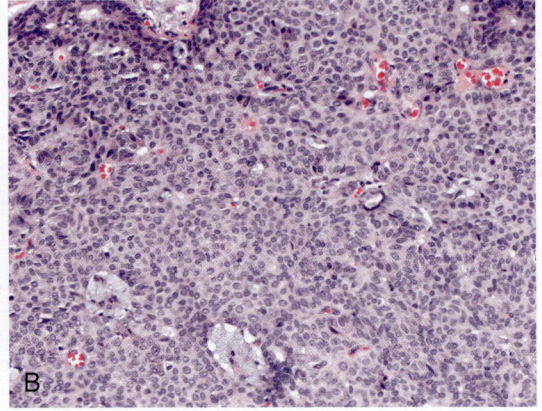

Figure 9-24 A, Dense, hyalinized collagenous fronds form the stromal cores of many solid papillary carcinomas. **B,** Delicate, dilated capillaries contribute to the papillary stromal skeleton.

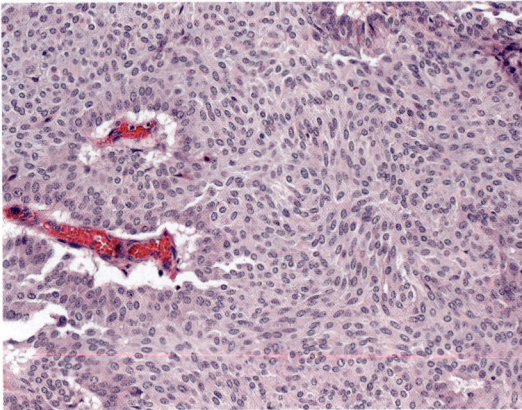

Figure 9-25 The cells in the upper left have polygonal shapes, whereas those in the center exhibit fusiform configurations.

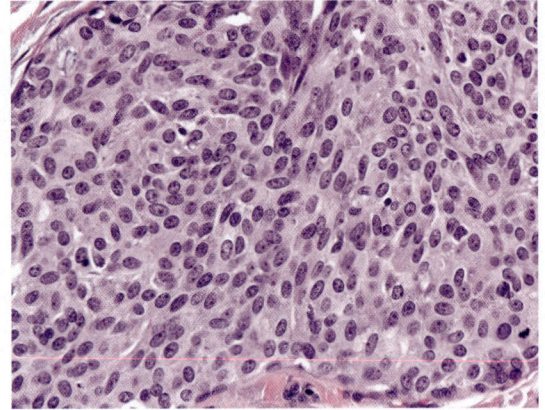

Figure 9-26 The nuclei of solid papillary carcinoma vary from round to spindle shaped.

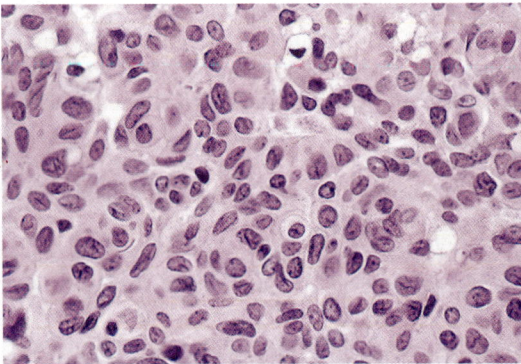

Figure 9-27 The nuclei may have irregular shapes and exhibit nuclear folds, grooves, and notches. The chromatin often appears slightly pale and granular, and many nuclei contain small nucleoli.

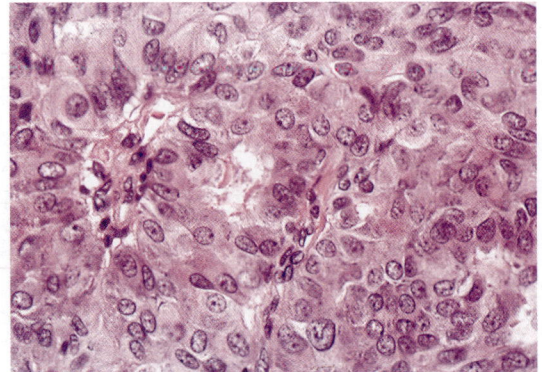

Figure 9-28 Many cells of this solid papillary carcinoma contain miniscule eosinophilic granules in their cytoplasm.

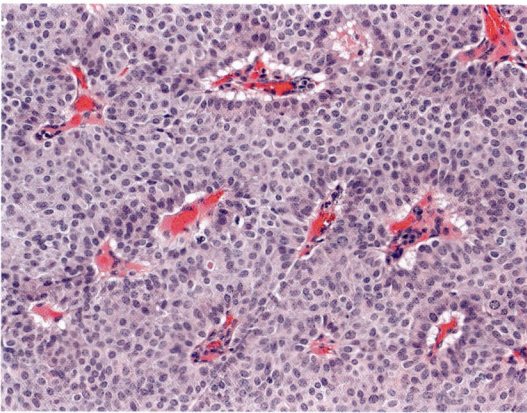

Figure 9-29 The nuclei of the cells adjacent to the stromal cores line up to create a palisade arrangement.

apex, the point of exit of mucin-secreting epithelial cells.

For many years, pathologists have mistaken this variety of papillary carcinoma for a papilloma harboring ductal hyperplasia; in fact, early writing used the term *atypical papilloma* to refer to certain examples of this tumor. One can understand the reasons for this confusion; the abundance of the stroma and its hyalinized quality do suggest the structure of a benign papilloma. Furthermore, the irregularities of nuclear contour, the granularity of the chromatin, and the presence of small nucleoli all seem more in keeping with hyperplastic nuclei than those of low-grade carcinoma cells. Figure 9-31 illustrates the similarity in nuclear characteristics between the cells of conventional ductal hyperplasia and those of certain cases of solid papillary carcinoma. Despite the presence of these common features, careful study yields several findings that point to the proper diagnosis. First, the presence of extremely spindly cells containing especially attenuated nuclei does not fit with the diagnosis of ductal hyperplasia (Fig. 9-32). One might mistake the spindled appearance of such cells as a manifestation of myoepithelial differentiation, but hyperplastic ductal cells virtually never adopt

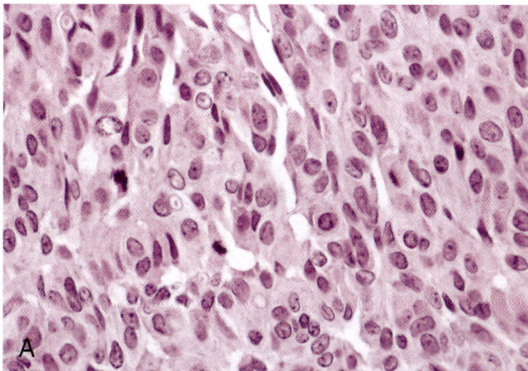

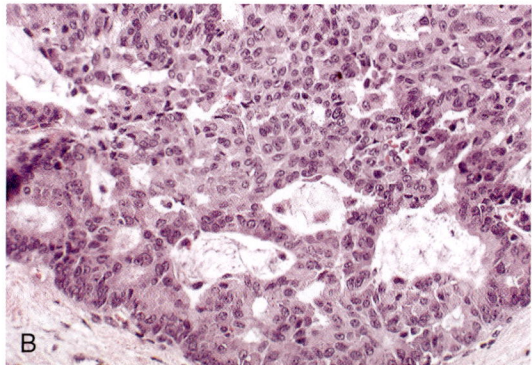

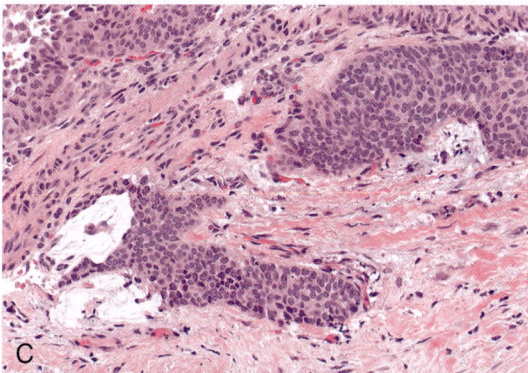

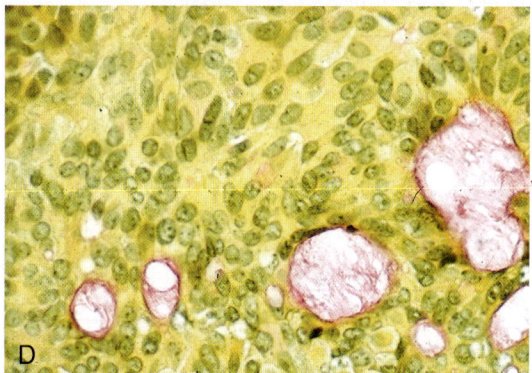

more mucin than one appreciates in conventionally stained sections (Fig. 9-30D). In foci of minimal stromal mucin extravasation, the mucin seems to first collect at the interface between the cells and the stroma. This appearance suggests that the mucin exits from the base of the cells, as dense core granules do from normal endocrine cells, rather than from the

Figure 9-30 A, Intracellular mucin collects as tiny droplets and small "targetoid" vacuoles. **B,** The mucin collects within neoplastic spaces or between the cells and their stromal skeleton and dissects into the stroma as seen in **C. D,** A mucin stain often reveals more mucin than one appreciates in conventionally stained sections.

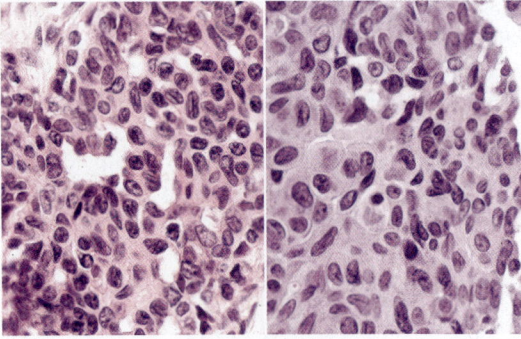

Figure 9-31 The nuclei of solid papillary carcinoma (*left*) appear virtually identical to those of conventional ductal hyperplasia (*right*).

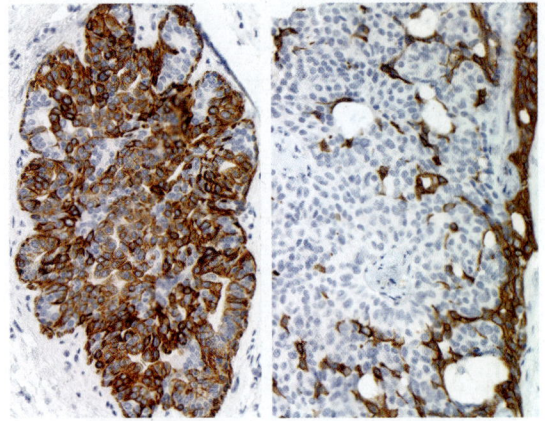

Figure 9-33 *Left,* Many cells in this focus of usual ductal hyperplasia stain for cytokeratin 5/6. *Right,* The tumor cells of this solid papillary carcinoma do not stain, although they entrap positively stained benign cells.

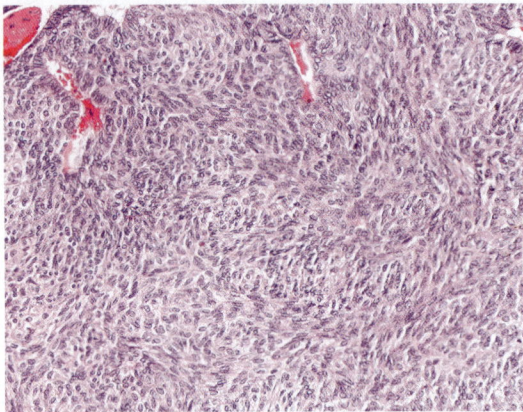

Figure 9-32 The cells of this solid papillary carcinoma have very long, spindly shapes.

such a spindly configuration. Second, hyperplastic cells only rarely produce mucin, so its presence, especially in the stroma, should alert pathologists to the likelihood of another diagnosis. Well-developed nuclear palisades, frequent mitotic figures, or eosinophilic cytoplasmic granules do not characterize ductal hyperplasia, so their presence should prompt one to consider the diagnosis of solid papillary carcinoma. Finally, uncomplicated examples of ductal hyperplasia do not contain the stromal cores or capillary skeleton seen in solid papillary carcinomas.

Although these differences allow one to distinguish most cases of solid papillary carcinoma from foci of usual ductal hyperplasia, the distinction between solid papillary carcinoma and usual ductal hyperplasia involving a papilloma presents special difficulties, because both lesions have an underlying papillary architecture. When evaluation of hematoxylin and eosin–stained sections of a problematic lesion of this type does not permit a secure diagnosis, one can obtain additional information from the results of immunohistochemical staining

for cytokeratin 5/6. The majority of hyperplastic ductal cells stain for this cytokeratin molecule, but malignant ductal cells rarely do (Fig. 9-33). The interpretation of this stain requires some care and experience, because the malignant cells of solid papillary carcinoma frequently entrap benign luminal and myoepithelial cells, thereby creating a complex mixture of stained and unstained cells. Attention to the location of the positively stained cells, their size, and the size and morphologic characteristics of their nuclei helps to clarify the populations in such a complicated situation. Entrapped luminal cells usually sit in the center of the mass of neoplastic cells and often abut the residual duct lumen. These benign cells appear smaller than the carcinoma cells, and they possess smaller nuclei that lack the atypia and pleomorphism characteristic of the carcinoma cells. Myoepithelial cells form a single layer adjacent to the basement membrane, but tangential sectioning can create an appearance that simulates stratification and proliferation. Like entrapped luminal cells, myoepithelial cells appear smaller than the carcinoma cells and display spindly, attenuated shapes and small, oval nuclei.

Besides having difficulty determining the malignant nature of solid papillary carcinomas, pathologists find it difficult to evaluate the possibility of invasion. The invasive carcinoma cells often produce mucin and grow as the cellular type of invasive mucinous carcinoma (Fig. 9-34). Another pattern arises when large, smoothly contoured nests of carcinoma cells cluster in an arrangement vaguely similar in appearance to that of distended ducts and terminal duct–lobular units. Pathologists seem to approach the evaluation of invasion with the bias that rounded

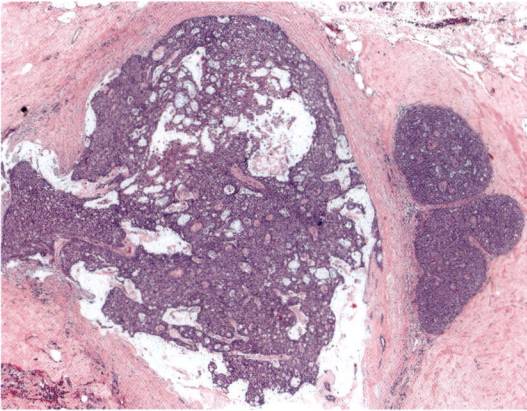

Figure 9-34 This carcinoma grows as noninvasive solid papillary carcinoma (*right*) and invasive cellular mucinous carcinoma (*left*).

nests like these represent noninvasive carcinoma; however, careful study of cases of solid papillary carcinoma elucidates the invasive nature of many such foci. Consequently, pathologists would do well to adopt the opposite point of view and assume that large, smooth nests represent invasive carcinoma until proven otherwise. One can get subtle hints

about the presence of invasion from the size, shape, and branching pattern of the nests, but one cannot rely on the impression formed from these features; instead, one must turn to the results of immunohistochemical staining for markers of myoepithelial cells such as p63 protein and myosin heavy chain. If these studies fail to disclose myoepithelial cells around the perimeter of these nests, one should conclude that invasion has occurred (Fig. 9-35). One sometimes observes myoepithelial cells surrounding only a portion of a nest. This finding probably indicates that a fraction of the cells remains within the confines of the duct but that others have penetrated the basement membrane and invaded the stroma.

Intracystic Papillary Carcinoma

Intracystic papillary carcinoma, the term introduced by Gatchell and colleagues,[2] refers to an uncommon type of papillary carcinoma presenting a distinctive macroscopic appearance: accumulated fluid distends the tissue surrounding the papillary tumor and thereby creates the appearance of a mass protruding into a cyst. The tumor adheres to the wall of the cavity by means of a broad base rather than a distinct stalk. Certain examples present a shaggy, obviously

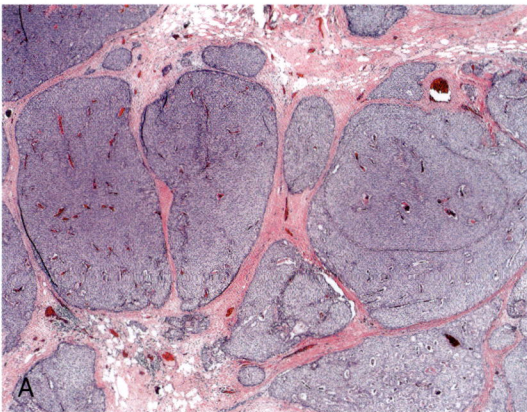

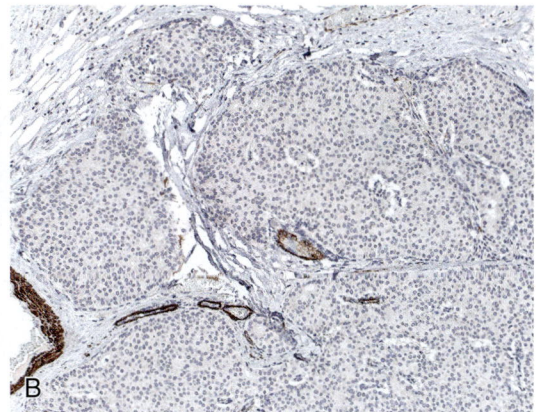

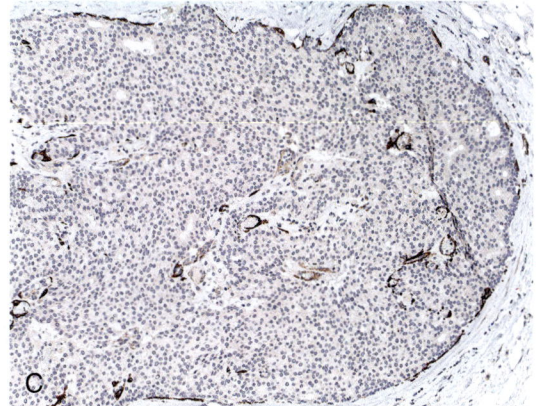

Figure 9-35 A, This solid papillary carcinoma grows in smoothly contoured nests of varying size, which resemble distended ducts. A stain for myosin heavy chain does not disclose myoepithelial cells around the nests of invasive carcinoma in **B** but reveals a few myoepithelial cells forming a discontinuous ring around the perimeter of the nest in **C**.

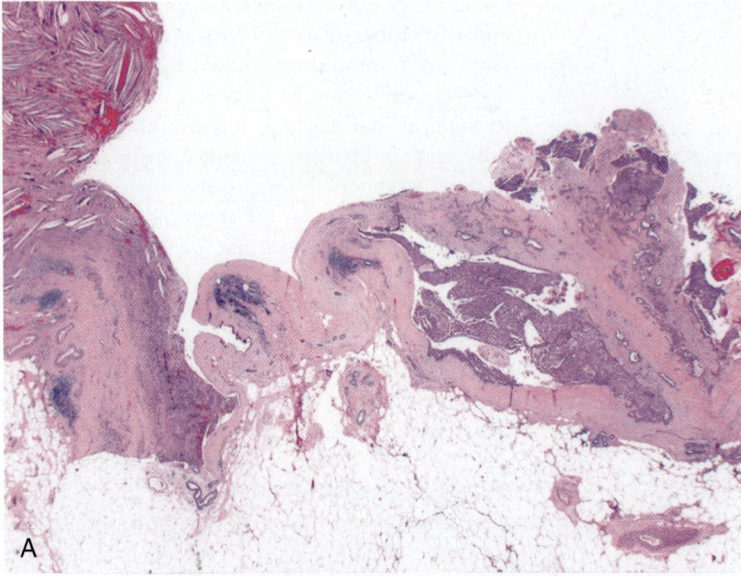

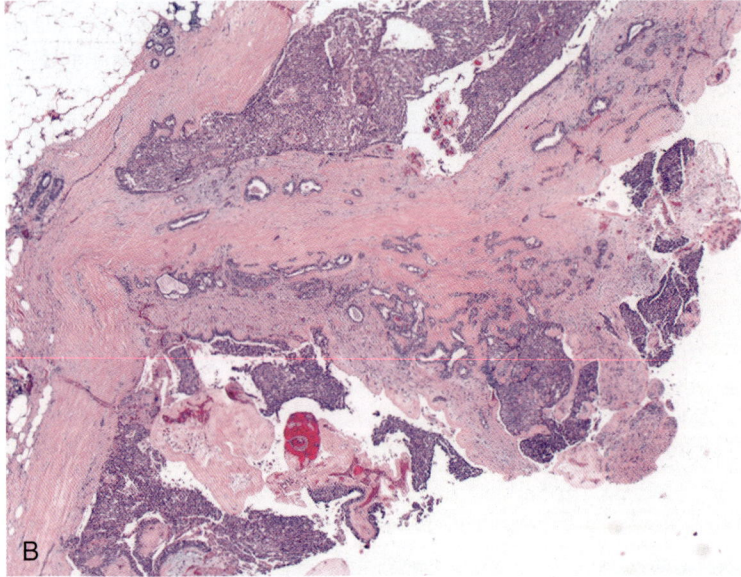

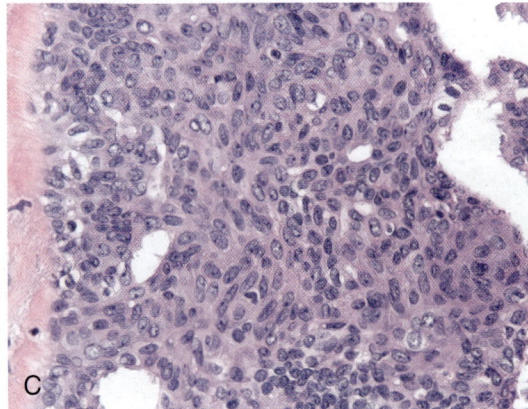

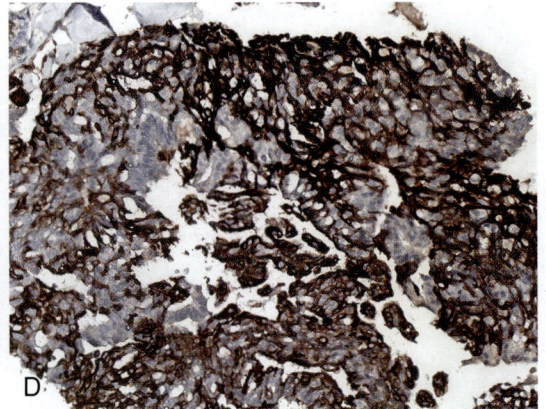

Figure 9-36 This papilloma grows on the wall of a blood-filled cavity in **A** and in the associated ducts in **B**. The proliferative epithelial cells display the cytologic characteristics of conventional ductal hyperplasia in **C**, and many stain for cytokeratin 5/6 in **D**.

papilloma projecting into a cyst.

papillary surface, whereas others grow as smooth, oval masses.

The histologic features of the lesion vary. The carcinoma often exhibits the delicate architecture of a conventional papillary carcinoma, but it can form a solid, compact mass with a polypoid macroscopic appearance. In the latter case, the malignant cells grow as large, thick sheets, and this abundance of epithelial cells obscures the underlying papillary architecture. The diagnosis of malignancy does not pose a problem in such tumors, because the cytologic atypism appears obvious, and the cells form clear-cut cribriform spaces. Less commonly, the mass comprises a papilloma involved by ductal carcinoma in situ or a solid papillary carcinoma. Because cases classified as intracystic papillary carcinoma exhibit a range of histologic patterns, one should probably regard this diagnosis as a description of a pattern of growth rather than as a reference to specific histologic appearance. Thus, the macroscopic characteristics of a lesion take on critical importance in the evaluation of the possibility of intracystic papillary carcinoma. One should not entertain the diagnosis of intracystic papillary carcinoma in the absence of an obvious fluid-filled cavity of macroscopic dimension containing a carcinoma that exhibits a papillary architecture. Moreover, this pattern of growth does not establish the diagnosis of malignancy, because a papilloma can also grow as a papillary tumor projecting into a cyst (Fig. 9-36).

Pathologists have traditionally believed that the cystic spaces occupied by intracystic papillary carcinomas represent distended ducts and that the lesion therefore constitutes a form of noninvasive carcinoma. The results of immunohistochemical staining for myoepithelial markers raise questions about this belief, because most intracystic papillary carcinomas lack myoepithelial cells entirely. Thus, it seems that intracystic papillary carcinoma represents an invasive carcinoma growing in an unusual papillary and cystic configuration rather than a form of noninvasive papillary carcinoma distending a cyst. To accommodate this conceptual change, certain writers suggest replacing the term *intracystic* with either *encysted* or *encapsulated*. Pathologists have not simply substituted one term for the other. It seems that many cases now classified as encysted or encapsulated do not exhibit the macroscopic characteristics of intracystic papillary carcinoma. They probably represent conventional papillary carcinoma invading in a blunt manner. It will take some time for pathologists to accept and to adjust to this new view regarding the manner of growth of these cystic and papillary carcinomas and to devise a more accurate and broadly accepted name for them.

Whatever the choice of terminology, pathologists should remind their clinical colleagues that intracystic papillary carcinoma has an especially favorable prognosis.

References

1. Lefkowitz M, Lefkowitz W, Wargotz ES: Intraductal (intracystic) papillary carcinoma of the breast and its variants: A clinicopathological study of 77 cases. Hum Pathol 1994;25:802-809.
2. Gatchell FG, Dockerty MB, Clagett OT: Intracystic carcinoma of the breast. Surg Gynecol Obstet 1958; 106:347-352.

Selected Readings

Carter D, Orr SL, Merino MJ: Intracystic papillary carcinoma of the breast after mastectomy, radiotherapy or excisional biopsy alone. Cancer 1983;52:14-19.

Collins LC, Carlo VP, Hwang H, et al: Intracystic papillary carcinomas of the breast: A reevaluation using a panel of myoepithelial cell markers. Am J Surg Pathol 2006;30:1002-1007.

Gatchell FG, Dockerty MB, Clagett OT: Intracystic carcinoma of the breast. Surg Gynecol Obstet 1958;106: 347-352.

Hill CB, Yeh IT: Myoepithelial cells staining patterns of papillary breast lesions: From intraductal papillomas to invasive papillary carcinomas. Am J Clin Pathol 2005;123:36-44.

Leal C, Costa I, Fonseca D, et al: Intracystic (encysted) papillary carcinoma of the breast: A clinical, pathological, and immunohistochemical study. Hum Pathol 1998;29:1097-1104.

Lefkowitz M, Lefkowitz W, Wargotz ES: Intraductal (intracystic) papillary carcinoma of the breast and its variants: A clinicopathological study of 77 cases. Hum Pathol 1994;25:802-809.

Maluf HM, Koerner FC: Solid papillary carcinoma of the breast: A form of intraductal carcinoma with endocrine differentiation frequently associated with mucinous carcinoma. Am J Surg Pathol 1995;19:1237-1244.

Mulligan AM, O'Malley FP: Metastatic potential of encapsulated (intracystic) papillary carcinoma of the breast: A report of 2 cases with axillary lymph nodes micrometastases. Int J Surg Pathol 2007;15: 143-147.

Tsang WY, Chan JK: Endocrine ductal carcinoma in situ (E-DCIS) of the breast: A form of low-grade DCIS with distinctive clinicopathologic and biologic characteristics. Am J Surg Pathol 1996;20:921-943.

10

Micropapillary Proliferations

The category of micropapillary proliferations consists of lesions forming microscopic papillary tufts and projections. It contains only two common entities, *micropapillary ductal hyperplasia* and *micropapillary ductal carcinoma in situ*.

MICROPAPILLARY DUCTAL HYPERPLASIA

Definitions and Clinicopathologic Characteristics

An uncommon pattern, micropapillary ductal epithelial hyperplasia occurs most often in cases of florid gynecomastia (Fig. 10-1). Less frequently, the proliferation accompanies other benign conditions, such as early stages in the formation of radial scars, pseudoangiomatous stromal hyperplasia, and fibrocystic disease (Fig. 10-2). In the last circumstance, the micropapillary component usually constitutes a minor fraction of the hyperplastic population and merges with conventional patterns of ductal hyperplasia (Fig. 10-3). Only rarely does ductal hyperplasia grow in an extensive, well-developed, and purely micropapillary pattern in women. Whatever the clinical setting, the lesion represents a proliferation of slightly variable, cohesive, non-polarized cells that exhibit the morphologic properties of hyperplastic ductal cells.

Histologic Characteristics

Degree of Glandular Distention

Micropapillary ductal hyperplasia causes only a modest distention of terminal duct–lobular units (Fig. 10-4). Usually they appear only a few times larger than their uninvolved counterparts (Fig. 10-5).

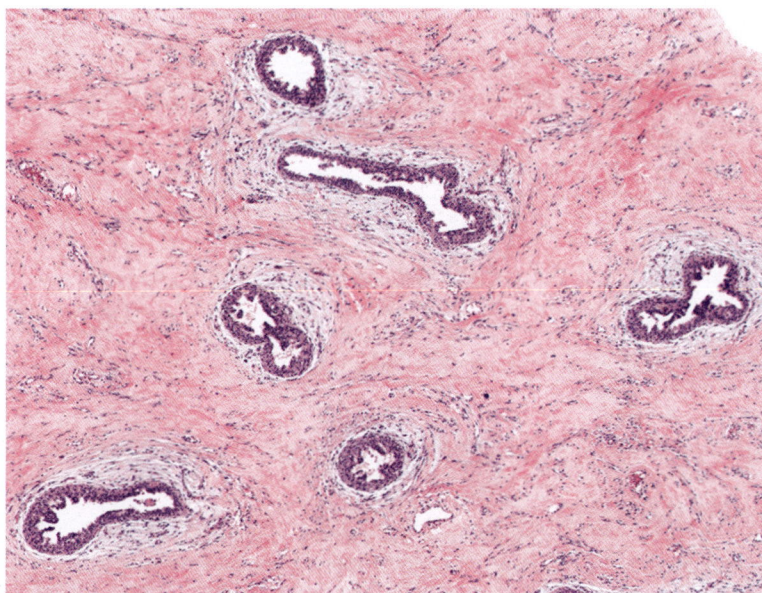

Figure 10-1 The epithelial proliferation in this case of gynecomastia has a micropapillary architecture.

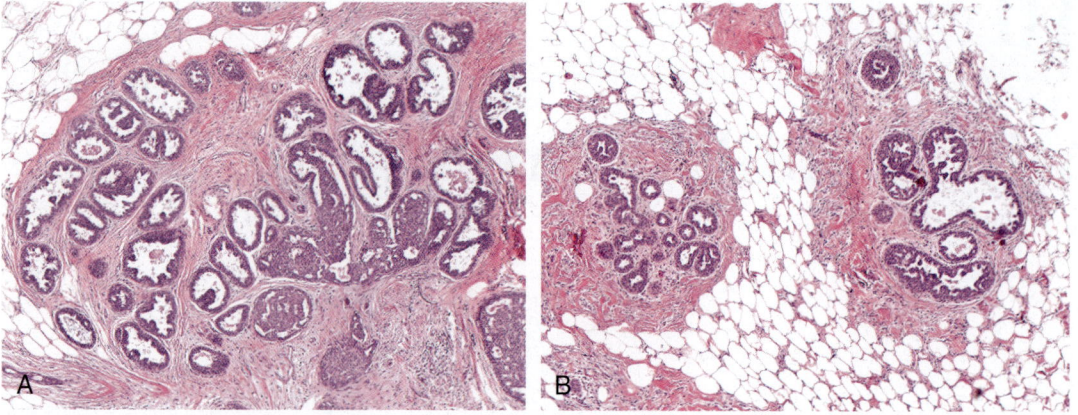

Figure 10-2 A, The corona of this radial scar contains a small region of micropapillary hyperplasia; so do the ducts trapped in this focus of fascicular pseudoangiomatous stromal hyperplasia shown in **B**.

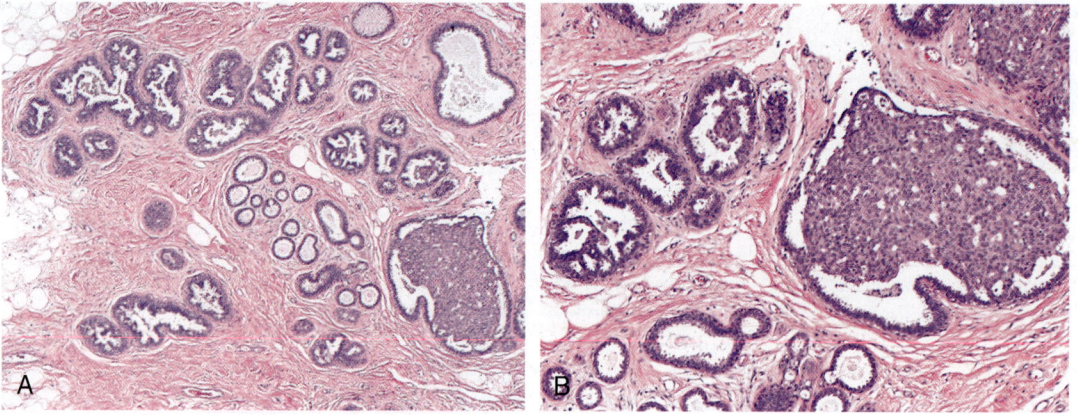

Figure 10-3 A and **B,** This small focus of micropapillary hyperplasia belongs to a large region showing usual ductal hyperplasia and other fibrocystic changes.

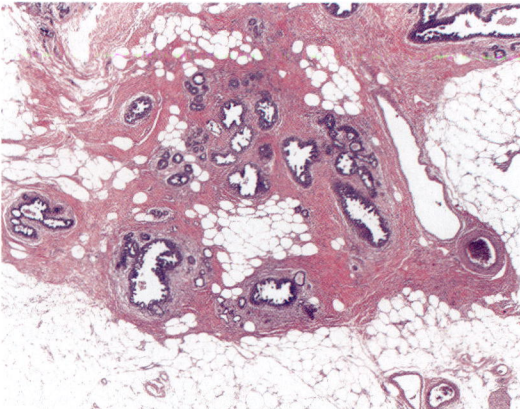

Figure 10-4 Micropapillary hyperplasia has distended these ducts to only a modest degree.

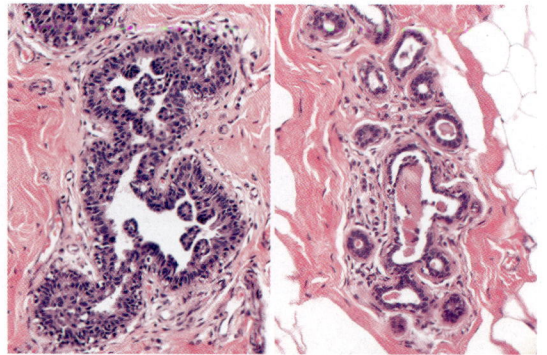

Figure 10-5 The duct harboring micropapillary hyperplasia (*left*) appears only slightly enlarged compared with the uninvolved duct (*right*).

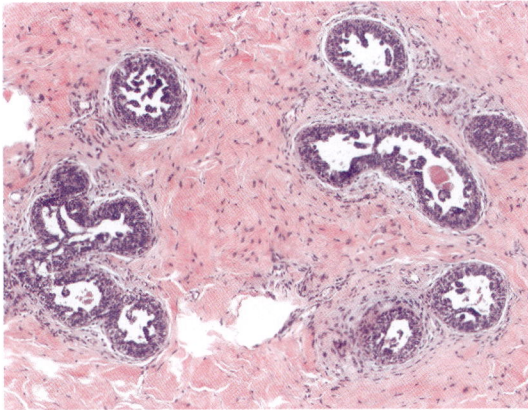

Figure 10-6 The micropapillary hyperplasia has distended these ducts to similar extents.

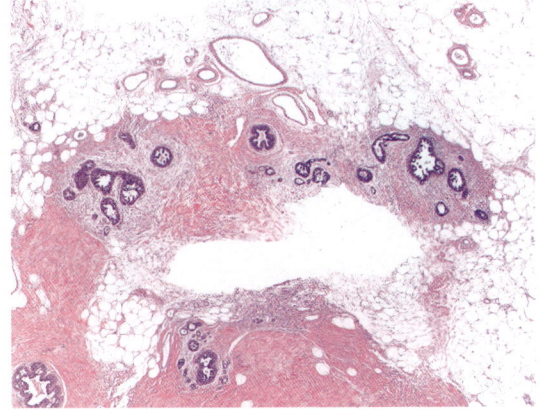

Figure 10-7 Edema enlarges the specialized stroma around the ducts containing this micropapillary ductal hyperplasia.

Furthermore, the extent of distention generally appears uniform from gland to gland (Fig. 10-6). The specialized stroma surrounding the altered ducts sometimes develops edema (Fig. 10-7), and a few pathologists refer to this pattern as *gynecomastia-like*.

Size and Configuration of the Micropapillae

The micropapillae have similar shapes and heights. Most look like tapering tufts, and they all project into the lumen for approximately the same distance. A line connecting the tips of the papillary projections roughly parallels the outline of the duct (Fig. 10-8).

Contents of the Duct Lumen

Because hyperplastic ductal cells stick together tightly, the duct lumens do not contain sloughed

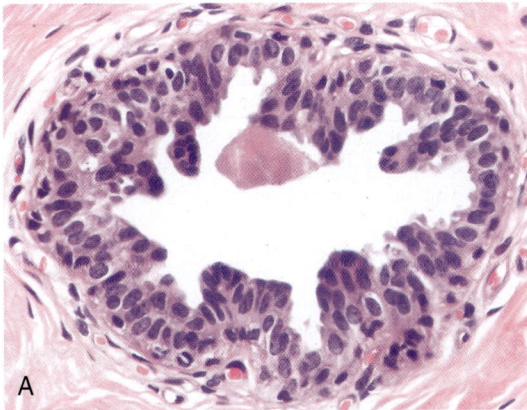

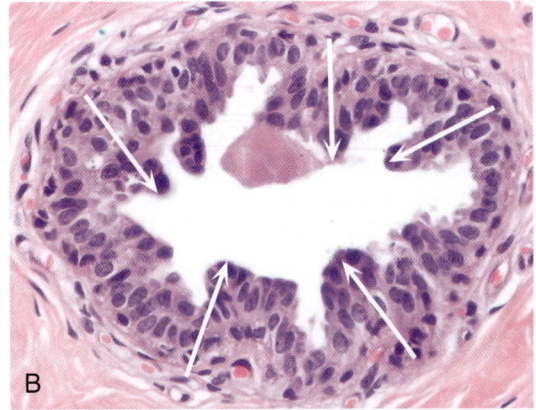

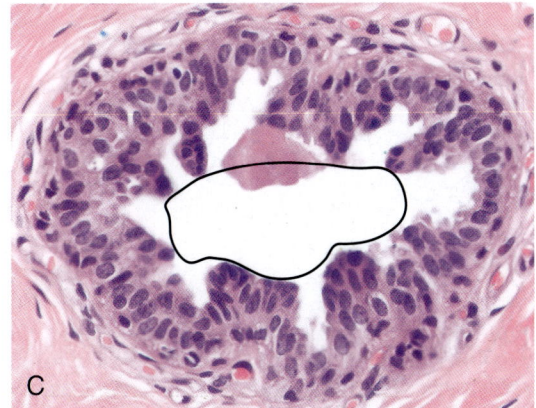

Figure 10-8 A, The papillae in this case of micropapillary ductal hyperplasia appear uniform in height and configuration. **B,** All the papillae extend for about the same distance above the basement membrane. **C,** A line connecting the tips of the papillae roughly parallels the basement membrane of the duct.

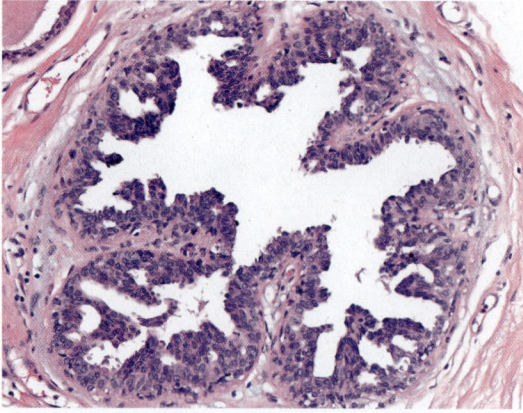

Figure 10-9 The lumen of the duct involved by micropapillary ductal hyperplasia appears empty.

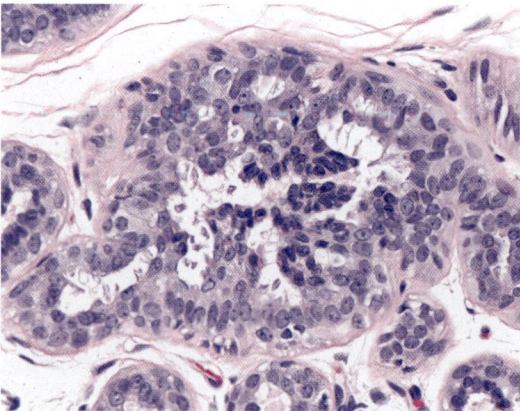

Figure 10-10 The cells of micropapillary ductal hyperplasia show the variability in nuclear placement, in nuclear shape, and in chromatin texture and the presence of small nucleoli that characterize conventional hyperplastic ductal cells.

epithelial cells or cellular debris. The glandular spaces might contain a few histiocytes or eosinophilic secretions; however, the lumens usually look empty (Fig. 10-9).

Cytologic Characteristics of the Cells

The cells of micropapillary hyperplasia display the cytologic characteristics of conventional hyperplastic ductal cells (Fig. 10-10). The nuclei have irregular placement and convoluted shapes and they possess granular chromatin, with some clearing and uniform nucleoli of a modest size. The nuclei of the cells at the tips of the micropapillae tend to sit immediately beneath the luminal aspect of the cell membrane, so one does not observe apical cytoplasmic compartments (Fig. 10-11). Furthermore, the nuclei of the cells bordering the lumen often flatten to form ovals

and arch along the curve of the papillary tip. This close apposition of the nucleus against the luminal border of the cell and the compression of the nucleus against the cell membrane reflect the marked cohesion of the cells and therefore serve as especially reliable indications of a benign proliferation.

Presence of Maturation

The cells at the tips of the papillary units appear inactive compared with the cells along the basement membrane. The cells in the former location look smaller, their nuclei more irregular and more darkly staining, and their cytoplasm denser and more eosinophilic in comparison with cells in the latter position (Fig. 10-12).

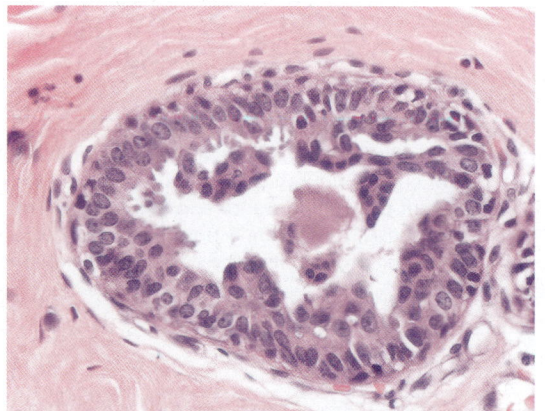

Figure 10-11 The nuclei of cells at the tips of the papillae sit immediately adjacent to the luminal cell membranes. One does not observe apical cytoplasmic compartments.

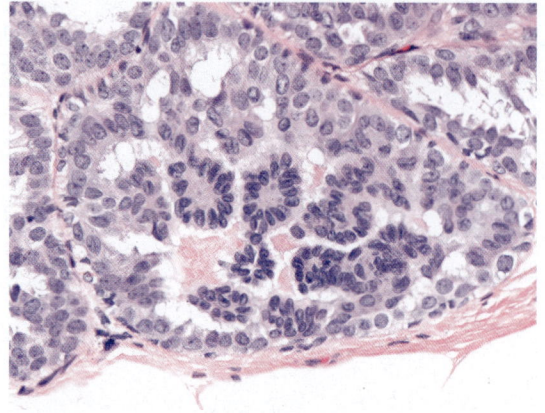

Figure 10-12 The cells at the tips of these benign micropapillae appear smaller than those along the basement membrane, and the former have smaller and darker nuclei and less cytoplasm than the latter.

MICROPAPILLARY DUCTAL CARCINOMA IN SITU

Definitions and Clinicopathologic Characteristics

In common with conventional ductal carcinoma in situ, micropapillary ductal carcinoma in situ represents a proliferation of dishesive, polarized cells. Most cases also display cribriform patterns, but an occasional example grows in a purely micropapillary architecture. The cells of the typical case appear monomorphic, and their nuclei exhibit features of low-grade atypia; less commonly, the cells appear pleomorphic and display anaplastic cytologic features. The lesion tends to occupy many ducts and terminal duct–lobular units. This form of ductal carcinoma in situ produces only small amounts of calcification; thus, the carcinoma often involves many more ducts and lobules than the patient's mammogram would indicate. Micropapillary ductal carcinoma in situ commonly coexists with lobular carcinoma in situ and tubular carcinoma (Box 10-1).

Histologic Characteristics

Extent of Glandular Distention

Terminal duct–lobular units involved by micropapillary carcinoma appear greatly dilated, and the level of dilatation varies from duct to duct (Fig. 10-13). Often the involved structures measure ten or more times the diameter of the uninvolved ones. Comparison with

> **Box 10-1**
>
> A good rule of thumb:
>
> • An extensive, well-developed micropapillary ductal proliferation in a woman usually represents carcinoma, whereas in a man it usually represents gynecomastia.

uninvolved glands makes the distention especially obvious (Fig. 10-14). This extreme and variable distention contrasts with the modest and uniform enlargement seen in cases of micropapillary hyperplasia (Fig. 10-15).

Size and Configuration of the Micropapillae

Unlike the micropapillae of hyperplasia, which appear uniform in structure, those of ductal carcinoma in situ vary greatly in shape and size. Tiny stubs sit next to long, graceful festoons, and these malignant micropapillae sometimes contain cribriform spaces (Fig. 10-16A). Certain pathologists assert that micropapillary structures with bulbous tips provide secure evidence of carcinoma, because benign hyperplastic cells only rarely give rise to papillae with this configuration. Other pathologists have pointed out that the micropapillae of micropapillary ductal carcinoma in situ often appear to point in the direction of the central ducts (Fig. 10-16B).

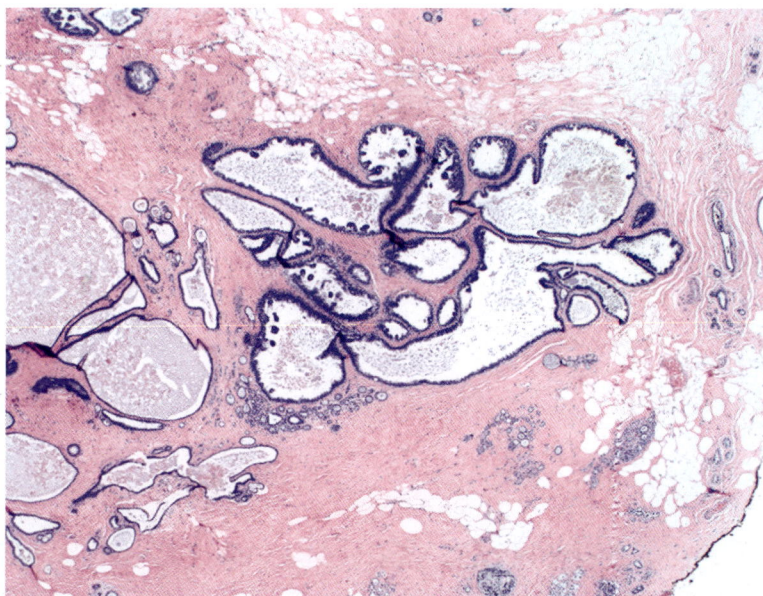

Figure 10-13 The growth of ductal carcinoma in situ in a micropapillary pattern has distended these ducts to an extreme and variable extent.

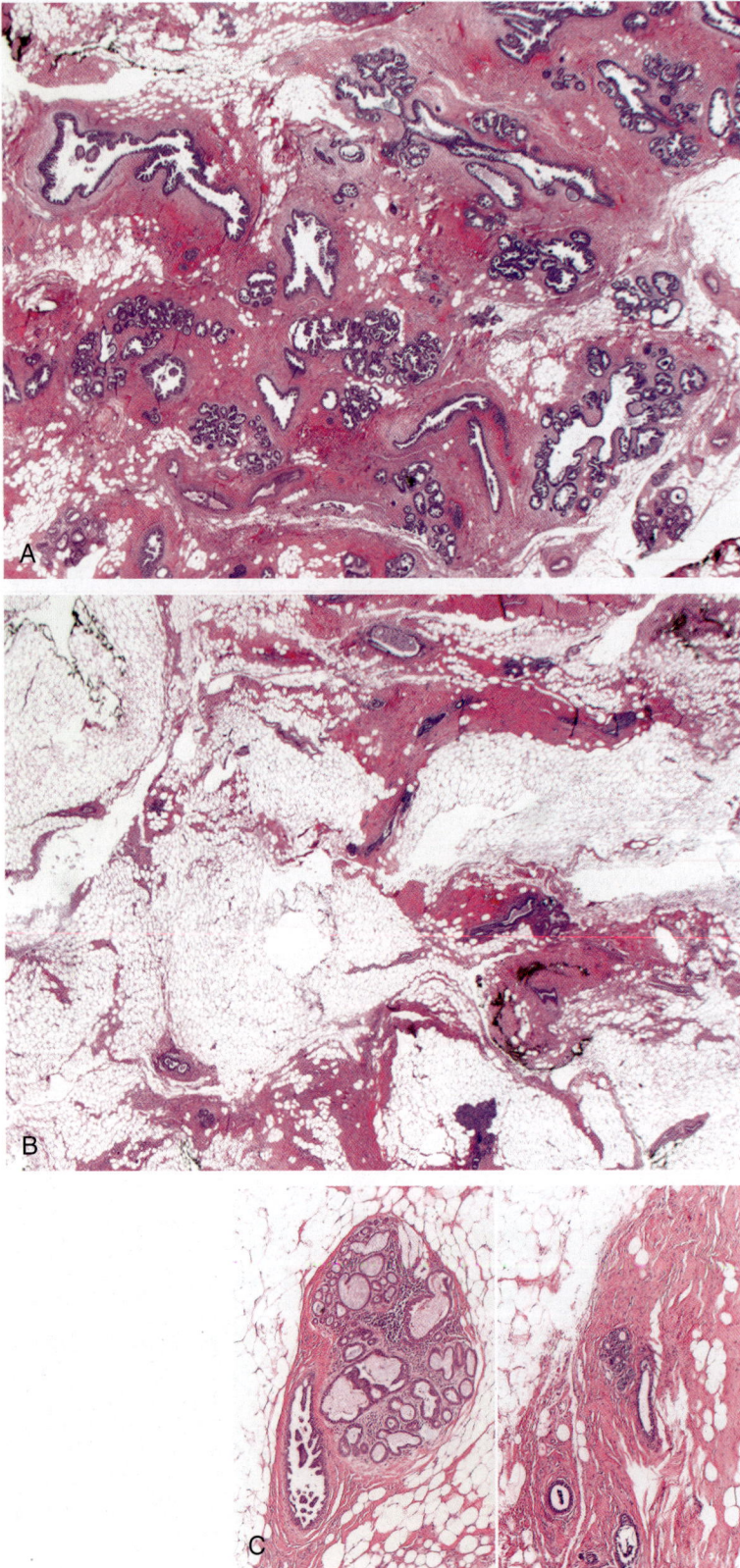

Figure 10-14 The glands involved by the micropapillary ductal carcinoma in situ shown in **A** do not seem greatly dilated until one contrasts them with the atrophic and nearly invisible structures in the uninvolved tissue in **B**. **C**, Higher magnification depicts a small duct and associated lobules involved by the carcinoma (*left*) and similar but uninvolved structures (*right*).

Figure 10-15 Micropapillary ductal carcinoma in situ distends ducts in **A** more than micropapillary ductal hyperplasia enlarges those in **B**.

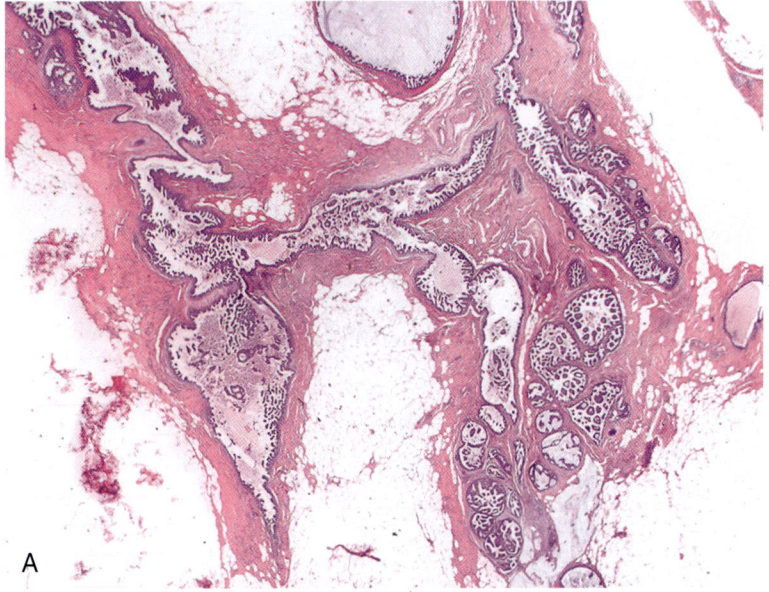

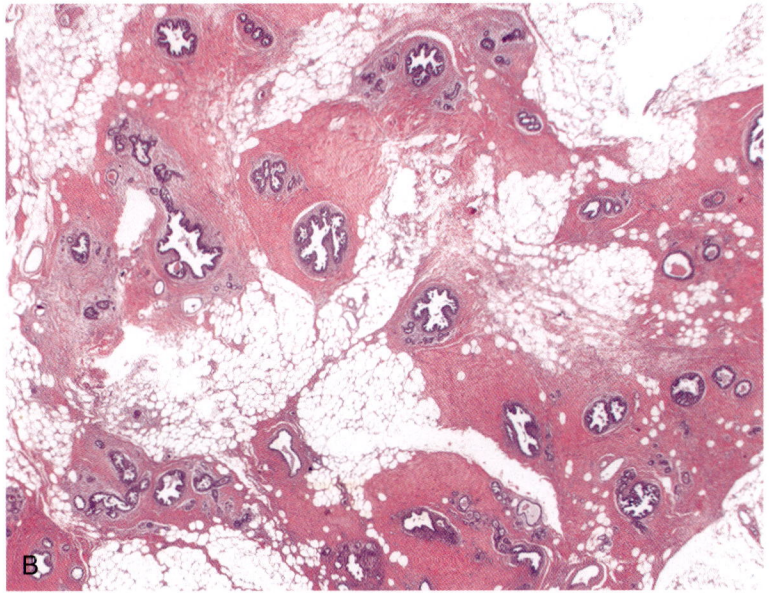

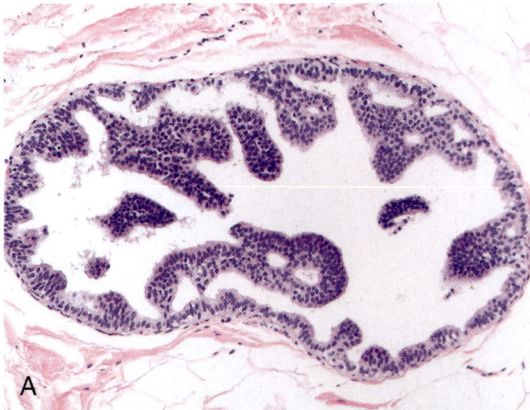

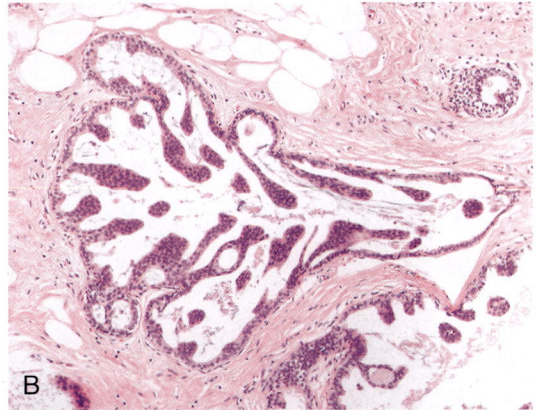

Figure 10-16 A, The papillary tufts of this micropapillary ductal carcinoma in situ vary in size and configuration. Several have internal cribriform spaces. **B,** Many papillary tufts in this example of micropapillary ductal carcinoma in situ point toward the draining duct to the right of the field.

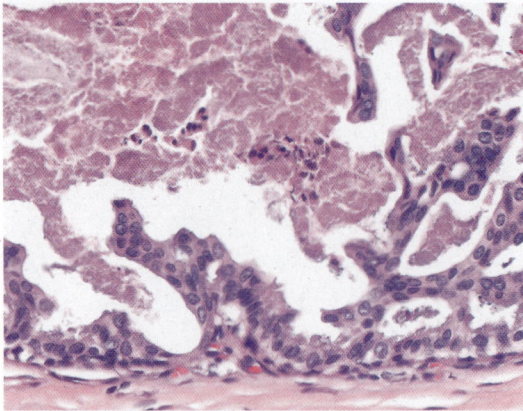

Figure 10-17 The lumen of the duct involved by micropapillary ductal carcinoma in situ contains degenerating, sloughed epithelial cells and cellular debris.

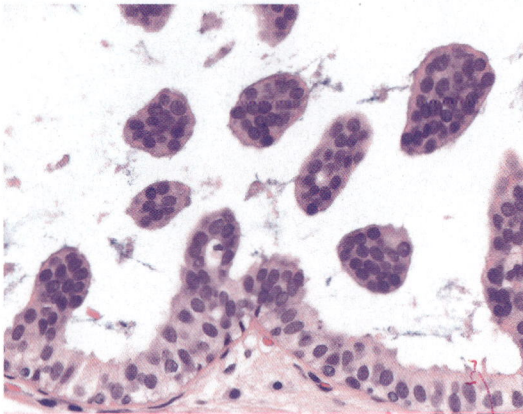

Figure 10-18 The cells have smoothly contoured, oval or round nuclei, homogeneous and dark chromatin, and inconspicuous nucleoli.

Contents of the Duct Lumen

Ducts and lobules harboring micropapillary ductal carcinoma in situ sometimes contain sloughed tumor cells and degenerating cellular debris (Fig. 10-17). Thus, the glandular lumens do not appear as clean as those in examples of micropapillary hyperplasia.

Cytologic Characteristics of the Cells

The cytologic characteristics of micropapillary ductal carcinoma in situ duplicate those found in the other patterns of low-grade ductal carcinoma in situ. The cells display uniform spacing, and their nuclei do not overlap. The latter have uniform, round or oval shapes, smooth contours, homogeneous chromatin, and inconspicuous nucleoli (Fig. 10-18). The cells exhibit the phenomenon of polarization, a feature that appears especially obvious in cells abutting the lumen, which have basal nuclei and well-developed apical cytoplasmic compartments (Fig. 10-19). The presence of these apical cytoplasmic compartments in the malignant cells contrasts with their absence in the benign cells of micropapillary hyperplasia. Figure 10-20 contrasts the cellular features of micropapillary carcinoma and micropapillary hyperplasia.

Presence of Maturation

The cells of micropapillary ductal carcinoma in situ do not exhibit the phenomenon of maturation seen in examples of ductal hyperplasia. Those at the tips of the papillae have the same morphologic characteristics as the ones along the basement membrane (Fig. 10-21). Figure 10-22 contrasts the appearance resulting from the lack of maturation in micropapillary carcinoma

Figure 10-19 The cells in the malignant micropapillae have clear-cut apical cytoplasmic compartments.

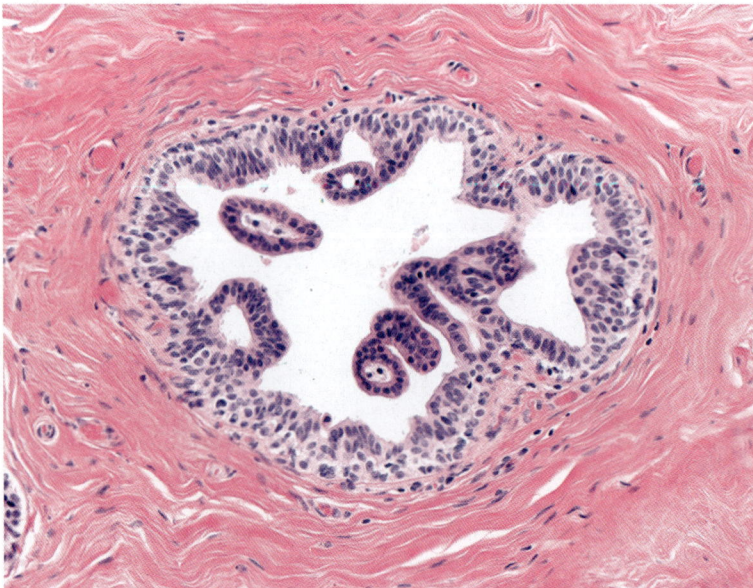

CA   *Hyperplasia*

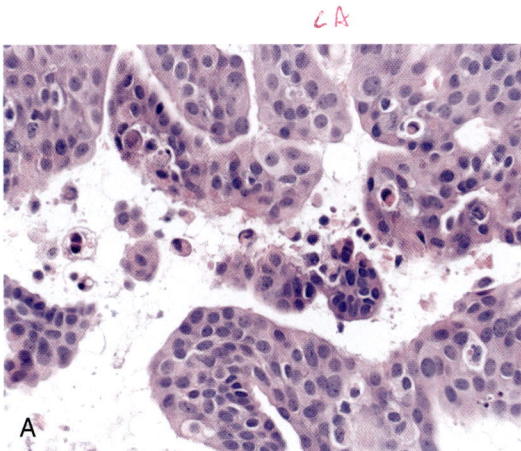

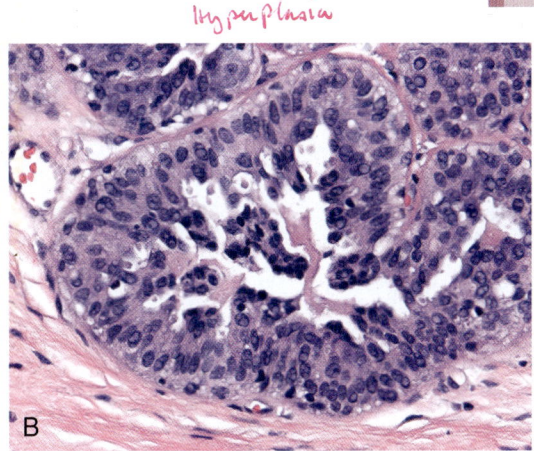

Figure 10-20 A, The cells of micropapillary carcinoma in situ exhibit the cytologic atypia, architectural atypia, and dishesion characteristic of low-grade carcinoma. **B,** Those of micropapillary hyperplasia show the variability in nuclear placement, nuclear shape, and chromatin texture typical of hyperplastic ductal cells.

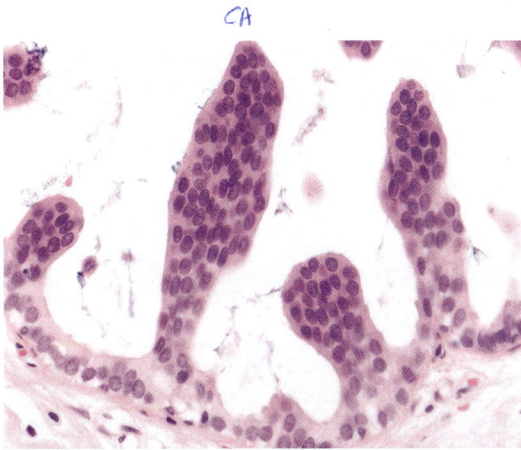

CA

Figure 10-21 The nuclei in the cells at the tips of these papillary structures appear nearly identical to those in the cells along the basement membrane.

No maturation

with the pattern produced by the maturation of hyperplastic cells. Immunohistochemical staining for cytokeratin 5/6 usually shows that the most superficial cells in the hyperplastic micropapillae stain, but none of the carcinoma cells do (Fig. 10-23). Like other types of ductal carcinoma in situ, the micropapillary variety can show cellular dimorphism (Fig. 10-24), and one must not misinterpret this pattern as a manifestation of maturation. Noting the round shape of the nuclei, the dispersed texture of the chromatin, and the presence of apical cytoplasmic compartments in the cells throughout the micropapillae helps to avoid this mistake.

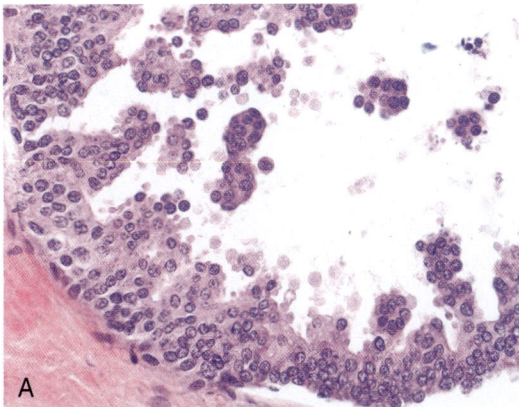

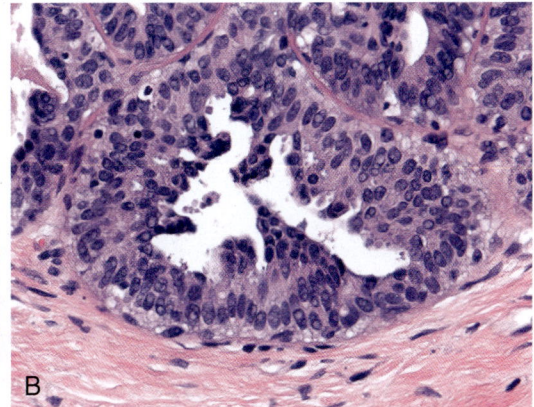

Figure 10-22 A, The malignant cells do not mature, and they fall apart. **B,** The benign cells show maturation and cohesion.

CA   *Hyperplasia*

Dont forget floral papillomatosis of the nipple - Has necrosis See Rosen p.116
See Page p.108-111

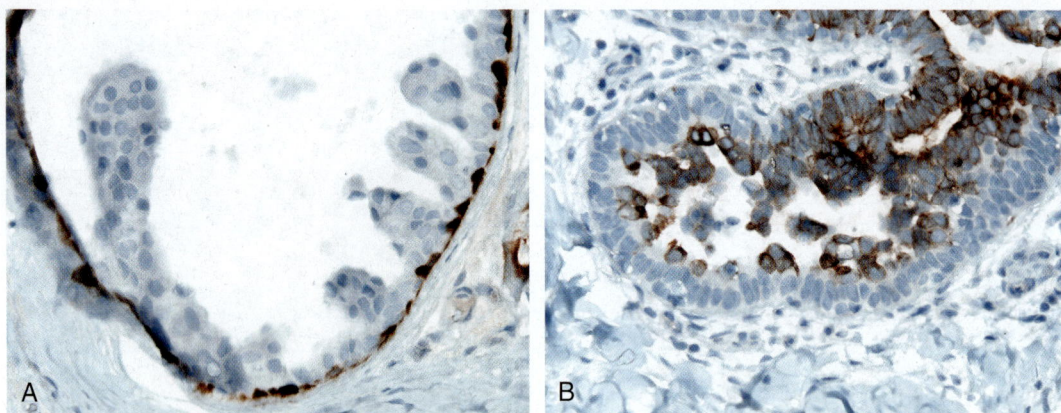

Figure 10-23 A, The cells of micropapillary carcinoma do not express cytokeratin 5/6. **B,** Those at the tips of the micropapillae in micropapillary hyperplasia do so.

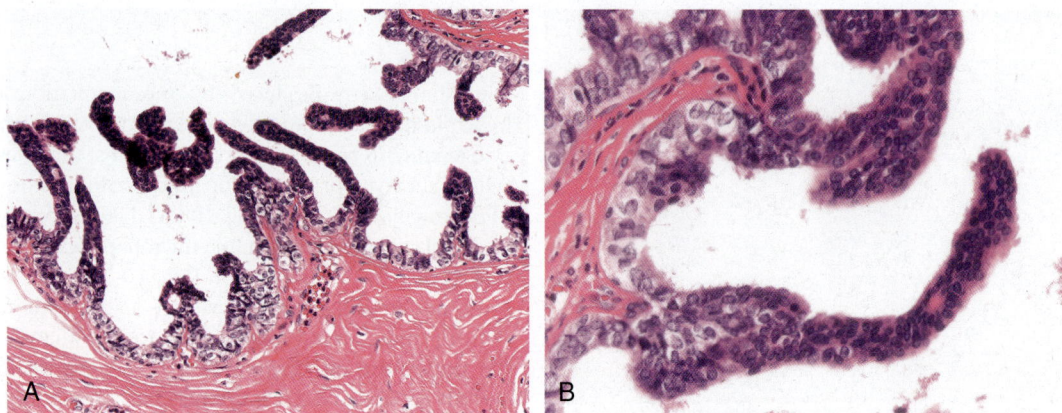

Figure 10-24 A, The malignant cells along the basement membrane of this dimorphic micropapillary ductal carcinoma in situ appear larger than the others and they contain larger, paler nuclei and pale cytoplasm. **B,** The cells at the tips of the micropapillae display obvious apical cytoplasmic compartments.

SUMMARY

Micropapillary proliferations represent varieties of conventional ductal hyperplasia and ductal carcinoma in situ characterized by the formation of small tufts and filiform strands of cells. These micropapillary versions exhibit all the essential characteristics of the corresponding lesions growing in conventional patterns (Table 10-1).

Table 10-1 Histologic Features of Micropapillary Hyperplasia and Micropapillary Carcinoma In Situ

	Micropapillary Hyperplasia	Micropapillary Carcinoma In Situ
Extent of glandular distention	Modest	Marked
Size and configuration of micropapillae	Uniform size and shape	Markedly variable in size and shape
Contents of the duct lumen	Empty, histocytes, or secretion	Degenerating epithelial cells
Cytologic characteristics of the cells	Benign	Atypical
Maturation	Present	Absent

Selected Readings

Holland R, Hendriks JH, Verbeek AL, et al: Extent, distribution, and mammographic/histological correlations of breast ductal carcinoma in situ. Lancet 1990;335:519-522.

Lagios MD, Margolin FR, Westdahl PR, et al: Mammographically detected duct carcinoma in situ: Frequency of local recurrence following tylectomy and prognostic effect of nuclear grade on local recurrence. Cancer 1989;63:618-624.

Part III

SCLEROSING LESIONS

11

Concepts Basic to the Diagnosis of Sclerosing Lesions

Benign entities commonly grouped under the heading of sclerosing lesions include sclerosing adenosis, sclerosing papilloma, radial scar, and subareolar sclerosing duct hyperplasia. One has difficulty justifying this grouping on biologic grounds, because the lesions do not seem to share pathogenetic pathways. Sclerosing adenosis looks like an alteration of preexisting lobules in which intralobular epithelial and myoepithelial cells proliferate in a fashion that creates a characteristic concentric, swirling pattern. Sclerosing papilloma, on the other hand, represents a neoplasm that arises in the wall of a duct and provokes intense scarring and entrapment of the surrounding ducts and terminal duct–lobular units. Radial scars and subareolar sclerosing duct hyperplasia may develop as reparative responses to tissue damage. Despite these seeming differences in pathogenesis, the lesions do share certain morphologic attributes. Proliferation of glands and stromal cells and distortion of the mammary architecture characterize all four processes. The glandular distortion common to all four gives rise to another shared attribute and a pragmatic reason for grouping them together—the ability to mimic low-grade invasive carcinomas. Most such carcinomas consist of polarized cells forming small glands or tubules and containing bland nuclei that lack noticeable mitotic activity. They usually represent well-differentiated invasive ductal carcinomas of no special type (NOS); however, two special types of invasive ductal carcinoma, tubular carcinoma and low-grade adenosquamous carcinoma, can also mimic a sclerosing lesion, and so can invasive lobular carcinoma.

The chapters in this section contrast the characteristics of certain problematic sclerosing lesions with those of masquerading carcinomas. Chapter 8, which discusses papillomas, describes the entity sclerosing papilloma. There, the reader will find a few points to aid in distinguishing this benign lesion from a carcinoma. Subareolar sclerosing duct hyperplasia exhibits all the characteristics of a radial scar; only its location in the subareolar tissue sets it apart from conventional radial scars. These two entities probably represent two faces of a single lesion, and pathologists can approach the analysis of the two in the same way. The discussion that follows therefore focuses on the two remaining basic types of sclerosing lesions: sclerosing adenosis and radial scar, and their most common mimics, well-differentiated invasive ductal carcinoma, including tubular carcinomas and low-grade adenosquamous carcinomas, and invasive lobular carcinoma.

Attention to the following four attributes of a sclerosing lesion usually reveals the information necessary for its proper classification: its shape, its internal structure, the characteristics of its peripheral epithelial elements, and the characteristics of any associated epithelial proliferation.

SHAPE OF THE LESION

Although sclerosing processes can assume a variety of shapes, most have either a globular or a stellate configuration. The presence of a round or oval shape and a smooth contour usually indicates a benign lesion; only rarely do carcinomas grow in this pattern. Lesions described as stellate or spiculate possess bands of tissue that radiate from a central point much like light radiates from a star or spines cover the coating of a seed. One cannot generalize about the nature of lesions with a stellate shape, because several types of benign lesions and most carcinomas have this appearance.

To determine the nature of such an abnormality, one must look beyond its shape and determine the mechanism responsible for the formation of the radiating bands. They can arise through two mechanisms. A lesion characterized by tissue loss puckers the underlying parenchyma and thereby draws bands of parenchyma toward the region of tissue loss; this puckering of the parenchyma creates the stellate configuration. A lesion that adds tissue to the breast, in contrast, forms a central nodule with tentacle-like extensions penetrating the surrounding parenchyma. Radial scars create their stellate shape via the first mechanism, whereas carcinomas do so via the second mechanism. When studying the shape of a sclerosing lesion, the pathologist might find it helpful to determine whether the lesion has the retracted configuration that would indicate a loss of tissue in the center or the bulging, space-occupying appearance characteristic of a neoplastic proliferation.

STRUCTURE OF THE LESION

Benign sclerosing lesions differ fundamentally in their pathogenesis from carcinomas. The former arise through a process of distortion of preexisting, normally formed mammary tissue, whereas the latter represent disordered proliferations of neoplastic glands, which by their nature overrun the underlying components of the breast. Consequently, benign sclerosing lesions have characteristic structures, but carcinomas do not. In foci of sclerosing adenosis, for instance, one observes compressed acini swirling around a central, small ductule; radial scars exhibit a zonal arrangement of components. Careful study of these benign lesions allows one to appreciate the preservation of the anatomic organization of the underlying tissue components and the orderly relationship among them. Carcinomas, in contrast, lack a distinctive internal organization. By studying the structure of a sclerosing lesion and, especially, its internal organization, one can usually identify the process that created it and, thereby, the diagnosis.

CHARACTERISTICS OF THE PERIPHERAL EPITHELIAL ELEMENTS

The center of a sclerosing lesion can present the pathologist with a confusing and worrisome set of findings, because this region of a benign focus can look nearly identical to an invasive carcinoma if examined out of context or at high magnification. Pathologists will find that the study of the epithelial structures in the outermost regions of sclerosing foci provides the clearest view of the nature of the abnormality. Two aspects of the peripherally situated glands merit close attention: their histologic characteristics and their relationship with the adjoining tissue. The glands at the edge of a benign sclerosing lesion exhibit a smooth contour, usually of a round or oval shape, a two-layered epithelium composed of cells without atypical characteristics, and a basement membrane; the epithelial nests of an invasive carcinoma lack certain of these features and sometimes all of them. Furthermore, the peripheral glands of benign lesions do not disrupt the organization of the surrounding tissue. They do not percolate through lobules or encircle ducts, nor do they disturb the flow of the collagen bundles. Invasive carcinomas, in contrast, always infiltrate the mammary parenchyma.

Pathologists have come to regard the extension of the epithelial aggregates into adipose tissue as the *sine qua non* of invasion, but the destructive growth of malignancies has other manifestations. When carcinomas encounter preexisting components of the breast, the malignant cells do not respect the integrity of the underlying structures. If the neoplastic cells do not obliterate the preexisting elements, they infiltrate them in a destructive fashion, which takes the form of malignant cells penetrating lobules, surrounding acini, and encircling ducts and blood vessels (Figs. 11-1 and 11-2). This invasion of fibrous connective tissue and glands does not stand out as obviously as invasion of fat does, but it provides equally conclusive evidence of malignancy. Disruption of the orderly structure of the stromal collagen bundles is an even subtler sign of invasion. The collagen of the normal mammary stroma consists of compact bundles flowing smoothly around the ducts and acini; infiltration by malignant cells interrupts this pattern of organization. One might observe fragmentation, fraying, splitting, angulation, or abrupt termination of collagen bundles, for example, and small bits of collagen can become trapped within epithelial clusters (Fig. 11-3). All of these findings reflect the malignant nature and destructive properties of the carcinoma. The ability to detect these histologic findings and to recognize them as conclusive evidence of invasion pays handsome rewards when one is analyzing sclerosing lesions.

CHARACTERISTICS OF THE ASSOCIATED DUCTAL EPITHELIAL PROLIFERATION

Noninvasive proliferations of ductal epithelial cells frequently coexist with sclerosing lesions, and the character of such proliferations provides limited evidence about the nature of the sclerosing process. The presence of ductal carcinoma in situ, for example, should prompt one to consider the possibility that a nearby collection of disorderly glands represents

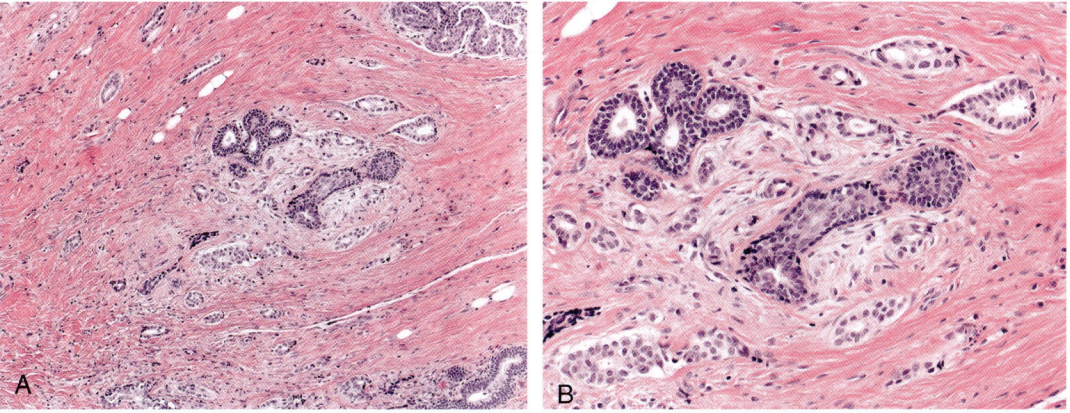

Figure 11-1 A, Clusters of carcinoma cells invade the tissue in the region of this terminal duct–lobular unit. The malignant glands grow without regard to the structure of this lobule. **B,** One can see the neoplastic glands encircling the benign ductules.

Figure 11-2 The invading clusters of malignant cells encircle a duct in **A** and grow between and within the lobules in **B**.

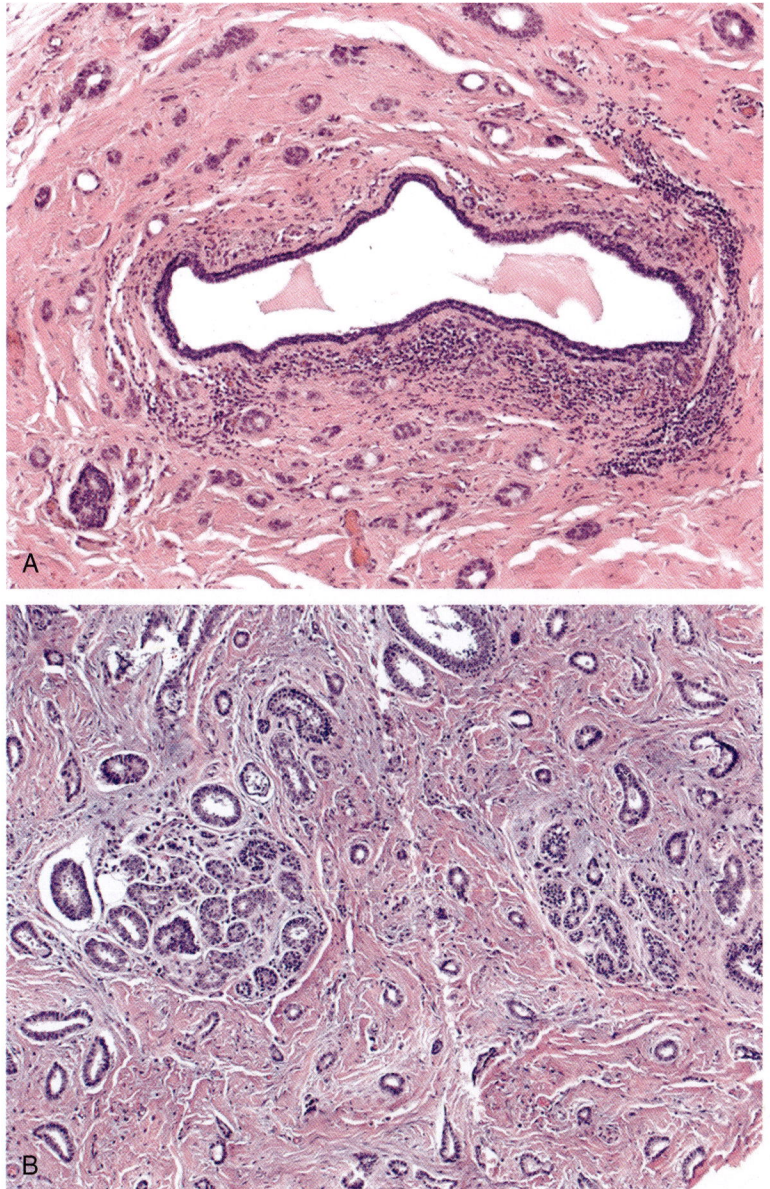

Bit of villus trapped in epitheloid structure

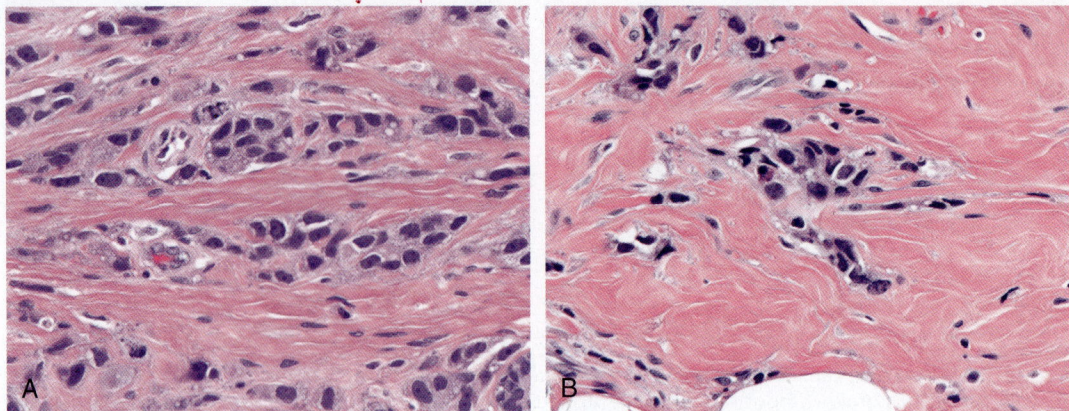

Figure 11-3 A and **B,** The malignant cells have disrupted the pattern of the collagen bundles. The cells separate the bundles and cause them to become frayed and fragmented. These alterations are obvious in **A** but subtle in **B**.

an invasive ductal carcinoma. This line of reasoning has its limits. Invasive carcinomas can lack a noninvasive component, so the absence of carcinoma in situ does not exclude the diagnosis of invasive cancer. On the other hand, carcinomas in situ can populate an otherwise benign sclerosing lesion; thus, the mere presence of a noninvasive carcinoma does not guarantee that associated disorderly glands constitute invasive carcinoma. Despite these limitations, one should not disregard the presence of a coexistent ductal proliferation when evaluating a sclerosing lesion.

Selected Readings

Fenoglio C, Lattes R: Sclerosing papillary proliferations in the female breast: A benign lesion often mistaken for carcinoma. Cancer 1974;33:691-700.

Rosen PP: Subareolar sclerosing duct hyperplasia of the breast. Cancer 1987;59:1927-1930.

Taylor HB, Norris HJ: Well-differentiated carcinoma of the breast. Cancer 1970;25:687-692.

Urban JA, Adair FE: Sclerosing adenosis. Cancer 1949;2:625-634.

12

Sclerosing Adenosis

DEFINITIONS AND CLINICOPATHOLOGIC CHARACTERISTICS

Sclerosing adenosis, once regarded as exotic and as a diagnostic challenge for even the experienced pathologist, has for the most part become a well-characterized and easily recognized lesion. Unlike certain other forms of adenosis, this variety seems to originate in preformed terminal duct–lobular units. It develops from the multiplication and elongation of filiform tubules in the centers of lobules. The sclerosis that characterizes the lesion develops because the myoepithelial cells deposit basement membrane proteins, which encase and compress the glands. This distortion creates an appearance that superficially resembles the pattern of invasive carcinoma.

Sclerosing adenosis is common, usually affecting women in their reproductive years. At least 10% of mastectomy specimens showing only benign changes also harbor sclerosing adenosis. The process typically occurs as scattered microscopic foci, which often serve as sites of calcification. Detection of these calcifications can provoke a biopsy; however, sclerosing adenosis more often represents a clinically silent lesion evident only to the pathologist at the time of histologic examination. In rare circumstances, small regions of sclerosing adenosis merge to create a mass referred to as an *adenosis tumor* or *nodular adenosis*. This nodular variety of sclerosing adenosis tends to afflict women about 10 years younger than those with the incidental, microscopic form. *see p. 227*

Although lobular neoplasia often coexists with sclerosing adenosis, researchers have not discovered a direct morphologic link between sclerosing adenosis and breast cancer, so clinicians usually disregard the presence of the adenosis. Pathologists, on the other hand, do not have this luxury. They must study the lesion's histologic features carefully and learn to evaluate those findings that differentiate it from invasive carcinoma. Only through careful study of the *see p. 228*

contrasting characteristics of these two lesions can pathologists avoid this disastrous error.

HISTOLOGIC CHARACTERISTICS

Shape of the Lesion

Sclerosing adenosis usually forms smoothly contoured, round or oval nodules of closely packed glands. The lesion originates in preexisting lobules and consists of the proliferation of ductules and the deposition of basement membrane–like material between them. The process often enlarges the terminal duct–lobular unit modestly, but it usually does not alter the round or oval configuration of the lobule (Fig. 12-1). Thus, the individual foci of sclerosing adenosis look like compact glandular aggregates demonstrating the approximate size and shape of a terminal duct–lobular unit. Occasional examples deviate from the expected round or oval outline. They can exhibit scalloped contours, for instance, if either the fibrous connective tissue or the peripheral acini undergo atrophy. In the former instance, stromal fibroblasts along the perimeter of the lobules transform into adipocytes. The fat cells accumulate lipids, enlarge, bulge into the lobule, and indent its contour, and the glands seem to extend into the septa between lobules of fat (Fig. 12-2). Atrophy of the peripheral acini also results in an irregular contour, as the remaining compact, central acini seem to extend into the nonspecialized stroma (Fig. 12-3). Despite such deviations from the usual rounded configuration, these foci exhibit the other typical features of sclerosing adenosis.

Structure of the Lesion

The classic example of sclerosing adenosis is a compact collection of glands that show a characteristic

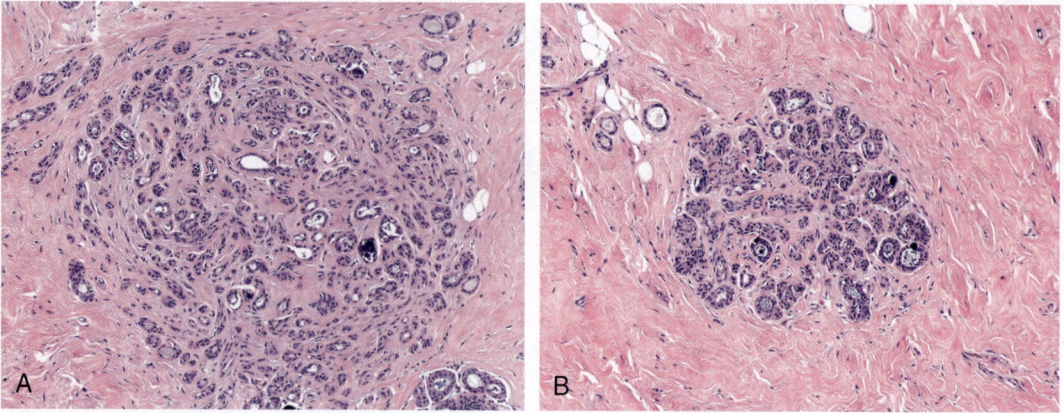

Figure 12-1 A, Sclerosing adenosis has enlarged the underlying terminal duct-lobular unit, but the focus retains the round shape and smooth contour of the unaffected lobule shown in **B**.

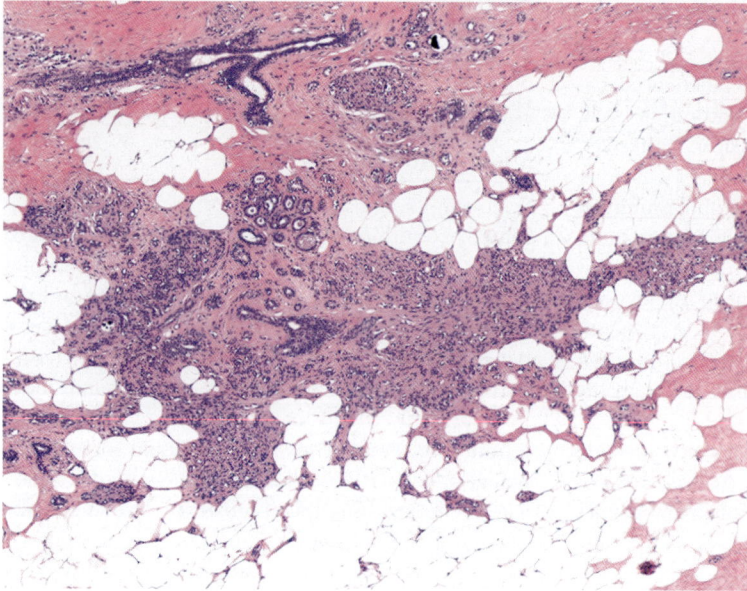

Figure 12-2 Atrophy of the peripheral nonspecialized stroma has given these lobules altered by sclerosing adenosis scalloped contours so that the compressed glands seem to extend into the adipose tissue.

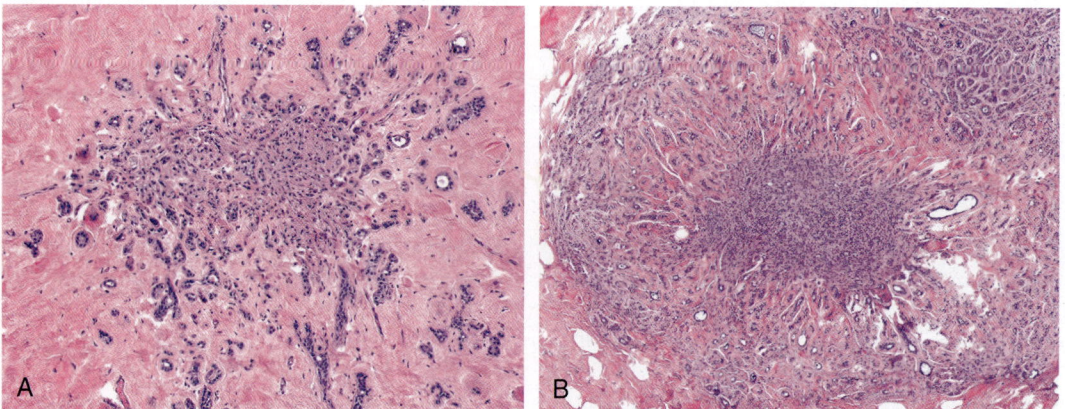

Figure 12-3 A and **B,** Deposition of collagen in the specialized stroma, thickening of the basement membranes, and acinar atrophy in the periphery of these lobules have made these foci of sclerosing adenosis look stellate.

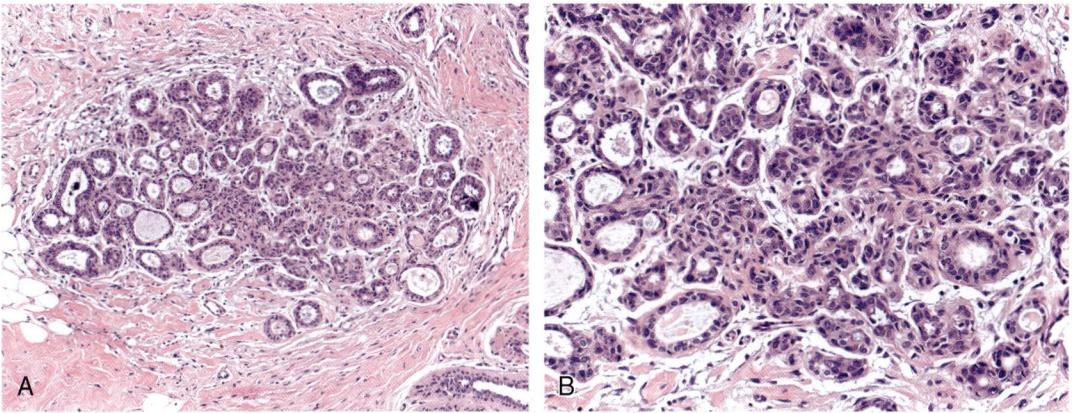

Figure 12-4 Sclerosing adenosis seems to begin in the center of the lobule in **A**, where tiny cords of epithelial cells proliferate among existing acini in **B**.

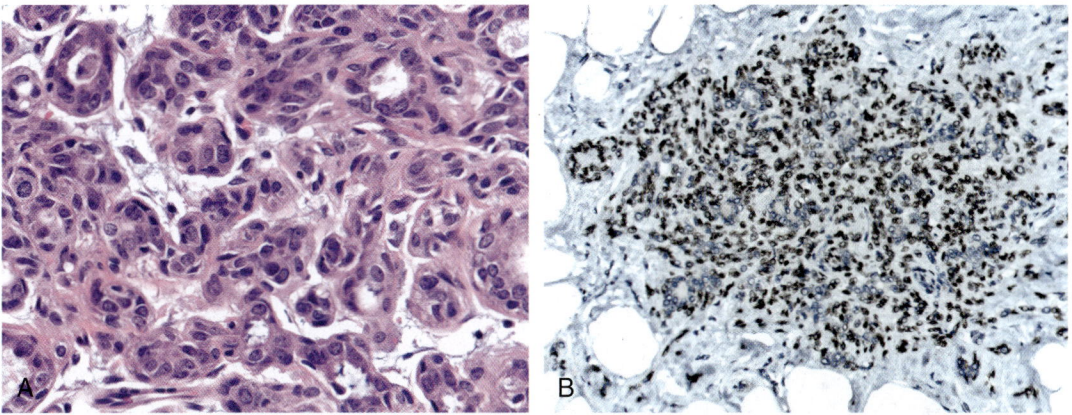

Figure 12-5 A, The proliferative cells in sclerosing adenosis include both epithelial and myoepithelial types. The epithelial cells appear slightly larger than the myoepithelial cells. The former have oval or round nuclei, pale chromatin, small nucleoli, and a modest amount of eosinophilic cytoplasm. Most of the latter possess small, flattened nuclei, dark chromatin, and scant cytoplasm. **B,** A stain for p63 protein highlights the myoepithelial cells.

internal structure. The lesion seems to begin as tiny epithelial clusters in the center of lobules proliferate and encase the intralobular terminal ductule (Fig. 12-4). The proliferative cells consist of two types. The luminal cells have polygonal shapes and oval or round nuclei, and the myoepithelial cells display elongate shapes and small, oval, hyperchromatic nuclei (Fig. 12-5). As the process evolves, the cells grow into slender cords and filiform tubules (Fig. 12-6). The minute diameter and the close packing of these epithelial cords usually obscure their glandular nature, but expansion of these tubules, for instance by a proliferation of neoplastic cells, makes their glandular architecture obvious (Fig. 12-7).

The extent of cellular proliferation typically diminishes in the outer reaches of the terminal duct–lobular unit, and the extent of the glandular

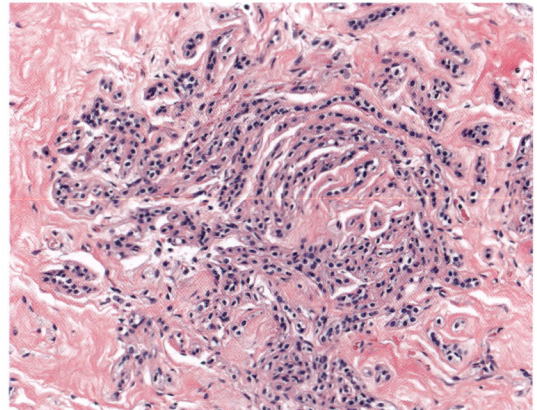

Figure 12-6 The proliferating glands in sclerosing adenosis form slender epithelial cords.

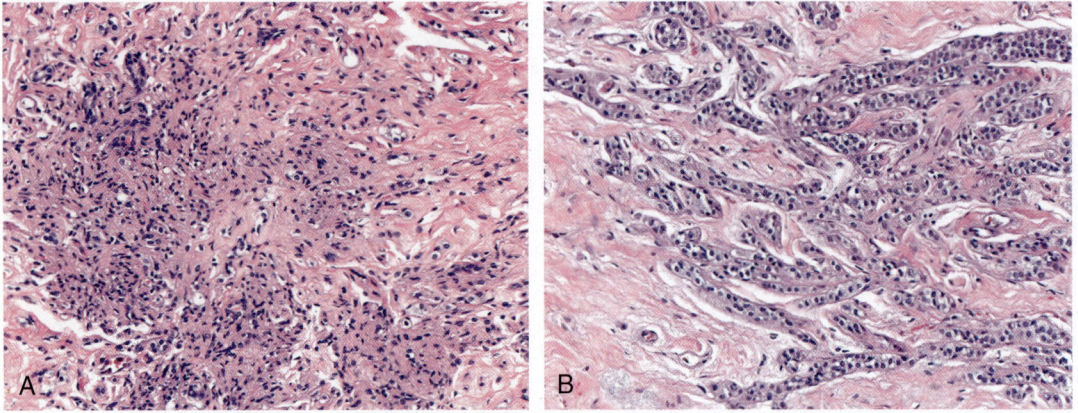

Figure 12-7 A, The close packing and small diameters of the tubules and the deposition of matrix proteins obscure the glandular nature of the proliferation. **B,** Expansion of the structures by neoplastic lobular cells brings out the anastomosing glandular structure of sclerosing adenosis.

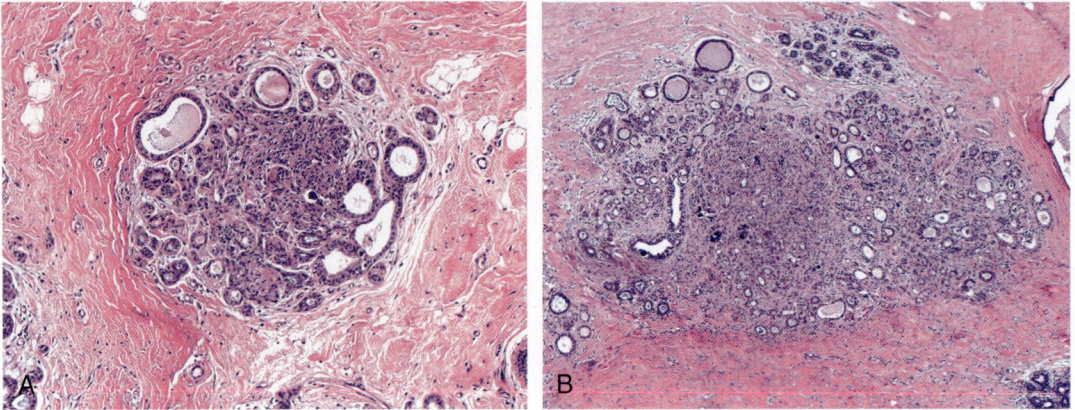

Figure 12-8 The peripheral acini in foci of sclerosing adenosis appear round and they have cuboidal cells and open lumens. **A** illustrates a modestly altered lobule, and **B** a lobule with marked sclerosing adenosis.

distortion decreases proportionately. Acini at the periphery of the lobule show the least alteration. They appear larger than the central ones and tend to have round shapes, cuboidal acinar cells, and open lumens, which contrast with the compressed contours, attenuated luminal cells, and compromised lumens of the central acini (Fig. 12-8). Acini in an intermediate position, those between the central proliferative zone and the periphery, usually maintain their round shape; however, they sometimes develop thick basement membranes (Fig. 12-9). In examples of florid sclerosing adenosis, the changes can overrun the lobule so extensively that a few peripherally situated, round acini with intact lumens may remain as the only evidence of the underlying zonal organization (Fig. 12-10).

The luminal cells do not develop the morphologic features of robust glandular cells; instead, they remain small and flattened or barely cuboidal in their

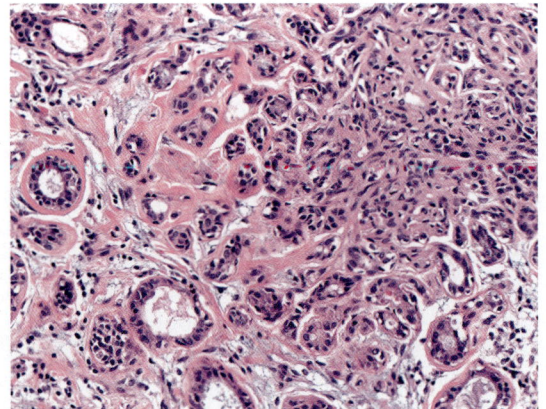

Figure 12-9 The upper right of the field depicts the central, compressed glands in a focus of sclerosing adenosis, and the lower left the peripheral acini. Glands in the middle of the lobule, which occupy the center of the field, have thick basement membranes.

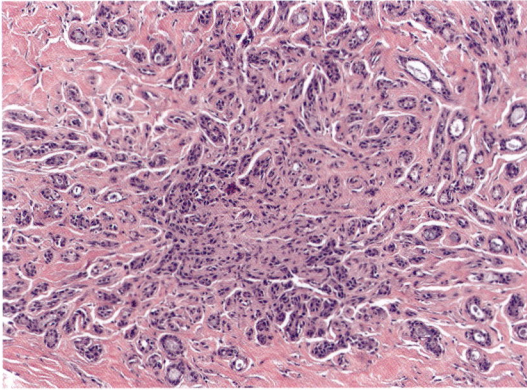

Figure 12-10 In this example of florid sclerosing adenosis, the presence of a few slightly dilated peripheral acini represents the only evidence of the typical zonal architecture.

configuration, and they possess small, oval nuclei, dark chromatin, and scant cytoplasm (Fig. 12-11). The myoepithelial cells, in contrast, display the cellular features of fully differentiated mature myoepithelial cells. They have spindly shapes; small, dark, oval nuclei; and scant cytoplasm. Reflecting the parallel arrangement of the cellular cords and tubules, the myoepithelial cells tend to run in similar arrays, which one can appreciate from the parallel arrangement of the long axis of their nuclei (Fig. 12-12). In certain examples, the myoepithelial cells appear especially myoid (Fig. 12-13). With the passage of time, the luminal cells atrophy and can disappear entirely; consequently, myoepithelial cells become the dominant type of cell in many examples of sclerosing adenosis.

Figure 12-11 The luminal cells appear rather anemic. They exhibit barely cuboidal shapes, small round nuclei, and small amounts of cytoplasm, which appears pale in this example. The myoepithelial cells look like conventional myoepithelial cells: they appear long and slender, and they contain flattened dark nuclei.

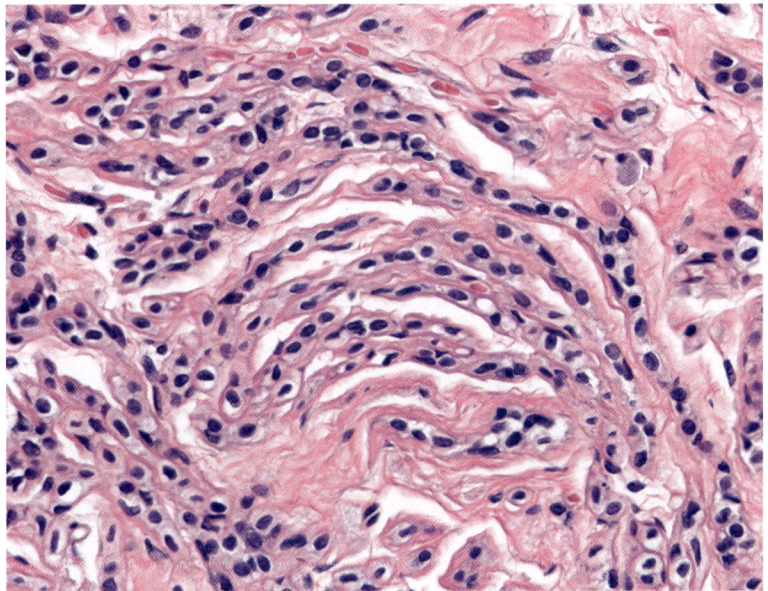

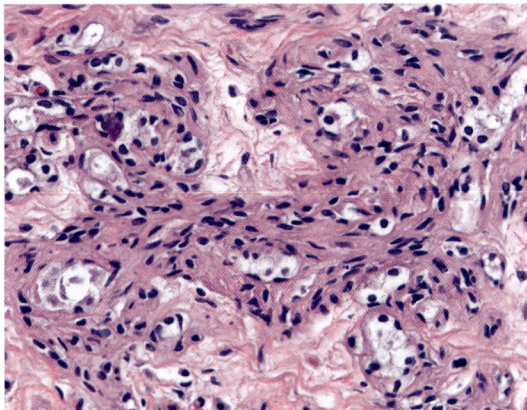

Figure 12-12 The parallel orientation of the myoepithelial cell nuclei reflects the parallel arrangement of the proliferative tubules.

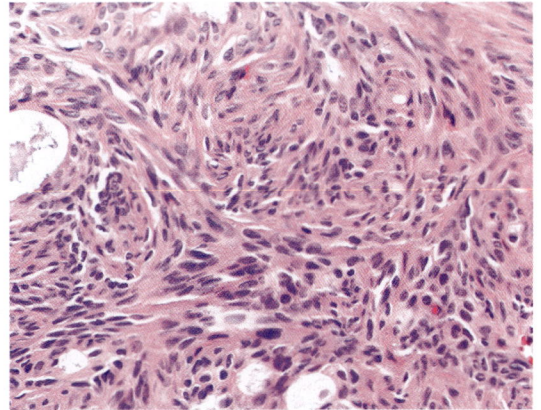

Figure 12-13 The fascicular arrangement and eosinophilic hue of the cytoplasm give these myoepithelial cells an especially myoid appearance.

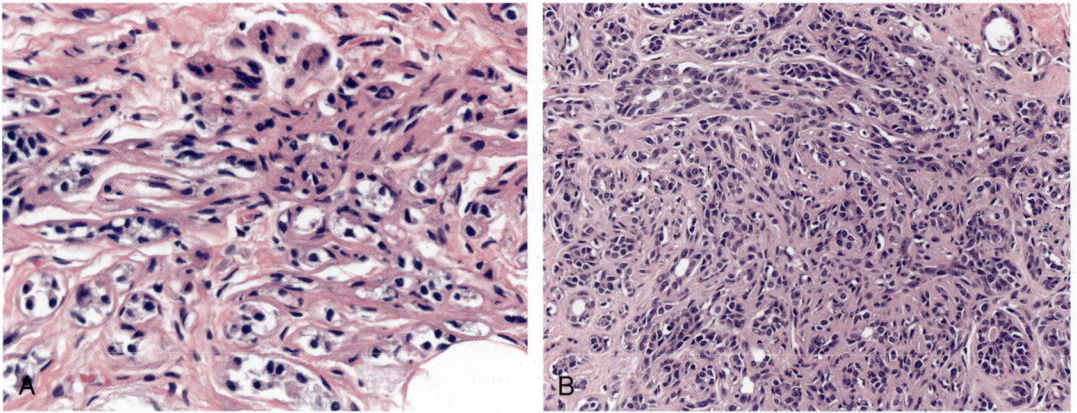

Figure 12-14 Deposition of matrix proteins thickens the basement membranes of the tubules in **A** and accumulates in the stroma between them in **B**.

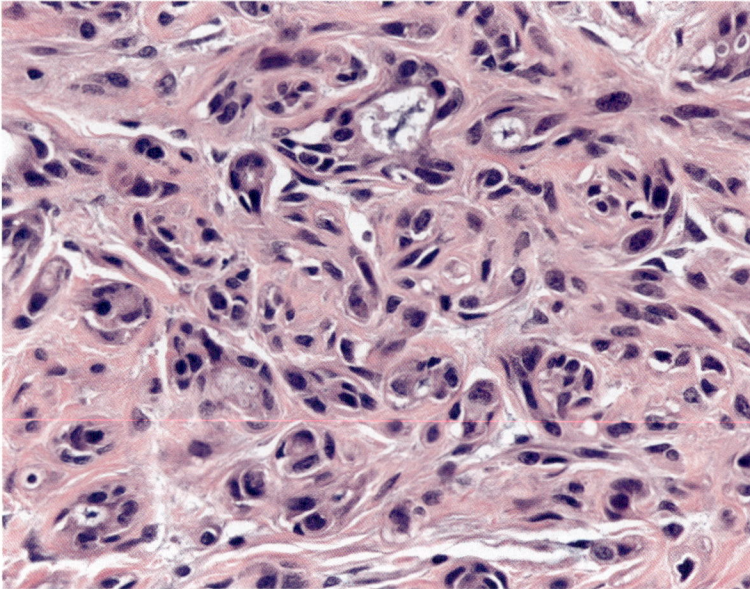

Figure 12-15 The smooth flow of the collagen bundles and the orderly relationship between the glandular cells and the stroma reflect the benign nature of this sclerosing process.

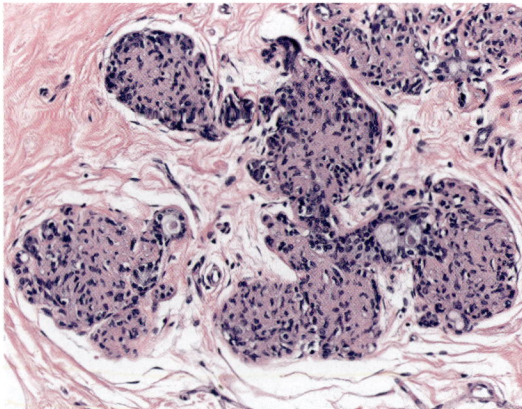

Figure 12-16 Myoepithelial hyperplasia superficially resembles sclerosing adenosis because of the common presence of numerous myoepithelial cells and abundant matrix proteins.

Besides the proliferation of tubules, sclerosing adenosis involves the deposition of eosinophilic material resembling basement membrane proteins. The matrix proteins can accumulate in thick rims surrounding the tubules or in linear deposits flowing along them (Fig. 12-14). This material narrows the tubules even more, but no matter how compressed the epithelial structures become, they maintain an orderly relationship with the collagen bundles and matrix proteins. The stromal elements sweep along the epithelial structures in uninterrupted bands, forming a pattern that reflects the benign nature of the process (Fig. 12-15).

Because of this myoepithelial cell proliferation and basement membrane protein deposition, nodules of sclerosing adenosis can resemble foci of intralobular myoepithelial hyperplasia (Fig. 12-16). Despite this resemblance, the two lesions probably

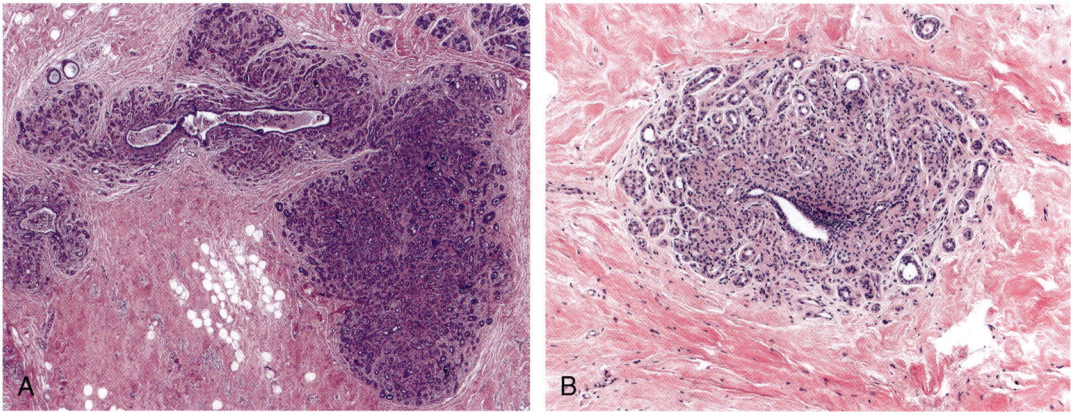

Figure 12-17 Sclerosing adenosis usually arises in relation to small ducts, shown in **A,** and ductules, seen in **B.**

Figure 12-18 Foci of sclerosing adenosis cluster along the length of a small duct.

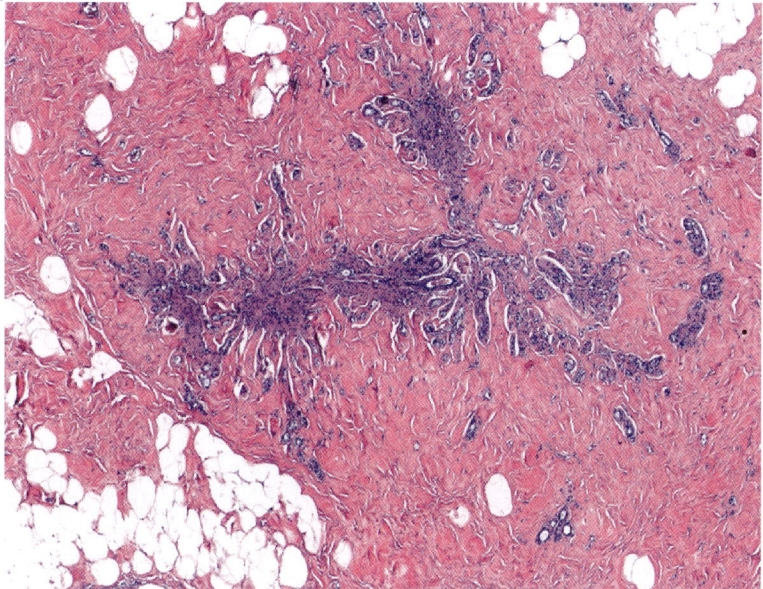

differ in pathogenesis. Sclerosing adenosis seems to result from the proliferation of entire glandular units, which contain both luminal and myoepithelial cells, whereas myoepithelial hyperplasia most likely represents a purely myoepithelial proliferation. One must keep an open mind about the reality of this distinction. Like many others, this conceptual difference might not have a counterpart in daily experience. Once pathologists develop a better understanding of the evolution of both sclerosing adenosis and myoepithelial hyperplasia, we may find that they have a common pathogenesis and represent different tissue manifestations of a single process.

Nodules of sclerosing adenosis often localize along the course of small ducts and extralobular ductules (Fig. 12-17). This linear distribution of regions of adenosis often serves as the only hint of the periductular distribution of the lesion (Fig. 12-18). The

process can also surround ducts of a medium caliber, and certain planes of section create the appearance of a nodule composed of glands and stroma bulging into the lumen of the duct (Fig. 12-19). Such foci recall the look of a papilloma and may account for the term *intraductal sclerosing adenosis,* which certain surgical pathologists used for papillomas in times gone by. Although not strictly speaking a structural characteristic of the individual foci, the arrangement of a sclerosing lesion in this distribution with respect to ducts and ductules argues strongly in favor of the diagnosis of sclerosing adenosis rather than invasive carcinoma. Individual nodules of sclerosing adenosis often coalesce to form small, multinodular aggregates; less commonly they unite in large, palpable nodules (Fig. 12-20). As previously mentioned, pathologists have referred to the latter condition as *nodular adenosis* or *adenosis tumor.*

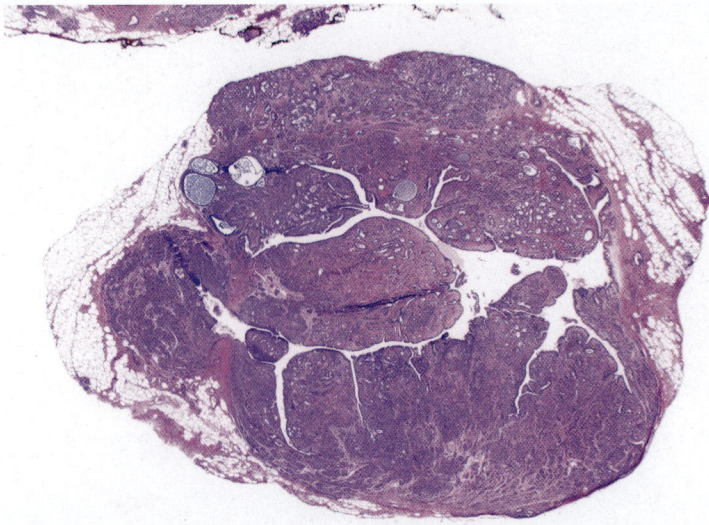

Figure 12-19 A, Sclerosing adenosis can also surround large ducts. **B,** Off-center planes of section can create the appearance of nodules bulging into the lumen of the duct.

A

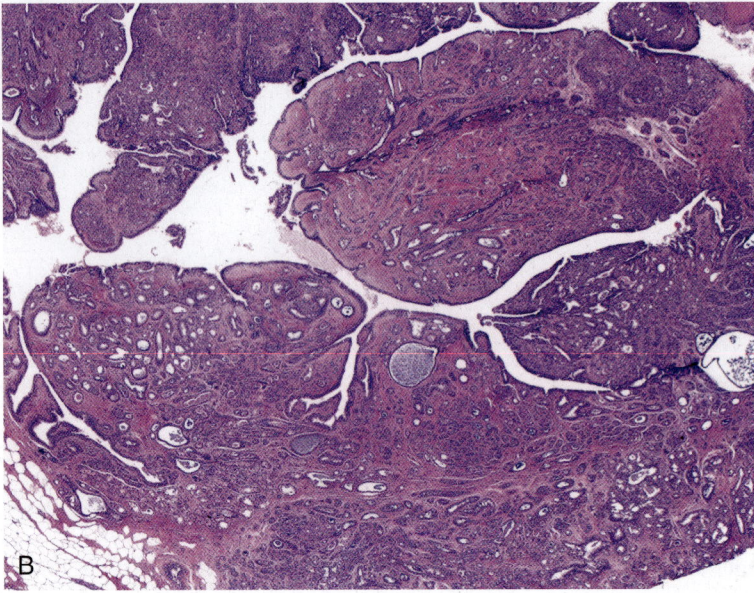

B

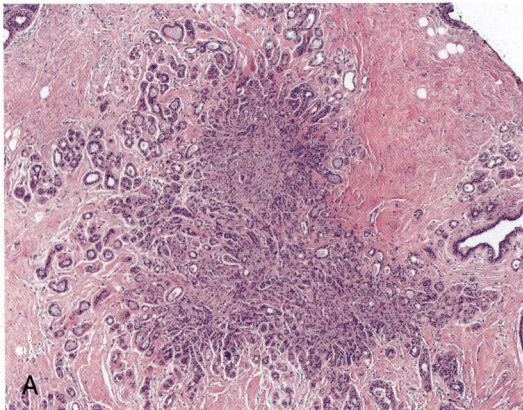

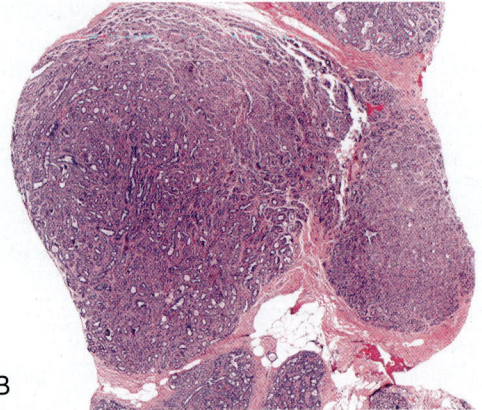

A   B

Figure 12-20 Lobules altered by sclerosing adenosis can coalesce to form small nodules in **A** or large masses in **B**.

Characteristics of the Peripheral Epithelial Elements

Study of the histologic characteristics of the peripheral glands and their relationship to the components of the surrounding tissue offers powerful evidence for the diagnosis of sclerosing adenosis. The smooth, round contours of the acini, the presence of luminal and myoepithelial cells in the expected two-layered arrangement, and the presence of a basement membrane all attest to the benign nature of these glands (Fig. 12-21). These features contrast with those of the invasive nests of carcinomas, which appear irregular in shape and consist entirely of cytologically atypical, neoplastic luminal cells. Furthermore, the peripheral glands of sclerosing adenosis have an orderly, cooperative relationship with the surrounding tissues. The glands

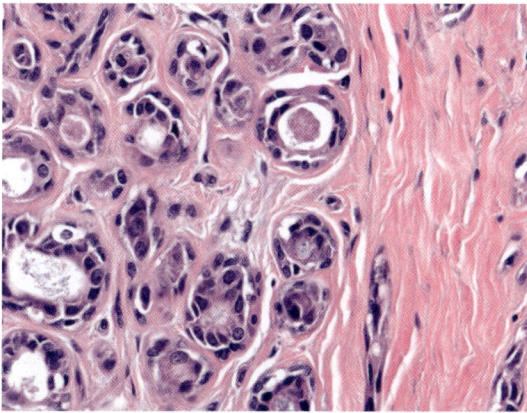

Figure 12-21 The acini at the edge of a focus of sclerosing adenosis appear round and smoothly contoured. They possess a two-layered epithelium composed of both luminal and myoepithelial cells, and a basement membrane encloses each acinus.

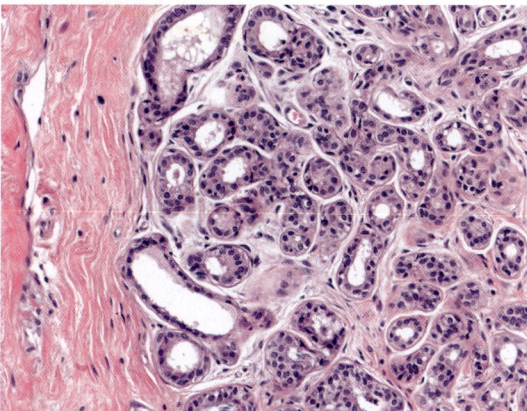

Figure 12-22 The peripheral glands at the edge of this focus of sclerosing adenosis do not disrupt the flow of the stromal collagen bundles, which flow smoothly around the glands.

do not penetrate into lobules, encircle ducts, or insinuate themselves between adipocytes, nor do they disrupt the flow of the collagen bundles (Fig. 12-22). Clusters of invasive carcinoma disrupt and destroy the mammary parenchyma in all these ways.

Characteristics of the Associated Ductal Epithelial Proliferation

Although helpful in the analysis of certain sclerosing lesions, the character of a coexistent ductal proliferation does not contribute to the analysis of a region suggestive of sclerosing adenosis. Ductal hyperplasia, for instance, frequently affects patients with sclerosing adenosis, but the two lesions do not seem to have either a close spatial relationship or a common etiology. Thus, one cannot use the presence of conventional ductal hyperplasia to buttress a diagnosis of sclerosing adenosis, nor can one rely on the absence of ductal hyperplasia to exclude the presence of sclerosing adenosis. The detection of ductal carcinoma in situ in a region of glandular disarray does not help in this regard, either. This finding would make one carefully consider the possibility that the glands represent invasive carcinoma, of course, but the presence of a carcinoma in situ itself does not establish the invasive nature of the irregular glands. Thus, in every situation, a secure diagnosis of sclerosing adenosis depends only on the presence of the appropriate structure of the region in question and the appropriate relationship between the peripheral glands and the tissues around them.

Summary

Sclerosing adenosis represents a proliferation of small glands and tubules within preexisting terminal duct–lobular units. In its characteristic form, the lesion gives rise to smoothly contoured, round or oval nodules about the size of lobules. They exhibit an orderly internal structure in which compressed glands sit in the center and slightly dilated acini rim the nodule. Throughout the focus, the glands and the stroma exhibit an organized relationship, which one can appreciate most easily by examining the periphery of the lesion (Box 12-1).

Box 12-1

Histologic characteristics of sclerosing adenosis:

- Smoothly contoured, round, compact aggregate of glands
- Compressed central glands and preserved outer glands
- An orderly relationship between the glands and the stroma

PROBLEMS IN THE DIAGNOSIS OF SCLEROSING ADENOSIS

When pathologists consider alternatives to the diagnosis of sclerosing adenosis, they usually think of well-differentiated invasive ductal carcinoma first. Although gland-forming carcinomas do look like certain varieties of adenosis, such as florid adenosis and tubular adenosis, they do not closely resemble foci of sclerosing adenosis unless artifacts of tissue handling compromise the analysis or there is only a small sample of the lesion to study. The distinction from invasive lobular carcinoma, on the other hand, poses a more common and an especially difficult problem, because the diminutive cords of cells in the middle of foci of sclerosing adenosis duplicate the classic, single-file arrangement of the cells of invasive lobular carcinoma.

The diagnosis of epithelial proliferations involving tissue altered by sclerosing adenosis poses certain challenges, also. The presence of atypical apocrine cells in foci of sclerosing adenosis characterizes the entity known as *atypical apocrine sclerosing lesion*. The evaluation of epithelial proliferations involving terminal duct–lobular units altered by sclerosing adenosis presents difficulties, because the distortion of ducts and lobules by the sclerosing process can obscure the architectural characteristics of the glands and can even make it difficult to determine the extent of epithelial proliferation and the nature of the proliferative cells. Moreover, the distortion of the glandular architecture impairs the detection of invasion. The parenchymal scarring associated with sclerosing adenosis can entrap nerves and blood vessels, and the presence of glands within a nerve always suggests the presence of an invasive ductal carcinoma. The following paragraphs offer guidance for the solution of these problems.

Invasive Lobular Carcinoma

The slender columns of small cells that occupy the center of a focus of sclerosing adenosis can look nearly identical to the cells of invasive lobular carcinoma when examined out of context or at high magnification (Fig. 12-23). The most reliable diagnostic clues to differentiating these two lesions come from the structural characteristic of the focus in question. Foci of sclerosing adenosis typically create smoothly contoured, compact nodules; in contrast, regions of

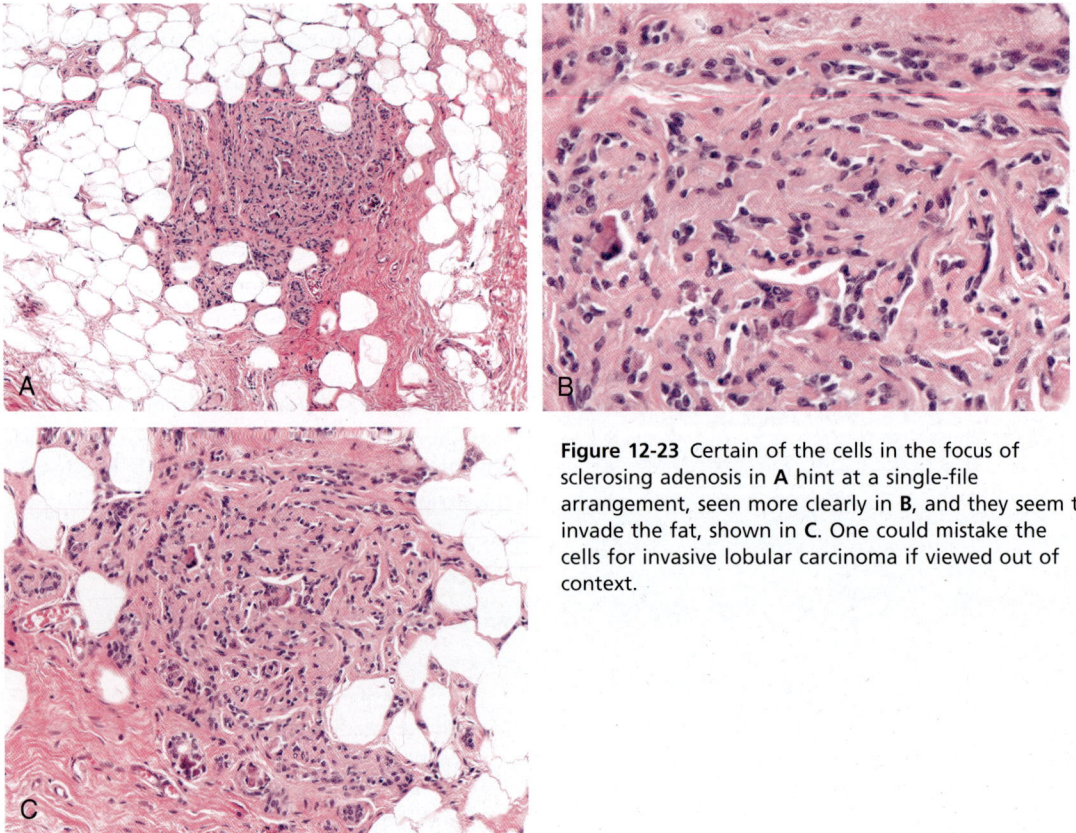

Figure 12-23 Certain of the cells in the focus of sclerosing adenosis in **A** hint at a single-file arrangement, seen more clearly in **B**, and they seem to invade the fat, shown in **C**. One could mistake the cells for invasive lobular carcinoma if viewed out of context.

invasive lobular carcinoma usually have shaggy contours, and the cells within them appear somewhat loosely arranged (Fig. 12-24). Inspection of the periphery of an example of sclerosing adenosis reveals that the proliferative cells do not invade into glandular tissue or fat; furthermore, even within the region of sclerosing adenosis, the cells do not disrupt the pattern of the collagen bundles. Invasive lobular carcinomas cannot hide their invasive properties. They always disrupt the structure of the underlying fibrous connective tissue (Fig. 12-25), and as they enlarge, they overrun any glandular tissue or fat in their vicinity.

Pathologists usually find this distinction achievable when they can study the entirety of a focus, especially using low magnification. Core biopsy specimens do not provide this opportunity, and neither do samples compromised by artifacts of specimen handling. In such suboptimal circumstances,

pathologists must turn to even more subtle characteristics, the cytologic properties of the suspect cells. The proliferative cells in a small nodule of invasive lobular carcinoma consist entirely of carcinoma cells. They are usually round, oval, or polygonal and have a small amount of pale or eosinophilic cytoplasm. The nuclei look slightly pleomorphic, often exhibit slight irregularity of their contour, and typically have an eccentric position in the cell. The chromatin often appears finely granular (Fig. 12-26). The cells within a region of sclerosing adenosis, in contrast, consist of both epithelial and myoepithelial cells, and the latter typically predominate. Neither type of cell appears atypical. In many cases, these differences prove so slight that one cannot rely on them to distinguish the lesions; however, immunohistochemical staining for proteins present in myoepithelial cells and for E-cadherin clarifies the diagnosis in these

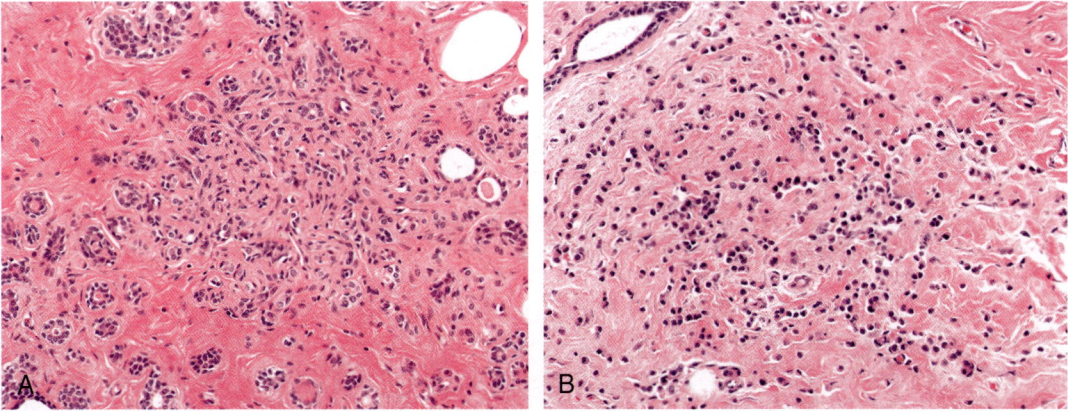

Figure 12-24 Foci of sclerosing adenosis in **A** appear well defined and compact compared with the shaggy and loosely formed collection of invasive lobular carcinoma cells shown in **B**.

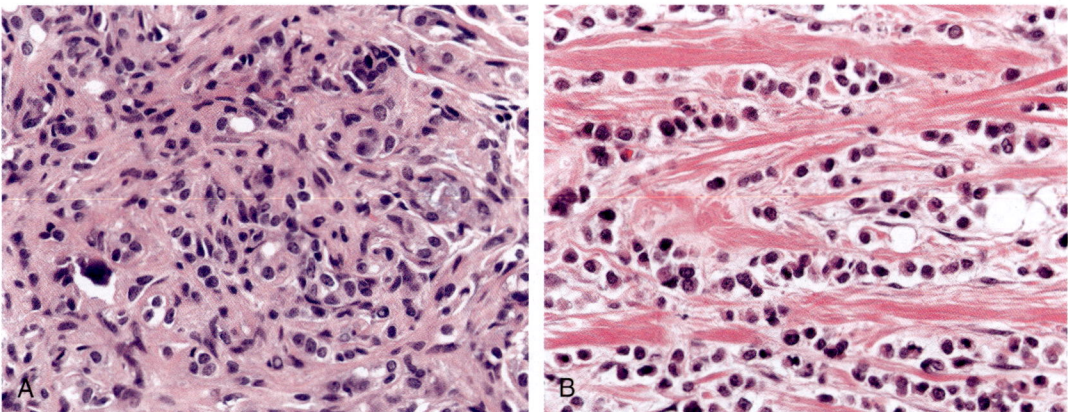

Figure 12-25 A, The cells of sclerosing adenosis exhibit a nondestructive relationship with the stroma; the glandular cells do not interrupt the flow of the collagen bundles. **B,** Invasive lobular carcinomas disrupt the organization of the stroma.

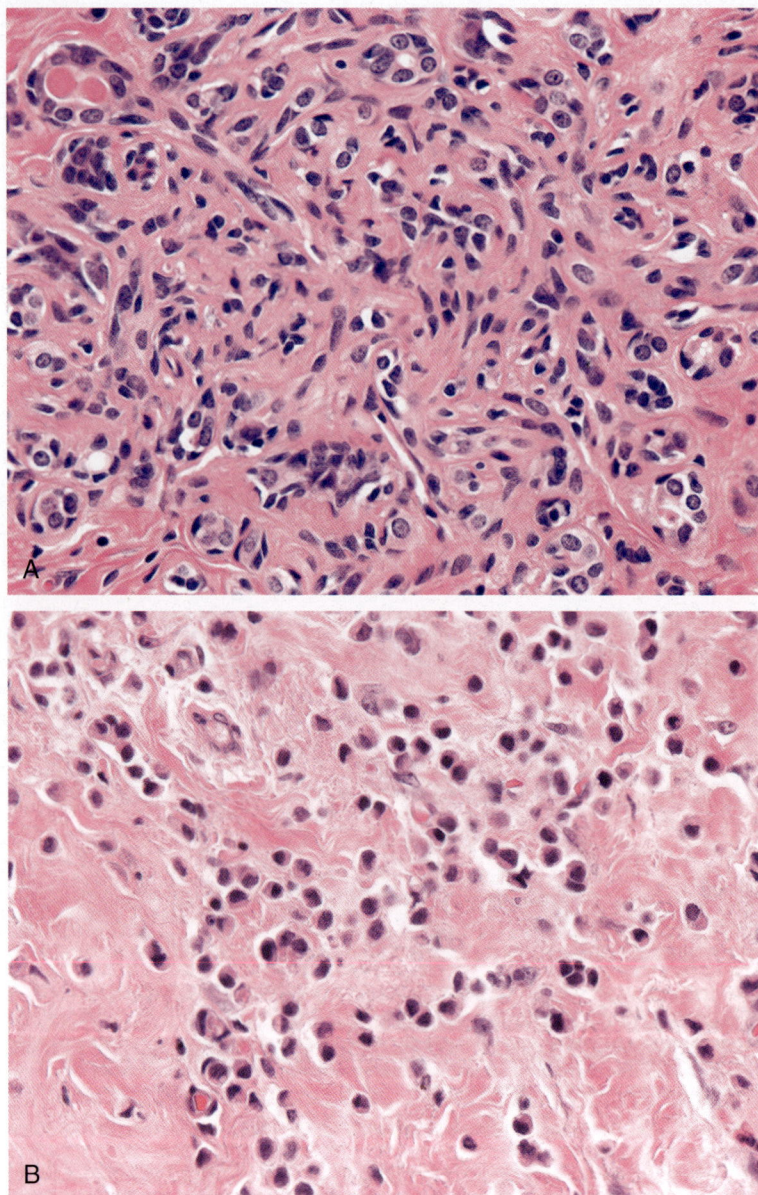

Figure 12-26 A, Bland cells of both epithelial and myoepithelial type compose the focus of sclerosing adenosis. **B,** Invasive lobular carcinoma consists of a single population of atypical epithelial cells.

ambiguous situations. Foci of sclerosing adenosis show staining for both myoepithelial markers and E-cadherin, whereas the neoplastic cells of invasive lobular carcinoma lack these proteins.

When lobular neoplasia involves a lobule already deformed by sclerosing adenosis, a particularly difficult diagnostic dilemma emerges. Extension of the neoplastic lobular cells into the deformed tubules recreates the single-file appearance of typical invasive lobular carcinoma. The malignant cells in this noninvasive form of lobular carcinoma do not disrupt the arrangement of the collagen bundles in the way that invasive carcinoma

cells do, nor do they provoke a stromal reaction. Chapter 5 discusses this problem in detail.

Atypical Apocrine Sclerosing Lesion

In the *atypical apocrine sclerosing lesion*, atypical apocrine cells populate a region of sclerosing adenosis (Fig. 12-27). The presence of large atypical cells irregularly disposed in the stroma creates a worrisome pattern, which one could mistake for invasive carcinoma. Chapter 3, devoted to the subject of apocrine proliferations, discusses this entity.

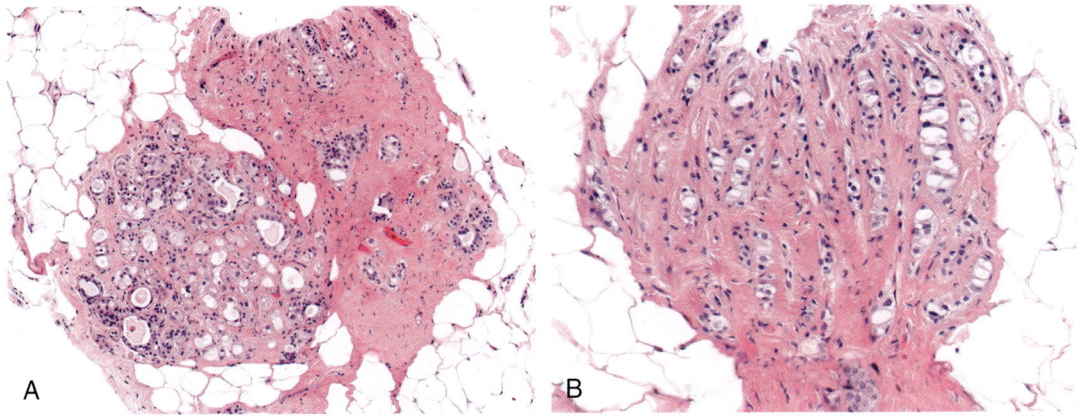

Figure 12-27 Atypical apocrine cells occupy a region of adenosis in **A** and sclerosing adenosis in **B**. **C,** Distortion of the underlying glands and atypia of the apocrine cells create an appearance resembling that of invasive carcinoma.

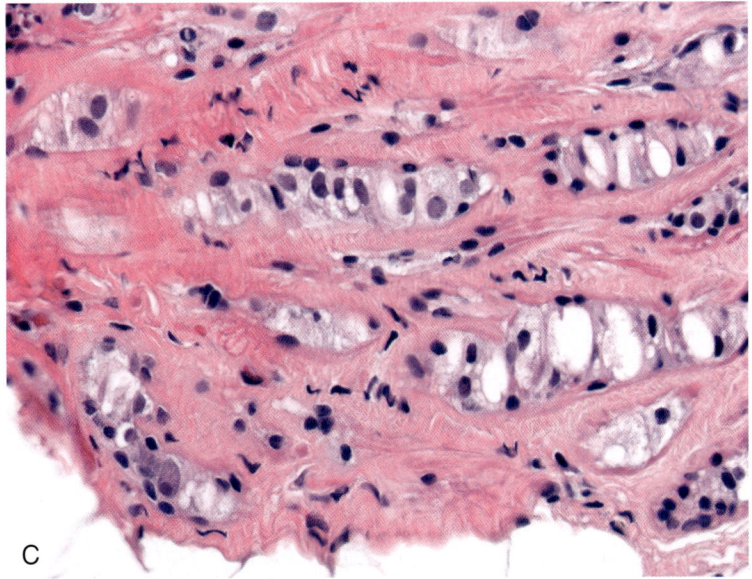

Carcinoma Involving Sclerosing Adenosis

The diagnosis of an epithelial proliferation within glands affected by sclerosing adenosis does not usually present a problem. The approach to the analysis of proliferations residing in otherwise unaltered ducts and lobules applies just as effectively to proliferations involving regions of adenosis, and the cytologic and architectural criteria used in the former situation do not require modification for use in the latter one, either. Thus, pathologists should not have much difficulty recognizing conventional ductal hyperplasia, ductal carcinoma in situ (Fig. 12-28), and lobular neoplasia (Fig. 12-29) when the disorders occur in glands altered by sclerosing adenosis. One must keep in mind that distortion of glandular profiles combined with off-center planes of section can create the appearance of proliferation where none

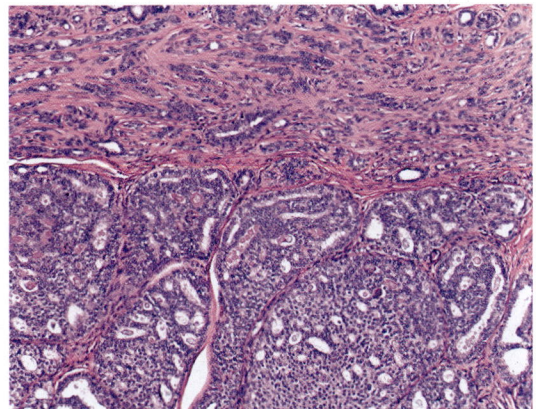

Figure 12-28 Cribriform ductal carcinoma in situ distends glands distorted by sclerosing adenosis.

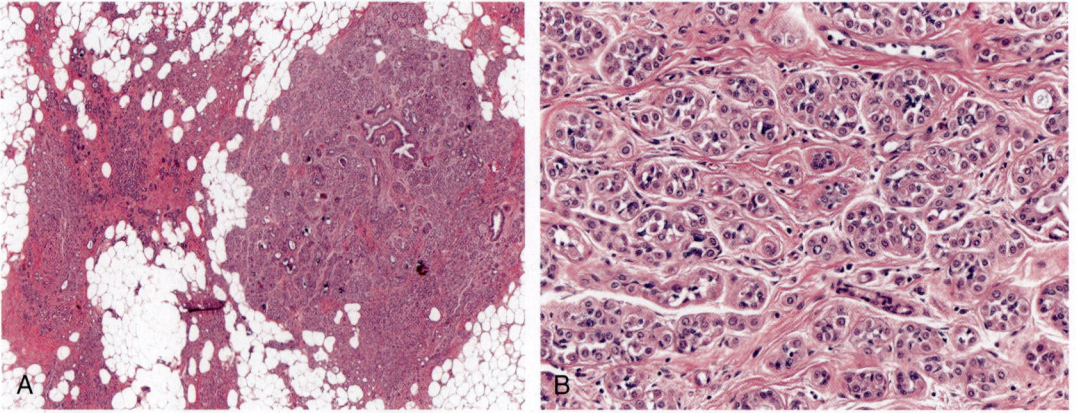

Figure 12-29 A, Lobular carcinoma in situ involves a region of sclerosing adenosis. Note the larger size of the involved glands (*right*) compared with their uninvolved counterparts (*left*). **B,** The neoplastic lobular cells distend the acini in the focus of adenosis.

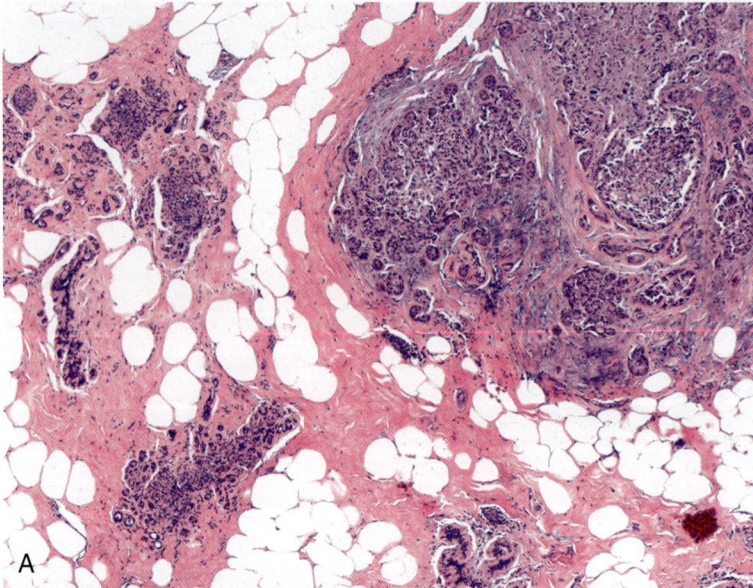

Figure 12-30 A, Colonization of a region of adenosis like the one on the left has produced a focus that looks like invasive ductal carcinoma on the right. **B,** The glands appear disorderly and the stroma shows reactive changes.

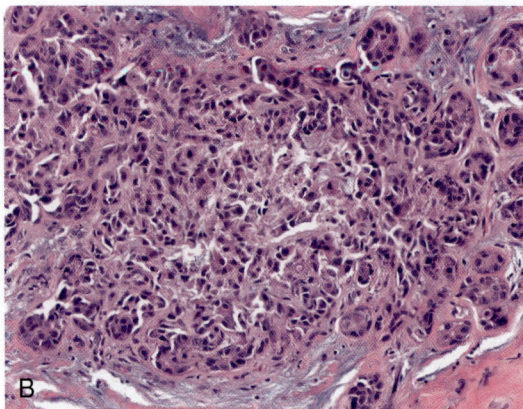

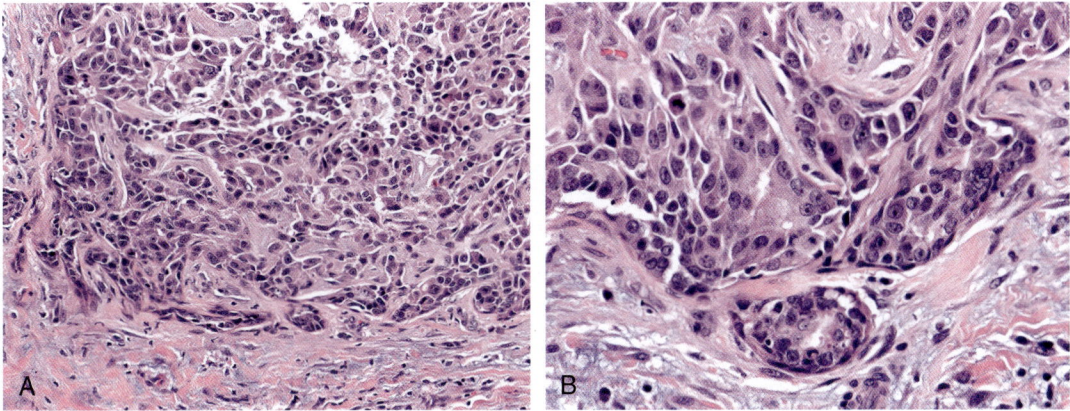

Figure 12-31 A, Ductal carcinoma in situ occupies a region of sclerosing adenosis. **B,** The irregular shapes of the groups and their haphazard disposition create the impression of invasion. Attenuated cells consistent with myoepithelial cells surround certain nests, but this finding seems somewhat debatable.

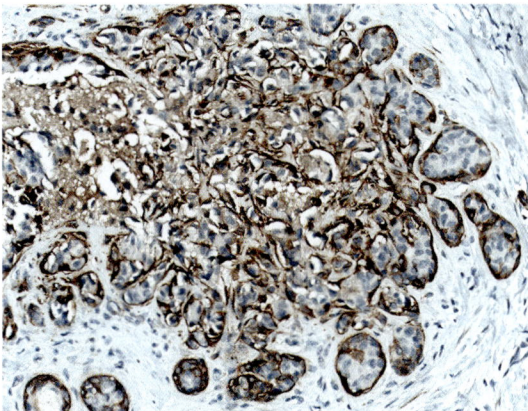

Figure 12-32 A stain for myosin heavy chain establishes the presence of myoepithelial cells and, thereby, the diagnosis of ductal carcinoma in situ involving sclerosing adenosis.

exists, so one should require the presence of unambiguous cellular proliferation, manifested as clear-cut glandular distention, before considering the diagnosis of carcinoma in situ in this setting.

The confluence of carcinoma and sclerosing adenosis presents the pathologist with two particularly difficult and sometimes insurmountable problems. First, the irregular shapes of the glands can easily cause one to mistake a region of sclerosing adenosis harboring carcinoma in situ for a focus of invasive carcinoma (Fig. 12-30). To avoid this misinterpretation, one can look for myoepithelial cells and basement membranes around the clusters of carcinoma cells (Fig. 12-31); however, confidently distinguishing myoepithelial cells from compressed carcinoma cells and stromal fibroblasts proves impossible in many cases. Pathologists should make liberal use of immunohistochemical staining for markers of myoepithelial cells to clarify these confusing situations (Fig. 12-32).

The parenchymal distortion that causes carcinoma in situ in sclerosing adenosis to mimic the appearance of invasive carcinoma also makes it nearly impossible to detect small nests of genuine invasive carcinoma. The search for microinvasion in regions of sclerosing adenosis begins with study of the conventional, hematoxylin and eosin–stained sections. The pathologist should look for regions in which the architectural pattern of the glands or the appearance of the stroma deviates from the expected. The detection of individual cells or small, irregular clusters, especially those growing in a myxoid stroma and disturbing the mammary parenchyma, should lead one to suspect the presence of invasion. Immunohistochemical staining of suspicious clusters for markers of myoepithelial cells usually clarifies the nature of these nests.

Neural Involvement by Small Glands

One occasionally encounters collections of small glands growing within nerves (Fig. 12-33). This finding does raise the possibility of neural invasion by a well-differentiated carcinoma; however, in the absence of an obvious cancer, these aggregates usually represent benign glands. Researchers have not determined the mechanism by which the glands come to reside within nerves, but the situation usually arises in the setting of a sclerosing lesion such as sclerosing adenosis or a radial scar. Writers have suggested that the scarring process entraps nerves and that, via some unspecified means, the glands find their way beneath the perineurium. Such an explanation obviously leaves many details unexplained. Whatever the mechanism of their displacement, these benign glands consist of normally structured epithelium composed of normally positioned myoepithelial cells and luminal cells (Fig. 12-34).

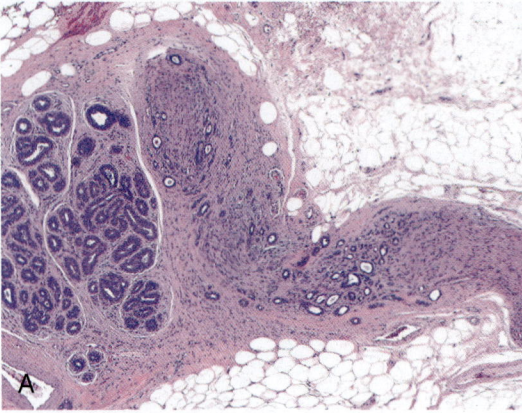

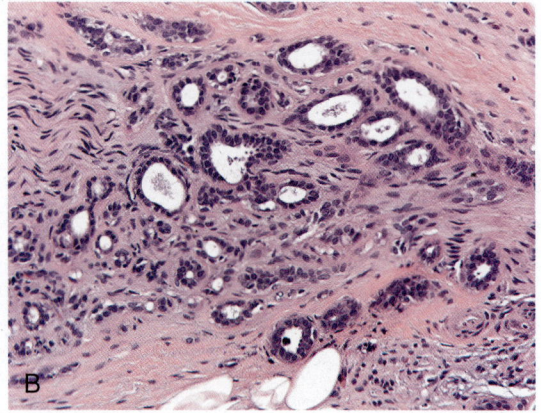

Figure 12-33 A and **B,** Small glands surround this nerve and penetrate within it.

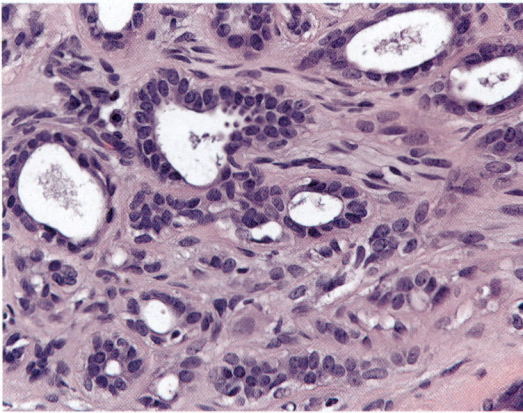

Figure 12-34 The glands consist of luminal and myoepithelial cells arranged in their normal two-layered structure.

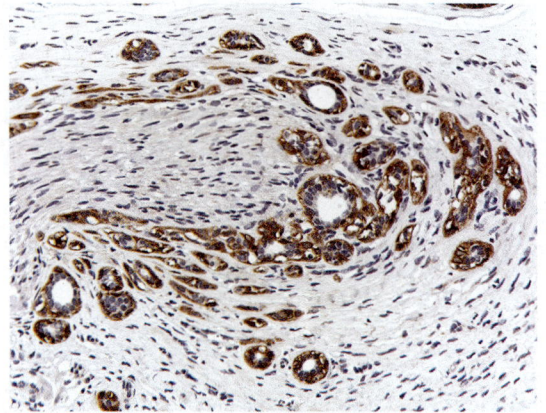

Figure 12-35 A stain for calponin highlights the myoepithelial cells in the benign glands within this nerve.

Careful study usually allows one to identify both types of cells, and immunohistochemical staining for markers of myoepithelial cells confirms the impression based on the hematoxylin and eosin–stained sections (Fig. 12-35).

Selected Readings

Davies JD: Neural invasion in benign mammary dysplasia. J Pathol 1973;109:225-231.

Fechner RE: Lobular carcinoma *in situ* in sclerosing adenosis: A potential source of confusion with invasive carcinoma. Am J Surg Pathol 1981;5:233-239.

Jensen RA, Page DL, Dupont WD, et al: Invasive breast cancer risk in women with sclerosing adenosis. Cancer 1989;64:1977-1983.

Lee KC, Chan JK, Gwi E: Tubular adenosis of the breast: A distinctive benign lesion mimicking invasive carcinoma. Am J Surg Pathol 1996;20:46-54.

Nielsen BB: Adenosis tumour of the breast—a clinicopathological investigation of 27 cases. Histopathology 1987;11:1259-1275.

Oberman HA, Markey BA: Non-invasive carcinoma of the breast presenting in adenosis. Mod Pathol 1991;4:31-35.

Taylor HB, Norris HJ: Epithelial invasion of nerves in benign diseases of the breast. Cancer 1967;20:2245-2249.

13

Radial Scar

DEFINITIONS AND CLINICOPATHOLOGIC CHARACTERISTICS

Radial scars look like regions of parenchymal distortion, but researchers have not determined either the etiology or the pathogenesis of this lesion. The histologic characteristics suggest that radial scars represent a reparative phenomenon occurring in response to tissue damage and loss, but this suggestion remains only hypothetical. The reported incidence of radial scars varies from 1.7% to 43%. The frequency of detection depends on the type of specimen studied, the method of detection, and the coexistence of other pathologic findings. The larger the specimens and the more intensive the examination, the greater the number of scars detected, and breasts containing fibrocystic changes harbor radial scars more frequently than breasts without these changes. Radial scars are usually multiple and often bilateral, and they sometimes cluster or follow the route of a single duct.

Radial scars of a visible size usually look like cancers to the unaided eye. They have stellate shapes and hard consistencies, and they seem to invade the surrounding parenchyma. On more than one occasion, even a seasoned pathologist has mistaken a scar for a carcinoma on the basis of the macroscopic characteristics. Partially developed scars usually form rubbery, ill-defined nodules that do not simulate cancers as closely as the well-established examples of this lesion.

The malignant potential of radial scar remains undefined. The superficial morphologic similarities between radial scars and small invasive carcinomas led certain writers to suggest that the former represent an early stage in the development of the latter. No study has provided convincing evidence to support this belief, but a few investigations suggest that the presence of a radial scar might indicate a heightened risk for the development of a carcinoma.

HISTOLOGIC CHARACTERISTICS

Shape of the Lesion

Radial scars usually exhibit a radially symmetric, stellate shape (Fig. 13-1). When observed in three dimensions, this appearance has reminded observers of the burs of the common burdock and certain varieties of sea urchin. The stellate configuration arises because of an apparent loss of tissue in the center. Fibrosis and retraction distort the peripheral tissues, drawing them toward the center and thereby creating the characteristic radiating appearance. Although most scars appear round, others have an oval or flattened configuration, and a few look lopsided or incomplete. Among the fundamental characteristics of radial scars, their shape offers the least secure diagnostic information, because most carcinomas also appear stellate. One can obtain information of a more persuasive nature by determining the process responsible for the spiculate shape of a sclerosing focus, because this configuration arises through different mechanisms in scars and carcinomas. The stellate shape of scar develops because of

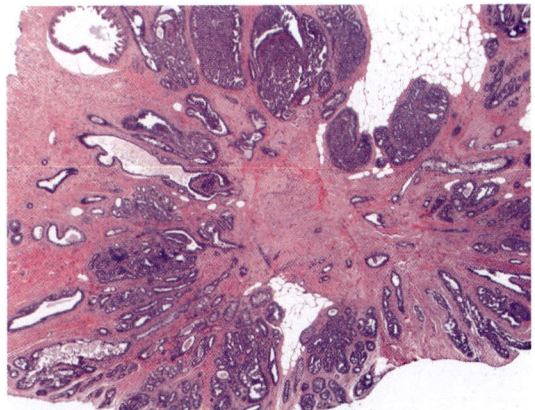

Figure 13-1 This typical radial scar has a radially symmetric, stellate configuration.

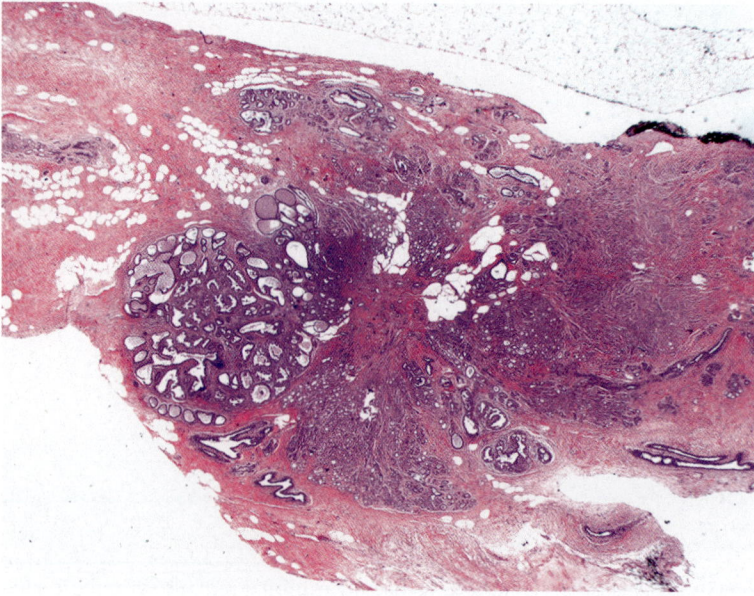

Figure 13-2 Radial scars exhibit a zonal arrangement: a rim of epithelial and glandular proliferation surrounds a central region of scarring.

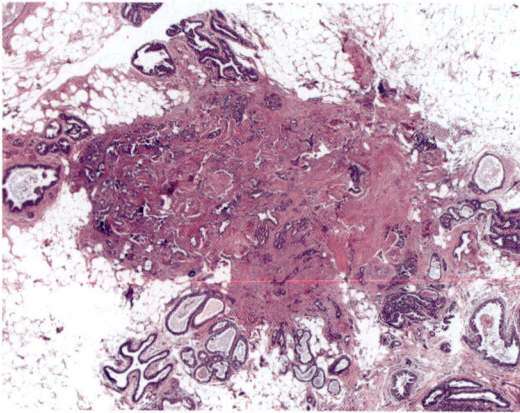

Figure 13-3 This radial scar has an unusually large nidus, which consists of stroma and entrapped glands.

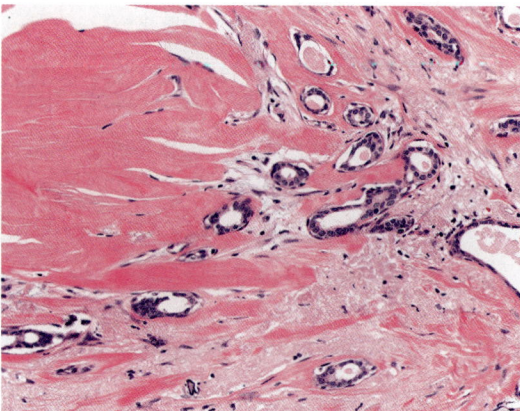

Figure 13-4 The stroma in the center of most scars consists of dense collagen and elastic tissue.

an apparent loss of tissue and puckering of the parenchyma, whereas malignant cells stream outward from a central mass in a spiculated carcinoma.

Structure of the Lesion

Fully developed scars display a characteristic zonal architecture (Fig. 13-2). One observes a central zone of scarring (the *nidus*) surrounded by a region of glandular proliferation (the *corona*). The tissue in the proliferative zone blends with the tissue beyond the lesion; consequently, the lesion appears discrete but unencapsulated. Each zone has a characteristic composition.

Nidus

The center of a fully developed scar consists of stroma and distorted epithelial elements (Fig. 13-3). Dense, eosinophilic collagen bundles, blue-gray elastic tissue, and a few spindle cells compose the stroma of typical scars (Fig. 13-4). The centers of loosely constructed scars can contain a few adipocytes (Fig. 13-5). The structure of the glandular elements varies. They usually consist of small tubules, but one can also find solid or fenestrated aggregates of polygonal cells, bundles of fusiform cells, tiny clusters of just two or three epithelial cells, and even isolated single cells. The tubular glands display irregular and inconsistent shapes (Fig. 13-6). Although they can appear round, the glands more often look flattened, hinting that they have become compressed by the fibrosis. Unlike the glands of sclerosing adenosis, those of a radial scar do not usually suggest a lobular configuration; rather, they appear

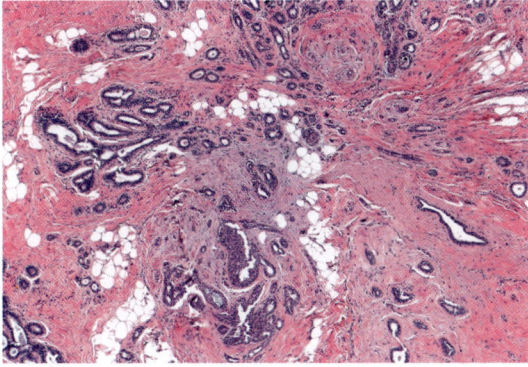

Figure 13-5 Fat occupies the center of this loosely formed scar.

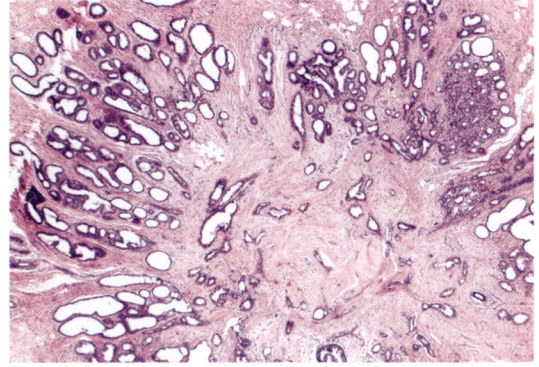

Figure 13-6 Tubular glands trapped in the nidus exhibit irregular and inconsistent shapes.

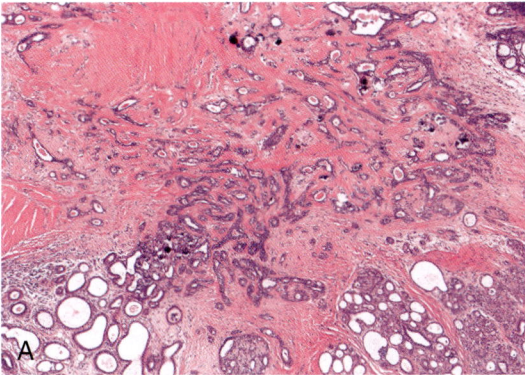

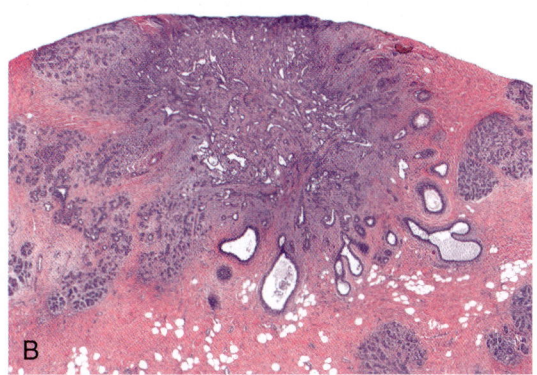

Figure 13-7 A and **B,** The glands in the nidus sometimes form an anastomosing network.

haphazardly distributed within the stroma of the nidus and they do not appear connected to one another. They may interconnect in small regions, and those in certain cases form a large complex network of interlacing channels (Fig. 13-7). The cells composing the tubules look bland, and one can discern both luminal and myoepithelial cells in most of them. The luminal cells appear of normal size and possess small nuclei, pale and granular chromatin, and small nucleoli. The appearance of the myoepithelial cells varies. Most often, they look flattened or even inconspicuous, and their small, oval, hyperchromatic nuclei run parallel to the basement membrane. Less commonly, the myoepithelial cells appear prominent and contain abundant clear cytoplasm and large pale nuclei (Fig. 13-8).

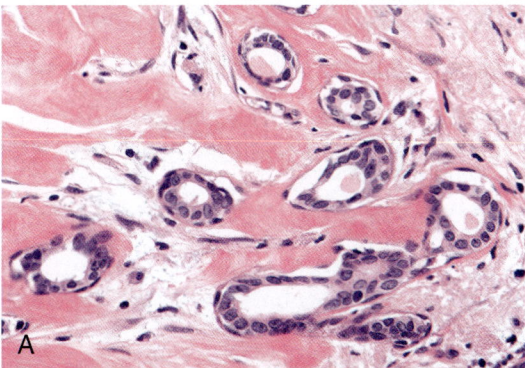

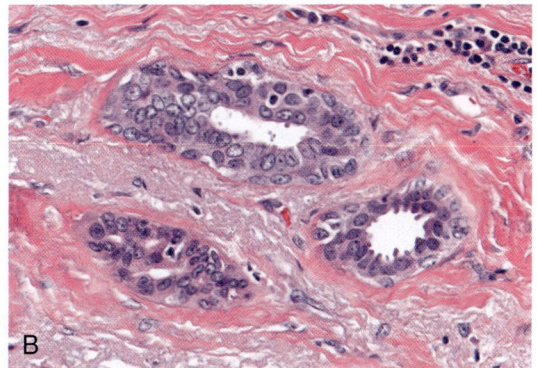

Figure 13-8 Small bland luminal cells and myoepithelial cells compose the tubules in the nidus of most radial scars. The myoepithelial cells usually look inconspicuous, as in **A,** but they occasionally appear plump and form a prominent layer, as seen in **B.**

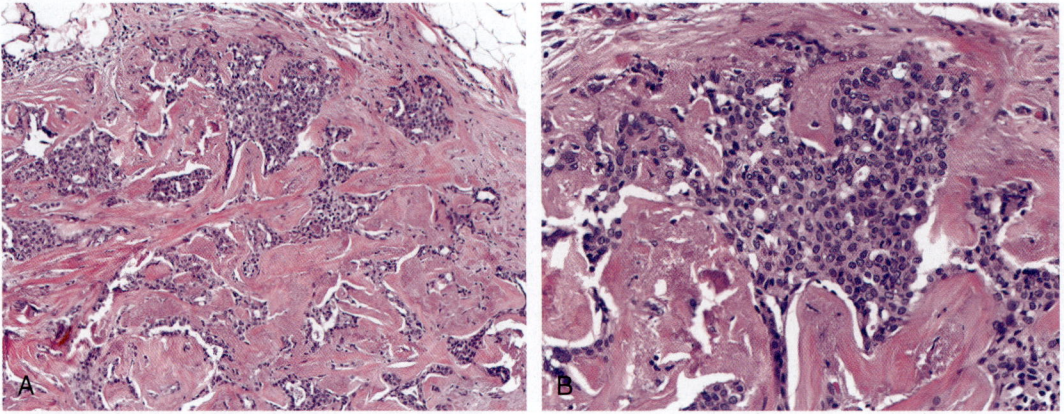

Figure 13-9 A, Irregular clusters of hyperplastic ductal cells occupy the nidus of this scar. **B,** The cells exhibit the cytologic characteristics of conventional ductal hyperplasia.

The glandular tissue in the nidus can take the form of solid or fenestrated nests of polygonal epithelial cells. Like the tubular elements, these groups vary in size and shape, and certain nests seem to penetrate between collagen bundles. The epithelial cells within the nests appear bland or exhibit the cytologic features of conventional hyperplastic ductal cells (Fig. 13-9). One can also observe small groups of fusiform cells, which often appear ill-defined and blend into the stroma (Fig. 13-10). Such cells possess eosinophilic cytoplasm and attenuated nuclei, which often stain darkly. The spindle shape of the cells, the deeply eosinophilic hue of the cytoplasm, and the hyperchromasia of the nuclei create the impression of squamous differentiation and bring to mind certain qualities of the cells in the epithelioid clumps seen in many spindle cell carcinomas. Finally, the formative stages of scars can contain clusters consisting of just a few glandular cells or even isolated single cells (Fig. 13-11).

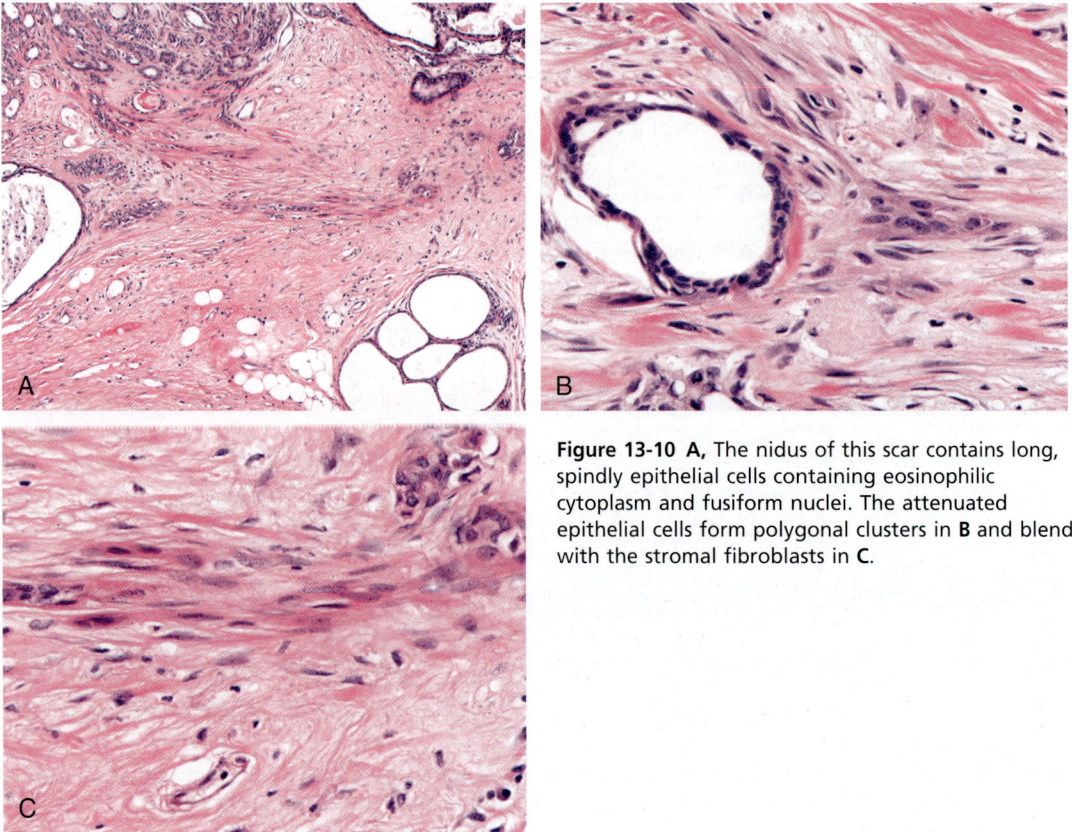

Figure 13-10 A, The nidus of this scar contains long, spindly epithelial cells containing eosinophilic cytoplasm and fusiform nuclei. The attenuated epithelial cells form polygonal clusters in **B** and blend with the stromal fibroblasts in **C.**

Of the potentially worrisome features of a typical radial scar, the disordered architecture of the central glandular tissue provokes the most confusion and anxiety for inexperienced pathologists. To understand the differences between this center of a scar and an invasive carcinoma, diagnosticians might find it worthwhile to contrast the causes of the glandular distortion in scars and carcinomas. The literature does not offer a cogent explanation for the disruption of expected, orderly arrangement of the glandular tissue in the center of radial scars, but daily experience demonstrates that the disturbance in the glandular architecture goes hand-in-hand with alterations in the structure and composition of the stroma. In fact,

one does not observe the former in the absence of the latter; furthermore, the distorted glands always sit within altered stroma. This observation establishes a spatial link between the distortion of the glandular tissue and the stromal fibrosis, and one could reasonably propose a cause-and-effect relationship between the two processes, also. The stromal fibrosis might disrupt the structure of preexisting ducts and lobules and thereby create the worrisome glandular pattern, for instance. The two phenomena need not have a causal relationship, of course; they could represent independent reactions to tissue damage. Whatever the relationship between the two phenomena, it seems clear that they consistently accompany each

Figure 13-11 A and B, Rare scars contain small clusters of cells or single epithelial cells devoid of myoepithelial cells and seemingly free in the stroma.

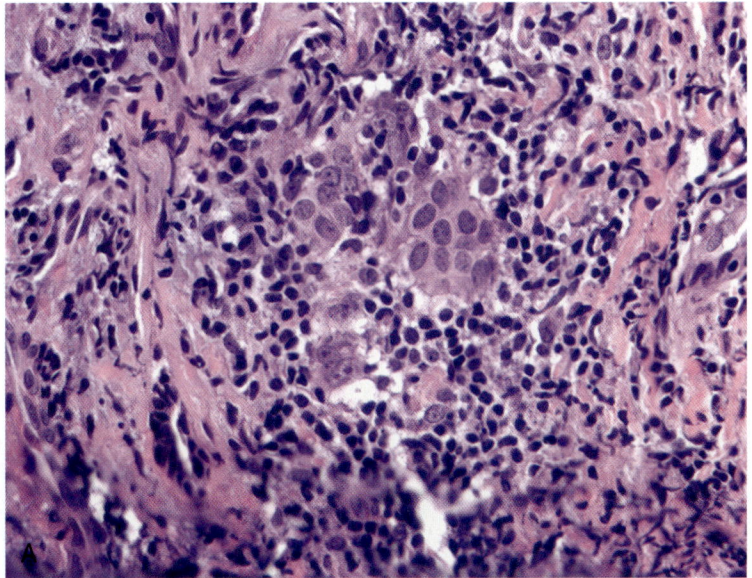

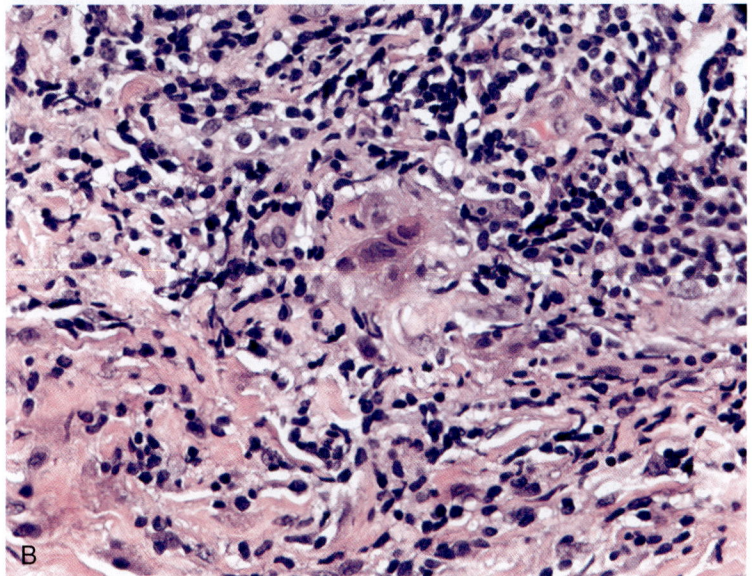

other in radial scars. The distortion of the glandular architecture does not take place in the absence of stromal alteration, and the distorted glands do not stray beyond the region of altered stroma.

The linkage of glandular distortion to stromal fibrosis does not hold in invasive carcinomas. The disarray in the structure of the glands of a carcinoma and the disorder in their disposition reflect the disorganization inherent in a malignant proliferation, not a secondary effect of a sclerosing process. Invasive carcinomas do evoke a stromal reaction in most cases; however, the periphery of the carcinoma often demonstrates irregular neoplastic clusters penetrating tissue that shows little or no stromal reaction. This uncoupling of the phenomena of glandular distortion and stromal alteration would not fit with a diagnosis of a radial scar.

Corona

The outer zone of altered glandular tissue consists of radially arranged, triangular clusters of ducts and terminal duct–lobular units, each cluster tethered at its apex to the scarred center (Fig. 13-12). The ducts and lobules within this zone exhibit benign alterations. The nature of these benign changes varies from case

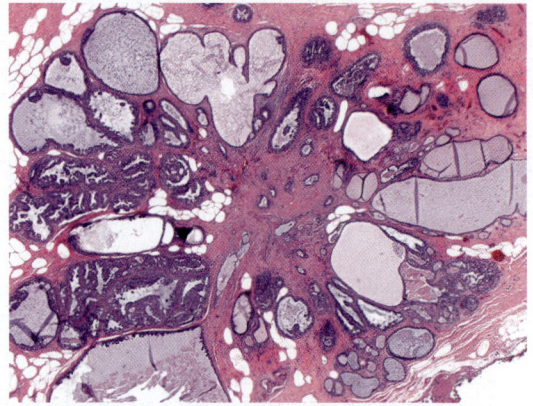

Figure 13-12 The corona of a radial scar consists of triangular aggregates of glandular tissue, each tethered at its apex to the nidus.

to case, but they can include fibrocystic changes, sclerosing adenosis, adenosis, blunt duct adenosis, collagenous spherulosis, and papilloma formation (Fig. 13-13). The variability in the nature and the extent of benign changes accounts for much of the variation in the appearances of radial scars and

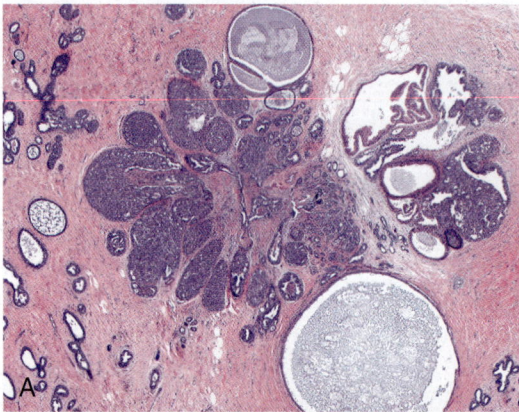

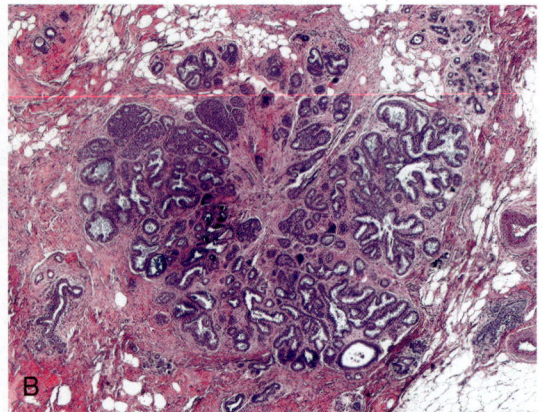

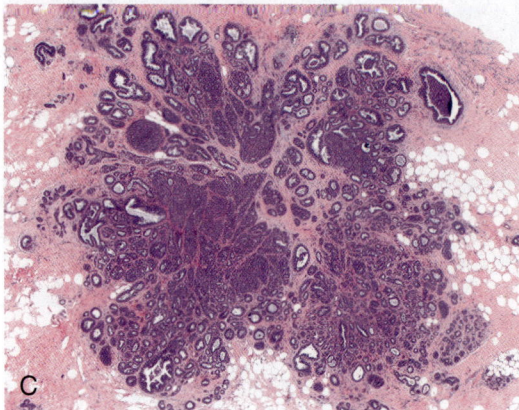

Figure 13-13 The glandular tissue of the corona usually exhibits proliferative changes such as conventional ductal hyperplasia in **A**, blunt duct adenosis in **B**, or florid adenosis in **C**.

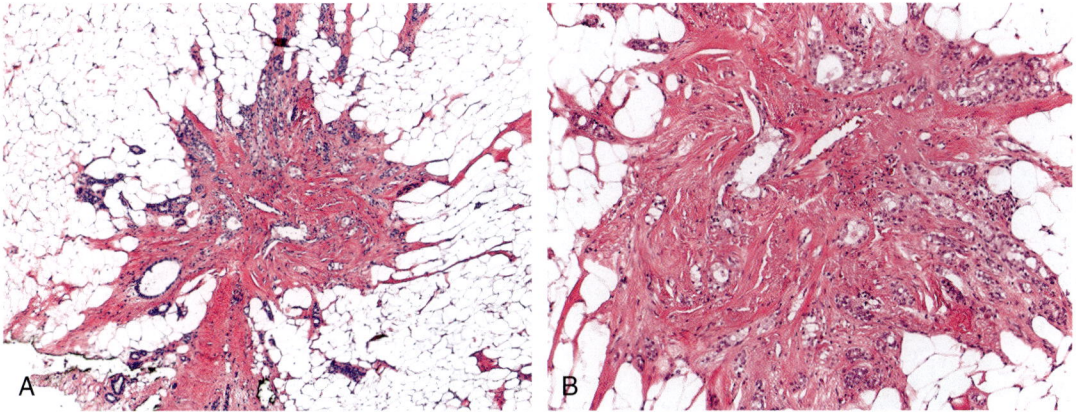

Figure 13-14 A, The corona of this radial scar has disappeared almost entirely. **B,** The proliferative region consists of a few radially oriented collections of acini.

the numerous diagnostic terms proposed for the lesion. The proliferative changes of the corona may represent a reaction of the mammary parenchyma to the loss of tissue in the nidus. The proliferation tends to appear more marked near the center and less florid in the periphery of the corona. The proliferative changes seem to abate with time; consequently, the size of the proliferative zone varies. The proliferative zone of most scars measures more than the nidus, but in ancient scars, the proliferative zone can vanish (Fig. 13-14).

Characteristics of the Peripheral Epithelial Elements

The corona of proliferative changes completely envelops the nidus in most scars and thereby separates the center of the lesion from the uninvolved tissue outside the scar. Because of this structure, the problematic, irregular epithelial aggregates remain confined to the altered stroma of the nidus; they do not extend to the periphery of the lesion (Fig. 13-15). This absence of suspicious glands and epithelial clusters

Figure 13-15 The corona completely envelops the nidus and separates the irregular glands from the surrounding uninvolved parenchyma.

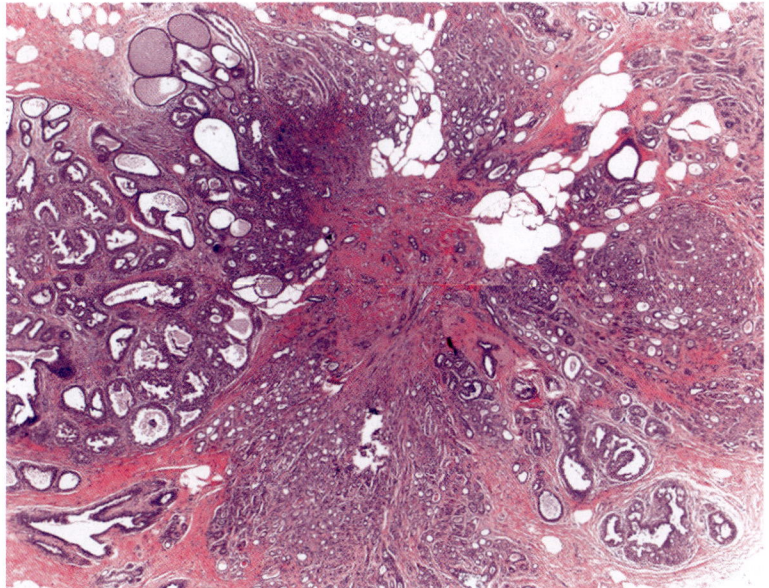

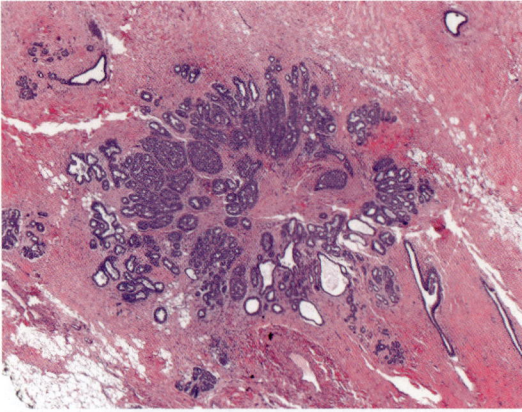

Figure 13-16 Although radial scars appear discrete, they do not have a capsule nor do they compress the parenchyma around them.

at the periphery of the mass represents the most helpful single feature to distinguish a radial scar from an invasive carcinoma.

Although radial scars appear discrete, they do not have a clearly defined boundary demarcating them from the surrounding tissue, nor do they compress the adjacent parenchyma (Fig. 13-16). Instead, the tissue of the corona merges uninterruptedly with the unaltered tissue beyond the borders of the lesion. The stroma of the corona flows into the surrounding parenchyma without a disturbance in the arrangement of its components, and the glands display a tapering in their proliferative qualities (Fig. 13-17). Because of this fading of proliferative glandular changes, the continuity of the stromal architecture, and the absence of compression of neighboring

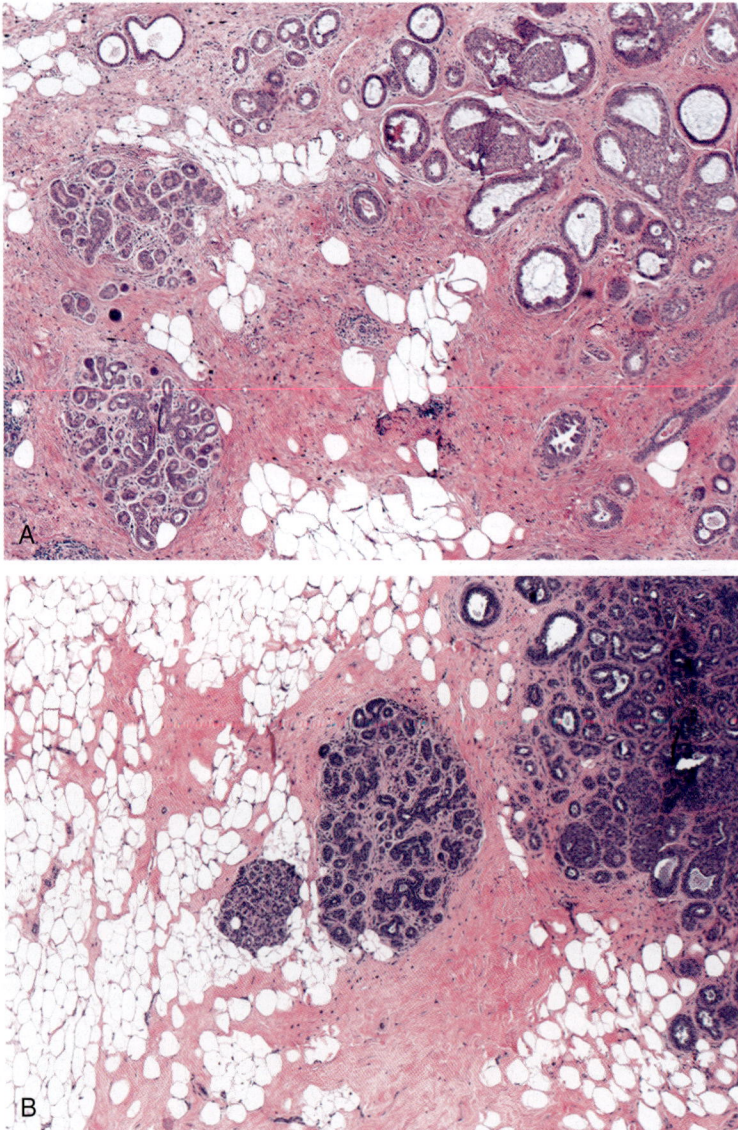

Figure 13-17 The corona merges with the tissue outside the scar without forming a distinct boundary. The cellularity of the stroma in **A** and the proliferative qualities of the epithelium in **B** in the corona fade away gradually.

structures, scars do not look like space-occupying lesions. Instead, these features, coupled with the radial orientation of the glands of the corona, create the impression of a region of tissue loss with secondary glandular proliferation and stromal scarring.

Characteristics of the Associated Ductal Epithelial Proliferation

Many radial scars contain foci of conventional ductal hyperplasia in their proliferative zones (Fig. 13-18). The presence of ductal hyperplasia provides suggestive but indirect evidence that a sclerosing lesion represents a radial scar rather than an invasive carcinoma; however, one cannot extend this line of reasoning very far. The absence of ductal hyperplasia does not exclude the diagnosis of radial scar, for example.

The corona of radial scars can display some of the most exuberant ductal hyperplasia that a pathologist will ever encounter (Fig. 13-19). These foci of intense proliferation include massive numbers of epithelial cells. The peripheral cells, those near the basement membrane, can appear large and immature, whereas the cells near the center of the duct sometimes become so small and flat that they flake off into the lumen and degenerate (Fig. 13-20). One sometimes observes genuine coagulative necrosis of the innermost cells; in this circumstance, the lumen contains proteinaceous debris and nuclear dust (Fig. 13-21). The presence of these uncharacteristic findings could lead one to misconstrue such examples of florid hyperplasia as ductal carcinoma in situ. To avoid this mistake, pathologists should study the cytologic attributes of the proliferative cells. Even in the presence of necrosis, hyperplastic ductal cells will display the typical cytologic features of usual ductal hyperplasia (Fig. 13-22), and one can rely on the cytologic findings to identify these proliferative foci as benign. Later sections will discuss the problems related to the recognition of atypical hyperplasia and carcinoma in the setting of a radial scar.

Figure 13-18 The ducts in the corona of this scar display florid conventional ductal hyperplasia.

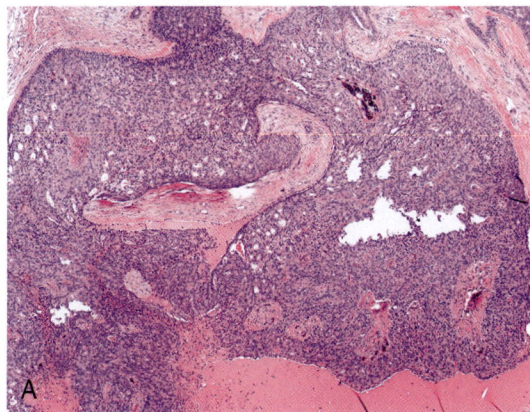

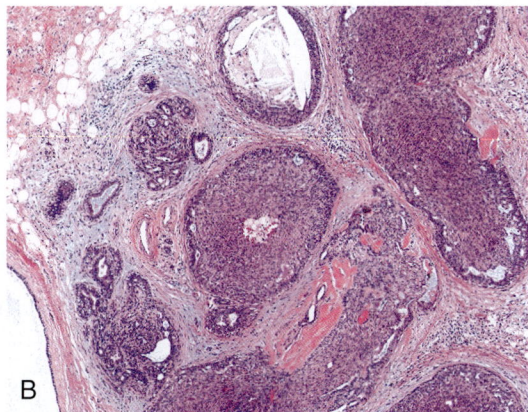

Summary

Radial scars seem to represent regions of tissue loss with reactive glandular changes. The lesion usually forms a distinct mass with a round shape and exhibits a radially symmetric internal architecture and a zonal structure. The nidus consists of altered stroma and entrapped glands, and a corona of proliferative glandular changes completely encloses it. At the periphery of the lesion, the stromal and glandular components of the corona blend with those of the uninvolved external parenchyma; never do the distorted glands of the nidus penetrate into unaltered tissue. Conventional ductal hyperplasia occupies the ducts associated with many radial scars (Box 13-1).

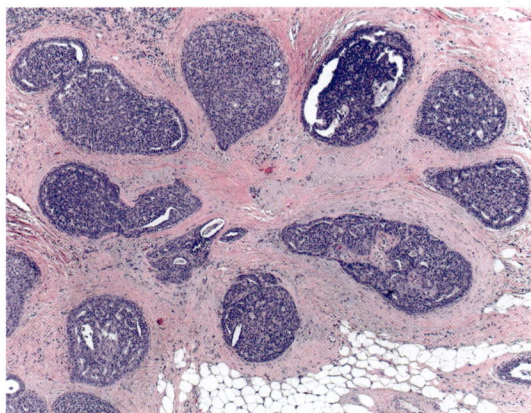

Figure 13-19 A and **B,** These two radial scars can harbor especially florid ductal hyperplasia.

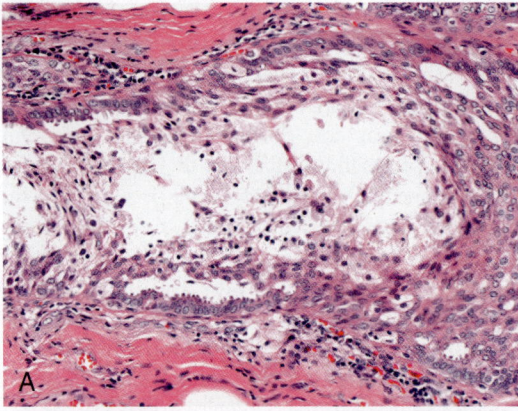

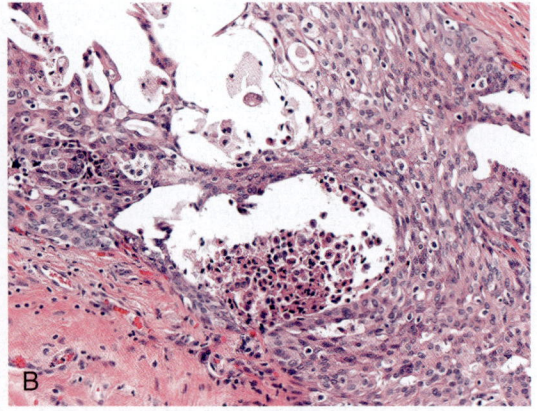

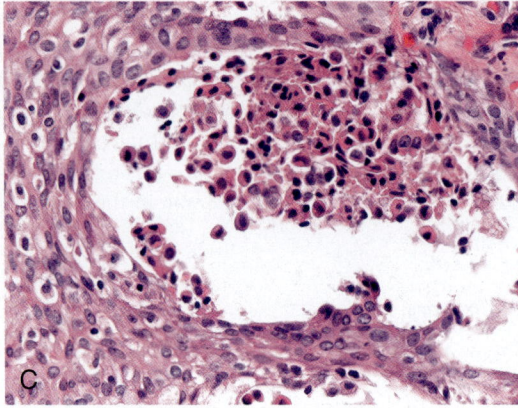

Figure 13-20 A and **B**, In regions of intense proliferation, the hyperplastic cells can flatten, separate from their neighbors, and fall into the lumen, as in **C**.

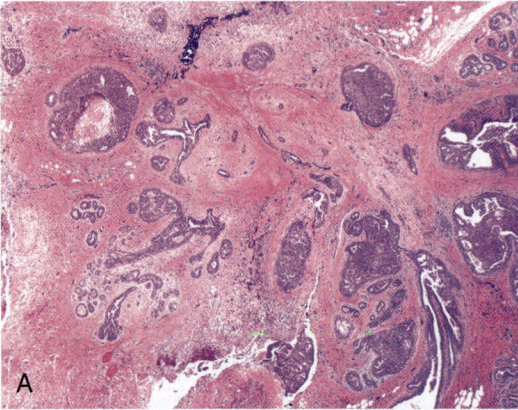

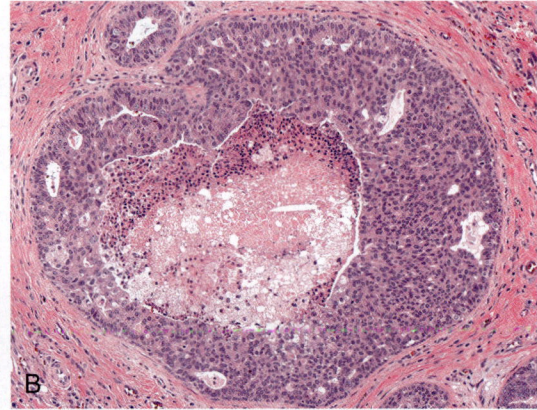

Figure 13-21 A and **B,** The hyperplastic cells in a radial scar can show genuine coagulative necrosis.

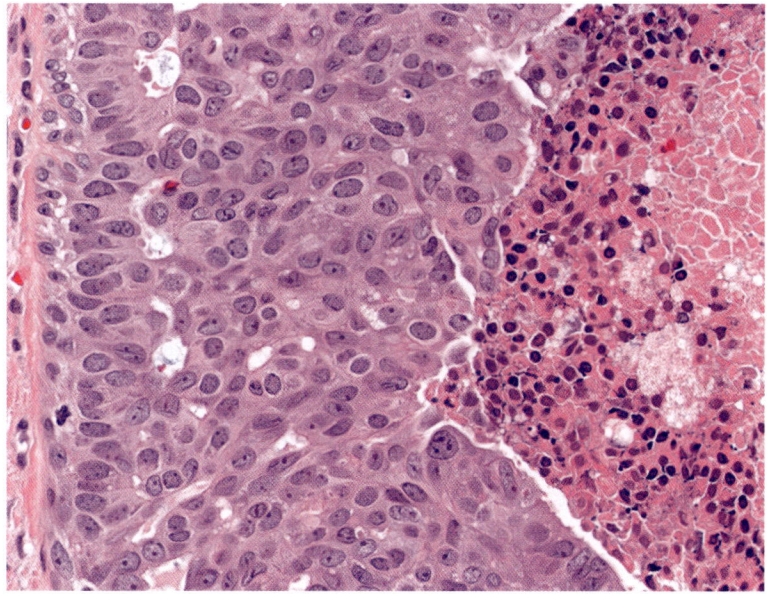

Figure 13-22 Despite the presence of cellular dishesion and necrosis, the proliferative cells exhibit the cytologic characteristics of hyperplastic ductal cells.

Box 13-1

Histologic characteristics of radial scars:

- Stellate shape
- Zonal structure
- Confinement of the irregular glands to regions of altered stroma
- An orderly relationship between the peripheral glands and the stroma

---

PROBLEMS IN THE DIAGNOSIS OF RADIAL SCARS

Typical radial scars do not cause diagnostic problems for experienced pathologists, but less characteristic examples provoke diagnostic uncertainty in several ways. First, scars regularly exhibit features that alarm pathologists when encountered in other settings. The presence of necrosis of the epithelial cells, for instance, would make one favor a diagnosis of carcinoma if observed in a proliferation of ductal cells within a terminal duct–lobular unit, and the proliferative ductal cells in the corona of scars can have modest cytologic atypia. Second, certain scars do not display the characteristic features. Such examples may not appear round or symmetric, or their centers may contain cellular, desmoplastic stroma rather than collagen and elastic tissue. Third, the dense collagen and elastic tissue of the nidus and the tubules trapped within them can radiate into the parenchyma rather than forming a compact mass in the center of the scar. Failure to recognize these lesions as variants of radial scars hobbles the pathologist's analysis of the foci and thereby sets the stage for an erroneous diagnosis. Fourth, carcinomas do take up residence in scars on rare occasions. Pathologists can find it difficult to differentiate carcinomas in situ from the reactive hyperplasia so commonly seen in scars; furthermore, the extension of a carcinoma in situ into the distorted glands of the nidus can produce a picture that closely resembles the appearance of an invasive carcinoma. The following sections address these and several other problems.

Scars with Epithelial Necrosis

The florid ductal hyperplasia occupying the corona of a radial scar sometimes exhibits necrosis. It can take the form of just a few degenerating cells sloughed from the surface of the proliferative epithelium or of large collections of amorphous protein and cellular debris. Necrosis of an epithelial proliferation usually signals the presence of a malignancy except in certain well-defined settings, one of which is a radial scar. Pathologists must not allow the presence of necrotic debris to dissuade them from the diagnosis of radial scar when the other features of a lesion point to that diagnosis. The cytologic and architectural characteristics of the proliferative cells establish the nature of the population. If the cells exhibit characteristics of hyperplastic ductal cells, one can safely overlook the presence of even abundant necrotic debris.

Minimal Cytologic Atypia in Scars

The proliferative ductal cells that occupy the corona of a radial scar can have minor levels of cytologic atypicality. In the most common examples, the cells display clearly defined cell membranes and appear somewhat evenly disposed. Their nuclei can have smoother contours, more finely dispersed chromatin, and smaller nucleoli than those of conventional hyperplastic cells (Fig. 13-23). Although these findings deviate from the usual characteristics of ductal hyperplasia, the cellular aberrations probably do not indicate that the population has a neoplastic nature. Careful inspection reveals focal clustering of nuclei, subtle variation in nuclear shape, irregularities in the nuclear contours, and variability in the staining and texture of the chromatin, features more in keeping with a hyperplastic proliferation than a neoplastic one. The cells can form a few spaces that suggest a cribriform architecture, but the cells creating the spaces do not display convincing cellular polarization (Fig. 13-24). A minority of examples displays the phenomenon of maturation (Fig. 13-25).

Researchers have not determined the clinical course of patients with radial scars showing these mildly atypical changes, so one cannot make secure statements about their clinical significance. Nevertheless, two observations influence the author's thinking about this topic. First, the literature does not contain convincing evidence of a pathogenetic relationship between radial scars and carcinomas, nor does daily practice suggest that such a relationship exists. Second, one finds minor levels of atypia in many scars. In light of these observations, one could regard this atypia as a reactive phenomenon reflecting the intense proliferation rather than a neoplastic process. It would seem safe to disregard such foci if they meet the following conditions:

1. The atypia appears low grade. Reactive cells create the impression of atypia by virtue of the modest enlargement and uniformity of their nuclei.

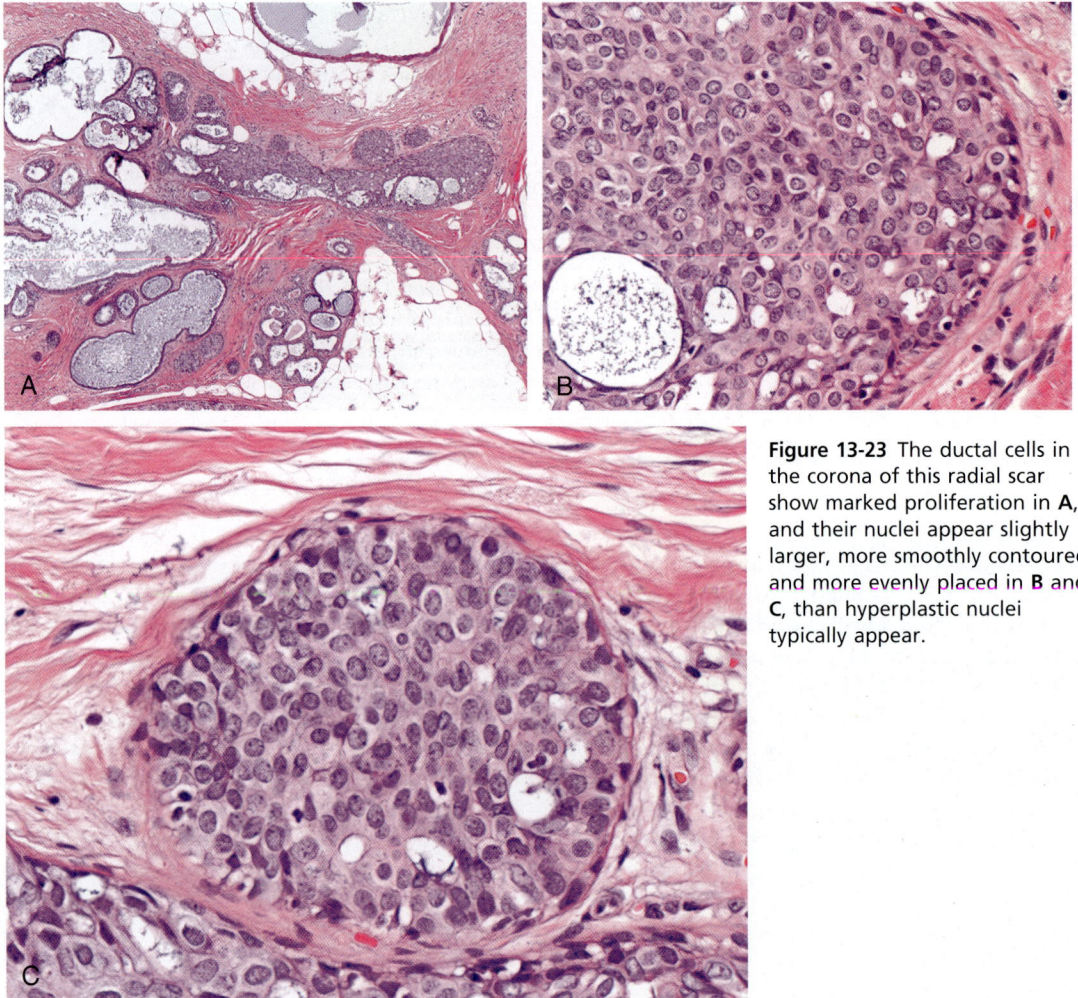

Figure 13-23 The ductal cells in the corona of this radial scar show marked proliferation in **A**, and their nuclei appear slightly larger, more smoothly contoured, and more evenly placed in **B** and **C**, than hyperplastic nuclei typically appear.

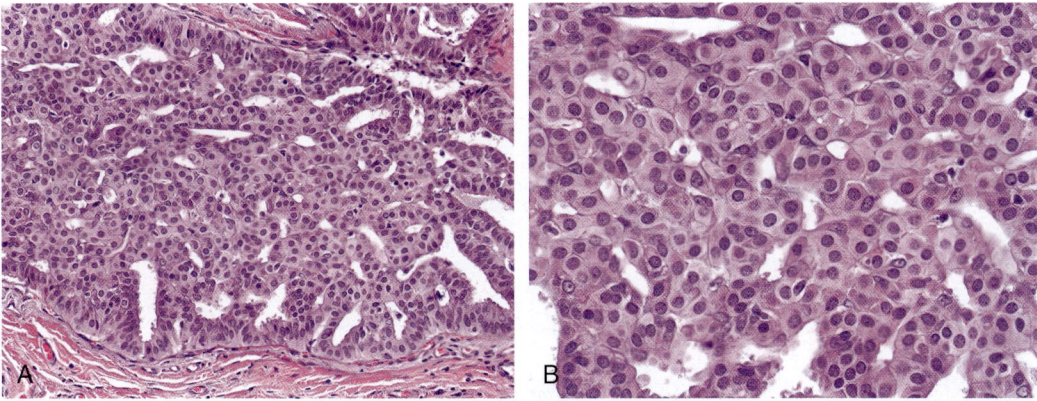

Figure 13-24 A, These ductal cells proliferate in a fenestrate sheet. **B,** They appear somewhat uniform in their morphologic characteristics; they possess pale cytoplasm and distinct cell borders, and they form a few vaguely cribriform spaces. **C,** Despite these unexpected findings, the cells exhibit the clustering of the nuclei, subtle variation in nuclear shape, irregularities in nuclear contours, and variability in the staining and texture of the chromatin that typify hyperplastic cells. They do not show clear-cut polarization.

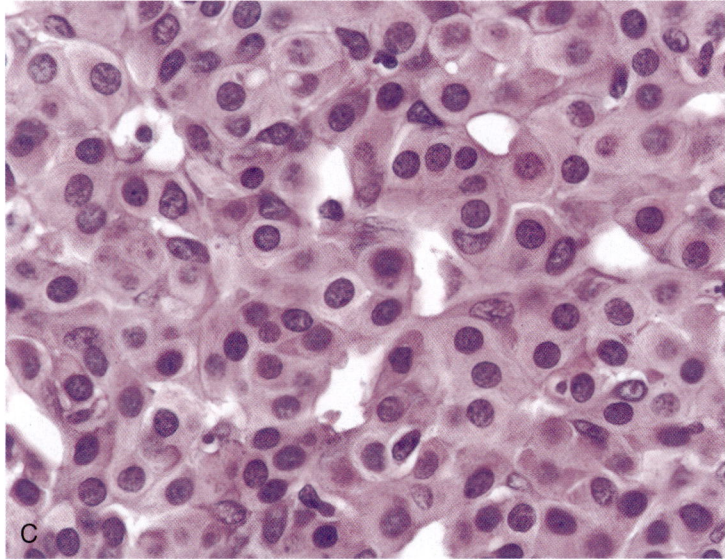

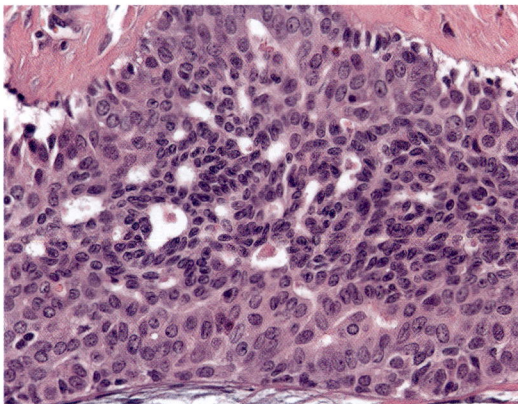

Figure 13-25 The ductal proliferation demonstrates the pattern of maturation: the peripheral cells appear larger than the central ones, and the former possess larger nuclei, paler chromatin, larger nucleoli, and more cytoplasm than the latter.

The presence of marked nuclear enlargement and obvious nuclear pleomorphism would favor the notion of a neoplastic proliferation rather than a reactive one.

2. The atypical cells display polygonal shapes and grow in several layers. If the atypical cells have columnar shapes and grow as a single layer, one must inspect them carefully, because the reactive cells in scars do not usually grow in this pattern. If such foci have the appropriate features, one should make the diagnosis of flat epithelial atypia (Fig. 13-26).

3. The atypical cells form a continuum with others that do not look atypical. Most scars harboring minimally atypical cells also contain conventional ductal hyperplasia, and the two populations typically merge.

4. The atypical cells do not display clear-cut architectural atypia (Fig. 13-27). The formation

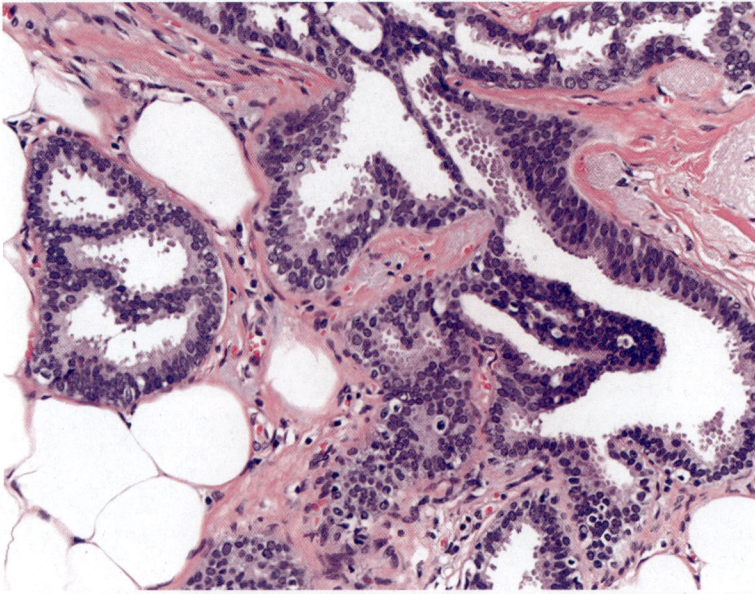

Figure 13-26 The corona of this radial scar harbors a population of columnar ductal cells growing in a single layer and displaying low-grade cytologic atypia. This proliferation merits the diagnosis of flat epithelial atypia.

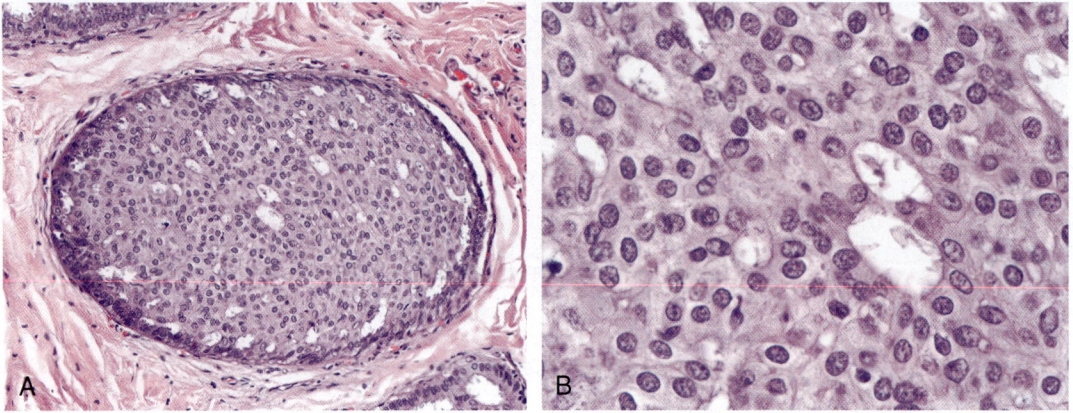

Figure 13-27 A and **B,** Although certain spaces formed by these ductal cells resemble cribriform spaces, the cells surrounding the spaces do not display clear-cut cellular polarization.

of obvious cribriform spaces, trabecular bars, or Roman bridges by atypical cells would signal the presence of a neoplastic proliferation (see Fig. 13-27).

5. The atypical cells do not extend beyond the proliferative corona of the scar. If one believes that the cellular atypia represents a reactive phenomenon, it stands to reason that the cells displaying these atypical changes should occupy only those glands within the corona of the scar. Extension of the atypical cells into ducts and lobules distant from the scar would not fit with the concept of a reactive process. Box 13-2 lists these criteria.

When examining specimens obtained by means of a core biopsy, one must adopt a more circumspect approach to the interpretation of these atypical cells, because the limited and fragmentary nature of the specimen precludes determining the location and extent of the atypical population. Because one cannot verify that the atypical cells occupy only the proliferative zone of the scar, one should probably classify

---

Box 13-2

Features of reactive atypia in radial scars:

- Cells of polygonal shape
- Merging of the atypical cells with hyperplastic cells
- Lack of architectural atypia
- Confinement to the proliferative zone

Figure 13-28 This core biopsy specimen of a radial scar in **A** contains a proliferation of ductal cells that appear atypical in **B**. Because one cannot verify that they remain confined to the corona, one should probably classify the population as atypical ductal hyperplasia.

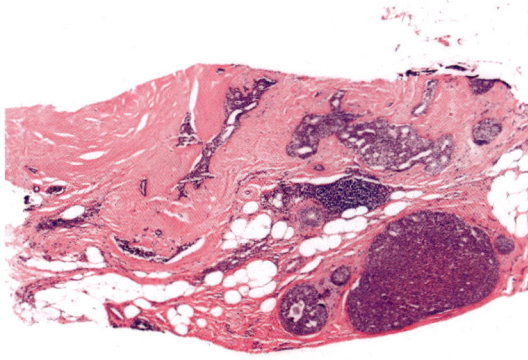

A

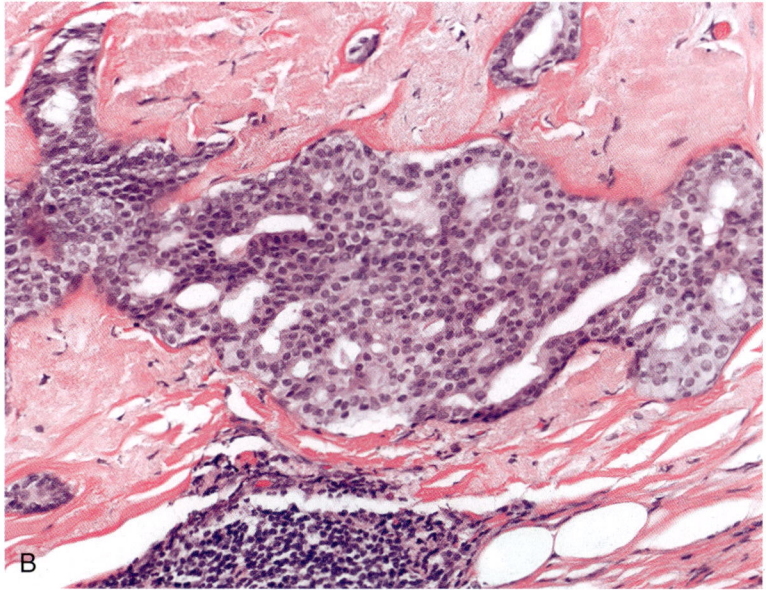

B

such proliferations as atypical (Fig. 13-28). Excision of the entire lesion allows one to base the diagnosis on a full evaluation of the cellular properties and the anatomic distribution of the population.

Misshapen Scars

Although most scars have a round and generally symmetric configuration, other, less common scars do not. Certain examples appear flattened and elongated, dumbbell shaped, or incomplete (Fig. 13-29). The formation of these irregular and unexpected shapes and the lack of symmetry by themselves do not commonly confuse the pathologist; however, the zonal architecture of these misshapen scars also looks disturbed, and this deviation from the classic structure creates problems. The nidus of entrapped glands, collagen, and elastic tissue in these malformed scars does not have the compact structure, the round shape, and the central location characteristic of classic examples. Instead, it forms linear bands tracking

along ducts and lobules and extending into the surrounding parenchyma (Fig. 13-30). Like the typical, centrally located nidus, these bands contain distorted glands, and the extension of these irregular epithelial elements around preexisting ducts and lobules and to the outer regions of the mass produces an appearance that superficially resembles that of invasive carcinoma (Fig. 13-31).

One can distinguish a scar with radiating central bands from an invasive carcinoma by paying attention to both the composition of the stroma surrounding the suspicious glands and the relationship between the glands and the altered stroma. The stroma in the radiating bands of a misshapen scar consists of tissue identical to that of the nidus, most commonly sparsely cellular, dense collagen and elastic tissue. These properties contrast with those of the stroma of invasive carcinomas, which often consists of desmoplastic connective tissue containing numerous fibroblasts and myxoid ground substances. Although this feature provides a certain

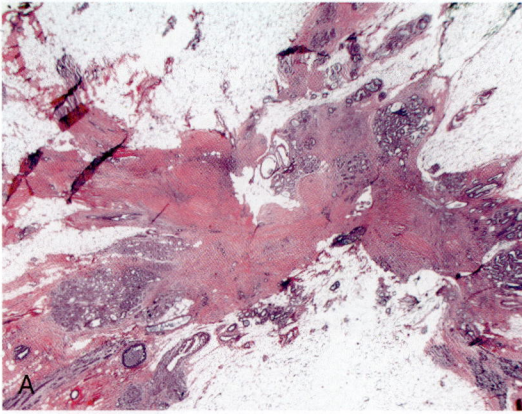

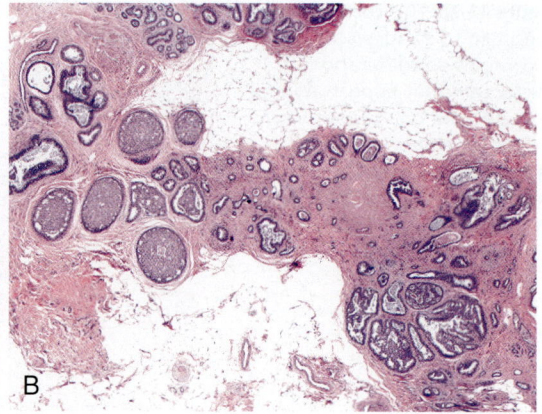

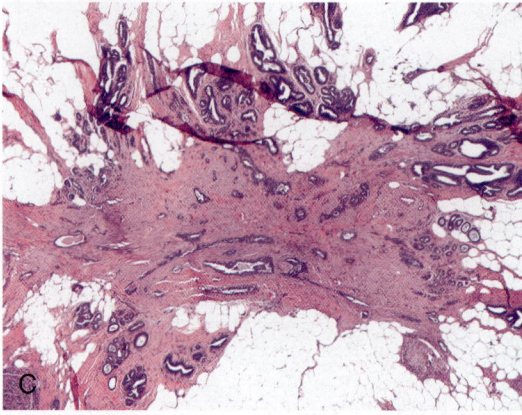

Figure 13-29 A to C, These three radial scars appear long, flat, and asymmetric rather than compact, round, and symmetric.

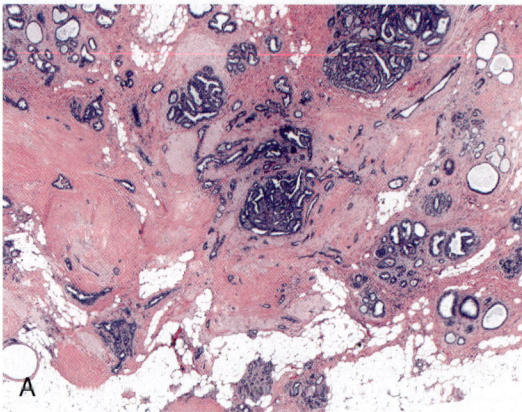

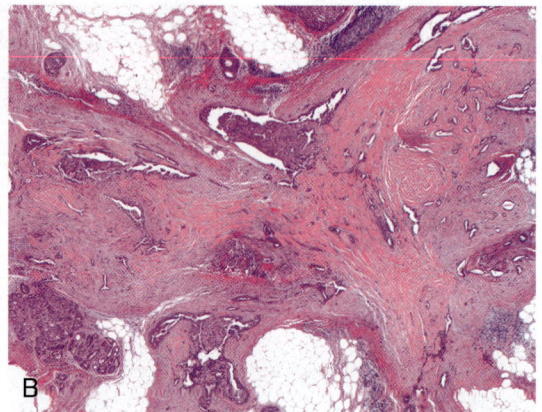

Figure 13-30 A and B, The collagen and elastic tissue of the nidus form bands that track along ducts and between lobules in these two misshapen radial scars.

amount of diagnostic guidance, it does not serve in every instance. Certain invasive carcinomas have dense collagenous and elastotic stroma not greatly different from the stroma of scars, and early stages in the formation of scars typically possess desmoplastic stroma similar to that seen in many carcinomas. Because of this overlap in the stromal characteristics of scars and carcinomas, one must also study the relationship between the distorted glands and the stroma. In conventional scars, the distorted glands always remain confined to regions of stromal alteration, and this generalization applies equally well to misshapen scars; never do the glands penetrate into unaltered tissue or invade otherwise undisturbed preexisting structures (Fig. 13-32). Carcinomas, on the other hand, invade normal tissue, and one can nearly always detect this process at the edge of the lesion.

Figure 13-31 The tracking of the components of the nidus around preexisting glandular structures and to the periphery of the radial scar in **A** and **B** creates a structure that mimics that of the invasive ductal carcinoma in **C**.

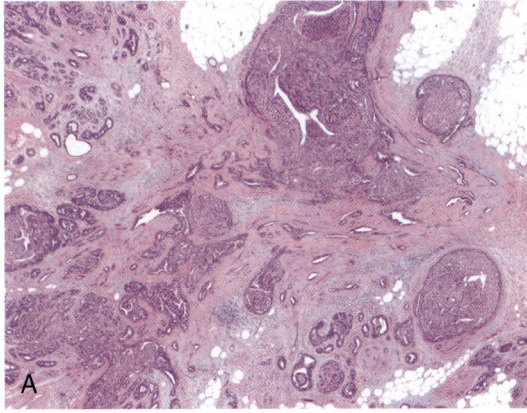

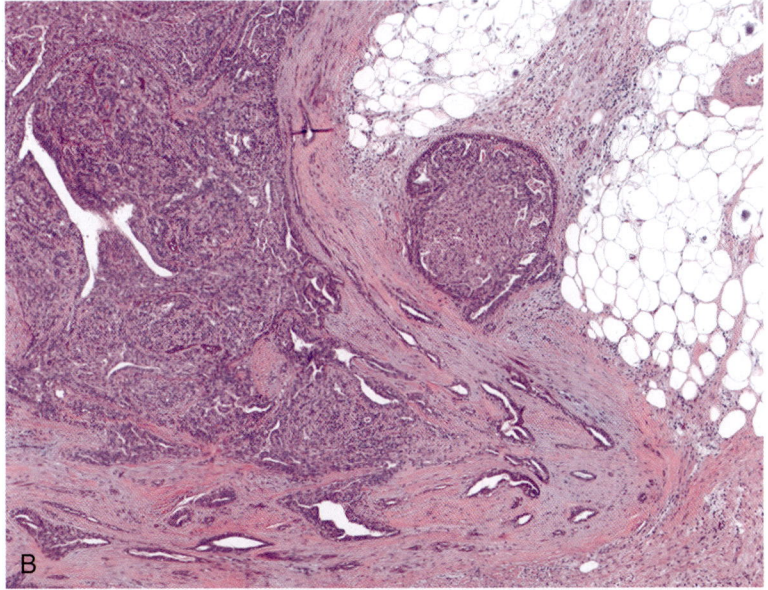

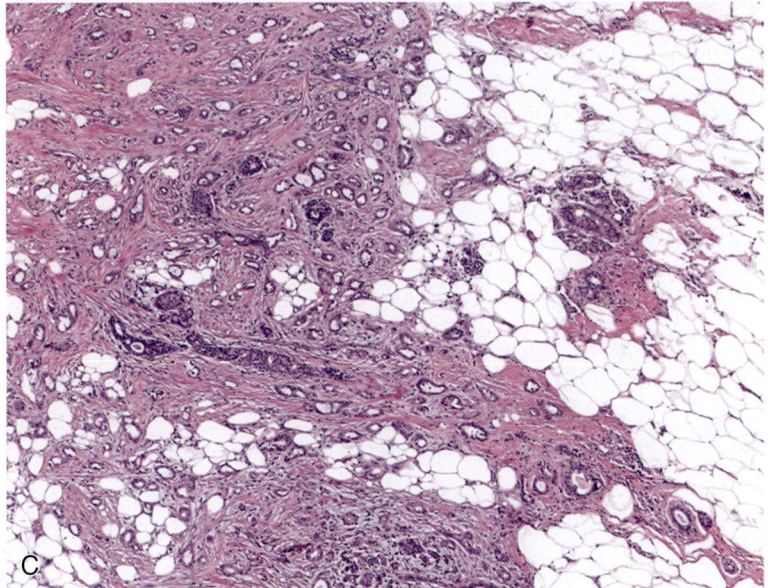

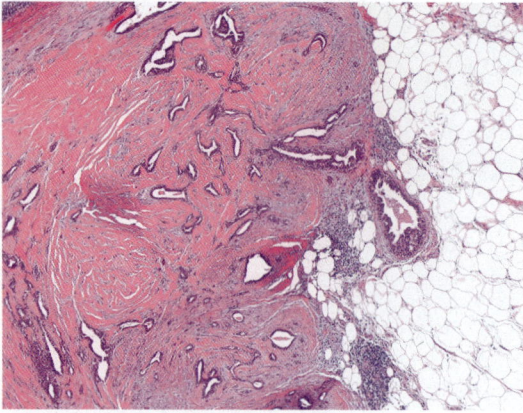

Figure 13-32 The irregular glands of a misshapen scar do not invade the fat.

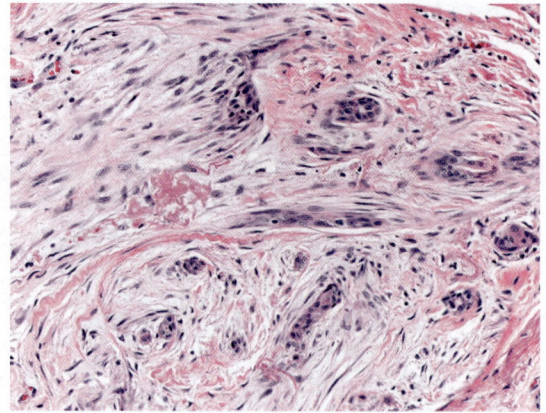

Figure 13-33 The stroma of this early radial scar consists of many fibroblasts and abundant myxoid ground substances.

Early Scars

Most discussions of radial scars focus on examples exhibiting the usual constellation of features, but everyday experience shows that scars vary in many of their histologic attributes. The lesion seems to pass through stages, and classic examples probably represent fully developed and mature lesions in the middle of this evolutionary process. The literature contains only the scantiest descriptions of the early stages in the formation of radial scars. Experience shows that these immature scars differ in several ways from their classic counterparts, and certain of these variant features would rightfully alarm pathologists if encountered in other settings. Failure to recognize the early lesions as a type of radial scar could therefore provoke an unwarranted diagnosis of ductal atypia or carcinoma.

Early scars differ from classic ones in several respects. First, the center of early radial scars includes a stroma rich in fibroblasts and myxoid ground substances (Fig. 13-33). These elements may compose the entirety of the stroma in the nidus (Fig. 13-34), or they may mix with the types of dense collagen and elastic tissue that characterize the stroma of mature scars (Fig. 13-35). Thus, the proportion of myxoid stroma in radial scars spans the entire range from exclusively myxoid to entirely collagenous and elastotic, and this blending of stromal components offers one piece of evidence that these foci represent stages in the evolution of a single entity. Second, lacking the distortion of the parenchymal architecture produced by the central scarring, early scars do not exhibit the retracted, stellate shape seen in mature scars (Fig. 13-36). These early lesions more commonly look like poorly defined, vague nodules to both the radiologist and the pathologist. Third, collections of lymphocytes and plasma cells mingle within the fibroblastic stroma and cluster at the interface between the fibrous connective tissue and the fat (Fig. 13-37).

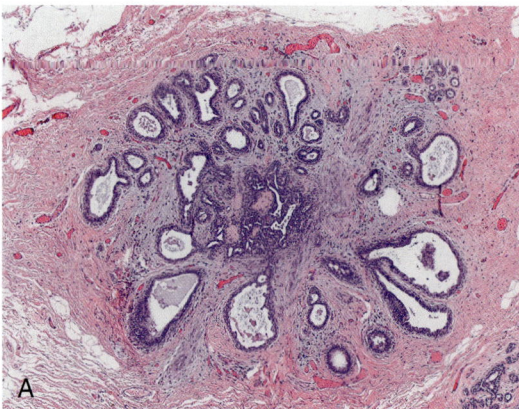

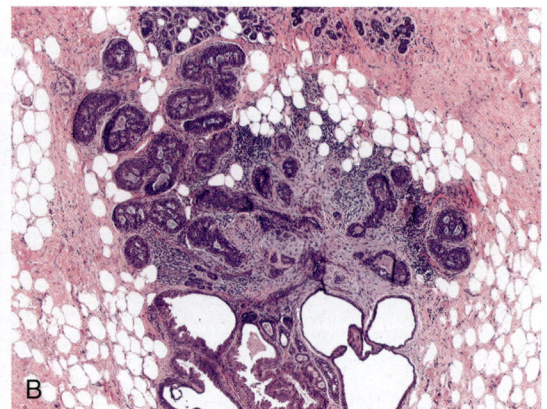

Figure 13-34 A and **B,** The stroma in the center of these two early radial scars consist entirely of fibroblasts and myxoid extracellular matrix.

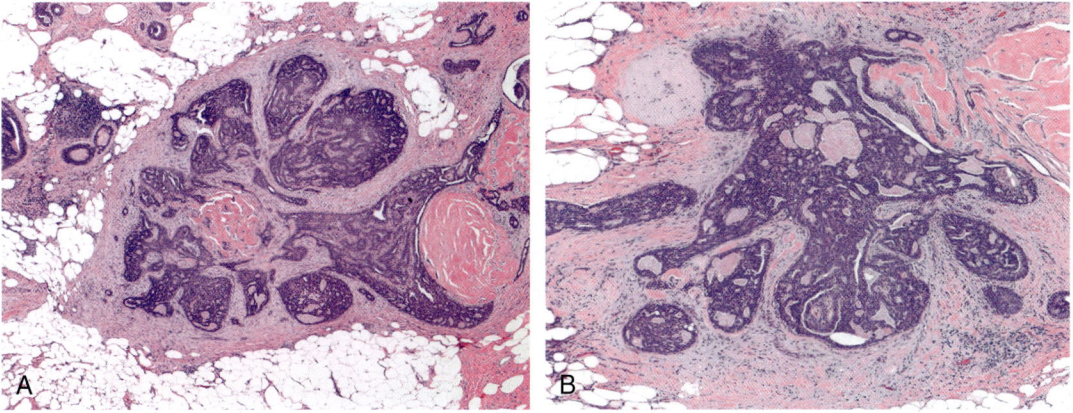

Figure 13-35 A and **B,** In both of these scars, the stroma of the nidus contains both myxoid material and dense collagen.

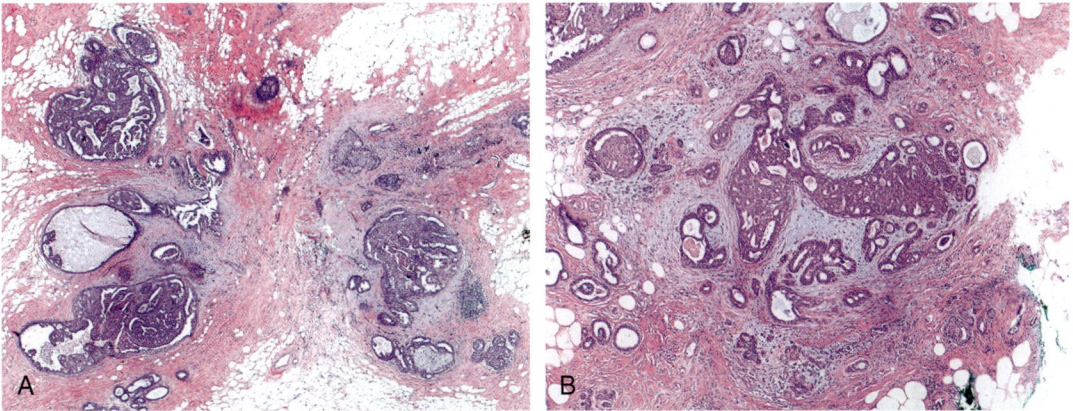

Figure 13-36 A and **B,** These two early radial scars have ill-defined, lobulated shapes rather than the retracted configuration seen in typical scars.

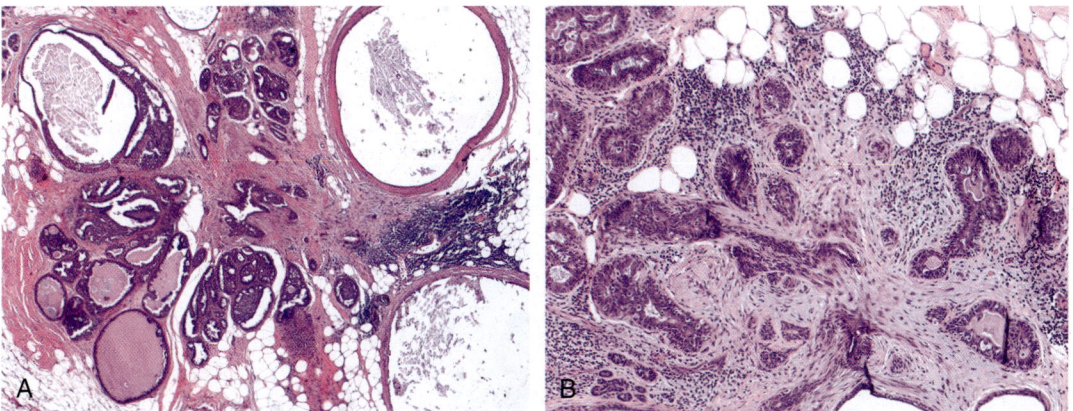

Figure 13-37 A and **B,** Lymphocytes and plasma cells cluster at the interface of the nidus and the fat in these two early radial scars.

Finally, early scars often demonstrate especially florid ductal hyperplasia. The proliferative ductal cells appear large and active; they possess large, pale nuclei and prominent nucleoli; one can sometimes find mitotic figures easily; and central, comedo-like necrosis can occur (Box 13-3).

Pathologists unfamiliar with the range of appearances seen during the evolution of radial scars can understandably fail to recognize the nature of these nodules. Furthermore, the presence of prominent epithelial proliferation, cellular enlargement, mitotic activity, and central necrosis can bring to mind diagnoses like atypical ductal hyperplasia and ductal carcinoma in situ. One can avoid this misinterpretation by paying attention to two pieces of evidence: the context of the epithelial proliferation and the cytologic characteristics of the proliferating cells. Recognizing that an underlying lesion represents a radial scar should always provoke a conservative approach to the diagnosis of a proliferation of ductal cells within it. Most often, such a proliferation represents a reactive process rather than a neoplastic one. The cytologic characteristics of the proliferative cells also offer important and persuasive diagnostic information, because the reactive hyperplastic cells within scars do not display the cytologic aberrations that one observes in neoplastic cells.

Scars Harboring Carcinomas

Although most radial scars only simulate carcinomas, rare examples actually contain malignant cells. Because scars so often harbor florid ductal hyperplasia, one might expect to have a difficult time distinguishing a carcinoma from the much more common reactive proliferation; however, most cases do not present this difficulty. When high-grade ductal carcinoma in situ involves a radial scar, for instance, the marked cellular enlargement and the pleomorphism of the nuclei and nucleoli identify the ductal cells as malignant rather than hyperplastic without much controversy (Fig. 13-38). High-grade carcinomas often display necrosis; however, this finding

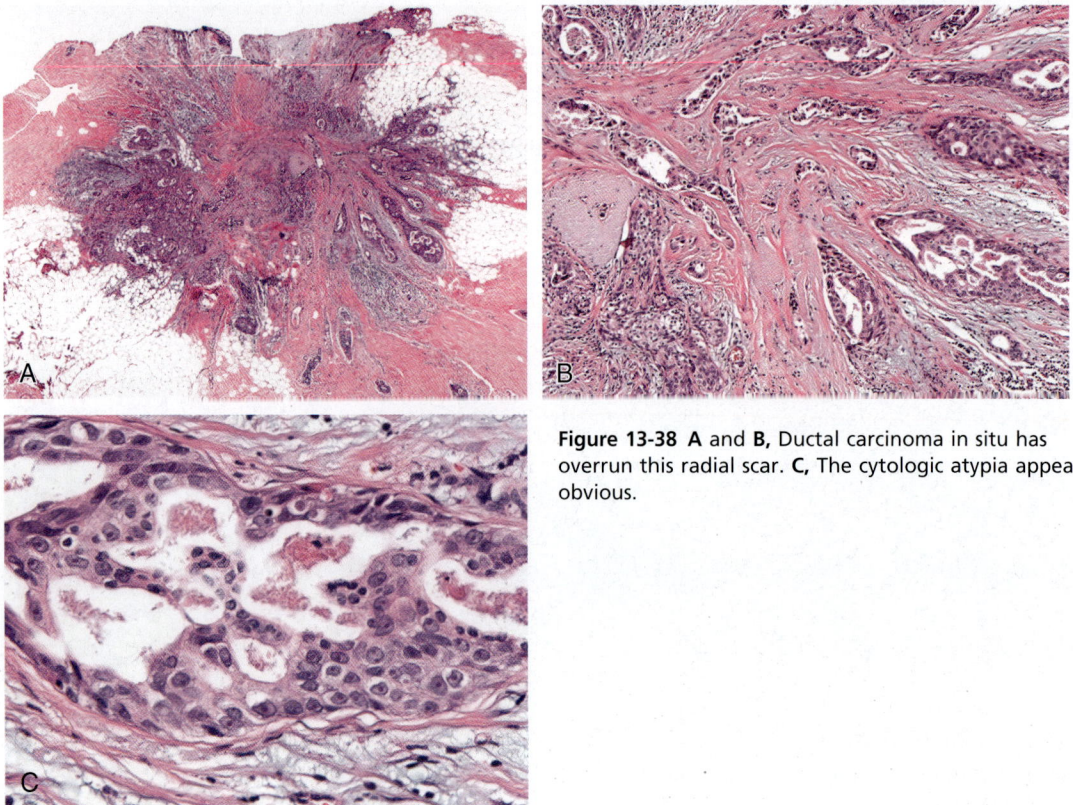

Figure 13-38 A and **B,** Ductal carcinoma in situ has overrun this radial scar. **C,** The cytologic atypia appears obvious.

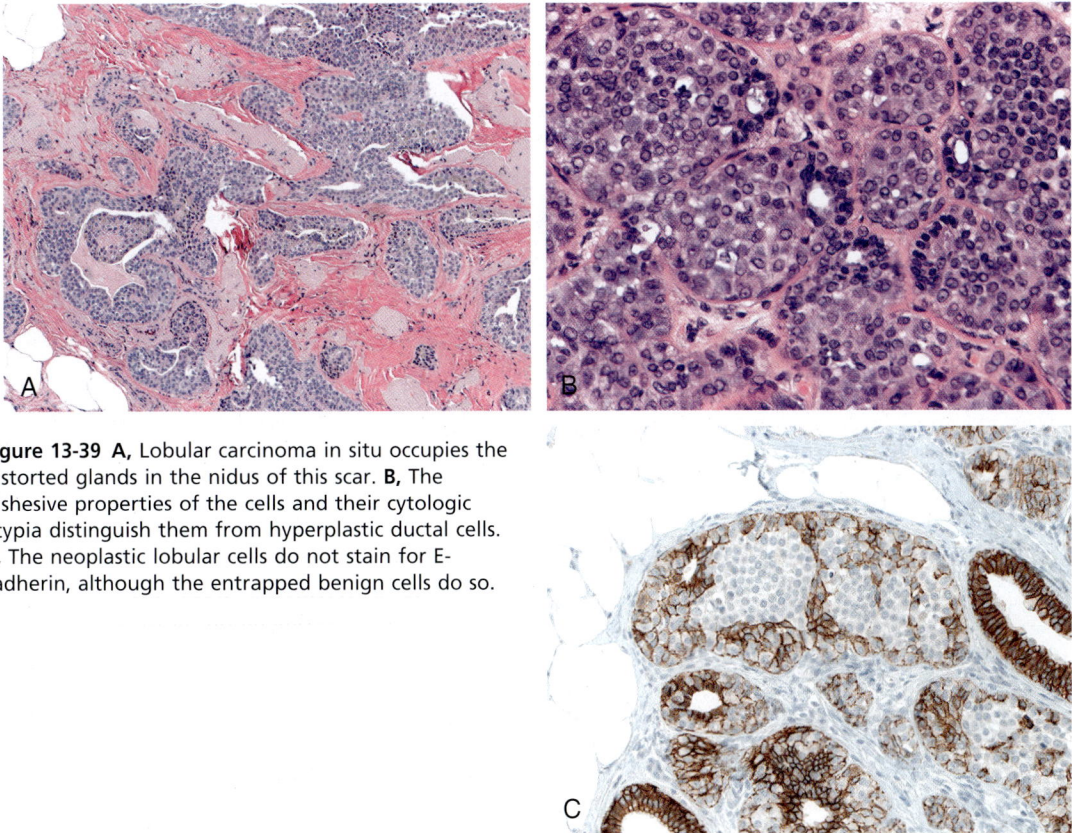

Figure 13-39 A, Lobular carcinoma in situ occupies the distorted glands in the nidus of this scar. B, The dishesive properties of the cells and their cytologic atypia distinguish them from hyperplastic ductal cells. C, The neoplastic lobular cells do not stain for E-cadherin, although the entrapped benign cells do so.

alone does not establish the diagnosis of malignancy in the setting of a radial scar, because hyperplastic cells can also undergo necrosis. In this background, the diagnosis of malignancy must rest on the presence of cytologic atypia.

The recognition of lobular neoplasia, too, does not create much of a problem. The dishesion and cytologic atypia of the lobular cells contrast with the obvious cohesion and lack of atypia of normal acinar cells (Fig. 13-39). Immunohistochemical staining for E-cadherin highlights the presence of the neoplastic population, whose cells lack the protein. The situation becomes more confusing if the radial scar also harbors conventional ductal hyperplasia and the two populations mingle. If one fails to recognize the dishesive properties of the lobular cells, one could easily misinterpret the proliferation as atypical ductal hyperplasia. Staining for E-cadherin clarifies the nature of the proliferation; the hyperplastic ductal cells stain, but the neoplastic lobular ones do not (Fig. 13-40).

Distinguishing low-grade ductal carcinoma in situ from the reactive atypia so commonly seen in scars, on the other hand, can present a formidable challenge. The following guidelines, which represent

---

Box 13-4

Findings favoring the diagnosis of low-grade ductal carcinoma in situ in a radial scar:

- Presence of a distinct population of atypical cells that does not merge with a hyperplastic population
- Presence of clear-cut architectural atypia
- Extension of the atypical population into glands beyond the scar

---

modifications of those used to recognize the cytological atypia in a scar as reparative, help pathologists to identify a neoplastic proliferation in this setting (Box 13-4):

1. The suspicious cells must differ obviously and unambiguously from any hyperplastic cells that occupy the corona of the scar. The florid and slightly atypical reactive cells of scars usually blend with ductal cells showing conventional cellular characteristics. Ductal carcinomas, in contrast,

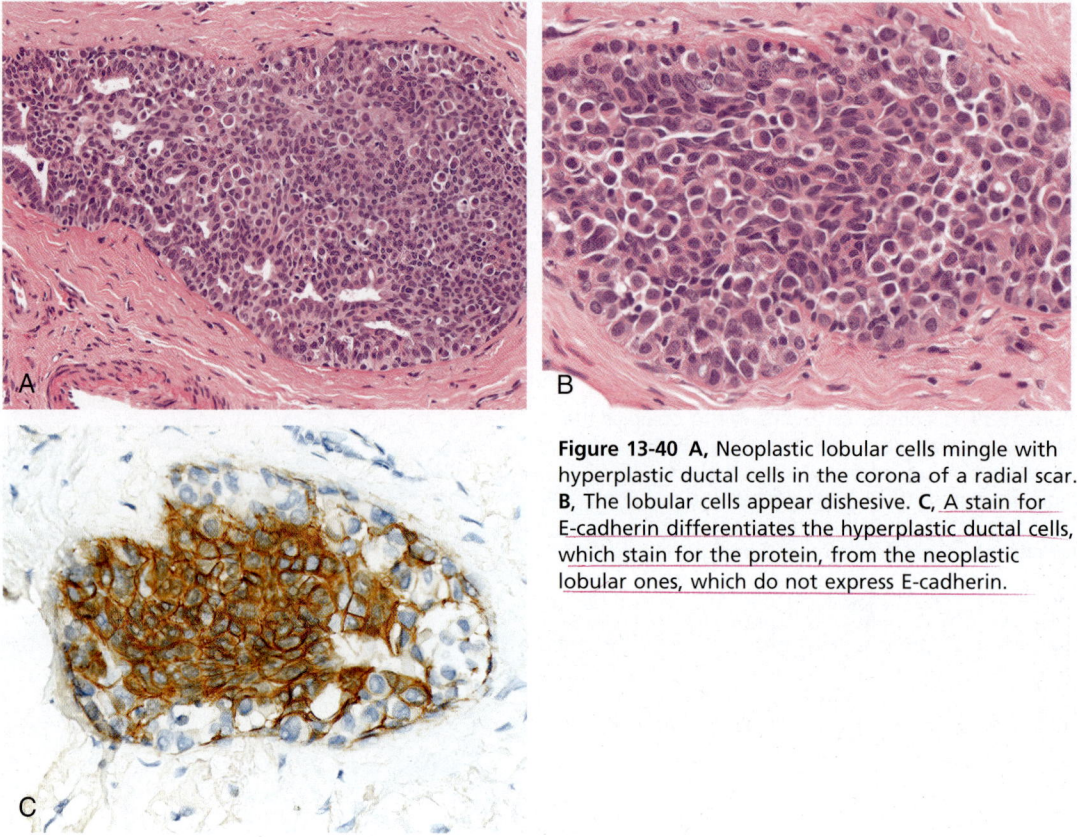

Figure 13-40 A, Neoplastic lobular cells mingle with hyperplastic ductal cells in the corona of a radial scar. **B,** The lobular cells appear dishesive. **C,** A stain for E-cadherin differentiates the hyperplastic ductal cells, which stain for the protein, from the neoplastic lobular ones, which do not express E-cadherin.

stand out as clearly different from any accompanying hyperplastic population (Fig. 13-41).

2. The suspicious region should have a substantial size and should demonstrate convincing architectural atypia (Fig. 13-42). Sclerosing lesions often distort the structure of lobules, and off-center planes of section of these distorted glands can create patterns that mimic the appearance of filled acini, papillary tufts, and cribriform spaces (Fig. 13-43). Pathologists would do well to insist on the presence of convincing cribriform spaces, trabecular bars, or Roman bridges involving clearly distended glands cut in transverse section and lacking internal stroma bands before making the diagnosis of low-grade ductal carcinoma in situ involving a radial scar.

3. When ductal carcinoma in situ involves a radial scar, the malignant cells usually also involve glands beyond the confines of the scar, often to a greater extent than the involvement of glands within the scar. This anatomic distribution contrasts with that of the inconsequential atypia seen in scars, which always remains confined to the proliferative zone. The incomplete involvement of glands of the corona and the extension into tissue outside the scar suggest that the malignant cells arose in ductules distant from the scar and later colonized the preexisting scar (Fig. 13-44).

The presence of carcinoma cells within a radial scar makes it especially difficult to exclude the diagnosis of invasive carcinoma. The distorted glands of the nidus in even the most pedestrian scar can simulate invasive carcinoma by virtue of their irregular shape and haphazard disposition, but attention to the benign cytologic characteristics of the epithelial cells lining these glands prevents this interpretative misadventure. When malignant cells replace the benign ones, these irregular glands populated by carcinoma cells resemble invasive carcinoma uncomfortably closely.

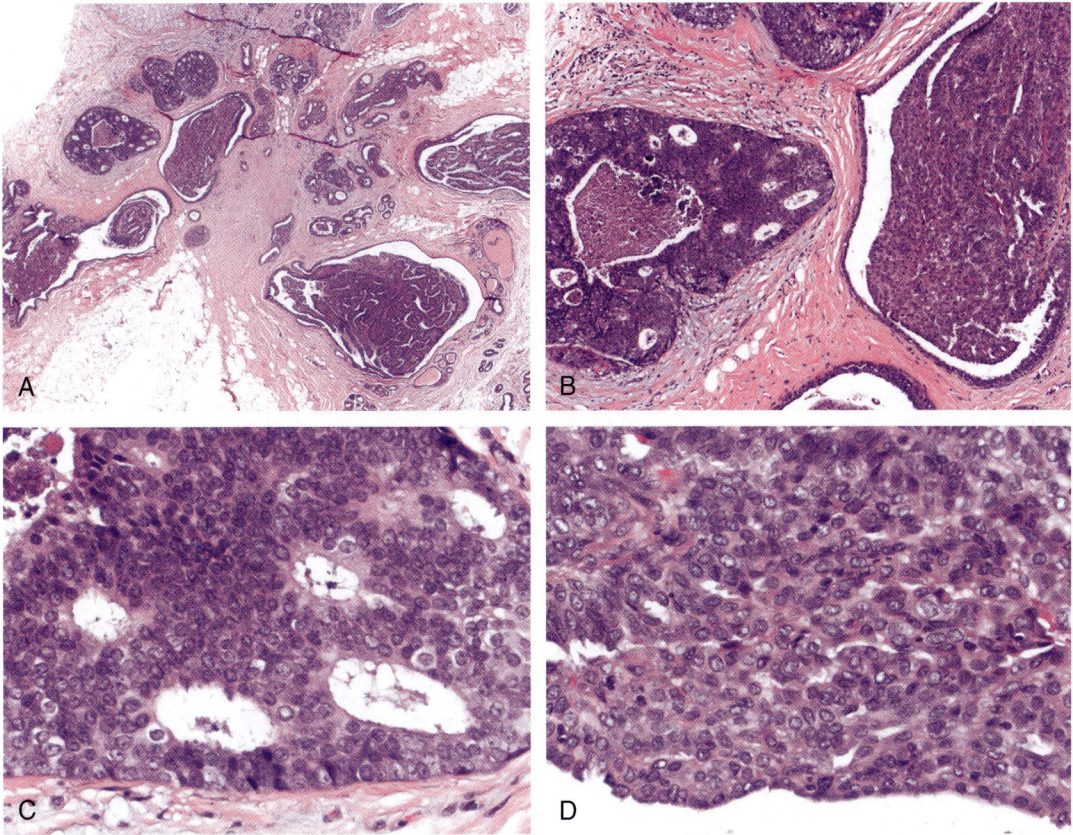

Figure 13-41 A, Ductal carcinoma in situ involves two ducts in this radial scar. **B,** The growth pattern of the malignant ductal cells differs from the architecture of the nearby benign cells. The cytologic features of the carcinoma cells in **C** differ from those of the hyperplastic cells in **D**.

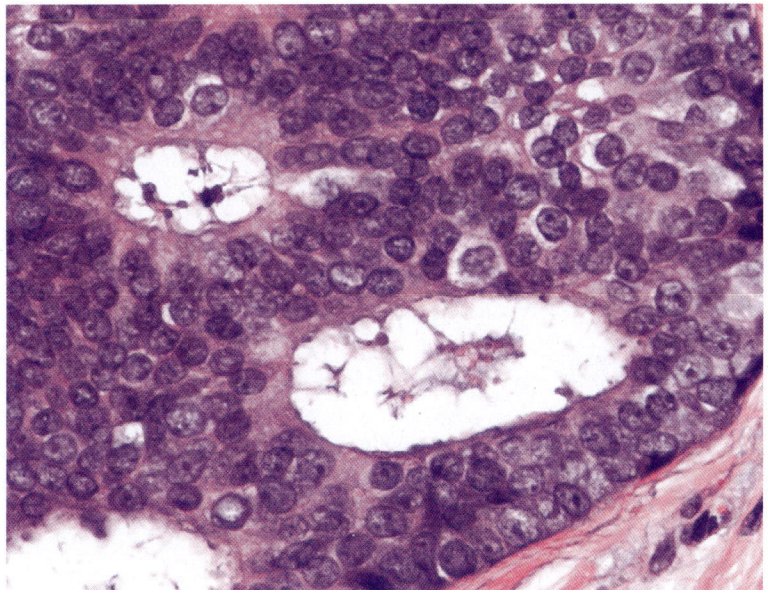

Figure 13-42 The malignant ductal cells display uncontroversial cribriform spaces.

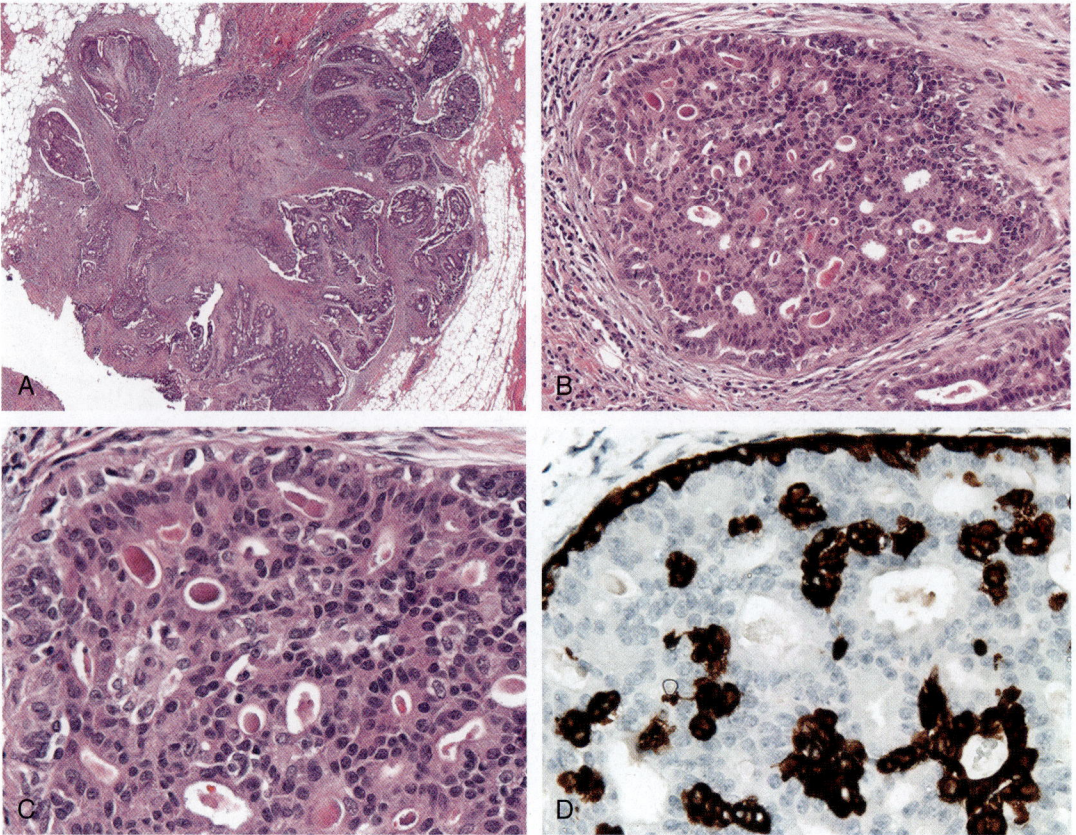

Figure 13-43 A, The corona of this early radial scar contains a distorted lobule, shown in **B,** which looks like a duct distended by atypical ductal cells. **C,** Close examination discloses stroma within the focus. **D,** A stain for myosin heavy chain brings out the presence of myoepithelial cells and makes it clear that the focus represents an altered lobule rather than a duct populated by neoplastic ductal cells.

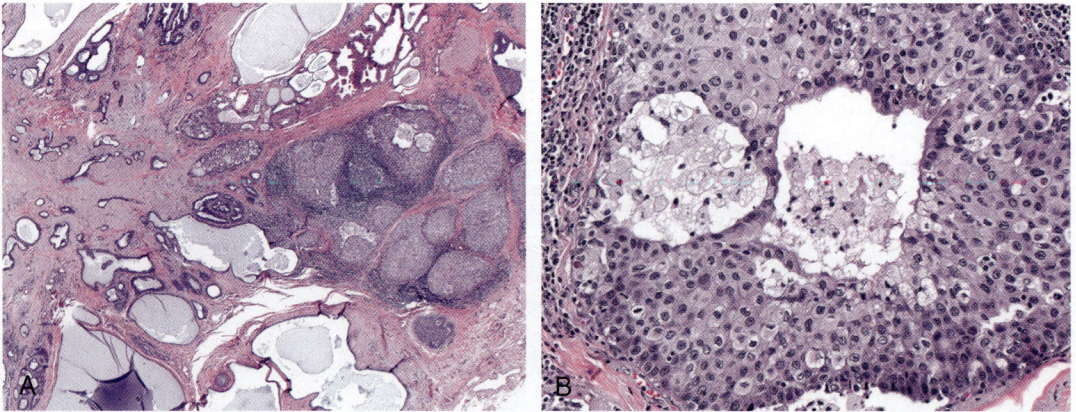

Figure 13-44 A and **B,** Ductal carcinoma in situ involves a few ducts in the corona of this scar and a few others in tissue beyond the lesion.

Figure 13-45 A, This radial scar harbors both in situ and invasive ductal carcinoma. **B,** Ductal carcinoma in situ involves glands in the corona. Entrapped benign glands sit in the nidus, but irregular clusters of invasive carcinoma percolate through the mass and extend to its periphery. The malignant clusters in **C** appear different from the entrapped glands in **D.**

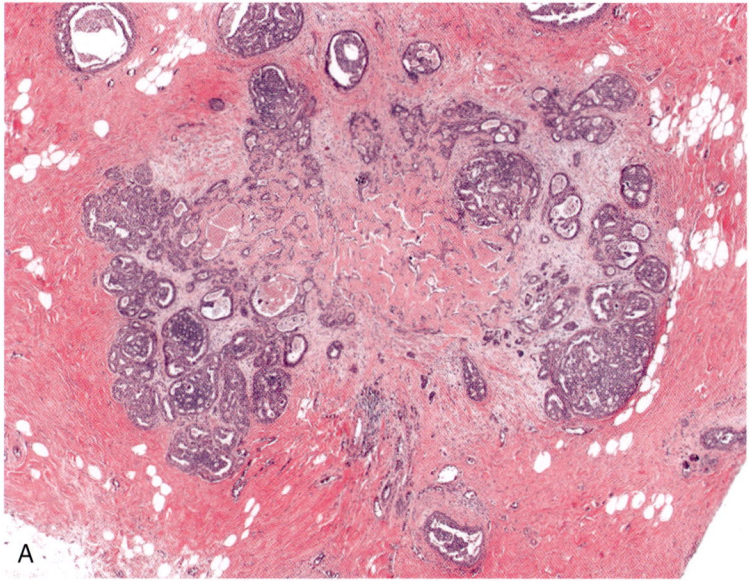

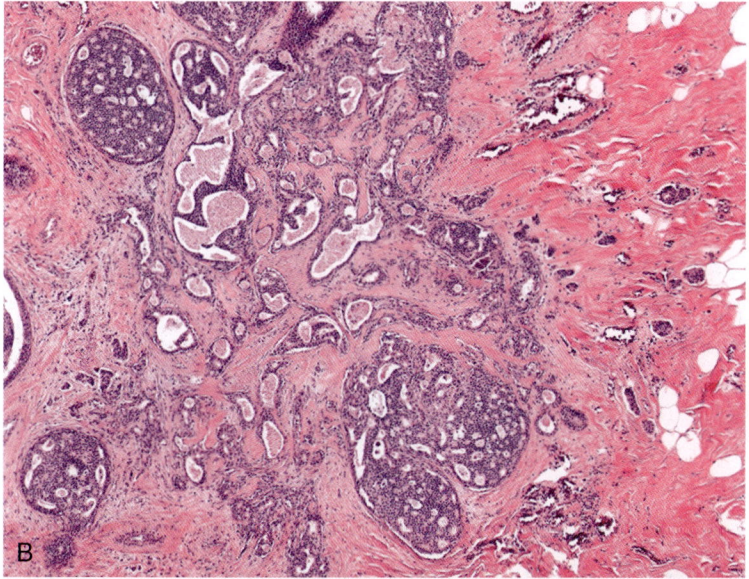

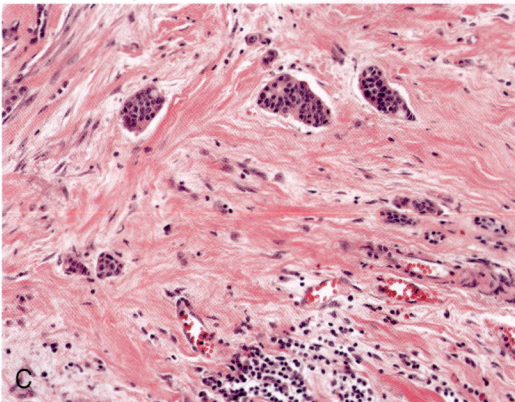

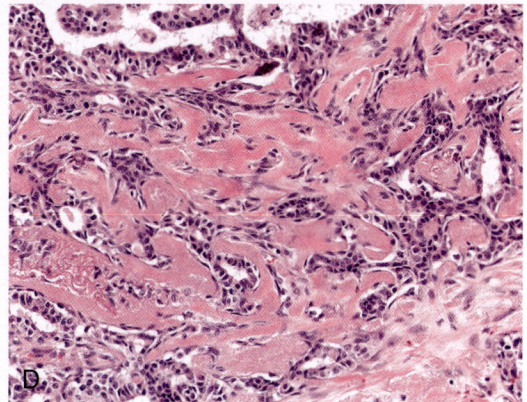

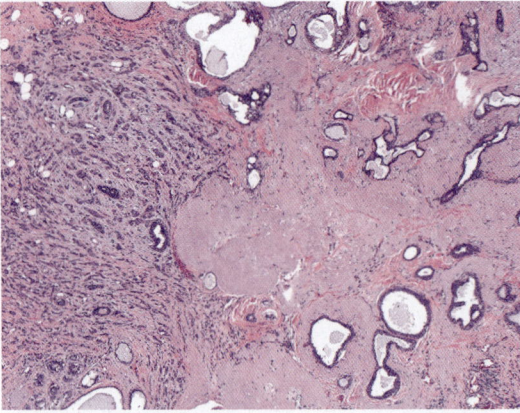

Figure 13-46 The pattern of glands of this invasive carcinoma (*left*) does not resemble the one produced by entrapment of benign glands in the nidus of the radial scar (*right*).

Several considerations allow diagnosticians to avoid misinterpreting a scar harboring carcinoma in situ as an invasive carcinoma. Attention to the structure of the mass provides an especially important clue. When carcinoma in situ involves a radial scar, the malignant population does not disturb the underlying zonal organization. Thus, the distorted glands harboring the carcinoma cells and simulating invasive carcinoma reside only in the nidus of the lesion; they do not penetrate the corona or invade unaltered parenchyma. When present, invasive glands create a destructive pattern, which differs from the appearance of benign glands entrapped by a scarring process (Figs. 13-45 and 13-46). The study of the shapes of the suspicious malignant clusters yields useful guidance in the setting of lobular neoplasia involving a scar, because invasive lobular carcinomas associated with scars grow in the typical single-cell pattern of infiltration (Fig. 13-47), which does not resemble the involvement

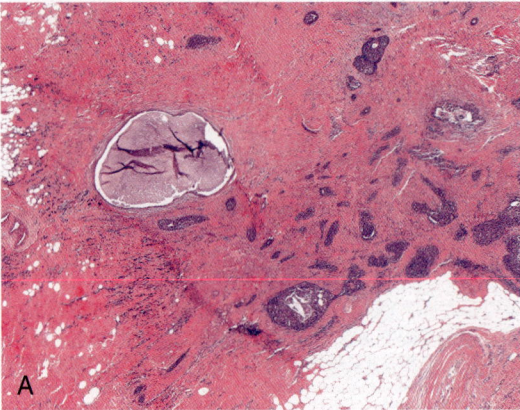

Figure 13-47 A, Invasive lobular carcinoma occupies the edge of the large, vague radial scar seen in the right. **B,** The carcinoma exhibits the single-file growth characteristic of lobular carcinomas.

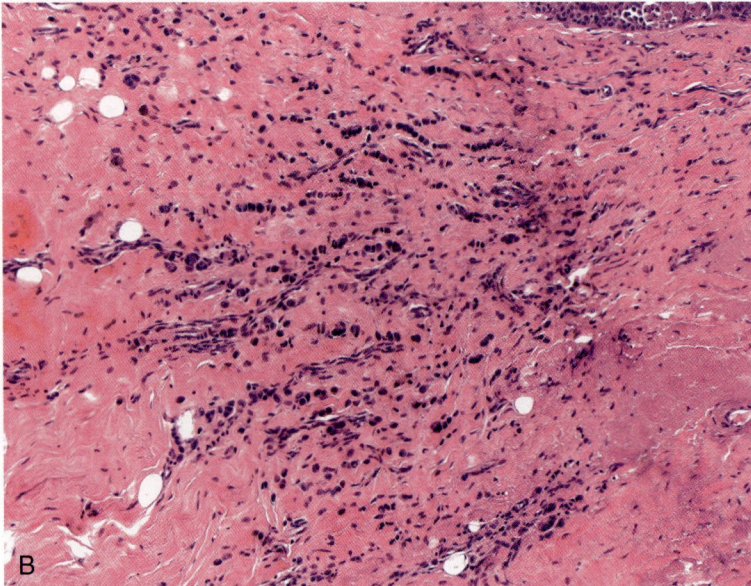

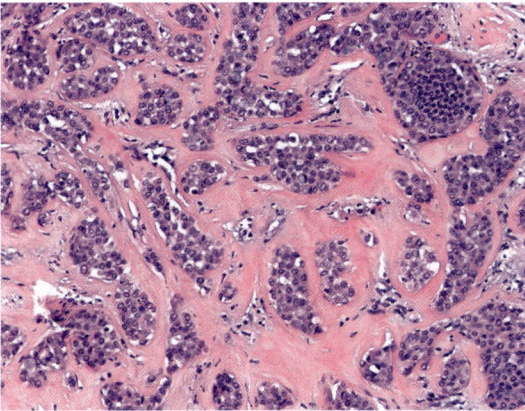

Figure 13-48 Extension of neoplastic lobular cells into distorted benign glands in the nidus of a radial scar results in clusters of malignant cells, not the single-file pattern usually seen in invasive lobular carcinoma.

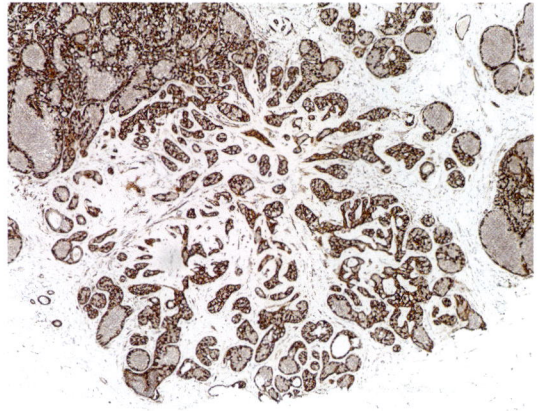

Figure 13-49 This immunohistochemical stain for calponin confirms the lack of invasion by the neoplastic lobular cells in the nidus of this radial scar.

of distorted glands by lobular carcinoma in situ (Fig. 13-48). Finally, immunohistochemical staining for myoepithelial proteins usually allows a clear distinction between carcinoma in situ involving distorted glands and genuine invasive carcinoma (Fig. 13-49).

Displaced Epithelium

Core biopsies of radial scars sometimes dislodge clusters of hyperplastic cells, which sit in the granulation tissue of the needle track (Fig. 13-50). These epithelial elements can exist as single cells, pairs, compact clusters, or even tiny glands. The displaced

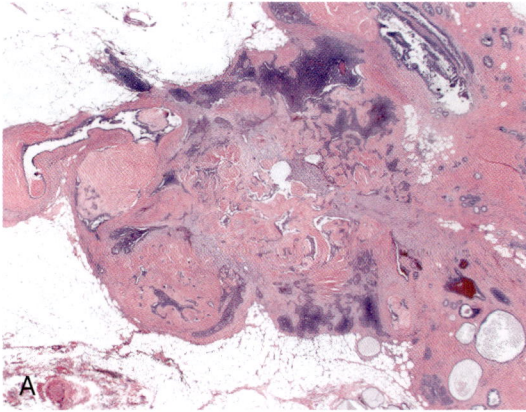

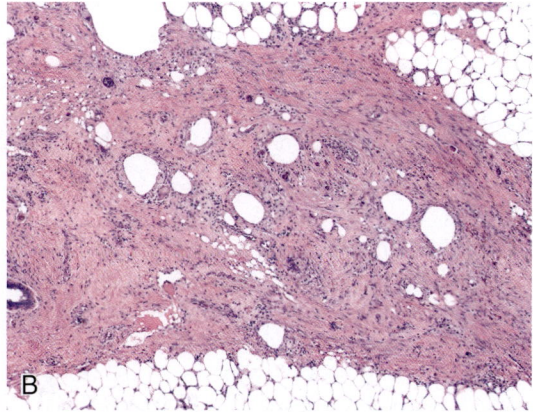

Figure 13-50 A, The core biopsy of this radial scar reveals florid ductal hyperplasia. The needle track of the excision specimen in **B** contains many single epithelial cells and others in small clusters shown in **C.**

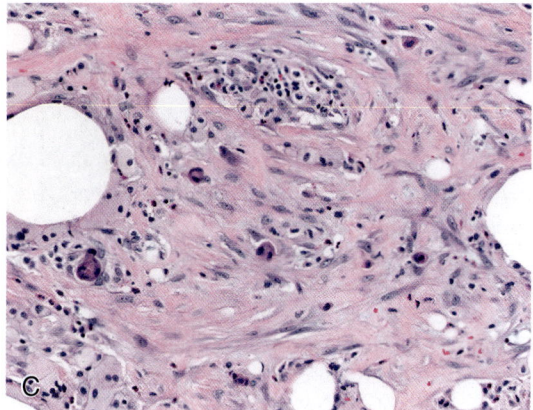

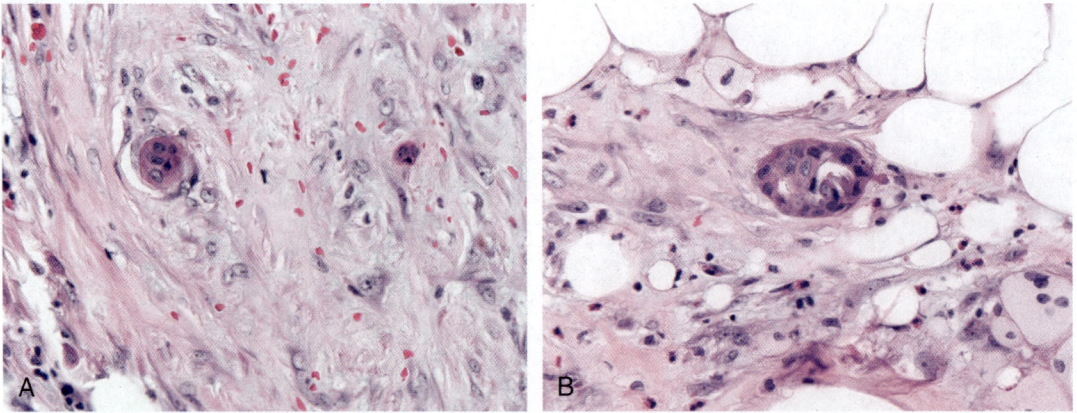

Figure 13-51 A, The presence of dense, eosinophilic cytoplasm gives certain of these displaced cells a squamous quality. **B,** Although the nuclei vary in size, shape, and chromatin quality, they do not appear atypical. The hyperchromasia probably represents a degenerative phenomenon.

cells often possess dense, eosinophilic cytoplasm, which imparts a squamous appearance. The nuclei can appear either small and bland or large and irregular in both shape and chromatin quality (Fig. 13-51). One sometimes observes mitotic activity; more often, however, the condensed nuclei reflect degeneration of the cell rather than cell division. Seeing these isolated clusters and single cells haphazardly disposed in the mammary stroma can prompt pathologists to entertain the diagnosis of invasive carcinoma, especially low-grade adenosquamous carcinoma, and an awareness of the frequent association of this type of carcinoma with sclerosing lesions only increases the likelihood of this erroneous diagnosis.

To prevent such a misinterpretation, pathologists should remember the following. First, displaced epithelial nests virtually never stray beyond the limits of the reactive stroma of the biopsy site. They do not penetrate into otherwise undisturbed tissue; rather, they remain embedded in a background of reactive fibroblasts, inflammatory cells, histiocytes, and blood. Second, the granulation tissue of a biopsy site differs from the stroma of an adenosquamous carcinoma in both its composition and its relationship with the epithelial elements. Granulation tissue contains inflammatory cells and tissue debris not present in the stroma of a carcinoma. Furthermore, the fibroblasts of granulation tissue appear loosely disposed and positioned without regard to the epithelial clusters. The spindle cells of an adenosquamous carcinoma encircle the epithelial nests in a compact, concentric arrangement. In fact, the two components of an adenosquamous carcinoma appear so intimately related that the epithelial clusters seem to emerge from the background spindle cells. Finally, one must pay attention to the context of the case. Displacement of benign epithelial cells usually occurs during the biopsy of tissue harboring florid ductal hyperplasia in the setting of an underlying benign lesion such as a radial scar, sclerosing papilloma, or conventional papilloma. Pathologists should take a particularly cautious approach to the diagnosis of malignancy when examining a case in which the prior specimen contained only benign cells and the current one shows florid ductal hyperplasia involving a sclerosing lesion or a papilloma. One cannot establish the diagnosis of invasive carcinoma simply by observing epithelial nests haphazardly disposed within the parenchyma of a biopsy site; a secure diagnosis rests on the presence of invasion of unaltered tissue.

As a final point of caution, pathologists must remember that displaced epithelial clusters show variable and inconsistent staining for markers of myoepithelial cells. Certain groups do not seem to possess myoepithelial cells no matter which of the usual stains one employs; others stain for one marker but not others. Thus, one cannot rely on immunohistochemical staining for p63 protein, calponin, and myosin heavy chain to distinguish clusters of displaced epithelial cells from malignant cells.

Scars in Core Biopsy Specimens

The recognition of radial scars in excision specimens usually does not pose problems once pathologists become familiar with the morphologic characteristics of such scars; however, the diagnosis proves more challenging when one is examining specimens obtained by a core biopsy. A confident assessment of the critical diagnostic findings requires a panoramic, low-magnification view of the entire lesion, which the slender tissue cores obtained during a needle biopsy do not provide. Nevertheless, studies

Figure 13-52 The radial scar in this core biopsy specimen displays the diagnostic characteristics clearly.

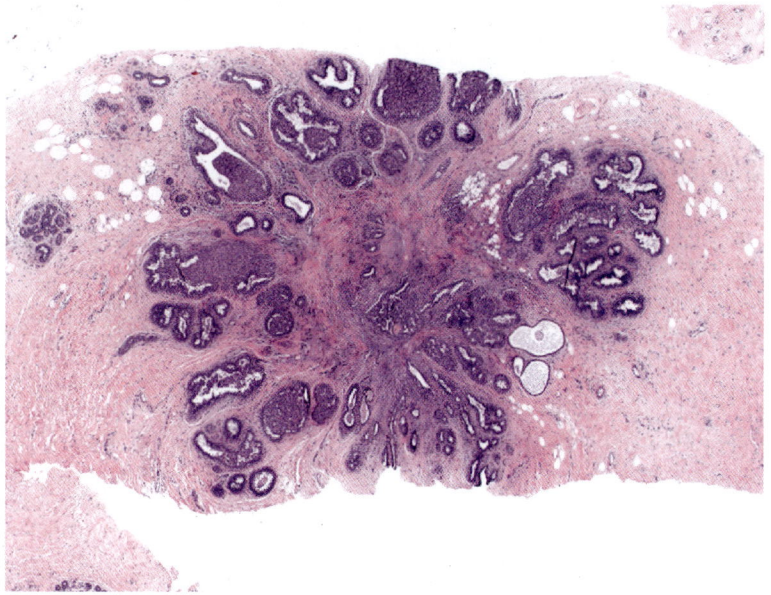

suggest that pathologists can usually recognize radial scars in needle biopsy specimens, and certain writers propose that radial scars diagnosed in this way do not require excision. If scars in core biopsy specimens always appeared as distinctive as the one pictured in Figure 13-52, pathologists could recognize them with confidence, and surgeons would not need to excise them; however, larger scars, misshapen scars, and early scars do not exhibit the classic diagnostic features so clearly (Fig. 13-53). Furthermore, the presence of a scar can camouflage other significant lesions (Fig. 13-54), and one has difficulty evaluating the significance of minimal cytologic atypia associated with a radial scar (Fig. 13-55). On the basis of these considerations, the author believes it prudent to excise lesions classified as radial scars in core biopsy specimens as frequently as the clinical details of the cases permit.

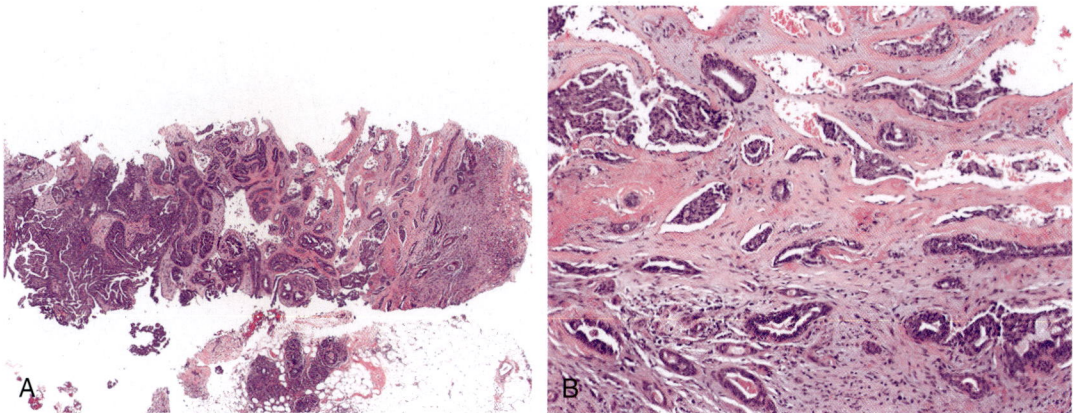

Figure 13-53 A and **B,** The zonal architecture of this large radial scar does not appear obvious.

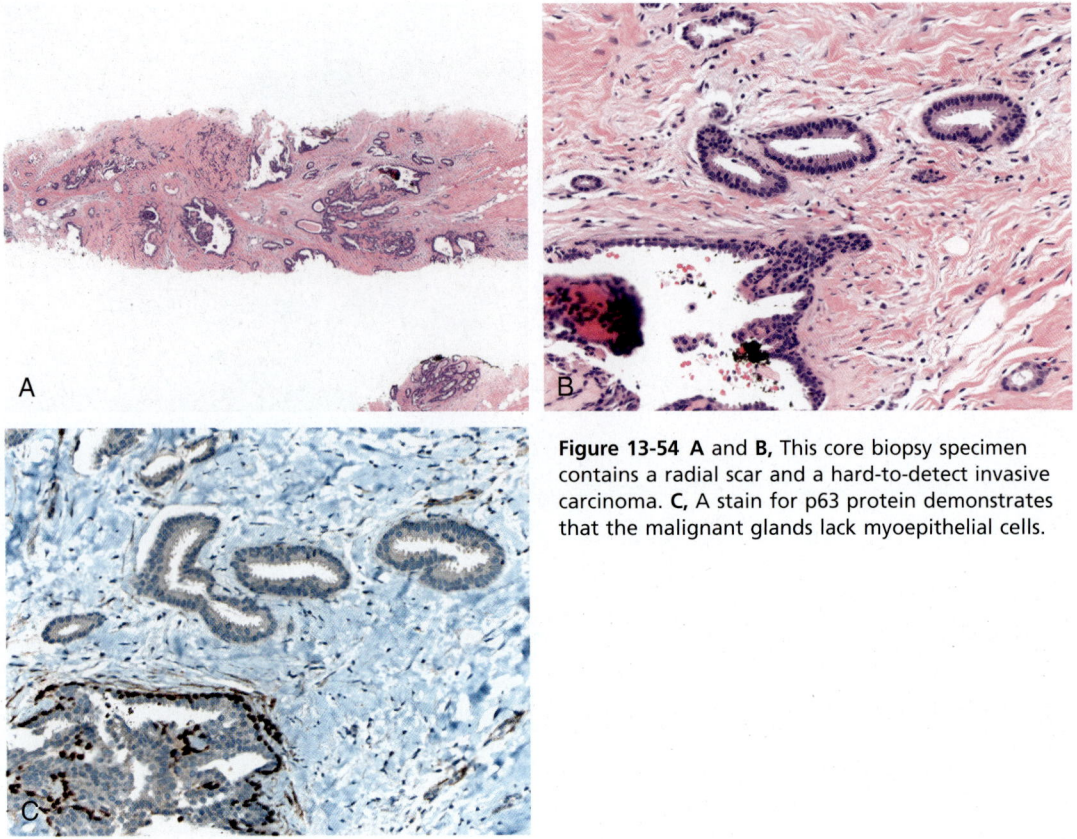

Figure 13-54 A and **B,** This core biopsy specimen contains a radial scar and a hard-to-detect invasive carcinoma. **C,** A stain for p63 protein demonstrates that the malignant glands lack myoepithelial cells.

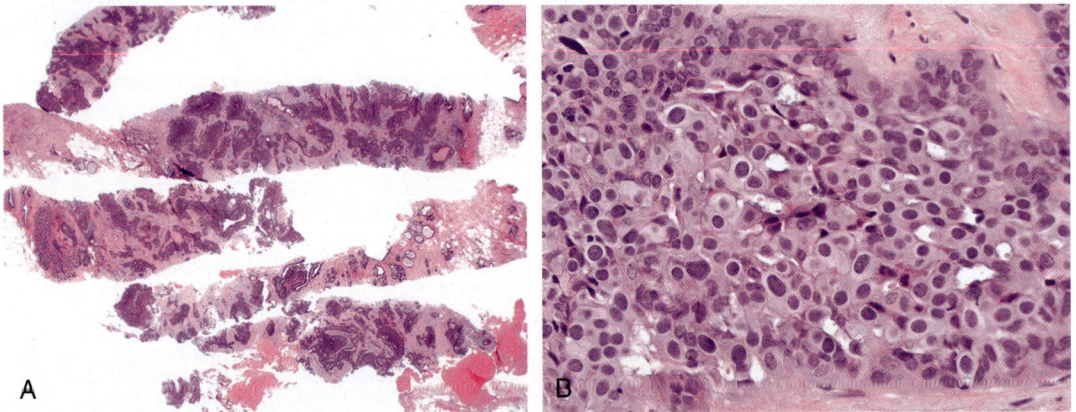

Figure 13-55 A and **B,** One cannot evaluate the significance of the atypical cells in this early radial scar. The excision did not show neoplastic atypia.

Selected Readings

Andersen JA, Gram JB: Radial scar in the female breast: A long-term follow-up study of 32 cases. Cancer 1984;53:2557-2560.

Anderson TJ, Battersby S: Radial scars of benign and malignant breasts: Comparative features and significance. J Pathol 1985;147:23-32.

Fenoglio C, Lattes R: Sclerosing papillary proliferations in the female breast: A benign lesion often mistaken for carcinoma. Cancer 1974;33:691-700.

Fisher ER, Palekar AS, Kotwal N, et al: A nonencapsulated sclerosing lesion of the breast. Am J Clin Pathol 1979;71:240-246.

Fisher ER, Palekar AS, Sass R, et al: Scar cancers: Pathologic findings from the National Surgical Adjuvant Breast Project (protocol No. 4) — IX. Breast Cancer Res Treat 1983;3:39-59.

Hamperl H: Strahlige narben und obliterierende mastopathie: Beiträge zur pathologischen histologie der mamma. XI. Virchows Arch A Pathol Anat Histol 1975;369:55-68.

Jacobs TW, Byrne C, Colditz G, et al: Radial scars in benign breast-biopsy specimens and the risk of breast cancer. N Engl J Med 1999;340:430-436.

Linell F, Ljungberg O, Andersson I: Breast carcinoma: Aspects of early stage, progression and related problems. Acta Pathol Microbiol Scand Suppl 1980; 272:1-233.

Nielsen M, Christensen L, Andersen J: Radial scars in women with breast cancer. Cancer 1987;59: 1019-1025.

Nielsen M, Jensen J, Andersen JA: An autopsy study of radial scar in the female breast. Histopathology 1985;9:287-295.

Rickert RR, Kalisher L, Hutter RV: Indurative mastopathy: A benign sclerosing lesion of breast with elastosis which may simulate carcinoma. Cancer 1981;47: 561-571.

Sloane JP, Mayers MM: Carcinoma and atypical hyperplasia in radial scars and complex sclerosing lesions: Importance of lesion size and patient age. Histopathology 1993;23:225-231.

14

Low-Grade Invasive Ductal Carcinoma

DEFINITIONS AND CLINICOPATHOLOGIC CHARACTERISTICS

Even beginning students of mammary pathology realize that invasive ductal carcinomas vary in their extent of differentiation and pattern of growth. Because most breast cancers consist of obviously atypical cells growing in disorganized masses, it does not demand much skill to recognize their malignant nature; however, challenging problems arise when the malignant cells look bland and invade in uncommon patterns. These well-differentiated carcinomas take several forms including papillary, mucinous, cribriform, and glandular. Earlier sections have discussed certain diagnostic problems associated with two of these patterns. This chapter focuses on those low-grade invasive carcinomas that form small glands or tubules.

The clinicopathologic characteristics of commonplace, low-grade, gland-forming carcinomas do not differ from those of higher-grade breast cancers, but certain special types of well-differentiated carcinomas have somewhat distinctive features. Tubular carcinomas rarely grow to a large size, and they often coexist with lobular neoplasia as well as low-grade ductal carcinoma in situ. Low-grade adenosquamous carcinomas frequently originate in the setting of a benign sclerosing lesion. Like other breast cancers, low-grade carcinomas usually form hard, spiculated masses.

HISTOLOGIC CHARACTERISTICS

Shape of the Lesion

Invasive ductal carcinomas look like expanding, space-occupying masses (Fig. 14-1). They develop as the multiplication of the malignant cells and the reaction of the mammary stromal cells to the presence of the carcinoma add new tissue to the breast. The shape of the resulting mass depends on the extent of both the glandular proliferation and the stromal reaction. Most carcinomas appear irregular or stellate because tongues of malignant glands penetrate into surrounding tissue (Fig. 14-2). If a stromal reaction ensues, the accumulation of collagen and fibroblasts enhances the irregularity of the mass's contour. The radiating architecture of certain carcinomas does recall the configuration of a radial scar, but the two lesions differ in their fundamental nature: carcinomas represent new growths, whereas scars look like regions of tissue loss. Thus, carcinomas have a bulging shape and often compress or separate the components of the mammary parenchyma around the periphery of the mass (Fig. 14-3). Radial scars, in contrast, draw the surrounding tissue toward the central region of scarring and tissue loss. Arising through different mechanisms, the two lesions also differ in internal structure, in the characteristics of the glands, and in the relationship between the glands and stroma.

Carcinomas do not always incite a reaction in the underlying tissue, and those that do not may not display the typical infiltrative shape. Although it might seem illogical to refer to carcinomas lacking a stromal reaction in a discussion of sclerosing lesions, these malignancies do resemble certain benign members of this family; consequently, consideration of these hard-to-recognize carcinomas fits most appropriately in this discussion. Such carcinomas can grow as smooth, round aggregates of glands that resemble altered lobules or foci of adenosis, and the malignant glands can simply infiltrate the mammary tissue without forming a distinct nodule at all (Fig. 14-4). Paying attention to the relationship between the glands and the surrounding tissue allows one to recognize the

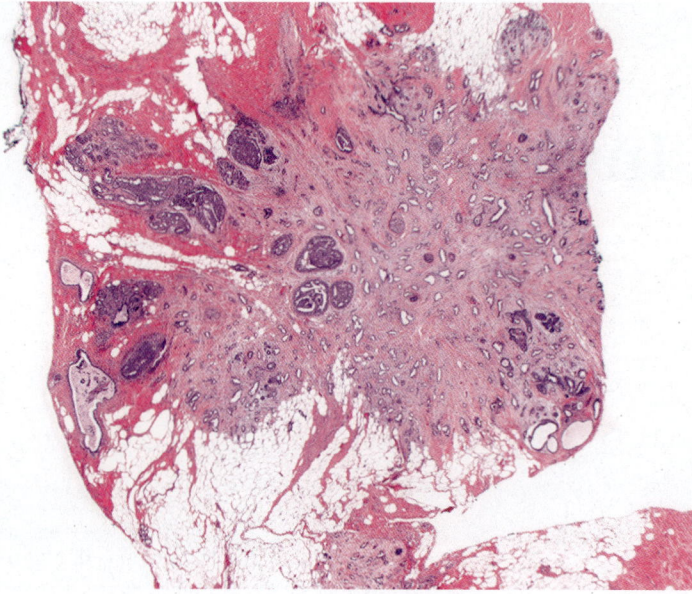

Figure 14-1 Because invasive carcinomas consist of new tissue, they look like space-occupying masses.

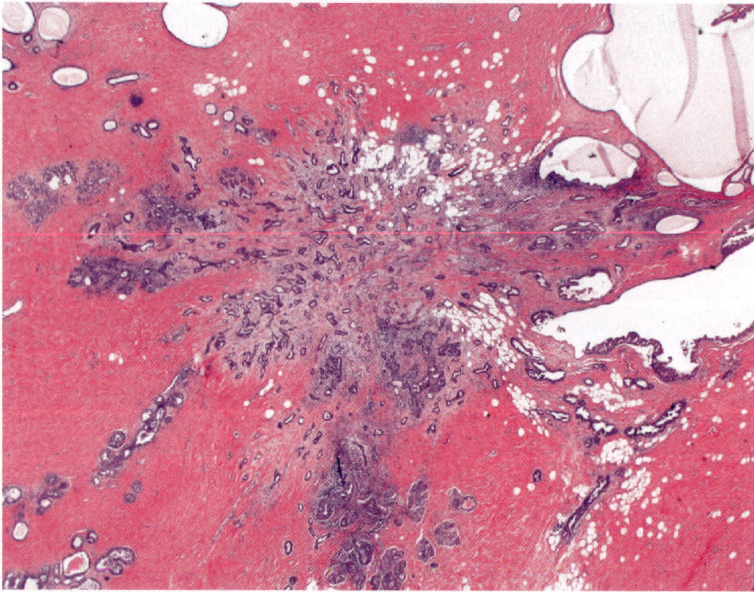

Figure 14-2 Infiltration of the malignant glands into the mammary parenchyma gives this invasive carcinoma an irregular, stellate shape.

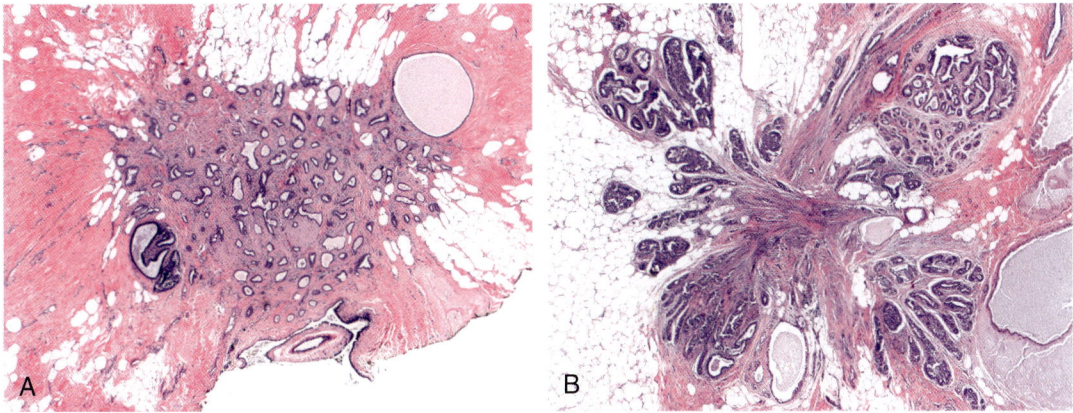

Figure 14-3 A, This invasive carcinoma forms a bulging nodule that compresses the surrounding tissue. **B,** This radial scar represents a region of tissue loss; scarring draws the surrounding tissue toward the nidus.

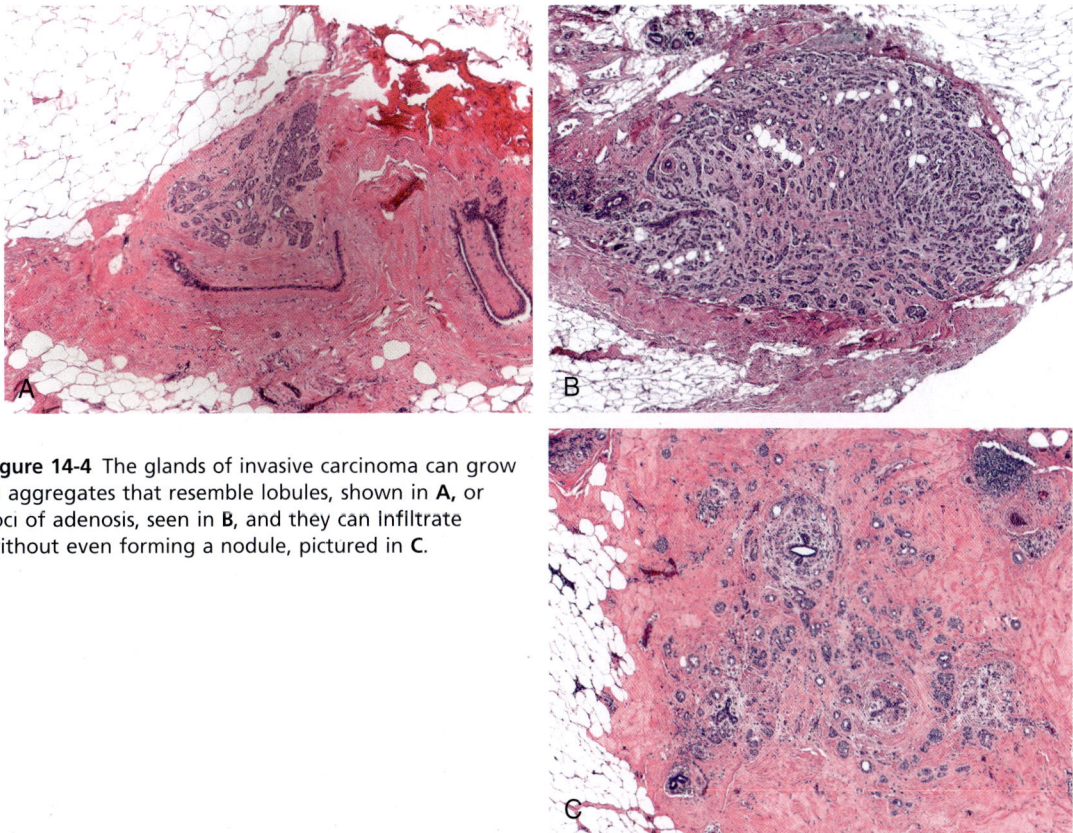

Figure 14-4 The glands of invasive carcinoma can grow in aggregates that resemble lobules, shown in **A,** or foci of adenosis, seen in **B,** and they can infiltrate without even forming a nodule, pictured in **C.**

invasive nature of the malignant glands and thereby to differentiate these carcinomas from benign lesions.

Structure of the Lesion

Well-differentiated invasive ductal carcinomas consist of a structureless mass of neoplastic glands and stroma intermixed with variable amounts of preexisting mammary parenchyma (Fig. 14-5). This absence of an internal structure differentiates carcinomas from most benign sclerosing lesions. For example, carcinomas do not display the underlying lobular organization seen in foci of sclerosing adenosis. The glands of most carcinomas do not seem as densely packed as the glands of adenosis; moreover, carcinomas do not show either the compression of the central acini or the preservation of the size and shape of the peripheral acini that typify foci of sclerosing adenosis (Fig. 14-6). The lack of an internal zonal architecture also distinguishes carcinomas from radial scars: carcinomas lack the central nidus and corona of proliferative changes that one sees in most radial scars (Fig. 14-7). Furthermore, the neoplastic glands occupy the entirety of a carcinoma, whereas the entrapped glands of a radial scar sit only in the regions of stromal alteration.

Like the lack of an internal structure, the characteristics of the epithelial and stromal components of these lesions differentiate carcinomas from benign sclerosing lesions. The neoplastic cells of well-

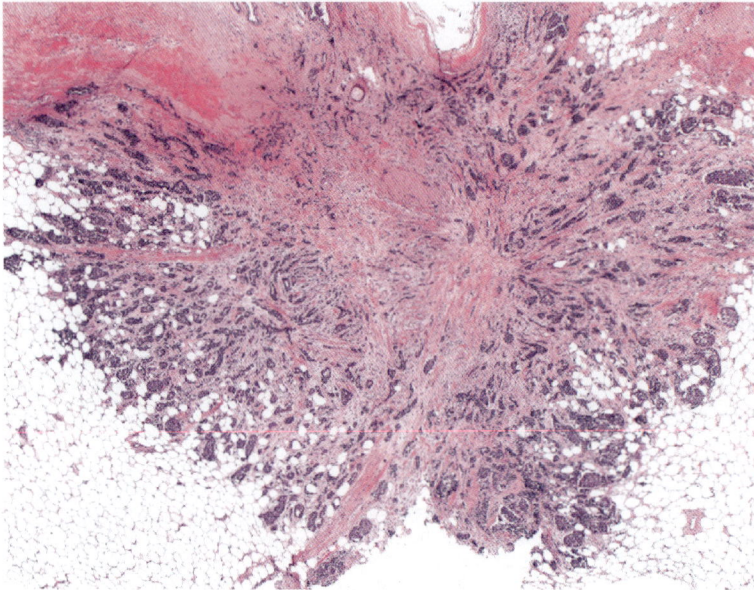

Figure 14-5 Invasive ductal carcinomas form a mass without an organized internal structure.

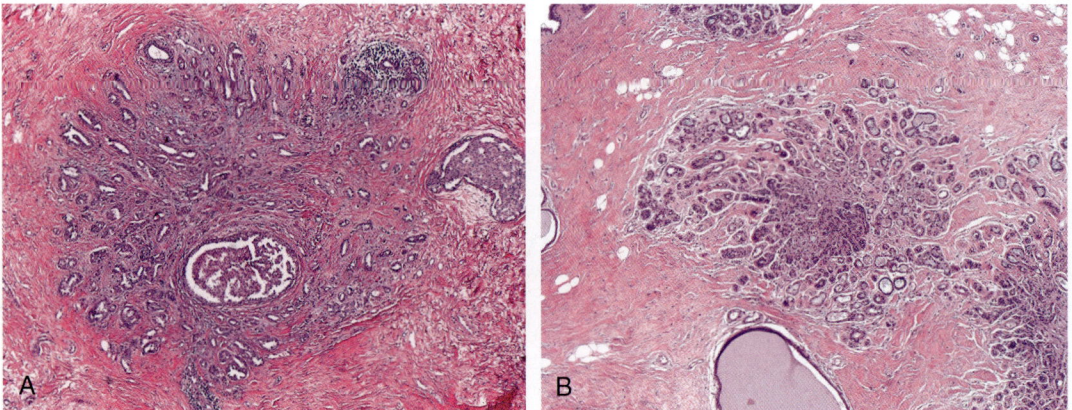

Figure 14-6 The glands of the invasive ductal carcinoma shown in **A** appear more loosely aggregated than those in the focus of sclerosing adenosis shown in **B**. Furthermore, the carcinoma does not display the compression of the central glands seen in the focus of sclerosing adenosis.

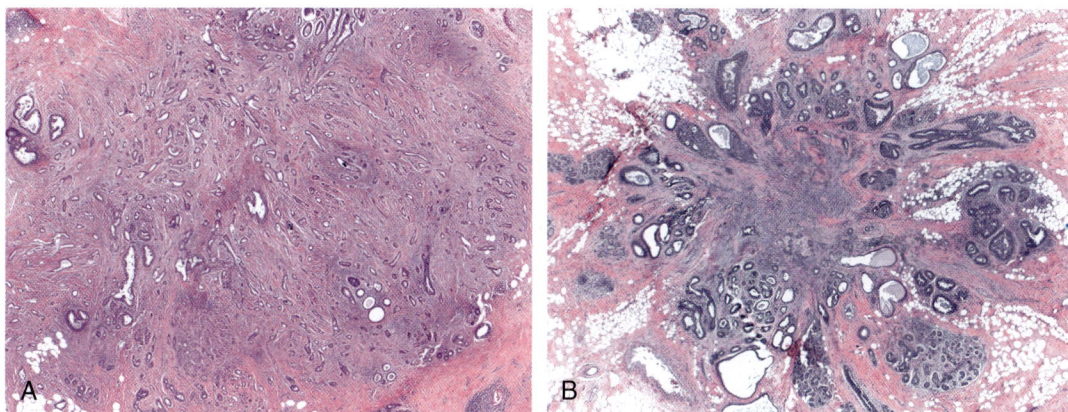

Figure 14-7 The invasive ductal carcinoma shown in **A** lacks the zonal structure of the radial scar shown in **B**.

differentiated ductal carcinomas usually form tubules and glands, but the cells can also grow in small clusters and as individuals. The glands vary in size and shape, and many have angulated ends and open lumens (Fig. 14-8). Although the geometric characteristics of the neoplastic glands can serve as helpful signs, they do not constitute fundamental properties of the malignant cells; therefore, pathologists may find it prudent to rely on other attributes of the glands to distinguish invasive ductal carcinomas from benign sclerosing lesions. The cytologic features of the cells composing the glands, for instance, provide diagnostic information of a more reliable nature, and so does the relationship between the glands and the neighboring tissue. Carcinoma cells appear slightly larger than their benign counterparts. The larger cell size results from an increase in both the amount of cytoplasm and the size of the nucleus; the latter contains homogeneous chromatin and

inconspicuous nucleoli. These alterations can seem subtle, and one might have difficulty appreciating them until one contrasts the neoplastic cells with normal cells in the same tissue section. Invasion of a lobule by the malignant glands brings the two types of glandular cells into close approximation; this side-by-side position facilitates an appreciation of the cytologic aberrations of the malignant cells (Fig. 14-9). Such a study usually makes obvious the relatively larger size of the neoplastic cells and their nuclei, the more finely dispersed character of their chromatin, the smaller size of their nucleoli, and the relative abundance of their cytoplasm.

The epithelial aggregates of conventional invasive carcinomas lack myoepithelial cells. Inexperienced pathologists frequently assume that this absence of myoepithelial cells establishes the presence of invasion by the epithelial cells and therefore their malignant nature. This assumption represents a serious flaw in reasoning. As an isolated finding, the lack of myoepithelial cells does not prove that the epithelial cells in question have transgressed the basement membrane, nor does it identify them as malignant. The distorted, benign tubules within the nidus of certain radial scars and the florid hyperplasia that occupies the corona of others sometimes lack myoepithelial cells, and so do the glands of microglandular adenosis, for instance. The author does not mean to dismiss the utility of immunohistochemical staining for myoepithelial cells in the analysis of sclerosing lesions; the results of such studies usually steer the pathologist in the direction of the proper diagnosis. Nevertheless, these results represent only one component of the analysis, and one must interpret them in the context of the conventional morphologic features. The diagnosis of invasive carcinoma always requires the presence of both cytologic atypia and conventional histologic evidence of

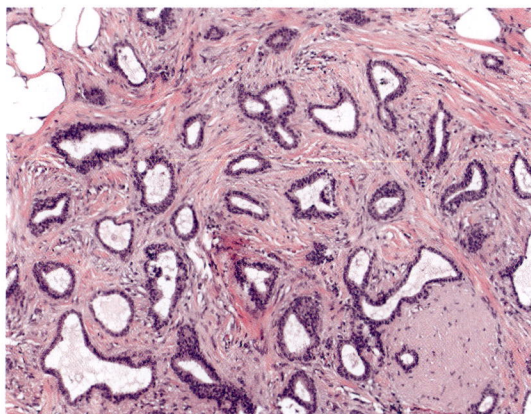

Figure 14-8 The glands of this invasive ductal carcinoma have irregular shapes and open lumens.

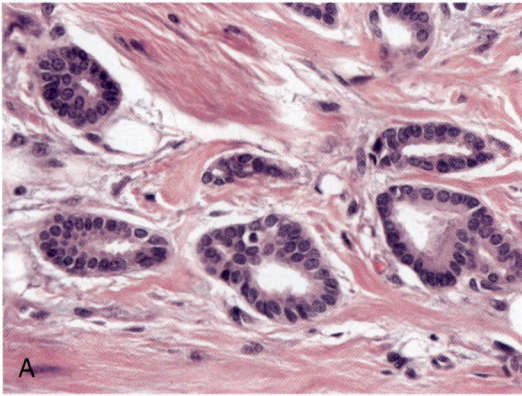

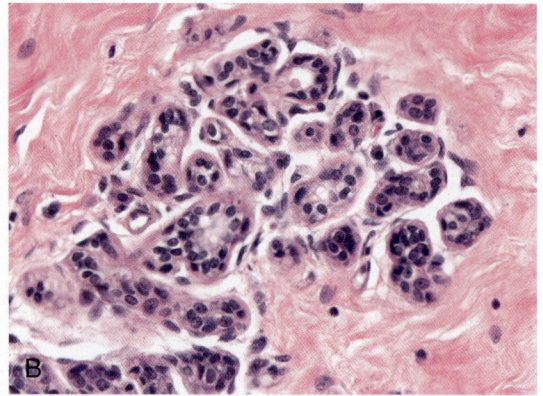

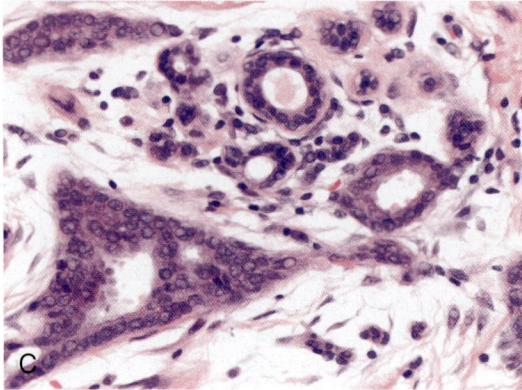

Figure 14-9 The malignant glands depicted in **A** consist of cells slightly larger than the ones of the normal lobule shown in **B**. The neoplastic cells have slightly larger nuclei and more cytoplasm than their benign counterparts. **C,** Invasion of a normal lobule by malignant cells brings the two types of cells in close approximation and facilitates the appreciation of the subtle cytologic differences between the benign and malignant populations.

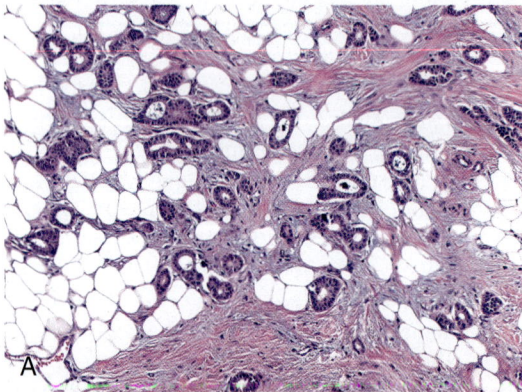

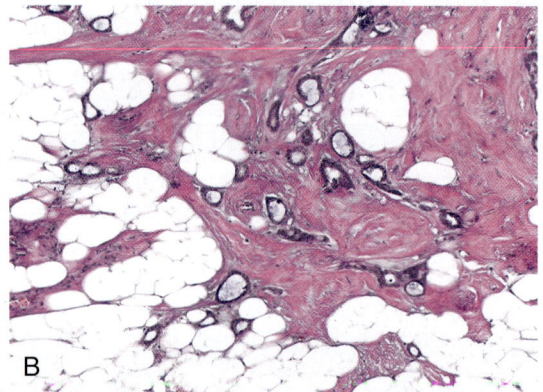

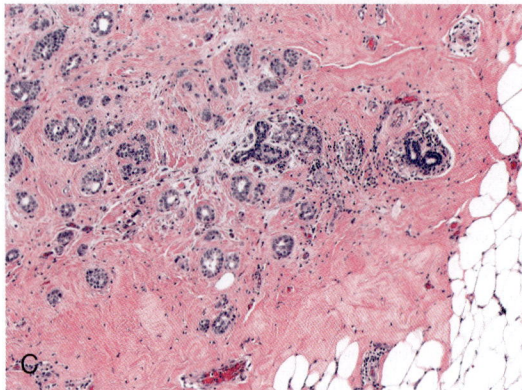

Figure 14-10 **A,** The stroma of most invasive ductal carcinomas shows desmoplastic changes. **B,** A minority of carcinomas have stroma composed of dense collagen, elastic tissue, and just a few stromal cells. **C,** Certain carcinomas do not provoke a stromal reaction.

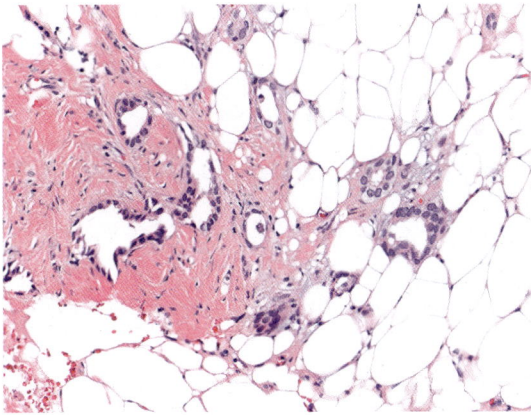

Figure 14-11 Invasion of adipose tissue by the carcinoma has caused necrosis of a few adipocytes.

destructive tissue invasion; never does the mere absence of myoepithelial cells establish the diagnosis of malignancy.

The amount and composition of the stroma in carcinomas vary from one example to the next (Fig. 14-10). Usually the fibrous connective tissue invaded by the carcinoma assumes a desmoplastic appearance. This type of reactive stroma consists of numerous fibroblasts sitting within myxoid ground substances and among collagen bundles. The presence of desmoplastic stroma helps distinguish carcinomas from both mature radial scars and well-established sclerosing adenosis, because the stroma of the two benign lesions does not display these reactive features. Dense collagen, elastic tissue, and just a few fibroblasts constitute the stroma of less commonly seen carcinomas, and certain cancers do not provoke any stromal reaction whatsoever. When the malignant glands penetrate into adipose tissue, the

reactive phenomena take the form of focal fat necrosis, inflammation, and fibrosis (Fig. 14-11). These stromal alterations aid in distinguishing malignant glands invading fat from benign acini stranded in adipose tissue as a consequence of stromal atrophy.

Characteristics of the Peripheral Epithelial Elements

The presence of the proliferative glands at the periphery of the lesion and their destructive invasion of the surrounding tissue provide the most consistent and the most persuasive evidence to establish the diagnosis of invasive carcinoma. All invasive carcinomas have these features, but no benign sclerosing lesion exhibits both of them. Most radial scars, for instance, have a proliferative corona enveloping the distorted glands and altered stroma of the nidus and thereby confining the epithelial elements to the center of the lesion. Never do the irregular glands of a scar escape the region of stromal alteration, but those of a carcinoma always extend to the edge of the mass (Fig. 14-12). Like invasive carcinomas, nodules of adenosis mostly consist of distorted glands occupying the entire nodule; however, the relationship of these glands to the surrounding stroma differentiates these two lesions. The peripheral glands in foci of adenosis maintain an orderly relationship with respect to the collagen and do not disrupt its flow, whereas malignant glands invade it in a destructive fashion (Fig. 14-13).

Several writers comment on the importance of invasion of fat in the identification of invasive carcinoma, but invasive carcinomas sometimes grow in fibrous and glandular tissue apart from the fat. Thus, one cannot depend on the presence of suspicious

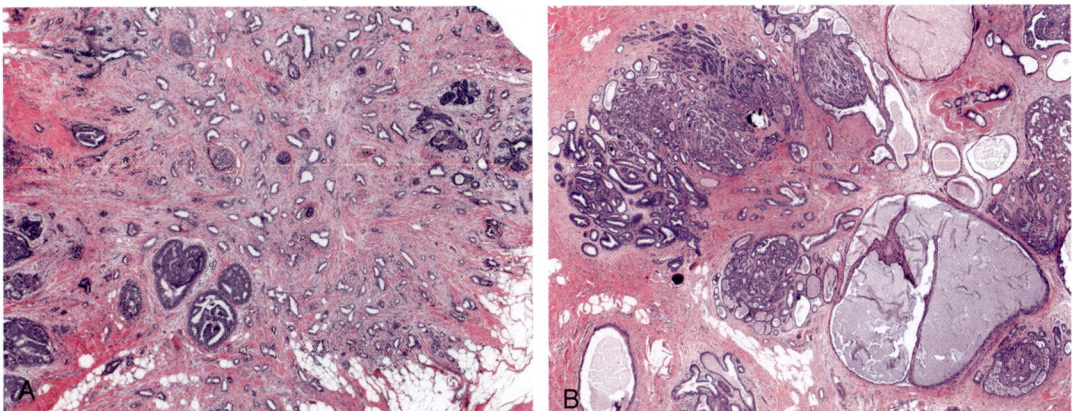

Figure 14-12 A, The glands of an invasive carcinoma extend to the periphery of the mass. **B,** In contrast, those of a radial scar remain confined to the altered stroma of the nidus.

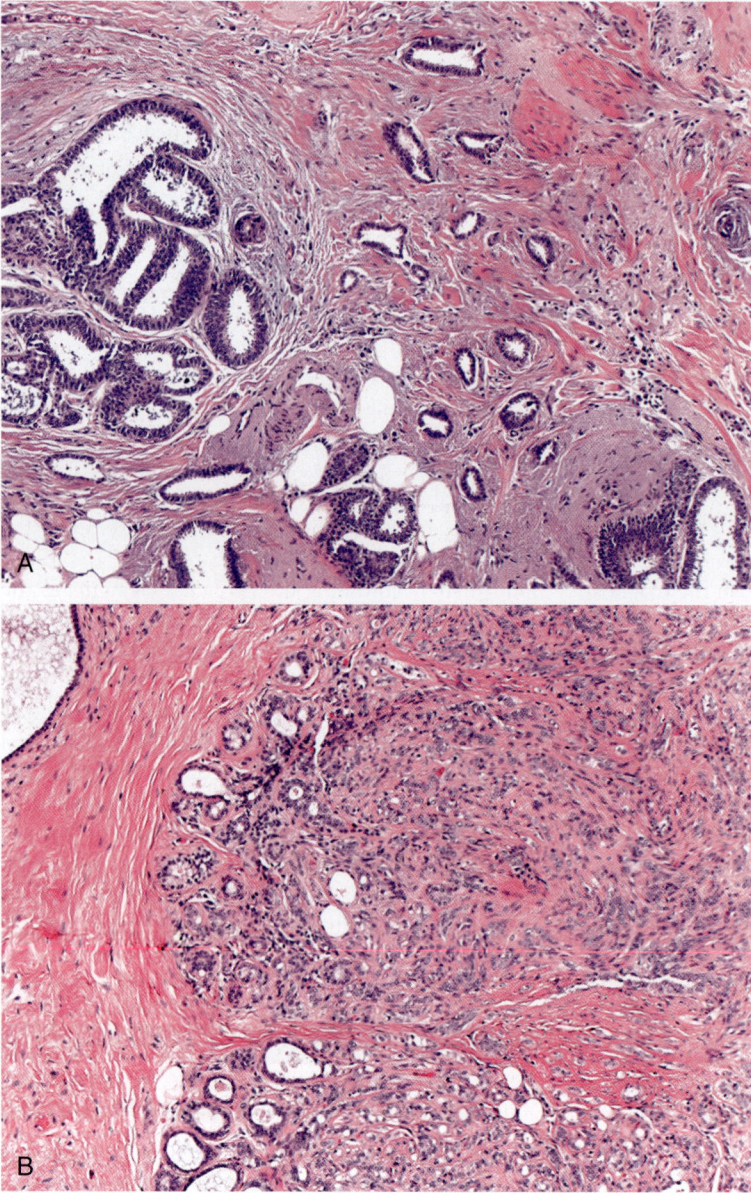

Figure 14-13 Malignant glands at the edge of a carcinoma interrupt the orderly flow of the collagen bundles in **A**, but the peripheral glands in a nodule of adenosis do not, as seen in **B**.

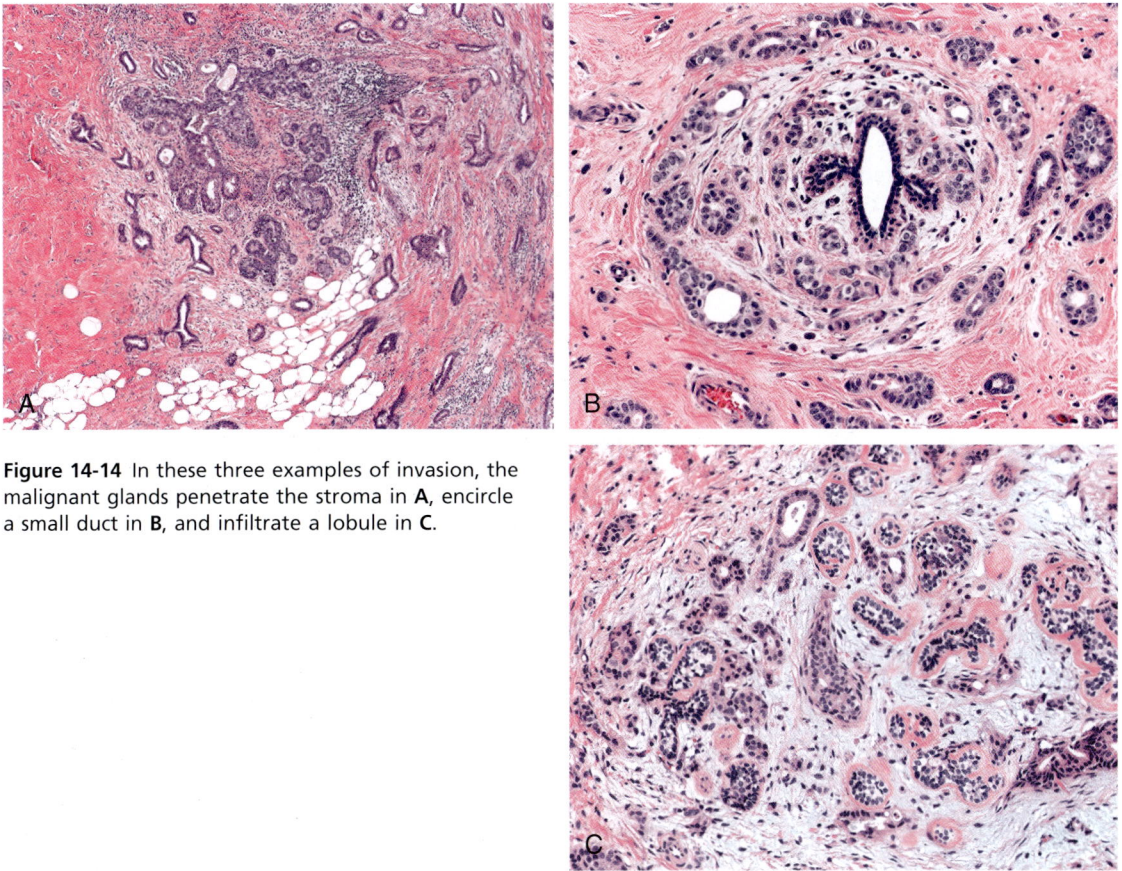

Figure 14-14 In these three examples of invasion, the malignant glands penetrate the stroma in **A**, encircle a small duct in **B**, and infiltrate a lobule in **C**.

glands in adipose tissue alone to establish the presence of invasion. Encirclement or penetration of preexisting, benign glandular structures and destruction of collagen bundles provide just as convincing evidence of malignancy as invasion of fat. Furthermore, invasion of glandular tissue or fibrous connective tissue occurs in every invasive carcinoma, whereas invasion of adipose tissue does not (Fig. 14-14). Pathologists will find that the ability to recognize this pattern of invasion proves an especially useful skill in the analysis of sclerosing lesions.

Characteristics of the Associated Ductal Epithelial Proliferation

In contrast to the conventional hyperplasia seen in the ducts of many scars, low-grade ductal carcinoma in situ occupies the ducts adjacent to the invasive carcinoma in the majority of examples. The presence of ductal carcinoma in situ does not establish the malignant nature of the irregular glands, of course, nor does the absence of ductal carcinoma in situ

exclude the diagnosis of invasive carcinoma; however, the nature of any associated noninvasive epithelial proliferation often confirms the pathologist's impression of the nature of the suspicious glands.

Summary

Invasive carcinomas create bulging infiltrative masses as the proliferation of the neoplastic glands and the reaction of the mammary stroma add tissue to the breast. The malignant glands usually form a compact central mass with radiating bands composed of neoplastic epithelial clusters and reactive stroma. Because carcinomas overrun the underlying mammary structures, they lack an internal organization, and the malignant cells extend to the periphery of the mass. This region of the mass offers the pathologist the best opportunity to detect the destructive and infiltrative properties of the malignant cells. Ductal carcinoma in situ occupies ducts and lobules in the vicinity of many invasive ductal carcinomas (see Box 14-1).

PROBLEMS IN THE DIAGNOSIS OF WELL-DIFFERENTIATED CARCINOMA

Once one learns to recognize the phenomenon of invasion with confidence, the diagnosis of well-differentiated invasive carcinomas does not give rise to many problems, because all invasive carcinomas demonstrate destructive invasion, which all benign lesions lack. Thus, certain forms of adenosis, such as florid adenosis and tubular adenosis, superficially resemble well-differentiated ductal carcinoma, but in neither lesion do the proliferative glands display characteristics of invasion. Two benign conditions can simulate the pattern of invasion more closely than these two forms of adenosis: atrophy and microglandular adenosis. Atrophy affects both the stromal and glandular components of the gland. When the stroma atrophies, adipose tissue replaces the fibrous connective tissue, leaving ductules and acini surrounded by fat. Atrophy of the acini can leave small clusters of epithelial cells seemingly dispersed within dense fibrous tissue. Microglandular adenosis consists of a proliferation of glands that permeate a region of the breast, and their lack of an anatomic arrangement mimics the pattern of invasion. Both of these lesions can look like an invasive carcinoma that has not incited a stromal reaction. Low-grade adenosquamous carcinoma stands out as the type of low-grade ductal carcinoma most easily confused with a benign sclerosing lesion. The bland cytologic characteristics of the neoplastic cells, the frequent association of this type of invasive carcinoma with sclerosing papillomas and radial scars, and the staining of the neoplastic cells for myoepithelial proteins all compound this confusion. Finally, pathologists frequently struggle with the distinction between well-differentiated invasive ductal carcinoma and tubular carcinoma. The following discussions examine these problems.

Adenosis

Two patterns of adenosis, florid adenosis and tubular adenosis, superficially resemble well-differentiated invasive ductal carcinoma; however, examination of the relationship between the glands and the stroma establishes the benign nature of these glandular proliferations (Fig. 14-15). The glands do not infiltrate the stroma in the way that carcinomas do and they possess myoepithelial cells, which carcinomas lack. In uncommon examples of adenosis and other sclerosing lesions, the myoepithelial cells may not stain in the expected pattern. They might express calponin and p63 protein but not myosin heavy chain, for example (Fig. 14-16). The existence of unexpected profiles such as this one makes it advisable to carry out a panel of immunohistochemical stains when searching for myoepithelial cells.

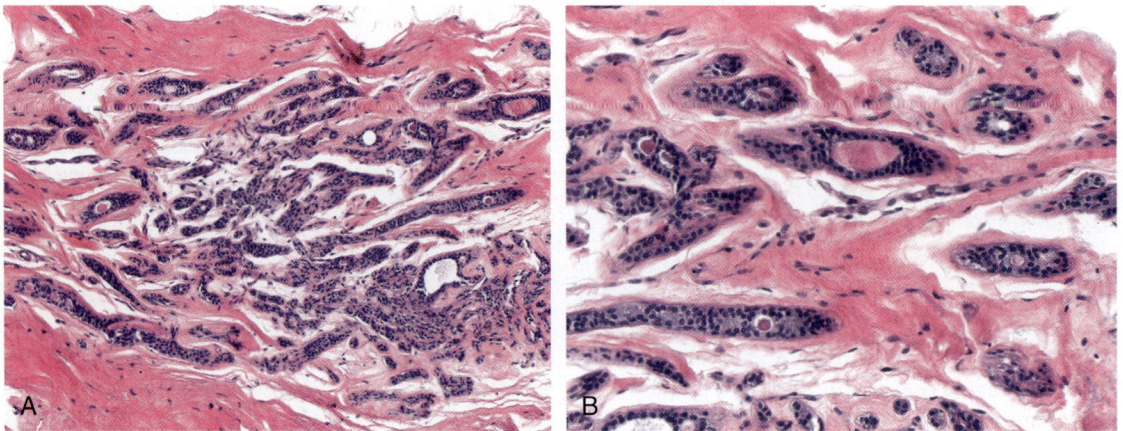

Figure 14-15 A, The irregular pattern and pointed ends of the tubules in the focus of tubular adenosis might make one consider the diagnosis of invasive carcinoma. **B,** However, the glands do not disrupt the arrangement of the collagen bundles.

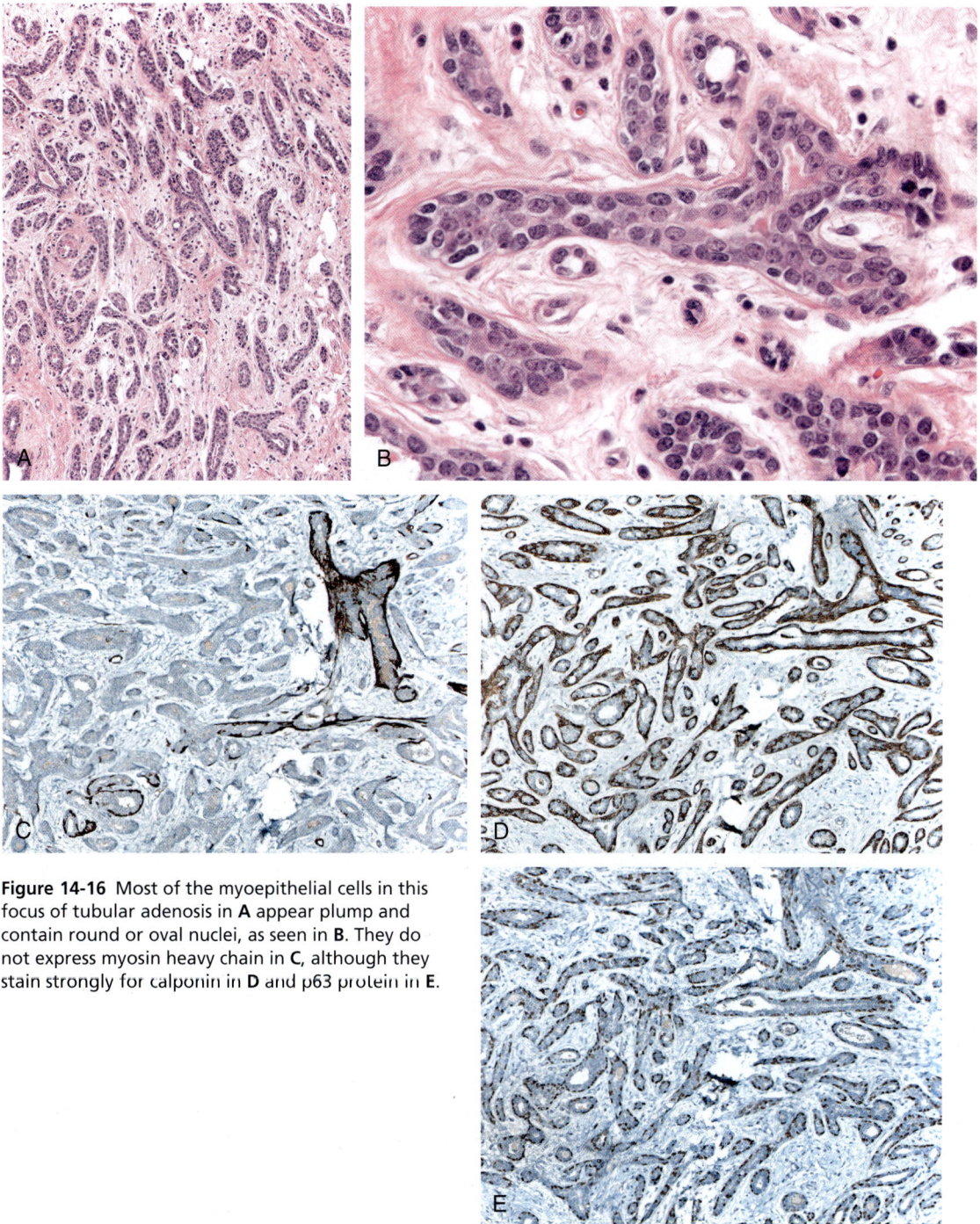

Figure 14-16 Most of the myoepithelial cells in this focus of tubular adenosis in **A** appear plump and contain round or oval nuclei, as seen in **B**. They do not express myosin heavy chain in **C**, although they stain strongly for calponin in **D** and p63 protein in **E**.

Atrophy

Conventional Atrophy

Conventional atrophy affects both the stroma and the glandular tissue. Stromal atrophy consists of replacement of fibrous connective tissue with fat. The process begins during the reproductive years, progresses at different rates from one woman to the next, and usually affects the nonspecialized stroma more than the specialized fibrous connective tissue, although uncommon cases demonstrate the opposite pattern (Fig. 14-17). Atrophy of the glandular tissue probably begins somewhat later, perhaps during the perimenopausal decade. The ducts remain generally unaltered, but the lobules show profound changes (Fig. 14-18). The acini vanish; consequently, the lobules come to consist of little more than

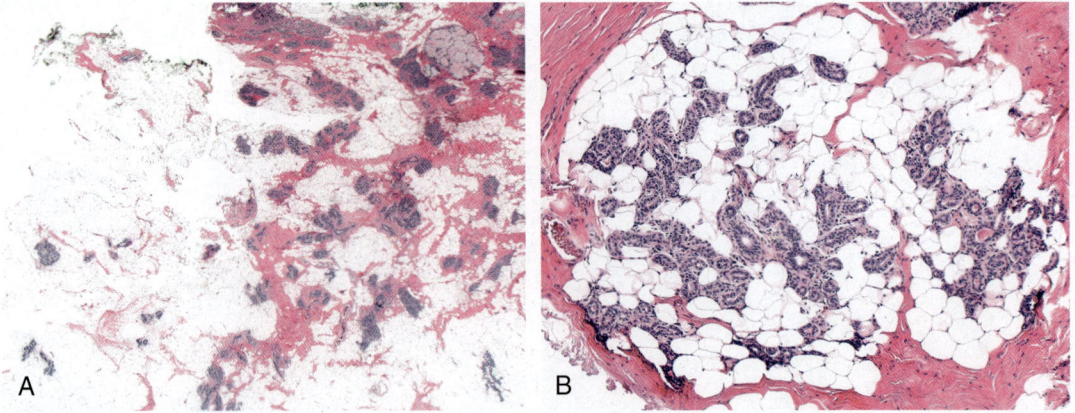

Figure 14-17 Fat has replaced much of the fibrous connective tissue of the nonspecialized stroma in **A** and the specialized stroma within the lobule in **B**.

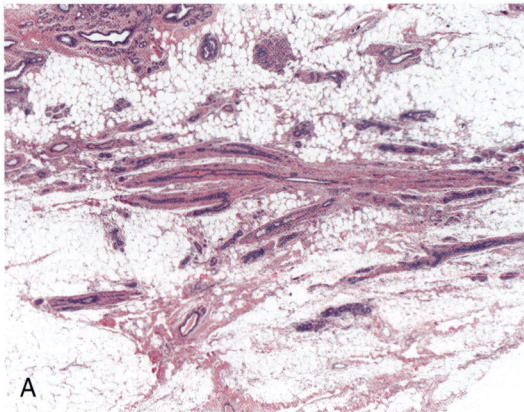

Figure 14-18 A, Glandular atrophy has caused most of the lobules in this region of the breast to disappear. **B,** The remaining lobules consist of terminal ductules and just a few acini. The stroma also displays marked atrophy.

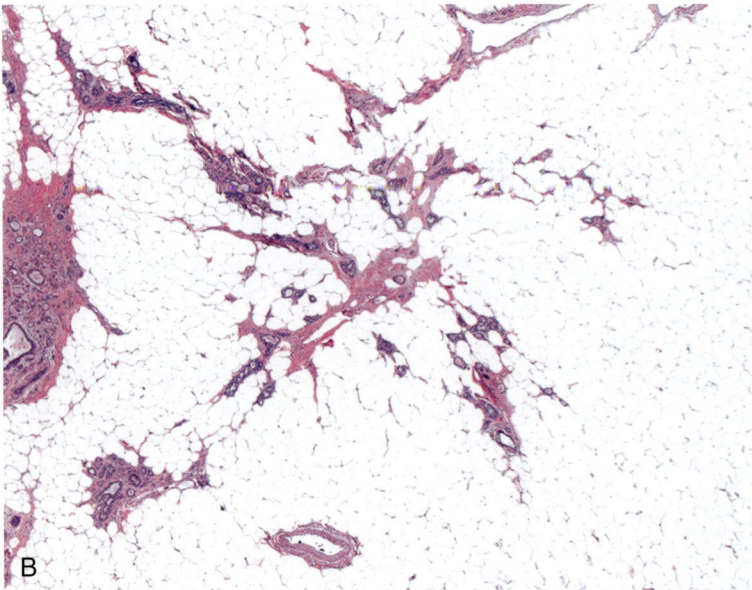

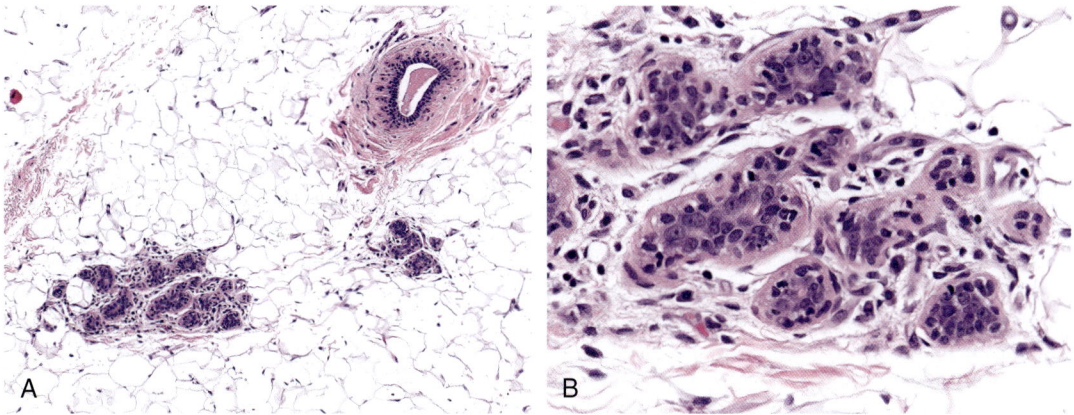

Figure 14-19 A, Atrophic lobules. **B,** At higher magnification, the lobules can be seen to consist of coiled intralobular terminal ductules supported by stroma containing a few fibroblasts, plasma cells, and lymphocytes. **C,** In extreme atrophy, most of the stroma disappears, too; just a few fibroblasts and a single capillary surround the gland.

intralobular terminal ductules surrounded by a few fibroblasts, capillaries, and plasma cells, and even these stromal components can nearly disappear in especially advanced examples (Fig. 14-19). The resulting close juxtaposition of small glands and adipocytes creates an appearance that superficially mimics the pattern of well-differentiated carcinoma invading adipose tissue with little or no stromal reaction. Several observations help pathologists differentiate these two conditions.

First, although glandular atrophy reduces the number of acini and thereby simplifies the lobules, it does not alter their architecture. They usually remain as localized, smoothly contoured clusters of orderly, evenly spaced glands of uniform size. Neoplastic glands, in contrast, do not form lobules; instead, they penetrate the adipose tissue in a haphazard fashion (Fig. 14-20). Variations from these generalizations occur. For instance, a plane of section through the edge of an especially atrophic lobule may

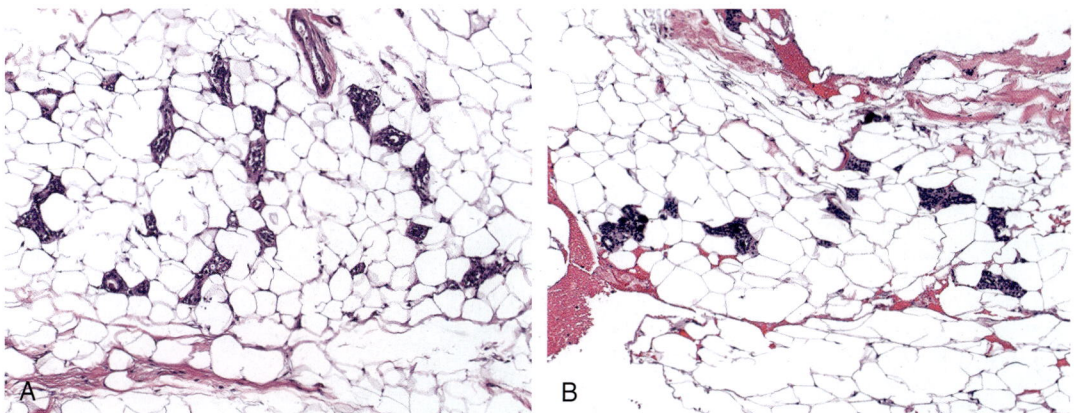

Figure 14-20 A, Despite the marked fatty atrophy of the specialized stroma, one can still recognize this collection of glands as a lobule because of their regular placement and the oval contour of the aggregate. **B,** The haphazard disposition of these glands and the irregular profile of the group reflect the malignant nature of the glands.

encompass so few acini that one would find it diffi-cult to recognize these lonely, isolated glands as com-ponents of a lobule (Fig. 14-21), and groups of carcinoma cells can cluster in round aggregates that resemble lobules (Fig. 14-22). Such masquerading foci exhibit other features that point to the proper diagnosis.

Second, thin sleeves of fibrous connective tissue sur-round the acini in atrophic lobules. This stroma either can contain a few fibroblasts and chronic inflammatory cells or can consist mostly of collagen (Fig. 14-23). From ductule to ductule, these fibrous sheaths appear uniform in composition and thickness, and they do not show reactive changes. Such orderly stroma does not surround the glands of an invasive carcinoma. If the carcinoma cells provoke a stromal response, the reac-tive tissue tends to incorporate them into a single mass (Fig. 14-24). This disorderly stromal reaction contrasts

with the organized stromal collars of atrophic ductules. In the absence of a stromal reaction, the malignant glands directly abut the adipocytes, and one can some-times observe the neoplastic clusters insinuated between fat cells (Fig. 14-25). Third, atrophic glands have round contours, a two-layered epithelium, and open lumens, whereas invasive carcinomas usually include at least a few small, irregular groups of cells that do not form lumens (Fig. 14-26). Finally, immu-nohistochemical stains for myoepithelial cells highlight their presence in atrophic acini and do not disclose such cells in most forms of invasive carcinoma.

Atrophy of the breast does not prevent the devel-opment of carcinomas. One might expect that the presence of carcinoma in situ in atrophic breast tissue would compound the difficulties distinguishing these glands from invasive carcinoma, but this com-plication does not usually develop. Although the acini

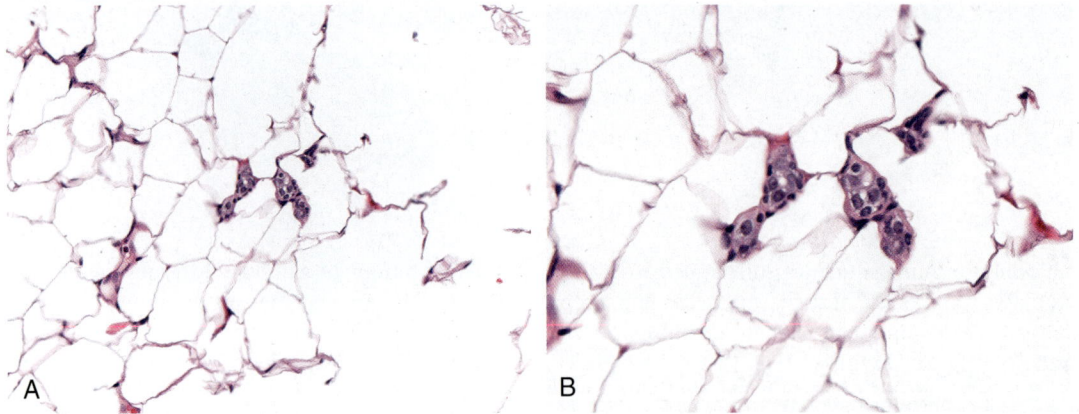

Figure 14-21 A, A plane of section through the edge of an atrophic lobule can create a picture of just a few glands isolated in the fat. **B,** One must carefully study the cytologic characteristics of the cells to recognize the glands as benign.

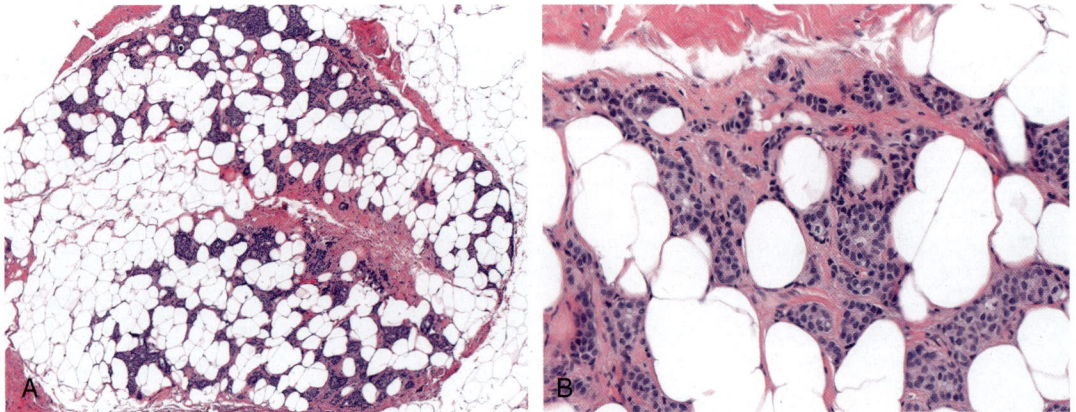

Figure 14-22 A, The round contour of this nodule of invasive carcinoma creates a pattern that superficially resembles the appearance of atrophy. **B,** Close study of the shapes of the individual groups reveals their invasive nature.

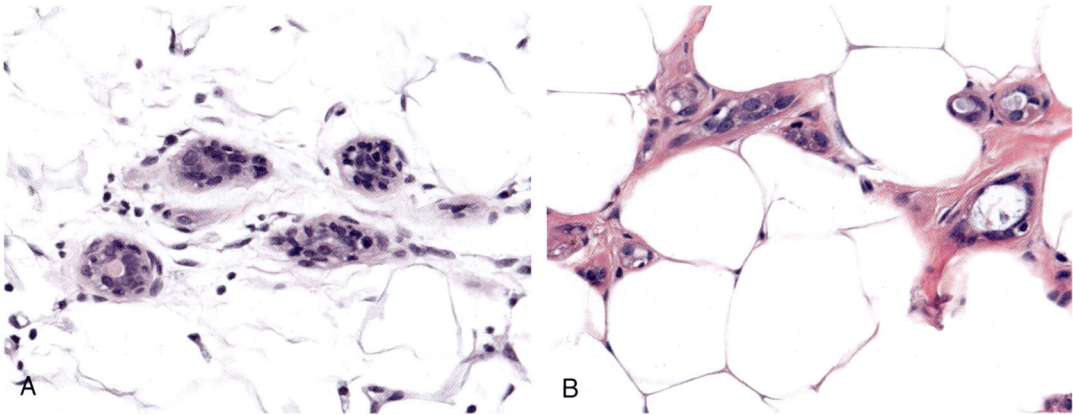

Figure 14-23 Uniform, thin sheaths of fibrous connective tissue surround atrophic ducts and acini. The fibrous connective tissue can appear slightly cellular, as seen in **A,** or collagenous, shown in **B**.

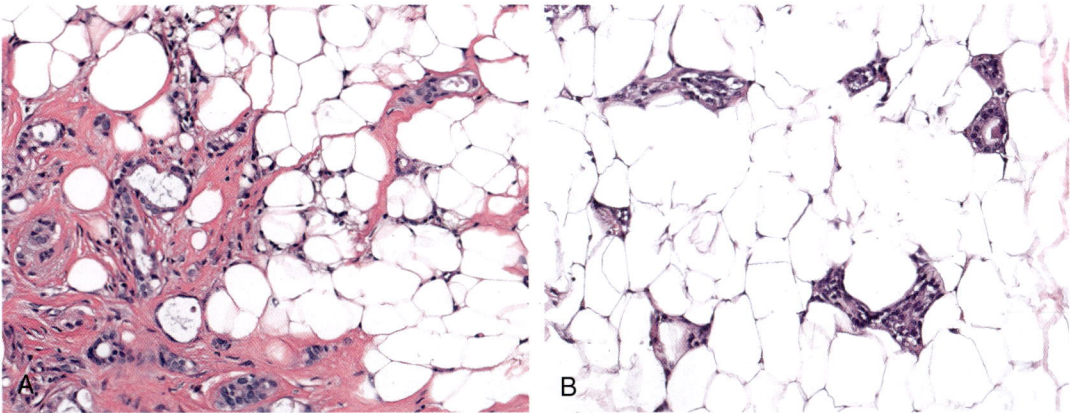

Figure 14-24 A, The collagen deposited in response to the malignant glands forms irregular collars and a confluent mass. **B,** Atrophic glands have uniform and distinct stromal coats.

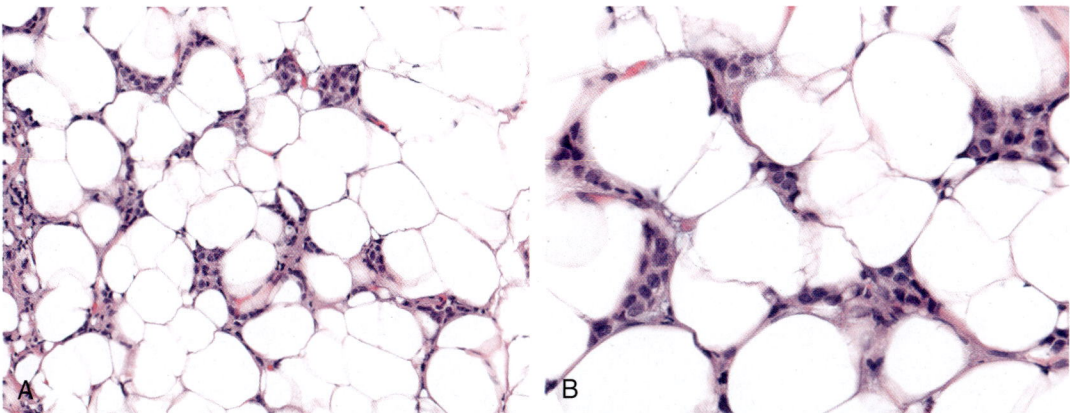

Figure 14-25 A, If invasive glands do not provoke a stromal reaction, the malignant cells directly abut the adipocytes. **B,** Miniscule groups of carcinoma cells dot the junctions of the fat cells.

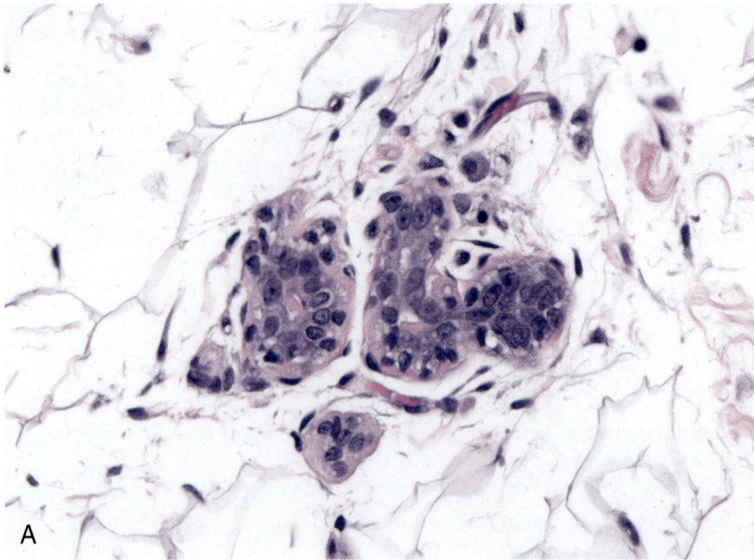

Figure 14-26 A, Atrophic glands consist of two layers of cells, luminal cells and myoepithelial cells, surrounded by a basement membrane, and the glandular lumen usually persists. **B,** Malignant glands consist entirely of epithelial cells.

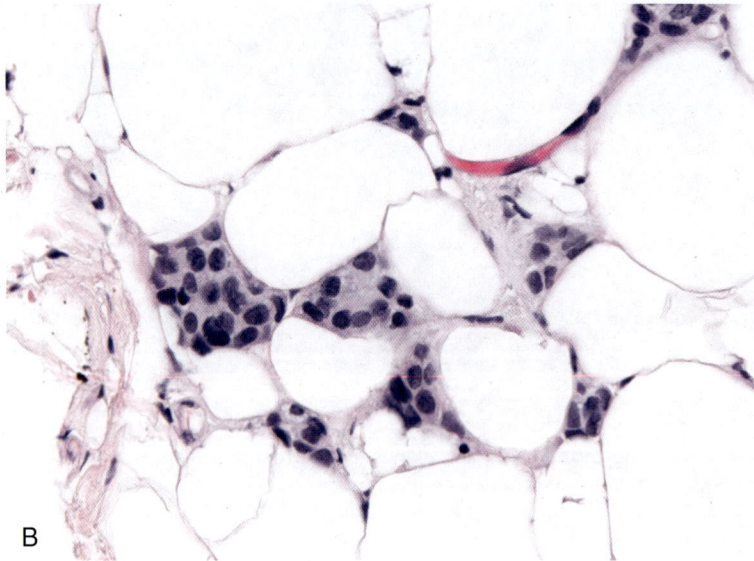

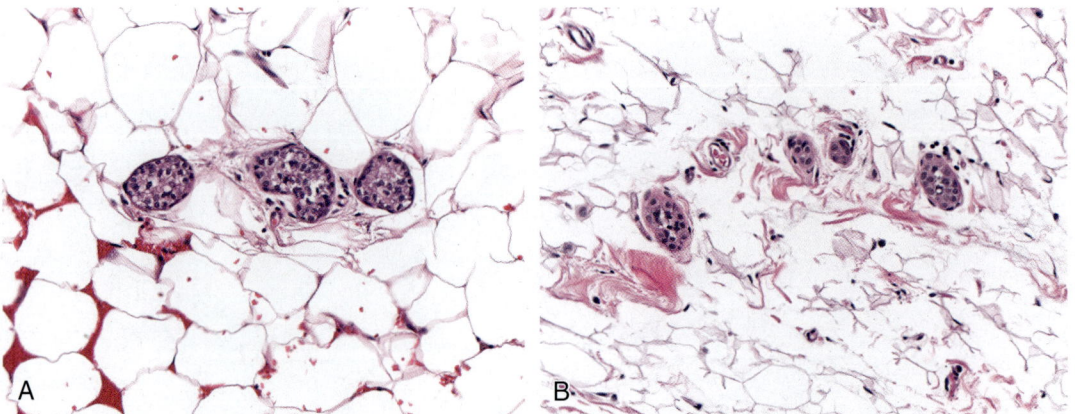

Figure 14-27 Colonization of atrophic glands by ductal carcinoma in **A** or lobular neoplasia in **B** does not alter the structural characteristics of atrophic glands. They have smooth contours, intact basement membranes, and delicate fibrous connective tissue sheaths.

harbor malignant cells and sit in a fatty stroma, they do not look like invasive carcinoma. Atrophic glands populated by malignant cells maintain the smooth, rounded contour, intact basement membranes, and delicate investment of fibrous connective tissue that typify uninvolved glands (Fig. 14-27). The presence of these findings distinguishes atrophic ductules containing carcinoma cells from nests of invasive carcinoma.

Glandular Atrophy and Stromal Fibrosis

Collagen deposition seems to underlie a variant type of atrophy. The basement membranes of the acini become thick, and in certain cases, nodules of basement membrane proteins replace entire acini. Residual acini may consist of just a few luminal cells and an accompanying myoepithelial cell or two. Dense collagen replaces the fibroblasts of the intralobular stroma. Perhaps because of this intralobular fibrosis, the surviving acini and intralobular terminal ductules become narrowed into long, slender tubules (Fig. 14-28); the same process may explain the frequent distortion of the lobular contour. Instead of their usual round or oval shape, the lobules can appear scalloped, as packets of spindly tubules and

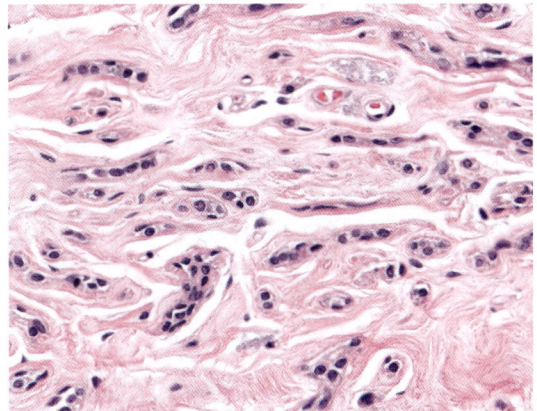

Figure 14-29 When viewed at high magnification, the compressed glands in this fibrosing type of atrophy simulate the appearance of invasive lobular carcinoma.

miniscule glands seem to flow into the adjacent fibrous connective tissue and fat. Extreme narrowing of the glands coupled with off-center planes of section can give rise to the appearance of invasive lobular carcinoma under high magnification (Fig. 14-29), and

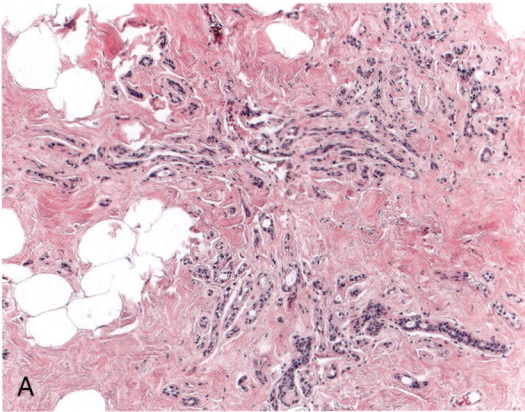

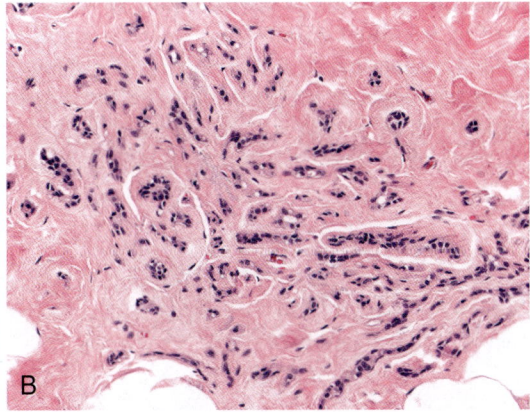

Figure 14-28 This lobule shows atrophy of the acini in **A**, thickening of the basement membranes and fibrosis of the intralobular stroma in **B**, and compression and distortion of the acini and ductules in **C**.

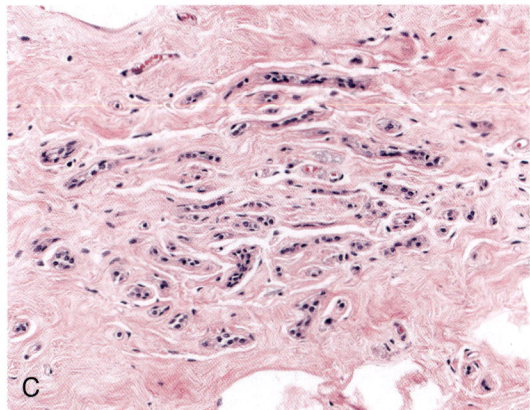

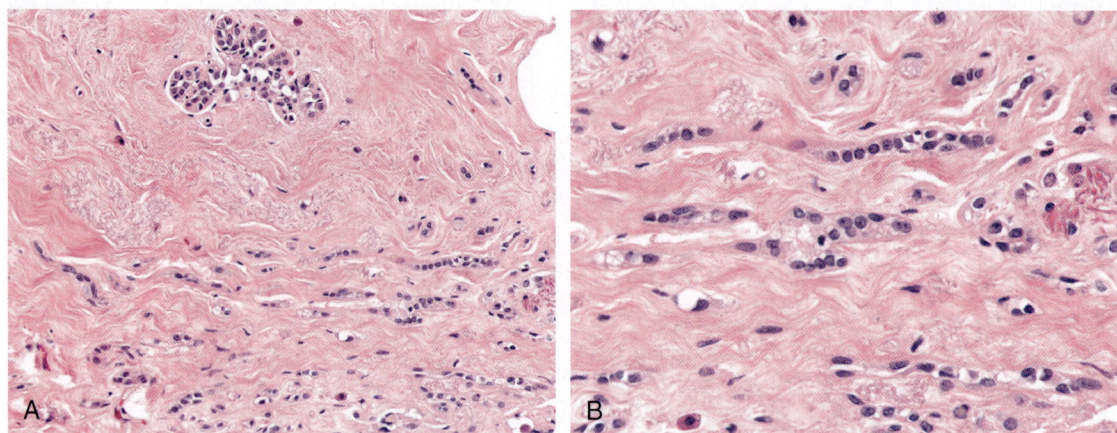

Figure 14-30 When neoplastic lobular cells like those in the ductule in the upper portion of **A** grow in the narrowed, atrophic glands in the lower portion, they simulate invasive lobular carcinoma, as shown in **B**.

the juxtaposition of this type of atrophy with lobular neoplasia increases the likelihood of an erroneous diagnosis of invasive carcinoma (Fig. 14-30). Attention to the nondestructive relationship between the epithelial cells and the stroma and to the consistent presence of myoepithelial cells prevents this mistake.

Stromal Atrophy and Sclerosing Adenosis

Atrophy of the stroma at the periphery of lobules altered by sclerosing adenosis can result in a pseudoinfiltrative appearance. Replacement of the slender stromal fibroblasts by massive adipocytes leaves the compressed glands apparently mingling with the fat (Fig. 14-31), but attention to the low-magnification view makes clear the nondestructive relationship between the glands and the fat. The former do not disrupt the structure of the latter. One does not observe compression of adipocytes or alteration of the pattern of the interlobular septa, nor does one see reactive changes such as fat necrosis and inflammation of the adipose tissue (Fig. 14-32). The cells in such foci appear bland (Fig. 14-33), and one can document the presence of myoepithelial cells by carrying out appropriate immunohistochemical staining.

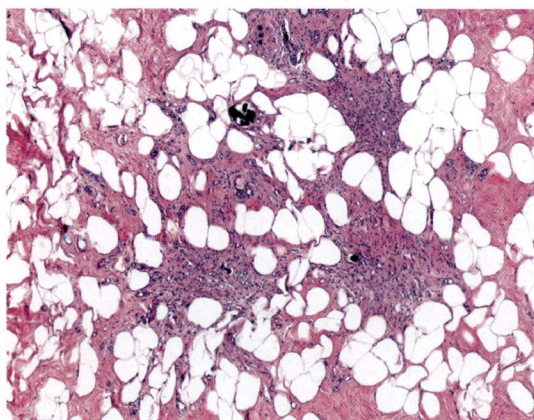

Figure 14-31 Atrophy of the nonspecialized stroma around these foci of sclerosing adenosis makes it seem like the glandular cells penetrate the fat.

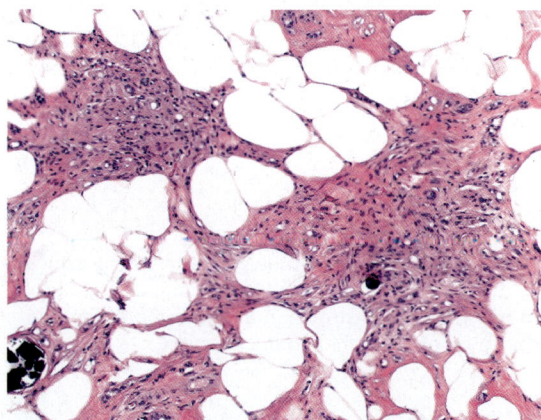

Figure 14-32 The epithelial cells do not disrupt the architecture of the fat. They do not deform the adipocytes, nor do they provoke a stromal response.

Figure 14-33 The epithelial cells display bland cytologic characteristics.

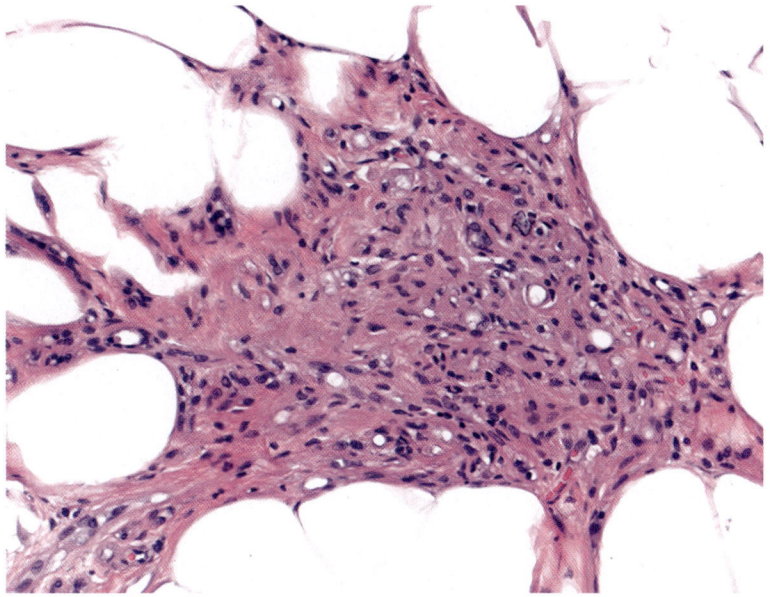

Microglandular Adenosis

Microglandular adenosis represents an unusual type of glandular proliferation in which small glands permeate a region of the breast. They grow within preexisting, normally formed mammary tissue without regard for the underlying stroma, ducts, and lobules (Fig. 14-34), and this manner of growth mimics the invasive growth pattern of a carcinoma. Mostly the glands grow as dispersed units; they can form a few aggregates, but these structures account for no more than a minor fraction of the glandular proliferation (Fig. 14-35). Thus, unlike certain other forms of adenosis, microglandular adenosis does not seem to have its roots in preexisting lobules. The glands typically exhibit round shapes, open lumens, eosinophilic secretions, a single layer of luminal-type epithelial cells, and a thin basement membrane (Fig. 14-36). The cells lining the glands possess round or oval nuclei, granular chromatin, small nucleoli, and pale, finely granular cytoplasm (Fig. 14-37). It sometimes contains eosinophilic, secretory droplets that resemble the eosinophilic substance present in the lumens. Occasional glands exhibit irregular contours, and a

Figure 14-34 Uniform, small round tubules occupy this region of the breast without regard for its underlying structure.

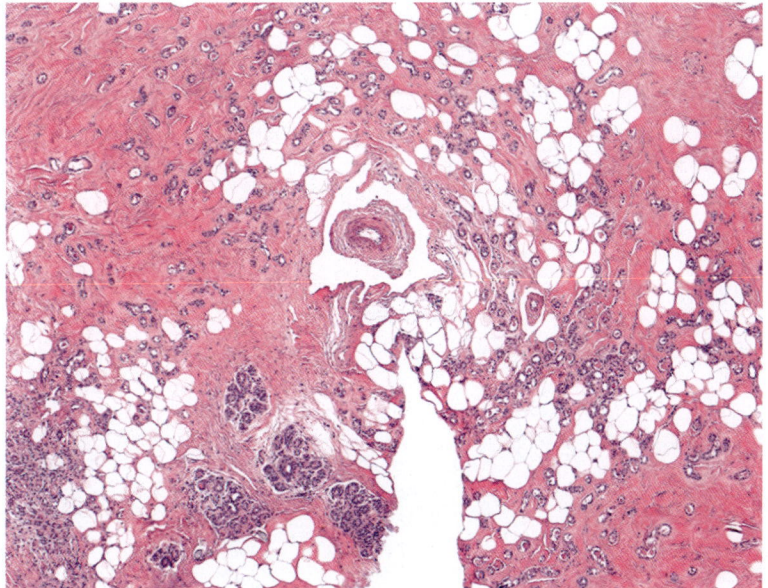

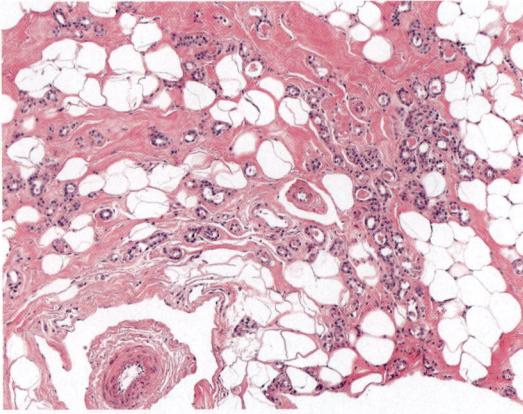

Figure 14-35 Most of the glands grow as dispersed units, but one can see a loosely formed aggregate in the right of the field.

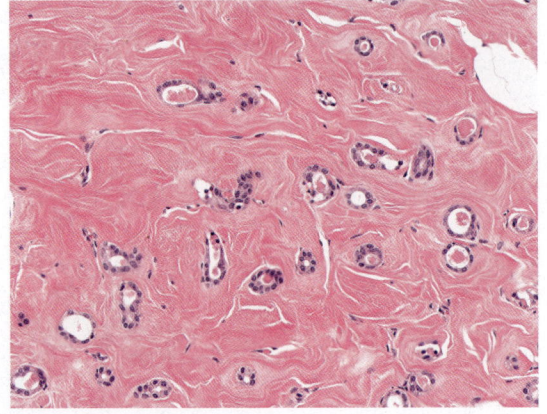

Figure 14-36 The glands have round shapes, open lumens, eosinophilic secretions, and a single layer of luminal-type epithelial cells.

Figure 14-37 The cells lining the glands have cuboidal or slightly flattened shapes, round or oval nuclei, granular chromatin, small nucleoli, and pale, finely granular cytoplasm in **A**, which can contain eosinophilic, secretory droplets in **B**.

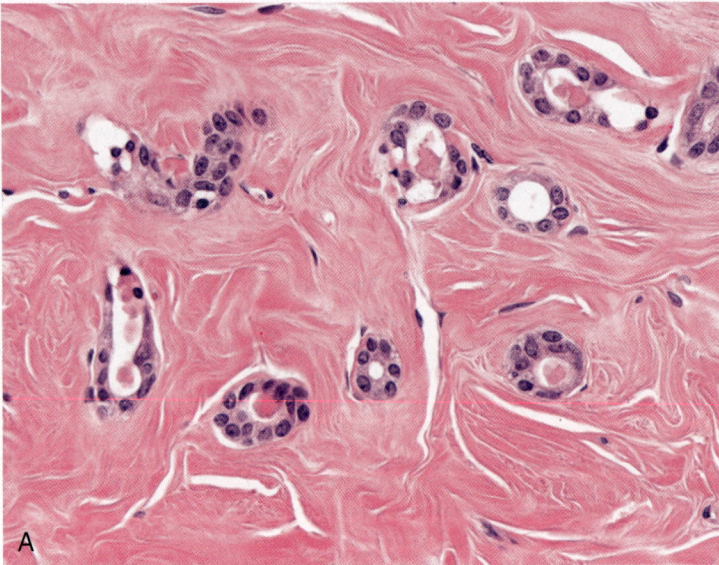

A

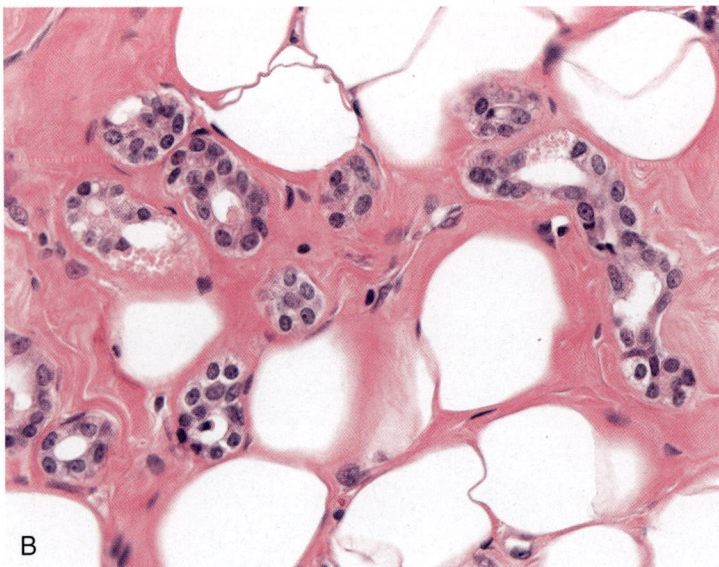

B

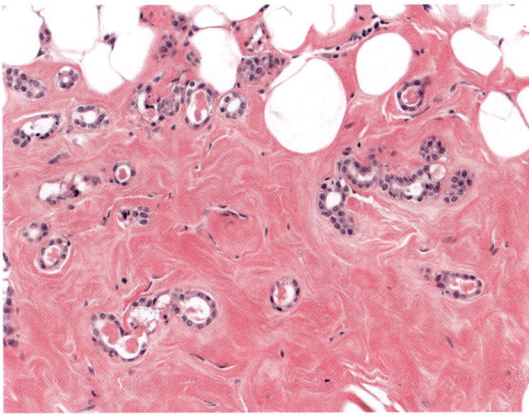

Figure 14-38 A few glands appear irregular in outline; others display a short tubular configuration.

few branch; one sometimes observes rare small solid clusters (Fig. 14-38). A thin basement membrane surrounds each gland. Despite the presence of this layer, the glands do not possess myoepithelial cells (Fig. 14-39).

The absence of myoepithelial cells and the haphazard disposition of the glands bring to mind the diagnosis of well-differentiated invasive ductal carcinoma, but several lines of evidence allow one to differentiate these two lesions. First, the cells of microglandular adenosis do not display the atypia present in carcinoma cells (Fig. 14-40). The cells of microglandular adenosis appear smaller than carcinoma cells, and the benign cells exhibit cuboidal or flattened shapes instead of the columnar configurations seen in the malignant ones. Consequently, the cells in microglandular adenosis do not appear as crowded or as closely packed as those composing the tubules of a carcinoma. The chromatin in

microglandular adenosis has a pale appearance and granular texture, whereas the chromatin in the malignant nuclei looks finely dispersed and dark. The cells of microglandular adenosis appear similar to the luminal cells of normal acini.

Second, the cells of microglandular adenosis grow almost entirely as well-structured, uniform, lumen-containing glands. Small solid groups represent only a tiny fraction of the epithelial structures, and those present number so few that one can dismiss them as glands cut in an off-center plane (Fig. 14-41). The tubules of well-differentiated carcinomas, on the other hand, vary in configuration, and many do not have a round profile; furthermore, most well-differentiated carcinomas have isolated single cells or aggregates of just two or three cells sprinkled among the glands. Third, the cells of microglandular adenosis do not express estrogen receptor protein or epithelial membrane antigen, whereas well-differentiated carcinomas typically express both proteins. Finally, pathologists should remember that well-differentiated carcinoma arises much more frequently than microglandular adenosis. When faced with a difficult case, one should probably favor the diagnosis of carcinoma until one can establish a diagnosis of microglandular adenosis by studying the entirety of the lesion and performing immunohistochemical staining.

The nature of microglandular adenosis remains open to study. The absence of myoepithelial cells in the proliferative glands and the lack of a lobular organization of the glands suggest that the pathogenesis of microglandular adenosis differs from that of other forms of adenosis. The infiltrative manner of growth and the subtle disruption of the pattern of collagen bundles (Fig. 14-42) lead this author to wonder whether the lesion could represent a distinctive type

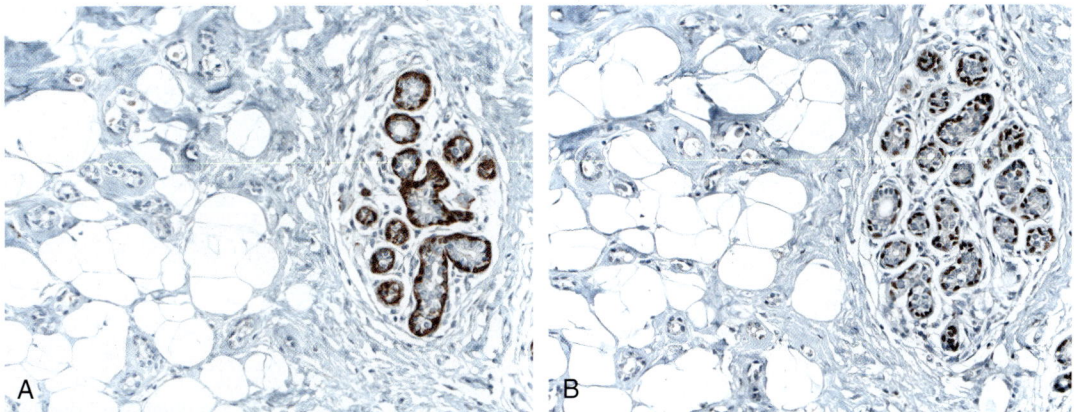

Figure 14-39 Immunohistochemical stains for calponin in **A** and p63 protein in **B** do not disclose myoepithelial cells in the glands of microglandular adenosis.

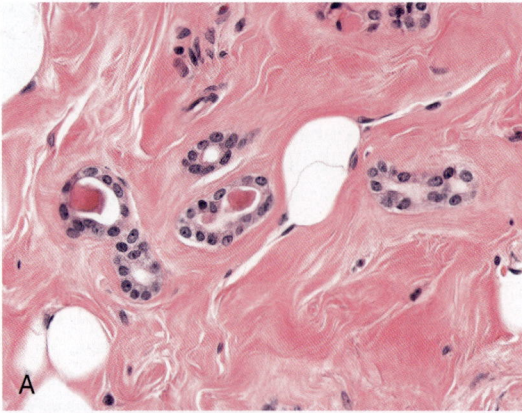

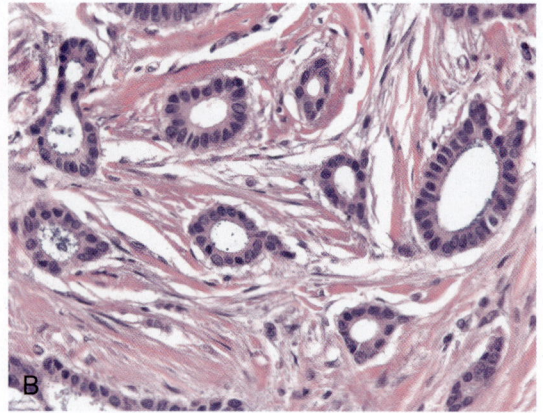

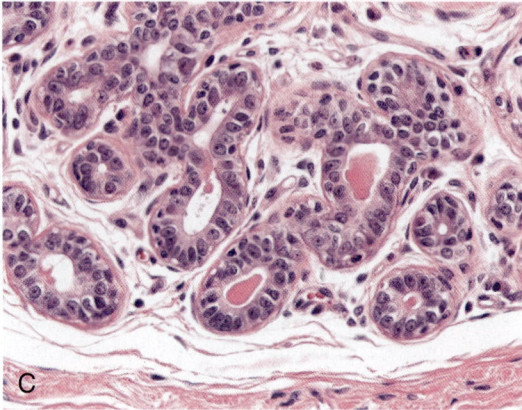

Figure 14-40 The cells of microglandular adenosis appear bland in **A** and do not exhibit the atypical cytologic features seen in carcinomas in **B**; instead, the cells of microglandular adenosis resemble the luminal cells of normal acini, shown in **C**.

of well-differentiated invasive carcinoma. The presence of secretory material within the glands and of eosinophilic droplets within the cytoplasm, as well as the similarity in the cytologic characteristics between the cells of microglandular adenosis and acinar luminal cells, raises the possibility that microglandular adenosis might constitute a carcinoma displaying features similar to those of normal estrogen-receptor-negative luminal cells. This unconventional thinking remains only a hypothesis until additional studies bring more information to light. Whatever the biologic nature of microglandular adenosis, clinical studies have not demonstrated that the proliferative glands have the potential for metastasis, although the lesion has

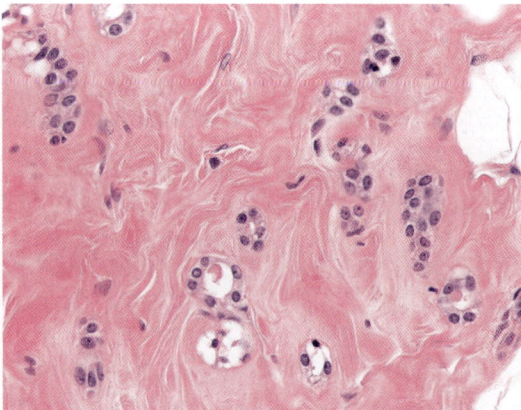

Figure 14-41 The few small clusters and solid nests that one occasionally sees in cases of microglandular adenosis may represent off-center sections of glands.

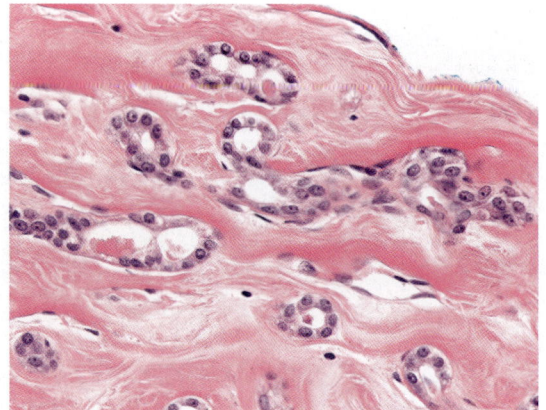

Figure 14-42 The glands of microglandular adenosis disrupt the pattern of the collagen bundles in a subtle fashion.

recurred in cases and may serve as the soil from which carcinomas, especially matrix-producing carcinomas, sprout. Pathologists and clinicians alike must keep this behavior in mind when devising a treatment strategy for patients with microglandular adenosis.

Low-Grade Adenosquamous Carcinoma

Classified as a variety of metaplastic carcinoma, the unusual type of low-grade invasive carcinoma known as *low-grade adenosquamous carcinoma* consists of tubules and small clusters of cells randomly disposed in a stroma composed of differing proportions of collagen and spindle cells (Fig. 14-43). The malignant cells typically grow in an especially infiltrative fashion, and one can observe them growing around ducts and within lobules at the periphery of the mass. The epithelial cells appear small, and their nuclei show only minor levels of atypia. As the name of the carcinoma implies, the neoplastic epithelial population consists of cells showing glandular characteristics and others exhibiting squamous features, the latter varying in both extent and degree (Fig. 14-44). The evidence of squamous differentiation may consist of a densely eosinophilic hue to the cytoplasm and a compact, stratified arrangement of the cells, the formation of squamous pearls (Fig. 14-45), or the creation of squamous-lined cysts. The stroma surrounding the squamous nests most often appears rich in spindle cells and intercellular

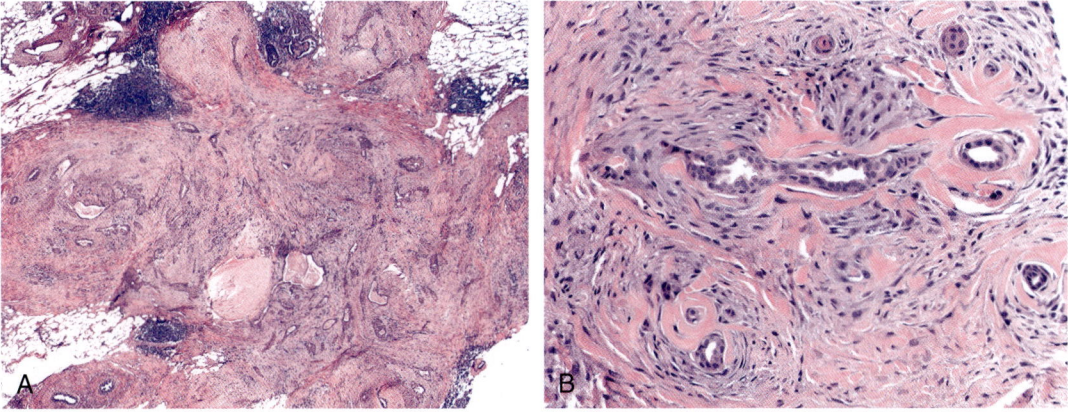

Figure 14-43 Low-grade adenosquamous carcinoma forms an irregular nodule in **A,** composed of glands embedded in a desmoplastic and collagenous stroma, as seen in **B.**

Figure 14-44 The neoplastic glands exhibit both glandular and squamous characteristics.

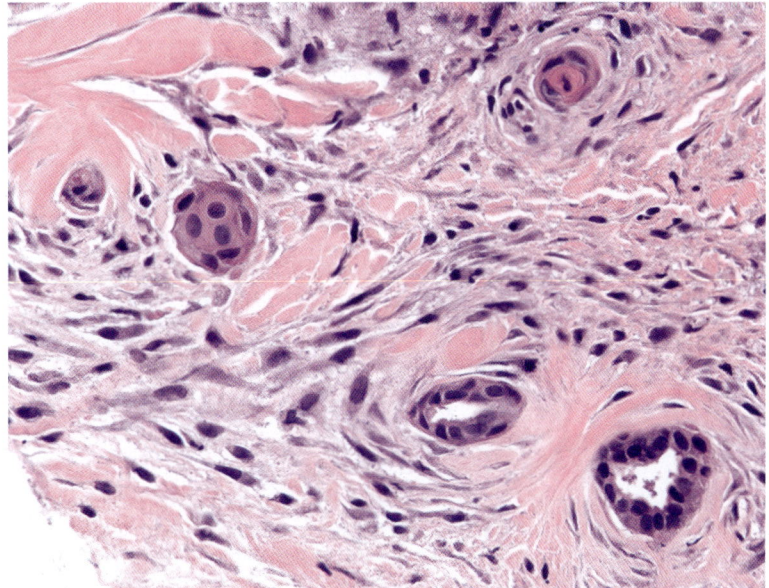

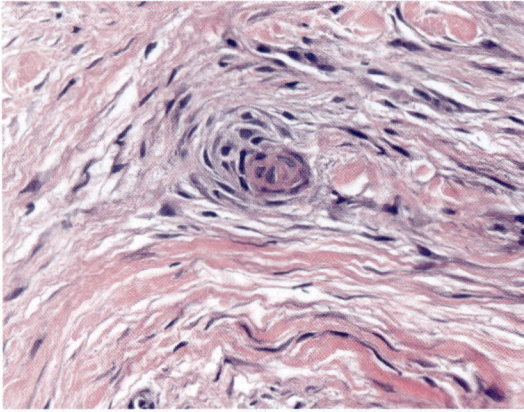

Figure 14-45 Squamous differentiation of the carcinoma cells accounts for the formation of squamous pearls.

ground substances, and the squamous cells may seem to emerge from the spindle cells. This phenomenon suggests that this lesion could represent a low-grade form of spindle cell carcinoma; however, the spindle cells do not usually express markers of epithelial cells, so the suggestion remains only a hypothesis. More distant from the epithelial cells, the stroma often has a collagenous matrix, and collections of chronic inflammatory cells commonly sit at the junction of the fibrous stroma and the fat.

Because these carcinomas frequently arise in the beds of sclerosing lesions such as radial scars and sclerosing papillomas (Fig. 14-46), pathologists may find it especially difficult to recognize the presence of the malignant glands. One could mistakenly attribute the desmoplastic appearance of the stroma to an early phase of the underlying sclerosing lesion

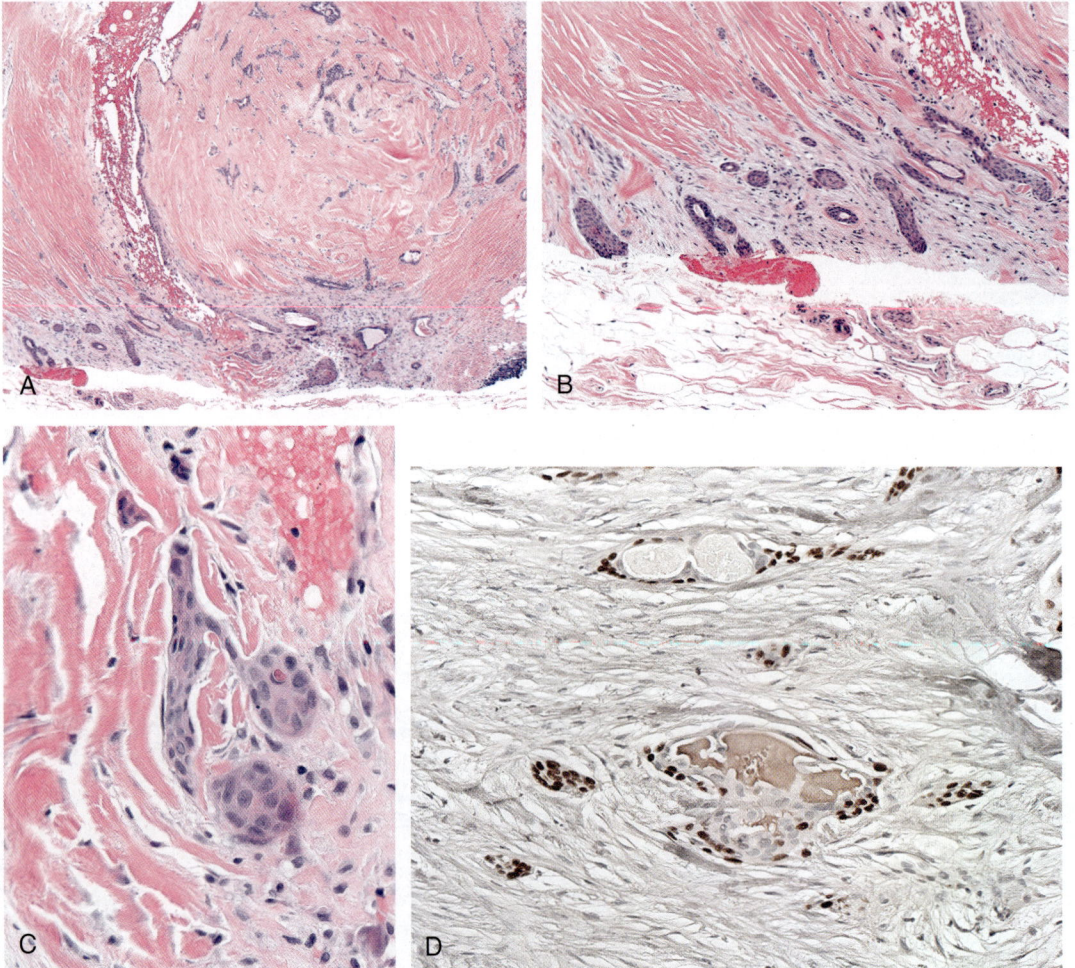

Figure 14-46 A, A sclerosing papilloma has spawned a low-grade adenosquamous carcinoma. **B,** A cellular stroma surrounds certain nests of carcinoma cells. **C,** Other clusters disrupt the collagen bundles. **D,** A stain for p63 protein documents the lack of myoepithelial cells and aberrant expression of the protein by the carcinoma cells.

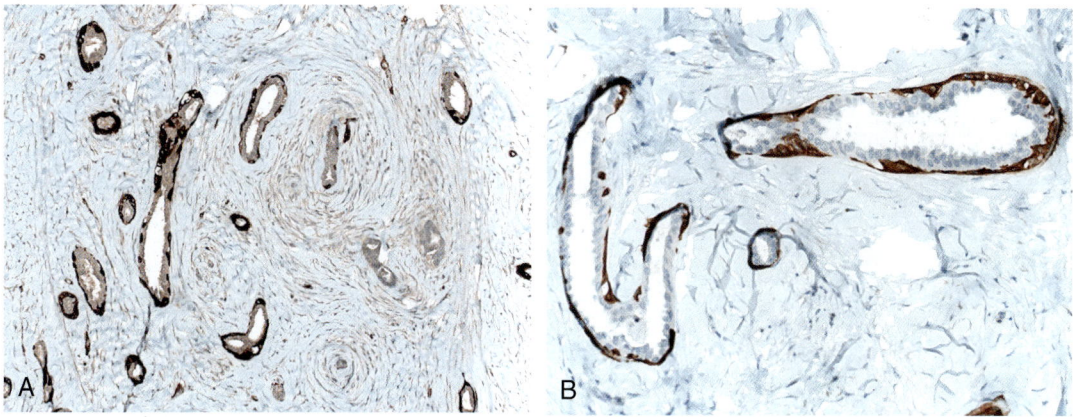

Figure 14-47 A, The glands of this adenosquamous carcinoma vary in their staining for myosin heavy chain. Certain glands contain many positive cells, whereas others do not have any at all. **B,** In a section stained for calponin, the positive cells vary in distribution within a single gland.

and the squamous characteristics of the glandular cells to a reactive phenomenon and thereby fail to appreciate the presence of the carcinoma. If one concluded that these features do not fit with the diagnosis of a sclerosing lesion, one might attempt to determine the nature of the clusters by carrying out immunohistochemical staining for proteins expressed by myoepithelial cells. This strategy may only confuse the situation, because the malignant cells of low-grade adenosquamous carcinomas usually stain for myoepithelial markers, and one might misinterpret this finding as evidence of the presence of myoepithelial cells and the benign nature of the glands. The staining pattern of the cells of adenosquamous carcinoma differs from that of normal myoepithelial cells in two ways. First, the glands do not show consistent staining. Expression of the proteins varies from gland to gland; certain glands contain many positive cells, and others none at all. The staining within a single gland also shows variation in the distribution and number of stained cells (Fig. 14-47). One also finds that staining for several markers does not yield consistent results: the malignant groups may stain for one myoepithelial protein but not another (Fig. 14-48). Second, the stained cells do not exhibit morphologic characteristics of myoepithelial cells (Fig. 14-49). Attention to these findings allows one to identify these groups as malignant cells and the lesion as a low-grade adenosquamous carcinoma.

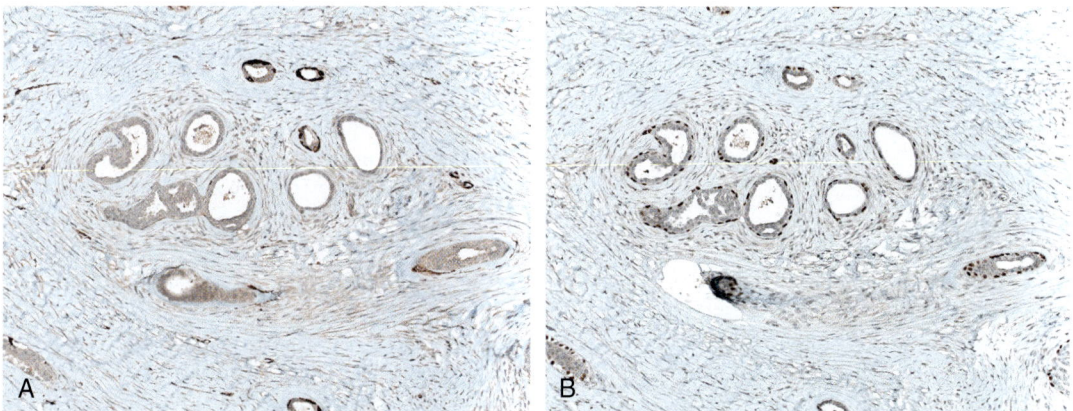

Figure 14-48 Cells in this collection of glands of an adenosquamous carcinoma do not stain for myosin heavy chain in **A,** but many in the same focus stain for p63 protein in **B.**

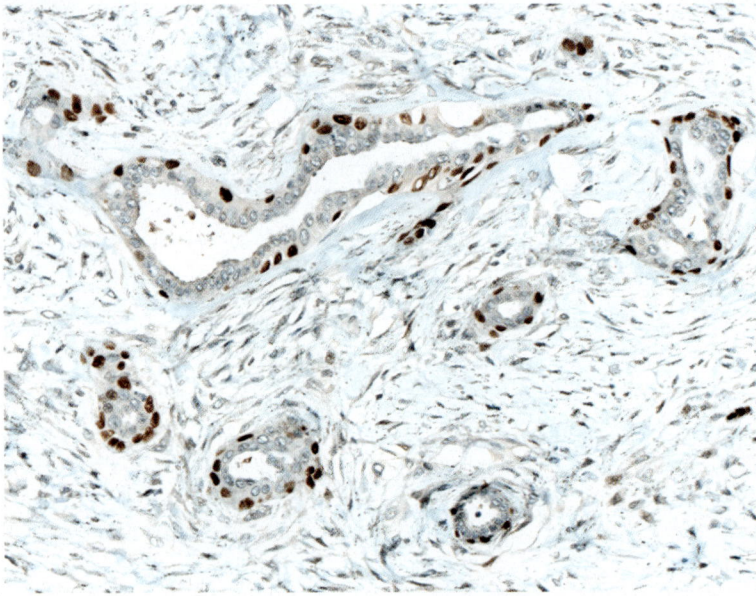

Figure 14-49 These cells stained for p63 protein do not have the flat shape and oval nuclei that normal myoepithelial cells display.

Criteria for the Diagnosis of Tubular Carcinoma

The category of well-differentiated invasive ductal carcinoma includes a special subtype designated tubular carcinoma. Authorities commonly cite a text by Drs. Victor Cornil and Louis Antoine Ranvier and another by Dr. James Ewing as the earliest references to this variety of carcinoma; however, neither of the descriptions presented in these works seems to fit with the current concept of this lesion. The first detailed account of this type of carcinoma appears in the writings of Drs. Taylor and Norris. These writers cite the following histologic features: "small gland-like or duct-like structures arranged haphazardly," "loose, cellular, desmoplastic stroma," "neoplastic epithelium made up of a single layer of uniform cuboidal cells," "little or no cytologic atypia," and "infrequent" mitotic figures.[1] They also comment on the following clinicopathologic associations: the small size of the mass, the frequent presence of low-grade ductal carcinoma in situ, the occasional presence of lobular carcinoma in situ, the limited tendency to spread to axillary lymph nodes, the tendency to involve only the low axillary lymph nodes, and the especially favorable prognosis (Box 14-2).

Studies conducted in the subsequent decade generally confirmed the original observations, although findings in certain cases deviate from the expected. Variation in the extent of tubule formation, the level of cytologic atypia, and writers' definitions of *tubule* probably accounts for much of the inconsistency in clinical behavior noted in these early publications. Subsequent investigations have demonstrated the

---

Box 14-2

Clinicopathologic characteristics of tubular carcinoma:

- Small size
- Limited metastatic potential
- Rare cause of death
- Frequent association with lobular neoplasia and flat epithelial atypia

---

importance of maintaining strict criteria for these properties, and the accumulated experience suggests that one should define *tubular carcinoma* as an invasive ductal carcinoma in which the majority of the malignant cells grow as tubules consisting of a single layer of cells characterized by low-grade cytologic atypia (Figs. 14-50 to 14-52). Pathologists differ in the requirement for the extent of tubule formation in this diagnosis. Purists would insist that at least 90% of the cells form typical tubules, but liberal observers would require that only 75% of the cells do so.

In studies using such criteria, most tubular carcinomas have shown three common attributes. First, they are small. Their mean diameter falls in the range of 1 to 1.5 cm; almost never do they span more than 3 cm. Second, tubular carcinomas have limited metastatic potential. Spread to axillary lymph nodes occurs in only about 15% of cases. The involvement usually consists of just one or two low axillary lymph nodes. Finally, this type of carcinoma rarely causes the patient's death. The literature contains only a few well-documented cases in

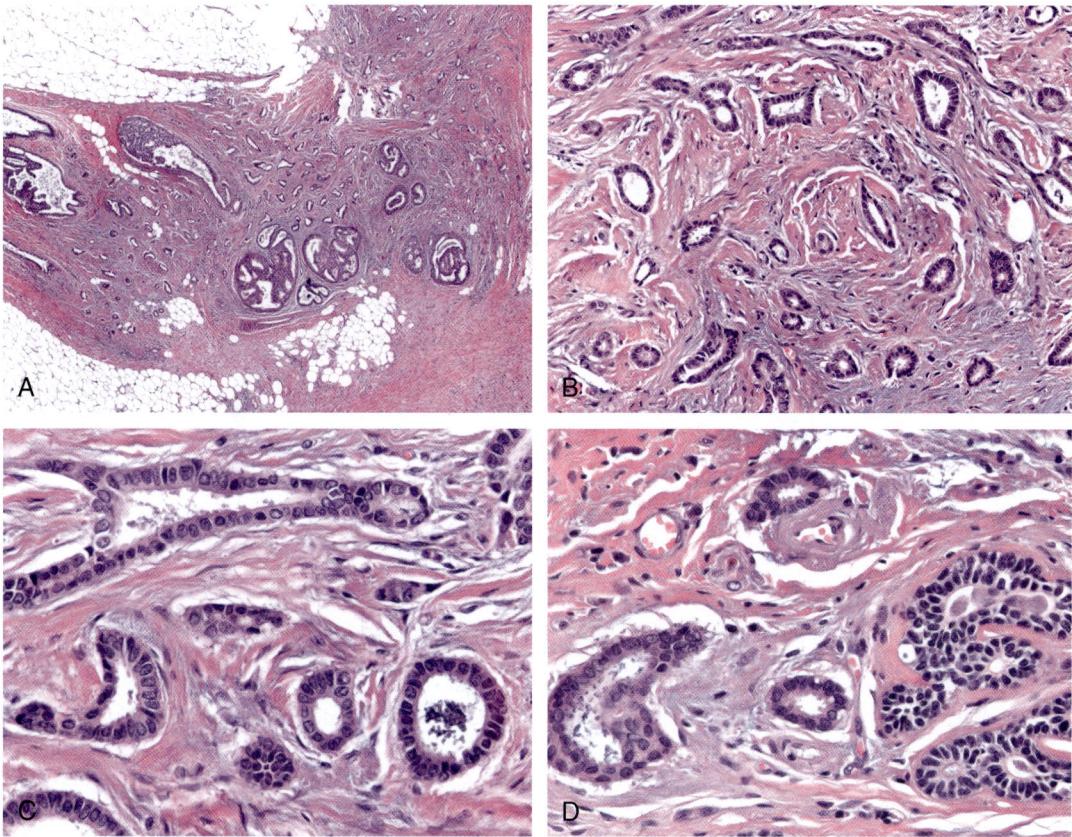

Figure 14-50 A, This carcinoma displays the characteristics of tubular carcinoma. It consists entirely of tubules formed from a single layer of cells showing only low-grade cytologic atypia in **B** and **C**, which appears obvious when one contrasts the malignant cells with entrapped benign ones, seen in **D**.

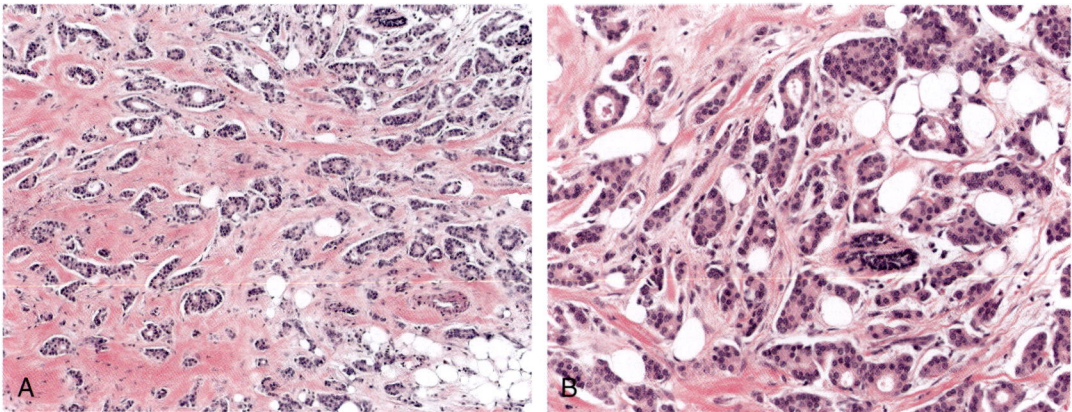

Figure 14-51 A and B, This low-grade ductal carcinoma does not form enough tubules to qualify for the diagnosis of tubular carcinoma.

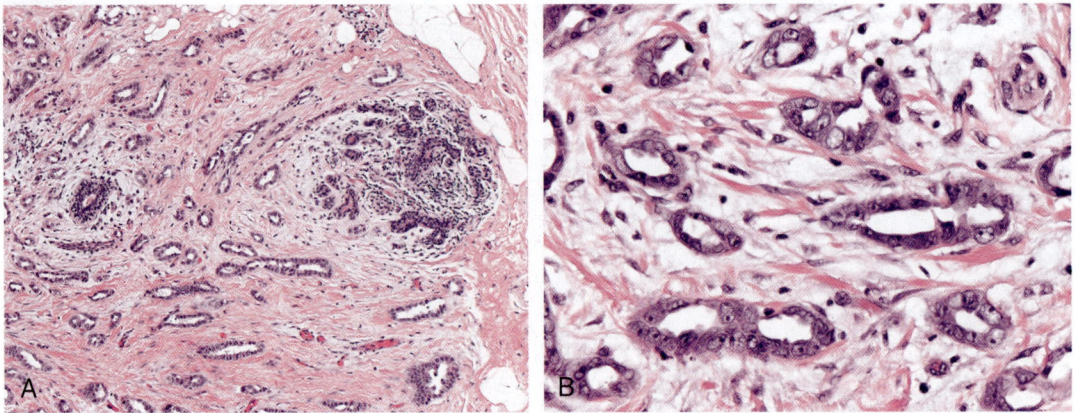

Figure 14-52 A and **B,** The degree of atypia shown by the cells of this tubule-forming invasive ductal carcinoma precludes the diagnosis of tubular carcinoma.

which patients died because of metastatic tubular carcinoma.

One must remember that these observations represent generalizations. Although they hold true in most cases, exceptions do occur. The literature contains reports of tumors as large as 6.2 cm, of others that had spread to many axillary lymph nodes, and of patients who died of disseminated tubular carcinoma. Thus, most tubular carcinomas represent small cancers with limited metastatic capability and even less potential for causing the patient's death, but unusual ones can prove deadly.

Tubular carcinomas frequently coexist with certain preneoplastic lesions and other forms of mammary carcinoma. Flat epithelial atypia accompanies tubular carcinomas so commonly that one writer once suggested the term *pretubular hyperplasia* for the former. Lobular neoplasia also stands out as an especially common companion of tubular carcinoma. The detection of any of these three lesions should prompt a search for the other two. Micropapillary ductal carcinoma in situ sometimes invades in the form of tubular carcinoma, and one can also find small, bland, invasive tubules associated with low-grade papillary carcinomas.

Reference

1. Taylor HB, Norris HJ: Well-differentiated carcinoma of the breast. Cancer 1970;25:687-692.

Selected Readings

Abdel-Fatah TM, Powe DG, Hodi Z, et al: High frequency coexistence of columnar cell lesion, lobular neoplasia, and low-grade ductal carcinoma in situ with invasive tubular carcinoma and invasive lobular carcinoma. Am J Surg Pathol 2007;31:417-426.

Carstens PHB, Greenberg RA, Francis D, et al: Tubular carcinoma of the breast: A long-term follow-up. Histopathology 1985;9:271-280.

Cooper HS, Patchefsky AS, Krall RA: Tubular carcinoma of the breast. Cancer 1978;42:2334-2342.

Deos PH, Norris HJ: Well-differentiated (tubular) carcinoma of the breast: A clinicopathologic study of 145 pure and mixed cases. Am J Clin Pathol 1982;78:1-7.

Diaz NM, McDivitt RW, Wick MR: Microglandular adenosis of the breast: An immunohistochemical comparison with tubular carcinoma. Arch Pathol Lab Med 1991;115:578-582.

Fernandez-Aguilar S, Simon P, Buxant F, et al: Tubular carcinoma of the breast and associated intra-epithelial lesions: A comparative study with invasive low-grade ductal carcinoma. Virchows Arch 2005;447:683-687.

Foschini MP, Pizzicannella G, Peterse JL, Eusebi V: Adenomyoepithelioma of the breast associated with low-grade adenosquamous and sarcomatoid carcinoma. Virchows Arch 1995;427:243-250.

Koenig C, Dadmanesh F, Bratthauer GL, et al: Carcinoma arising in microglandular adenosis: An immunohistochemical analysis of 20 intraepithelial and invasive neoplasms. Int J Surg Pathol 2000;8:303-315.

McDivitt RW, Boyce W, Gersell D: Tubular carcinoma of the breast: Clinical and pathological observations concerning 135 cases. Am J Surg Pathol 1982;6:401-411.

Parl FF, Richardson LD: The histologic and biologic spectrum of tubular carcinoma of the breast. Hum Pathol 1983;14:694-698.

Rosen PP: Microglandular adenosis: A benign lesion simulating invasive mammary carcinoma. Am J Surg Pathol 1983;7:137-144.

Rosen PP, Ernsberger D: Low-grade adenosquamous carcinoma: A variant of metaplastic mammary carcinoma. Am J Surg Pathol 1987;11:351-358.

Stalsberg H, Hartmann WH: The delimitation of tubular carcinoma of the breast. Hum Pathol 2000;31:601-607.

Taylor HB, Norris HJ: Well-differentiated carcinoma of the breast. Cancer 1970;25:687-692.

Tavassoli FA, Norris HJ: Microglandular adenosis of the breast: A clinicopathological study of 11 cases with ultrastructural observations. Am J Surg Pathol 1983;7:731-737.

Van Hoeven KH, Drudis T, Cranor ML, et al: Low-grade adenosquamous carcinoma of the breast: A clinicopathologic study of 32 cases with ultrastructural analysis. Am J Surg Pathol 1993;17:248-258.

FIBROEPITHELIAL LESIONS

15

Concepts Basic to the Analysis of Fibroepithelial Lesions

Fibroepithelial lesions form a heterogeneous group of processes, some neoplastic and others hyperplastic, united by the common presence of both glandular and stromal components. At times, writers have included lesions such as papilloma, adenomyoepithelioma, and even certain forms of metaplastic carcinoma in the family of fibroepithelial lesions; however, contemporary usage generally restricts the group to the entities discussed in this section: conventional fibroadenoma, myxoid fibroadenoma, fibroadenoma variant, phyllodes tumor (cystosarcoma phyllodes), hamartoma, and pseudoangiomatous stromal hyperplasia. The last entity most commonly creates an ill-defined area of stromal alteration, which pathologists would not usually consider a fibroepithelial lesion, but the process can also create a well-defined nodule containing both stroma and glands and resembling tumors such as fibroadenoma and phyllodes tumors. Expansion of the stromal compartment represents a common theme in all six lesions in this family. This process usually occurs because of proliferation of stromal cells, but accumulation of myxoid extracellular material can also account for the increase in the amount of stroma. In most lesions in this group, the glandular tissue represents preexisting ducts and terminal duct–lobular units entrapped by the enlarging stroma. Only in hamartoma and the related fibroadenoma variant do the glands represent newly created glandular units.

Because stromal cells play a central role in the pathogenesis of fibroepithelial lesions, discussions of the diagnosis of the entities usually emphasize the cellularity, cytologic characteristics, and growth pattern of the stroma as defining characteristics. These properties do represent important features, of course; however, this emphasis seems misplaced, because other histologic findings provide information equally important in reaching the diagnosis.

Such findings are the manner of growth of the tumor, the internal structure of the mass, and the structural and cytologic characteristics of the glands. Although these features might seem either unfamiliar or out of place in this context, they contribute important information to the analysis of fibroepithelial lesions, and students of mammary pathology will find themselves well rewarded for the time spent mastering an understanding of these additional aspects of fibroepithelial lesions.

CHARACTERISTICS OF THE STROMA

When examining the stroma of a fibroepithelial lesion, pathologists usually focus on several traditional and well-known characteristics: cellular density, nuclear morphology, and mitotic rate. These features do reflect certain important properties of the stromal cells and thereby aid in the diagnosis of these lesion, but they do not discriminate among certain fibroepithelial lesions except in the most obvious cases. Pathologists will find that the study of two other attributes of the stroma yield additional and helpful insights into the nature of the stromal proliferation: the nature of the extracellular matrix and the organization of the stroma.

Each type of mammary fibrous tissue, specialized and nonspecialized, produces a distinctive type of extracellular matrix. Specialized stromal cells grow in a background of faintly blue-staining mucopolysaccharides, whereas nonspecialized fibroblasts sit in eosinophilic collagen. Arising from specialized stromal cells, fibroadenomas and phyllodes tumors recall their heritage by producing a myxoid stroma, whereas pseudoangiomatous stromal hyperplasia, which originates from myofibroblasts of the nonspecialized stroma, has a collagenous matrix. Thus, the nature of the extracellular material in a fibroepithelial lesion helps identify the cell of origin.

Most fibroepithelial lesions contain both specialized and nonspecialized stroma, and the organization of these two stromal components also offers clues about the nature of the lesion. In cases of typical pseudoangiomatous stromal hyperplasia, the specialized stroma cuffs the glands in uniform, plump layers, and the nonspecialized stroma, which exhibits the pseudoangiomatous change, occupies the remainder of the mass. Fibroadenomas maintain an orderly relationship between the two types of fibrous stroma, but phyllodes tumors typically disrupt this organization. Many hamartomas do not have clearly defined specialized and nonspecialized stromal components. Determining the distribution of the stroma within the mass often points the pathologist in the direction of the proper diagnosis.

MANNER OF GROWTH

Fibroepithelial lesions can grow in three ways: within the specialized stromal compartment, within the nonspecialized stromal compartment, or without regard to either stromal compartment. The third category, growth without regard to either stromal compartment, has two subcategories, growth by displacement and growth by invasion.

Growth within the Specialized Stromal Compartment

The specialized stromal compartment consists of a continuous sleeve of fibrous connective tissue investing all the ducts and terminal duct–lobular units of the mammary tree. This layer of loose stroma occupies the region between the basement membrane of the epithelium and the dense nonspecialized stroma. Fibroblasts of the specialized stromal compartment give rise to tumors, and the neoplastic fibroblasts of certain of these tumors lack the ability to extend into adjacent tissues. Such neoplasms therefore expand the specialized stromal compartment and create a mass surrounding a segment of the ductal tree. Continuing enlargement of the mass sequentially envelops more and more lobules and ducts, and in the process, the glandular tissue becomes distorted in a characteristic fashion. Nonspecialized stroma, too, becomes engulfed within the mass, but adipose tissue usually does not. Because the specialized stromal compartment of one duct system does not communicate with that of any other duct system directly, these lesions lie within the distribution of a single major duct, usually with their long axis parallel to the main axis of the duct. Fibroadenomas and myxoid fibroadenomas exemplify

this manner of growth, and regions of many phyllodes tumors demonstrate this growth pattern, also.

Growth within the Nonspecialized Stromal Compartment

The nonspecialized stroma encases the specialized stroma and the glands held within it. The nonspecialized stroma adjacent to the specialized stroma consists of dense collagen; the more distant stroma consists of fat. Lesions of the nonspecialized fibrous connective tissue therefore entrap both the preexisting glands with their specialized stromal investment situated on one surface and the fat present on the opposite one. The engulfed glands sometimes grow, but they do not show the pattern of distortion characteristic of lesions growing within the specialized stromal compartment. Of the fibroepithelial tumors under consideration, only pseudoangiomatous stromal hyperplasia displays this pattern of growth.

Growth Unrelated to Either Stromal Compartment

Certain fibroepithelial tumors do not grow in either stromal compartment; instead, they either displace or invade the underlying parenchyma. Familiar to all pathologists, these two patterns of growth require only superficial description.

Growth by Displacement

Tumors that lack the capacity to invade grow by displacing the mammary parenchyma, which becomes compressed in a rim around the periphery of the tumor; consequently, all the tissues within the mass represent neoplastic tissue. In particular, the glands within a fibroepithelial tumor of this type constitute newly created, neoplastic structures rather than distorted preexisting ducts and lobules. Therefore, these neoplastic glands do not exhibit the expected anatomic structure of the mammary glandular tissues, nor do they show the pattern of distortion seen in lesions characterized by growth within the specialized stromal compartment. Fibroadenoma variants and hamartomas grow in this way exclusively.

Growth by Invasion

Growth by invasion creates an infiltrative appearance in which neoplastic cells encase or permeate preexisting structures such as ducts, lobules, and fat. Masses that grow in this way include both neoplastic and non-neoplastic tissues. Terminal duct–lobular units entrapped in the mass retain their proper microanatomic structure and do not display the pattern of distortion seen in tumors of specialized stroma. Among fibroepithelial lesions, only phyllodes tumors exhibit an invasive pattern of growth, and nearly all phyllodes tumors have invasive properties, at least in part.

INTERNAL STRUCTURE OF THE MASS

During their growth, fibroepithelial lesions such as fibroadenoma and pseudoangiomatous stromal hyperplasia distort the underlying mammary parenchyma, but they do not destroy the anatomic relationships of its components. The epithelium, specialized stroma, collagenous nonspecialized stroma, and fat remain in their proper topologic positions, and the internal structures of these lesions exhibit this organization. Thus, bands of nonspecialized stroma demarcate the preexisting ducts and lobules engulfed during the growth of a fibroadenoma, and uniform cuffs of specialized stroma outline the preexisting ductules and acini in nodular pseudoangiomatous stromal hyperplasia.

Phyllodes tumors, on the other hand, have invasive properties, and the process of invasion tends to obscure or even to obliterate the relationships among the tissue components. This disturbance in organization creates the heterogeneous appearance of phyllodes tumors. The distinction between specialized and nonspecialized stroma blurs, and the ratio of glands to stroma varies, as the neoplastic specialized stromal cells stray beyond their proper location and overpopulate regions of the tumor.

Hamartomas arise as developmental misadventures; from their onset, they lack the proper histologic relationship among their components. Acini might sit in nonspecialized stroma or fat, for example, or the stroma may not have clearly defined specialized and nonspecialized compartments. By analyzing the way in which the components of a fibroepithelial lesion interrelate, pathologists can derive important information about the pathogenesis of the mass.

Characteristics of the Glands

Because stromal abnormalities underlie the formation of most types of fibroepithelial lesions, many pathologists may think that study of the characteristics of the glands would not offer much insight into the diagnosis of these entities. This line of reasoning represents a misunderstanding; each type of fibroepithelial lesion has characteristic glandular alterations that provide diagnostic information as valuable as the properties of the stromal cells. Overlooking the characteristics of the glands only amplifies the difficulty of classifying fibroepithelial lesions.

When examining the glands of a fibroepithelial lesion, one must first determine whether they represent aberrant glandular tissue formed during the growth of the mass or entrapped preexisting ducts and lobules. Malformed glandular tissue sometimes resembles normal glandular tissue so closely that one can mistake it for normal tissue if one fails to pay close attention to the fine points of its organization. To aid in recognizing structural abnormalities in glandular tissue, pathologists might ask themselves the following questions:

- Does the nodule contain the expected numbers of "ducts" and "lobules"?
- Do the "ducts" and "lobules" display the expected anatomic relationship?
- Do the "lobules" have the expected size?
- Do the "lobules" appear discrete?
- Does each "acinus" unambiguously belong to one "lobule" or another?
- Does the nodule exhibit clearly defined "intralobular" and "extralobular" stroma?
- Do the vessels follow the course of the "extralobular" stroma?
- Do adipocytes mingle with the "acini" and "specialized stroma"?

If one answers many of the questions, except for the last one, in the negative, the glandular tissue probably represents malformed glands rather than lobules that formed normally and became distorted later. This conclusion narrows the diagnostic possibilities, because one observes malformed glandular tissue only in hamartomas and fibroadenoma variants. If one concludes that the glands within a fibroepithelial lesion represent entrapped, normally developed ducts and lobules, then one must identify the pattern of their alteration. Those in fibroadenomas and phyllodes tumors exhibit the well-known intracanalicular pattern, for example, whereas pseudoangiomatous stromal hyperplasia enlarges the lobules modestly, separates the ductules, and simplifies their branching pattern so that they look like primitive, type I lobules.

Besides considering the structural properties of the glands, one must evaluate the characteristics of their epithelium. Pseudoangiomatous stromal hyperplasia consistently induces ductal hyperplasia in the entrapped lobules, and phyllodes tumors do so in many cases. The canalicular epithelium of fibroadenomas, on the other hand, usually appears quiet and inactive.

Summary

The family of fibroepithelial lesions includes both neoplastic and hyperplastic entities characterized by the presence of stroma and glands. Proliferation of stromal cells underlies the growth of most types of fibroepithelial lesions, but overproduction of extracellular matrix gives rise to myxoid fibroadenomas. Depending on the type of fibroepithelial lesion, the stromal cells originate from either the specialized or

Table 15-1   Distinguishing the Types of Fibroepithelial Lesions

Lesion	Cell(s) of Origin	Glandular Tissue	
		Origin	Appearance
Fibroadenoma	Specialized fibroblast	Preexisting	Distorted
Myxoid fibroadenoma	Specialized fibroblast	Preexisting	Distorted
Phyllodes tumor	Specialized fibroblast	Preexisting	Distorted
Hamartoma	Stromal and epithelial cells	Newly formed	Disorganized
Fibroadenoma variant	Unknown	Unknown	Disorganized
Pseudoangiomatous stromal hyperplasia	Nonspecialized myofibroblast	Preexisting	Hyperplastic

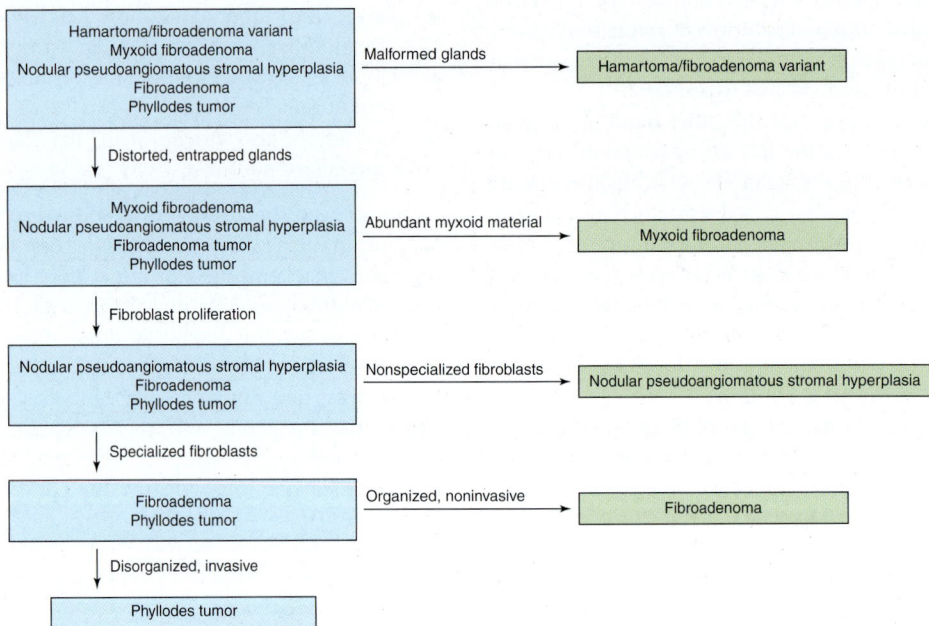

Figure 15-1 Diagram to aid in the diagnosis of fibroepithelial lesions.

the nonspecialized stroma. In most fibroepithelial lesions, the glands represent engulfed preexisting mammary duct and lobules, which become distorted in characteristic patterns. Both hamartomas and fibroadenoma variants contain neoplastic glandular tissue and stroma. Table 15-1 summarizes these concepts.

APPROACH TO THE DIAGNOSIS OF FIBROEPITHELIAL LESIONS

To analyze a fibroepithelial lesion, the pathologist may find it most helpful to examine three features of the nodule: its internal structure, the characteristics of its stroma, and the morphologic properties of its glands. The diagnosis of most fibroepithelial lesions is straightforward, but the classification of uncommon examples poses problems. To resolve these difficulties, the pathologist might find it helpful to consider the following questions:

- Do the glands look like distorted, entrapped, terminal duct–lobular units or like malformed ducts and lobules?
- Does the stroma contain abundant myxoid ground substance or proliferative fibroblasts?
- Does the stroma have the histologic characteristics of specialized or nonspecialized stroma?
- Do the fibroblasts grow in an orderly relationship with the glands and a noninvasive pattern with respect to the stroma?

Following the line of reasoning illustrated in Figure 15-1, the answers to these questions will help to classify cases of an uncertain nature.

Selected Readings

Arrigoni MG, Dockerty MB, Judd ES: The identification and treatment of mammary hamartoma. Surg Gynecol Obstet 1971;133:577-582.

Azzopardi JG: Problems in Breast Pathology. (Major Problems in Pathology, vol 11.) London, WB Saunders, 1979.

Carney JA, Toorkey BC: Myxoid fibroadenoma and allied conditions (myxomatosis) of the breast: A heritable disorder with special associations including cardiac and cutaneous myxomas. Am J Surg Pathol 1991;15:713-721.

Curran RC, Dodge OG: Sarcoma of breast, with particular reference to its origin from fibroadenoma. J Clin Pathol 1962;15:1-16.

Koerner FC, O'Connell JX: Fibroadenoma: Morphological observations and a theory of pathogenesis. Pathol Annu 1994;29:1-19.

Norris HJ, Taylor HB: Relationship of histological features to behavior of cystosarcoma phyllodes: Analysis of ninety-four cases. Cancer 1967;20:2090-2099.

Vuitch MF, Rosen PP, Erlandson RA: Pseudoangiomatous hyperplasia of mammary stroma. Hum Pathol 1986;17:185-191.

16

Fibroadenoma

DEFINITIONS AND CLINICOPATHOLOGIC CHARACTERISTICS

These benign tumors originate from fibroblasts of the specialized fibrous connective tissue. The smallest examples usually involve lobules and ductules (Fig. 16-1), so it seems that most conventional fibroadenomas arise in the stroma surrounding the small branches of the mammary glandular system (Fig. 16-2). As the neoplastic cells multiply, they engulf the nearby terminal duct–lobular units, ducts, and nonspecialized stroma and thereby form a compact mass. The proliferation and sustenance of these neoplastic stromal cells depend in some undefined way on the presence of nearby glandular epithelium. Never do the fibroblasts of fibroadenomas stray very far from glandular structures, nor do the stromal cells form large masses devoid of glands. One can therefore think of the fibroadenoma as a type of specialized stromal fibroma containing entrapped glands, a notion that underlies the term *adenofibroma*, which was originally applied to this lesion and is still preferred by certain purists. In certain circumstances, the fibroblastic proliferation appears so slight and dispersed that it creates a group of loosely aggregated small nodules instead of forming a distinct mass. Pathologists refer to this pattern as *fibroadenomatosis*, *sclerosing lobular hyperplasia*, and *fibroadenomatoid mastopathy* (Fig. 16-3).

Fibroadenomas most commonly arise in women in the second and third decades of life and typically measure a few centimeters. The tumors form solid, oval masses usually 3 cm or less and situated with their long axis radially oriented around the nipple. Macroscopic study of a typical fibroadenoma shows a well-defined, fleshy mass composed of uniform, whorled, gray-white tissue containing pinpoint yellow flecks. Tumors resected from older women usually feel firm and appear homogeneous and white.

If unresected, most fibroadenomas do not enlarge much after presentation; however, they can grow to a substantial size during pregnancy or as a consequence of other types of hormonal stimulation. Clinical histories that deviate from these generalizations would bring into question the diagnosis of fibroadenoma. For example, the history of the appearance of a new fibroepithelial tumor in a woman in her forties seems inconsistent with the diagnosis of fibroadenoma, and so does a mass containing cysts. The enlargement of a seemingly benign mass after a long period of constant size suggests the presence of a secondary process superimposed on an underlying fibroadenoma. Once excised, even if only by enucleation, fibroadenomas do not recur. In certain patients, especially those of African-American background, multiple, synchronous or successive fibroadenomas develop. One must take care to differentiate the development of multiple fibroadenomas from the recurrence of a primary tumor, because the regrowth of a fibroepithelial tumor in the bed of a previously resected one points strongly away from the diagnosis of fibroadenoma.

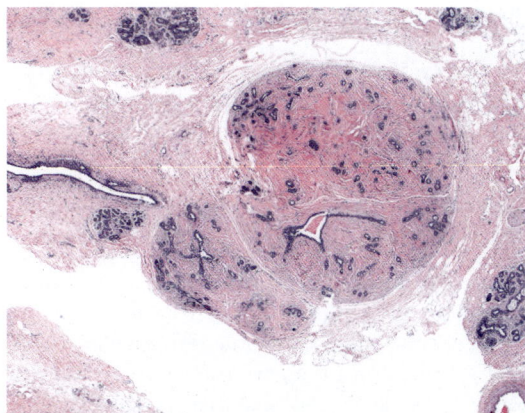

Figure 16-1 This tiny fibroadenoma surrounds a small duct and the associated terminal duct–lobular units.

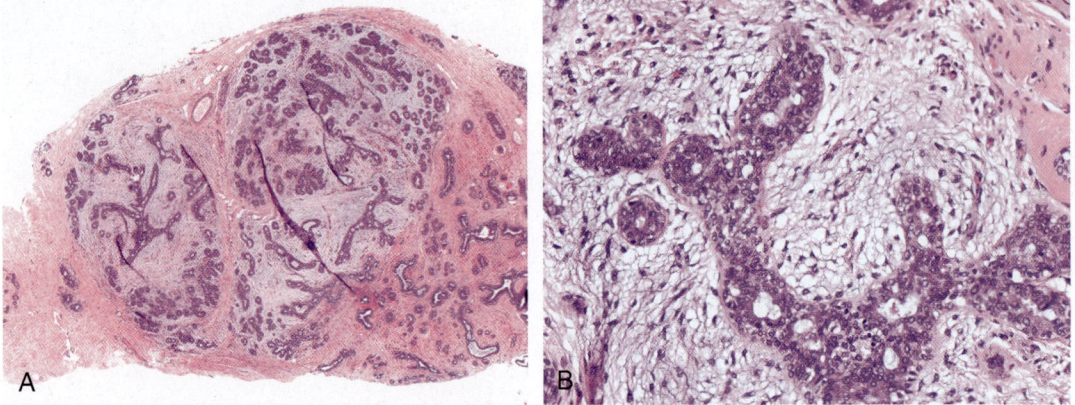

Figure 16-2 A, Proliferation of the specialized stromal fibroblasts surrounding several small ducts and terminal duct–lobular units has spawned a conventional fibroadenoma. **B,** High magnification reveals the presence of an increased number of stromal cells surrounded by myxoid ground substances.

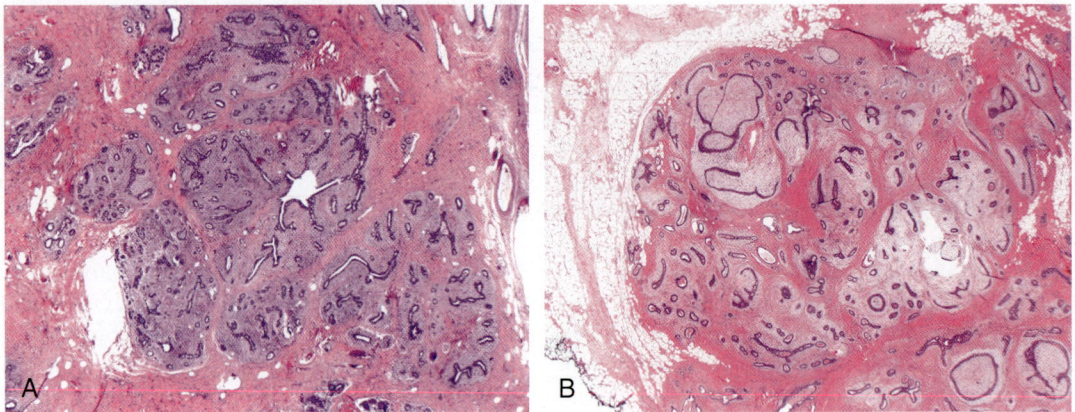

Figure 16-3 A, Proliferation of specialized stromal cells has given rise to a small fibroadenoma in the center of the field and less compact expansion of the specialized stromal compartment in the surrounding lobules. **B,** Some would classify this lesion as *fibroadenomatoid mastopathy*.

HISTOLOGIC CHARACTERISTICS

Uniformity of the histologic characteristics, organization of the tissue components, and harmony between the stromal and glandular elements characterize the conventional fibroadenoma.

Structure of the Mass

Commonplace fibroadenomas display a characteristic multinodular structure, which develops because the neoplastic fibroblasts grow only in the specialized stromal compartment. The tumors shown in Figure 16-4 show the characteristic organization. Each nodule within the mass represents a distorted terminal duct–lobular unit. The myxoid stroma constitutes the proliferative specialized stroma, and the canaliculi represent the elongated intralobular terminal ductules and acini of the engulfed terminal duct–lobular units. Entrapped nonspecialized stroma persists as bands of collagenous fibrous tissue running through the mass. A rim of compressed nonspecialized stroma encircles the nodule and separates the neoplastic fibroblasts from the adjacent adipocytes. The ability to appreciate this multinodular structure and organization greatly facilitates the recognition of fibroadenomas.

Although many fibroadenomas display the characteristic structural pattern clearly, others do not. Difficulties detecting the underlying architecture arise because pathologic processes alter the characteristics of either the specialized or the nonspecialized

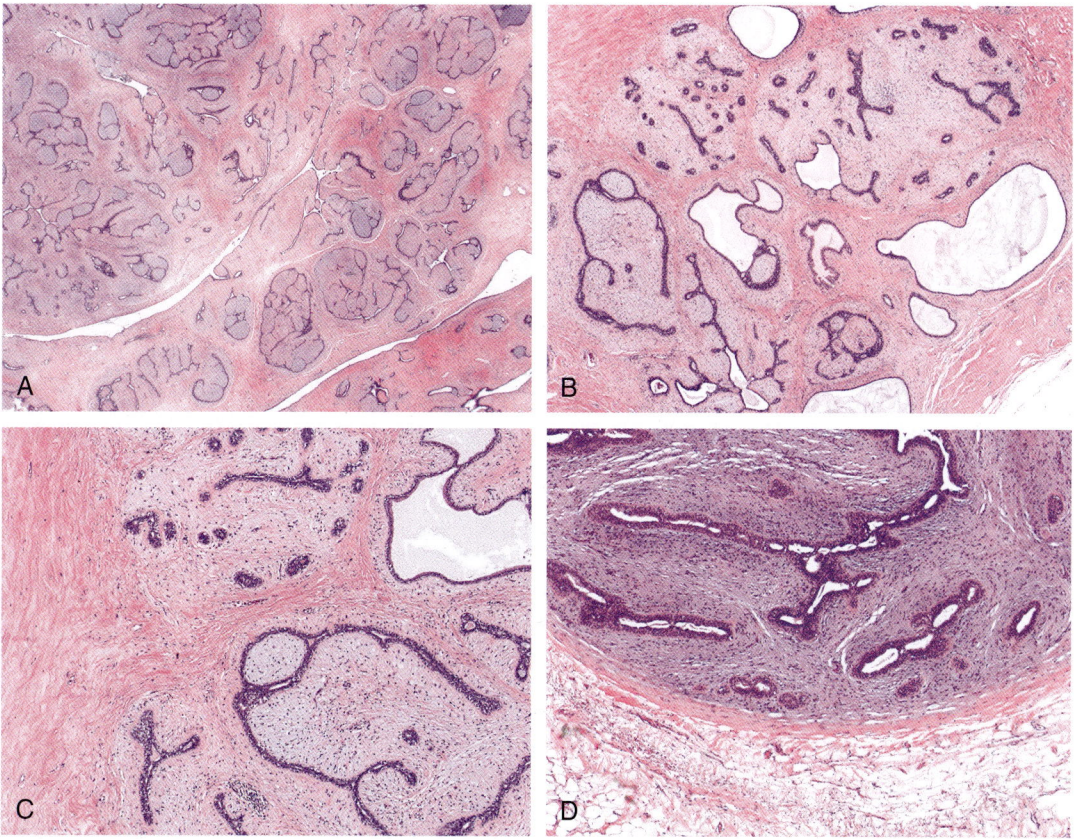

Figure 16-4 A, The multinodular nature of this conventional fibroadenoma stands out clearly. Each small nodule represents a terminal duct—lobular unit distorted by the proliferative myxoid specialized stroma. **B,** The bands of collagenous stroma coursing between the altered lobules in this tumor represent the nonspecialized stroma drawn into the enlarging mass. **C,** High magnification allows one to trace the continuity of the nonspecialized stromal bands from the exterior of the fibroadenoma (*left*) to its interior (*right*). **D,** A rim of compressed nonspecialized stroma separates the neoplastic fibroblasts from the surrounding adipocytes.

stroma in ways that blur the distinction between the two. For example, collagenization of the specialized stroma during involution causes it to become poor in cells and rich in collagen; thus, the specialized stroma comes to resemble the nonspecialized stroma, and the multinodular pattern becomes difficult to discern. Observation of subtle variation in the eosinophilia of the collagen and differences in the orientation of the collagen bundles helps differentiate the two types of stroma (Fig. 16-5). Help also comes from the identification of the small blood vessels that run in the nonspecialized stroma, because these vascular bundles reliably mark the location of the nonspecialized stromal bands (Fig. 16-6).

Occasional tumors from young women present the opposite difficulty; the nonspecialized stroma can become just as cellular as the neoplastic specialized stroma (Fig. 16-7). Once again, vascular bundles

mark the location of the internal stromal bands, and the presence of collagen between the stromal cells confirms this conclusion. Finally, fibroadenomas characterized by especially exuberant proliferation of the specialized stroma sometimes contain relatively few internal bands, perhaps because they become attenuated during the growth of the mass. Nevertheless, the small vessels persist and highlight the multinodular internal structure of the tumor.

Nonspecialized stroma also forms a layer around the perimeter of the tumor, where it separates the proliferating, specialized fibroblasts from the fat. The peripheral band of nonspecialized stroma sometimes becomes markedly attenuated; even then, however, it marks the limits of the tumor (Fig. 16-8). The presence of neoplastic fibroblasts or glands trespassing in the adipose tissue should lead one away from the diagnosis of fibroadenoma.

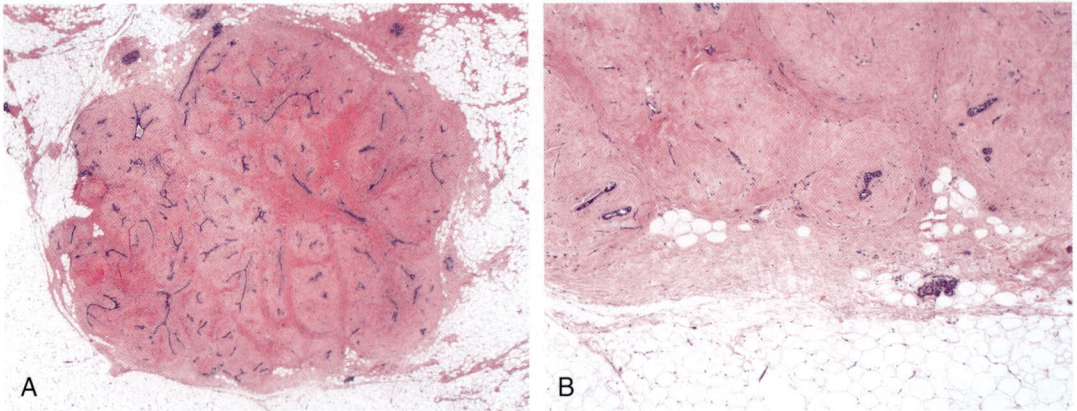

Figure 16-5 A, Because of collagenization, the specialized stroma in this conventional fibroadenoma resembles the nonspecialized stroma. **B,** Subtle differences in the degree of eosinophilia and the orientation of the collagen bundles allow one to distinguish the two types of stroma.

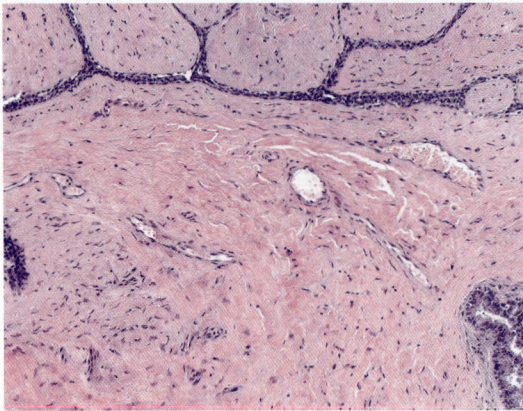

Figure 16-6 The presence of the small blood vessels (*center*) allows one to identify the surrounding stroma as a band of nonspecialized stroma.

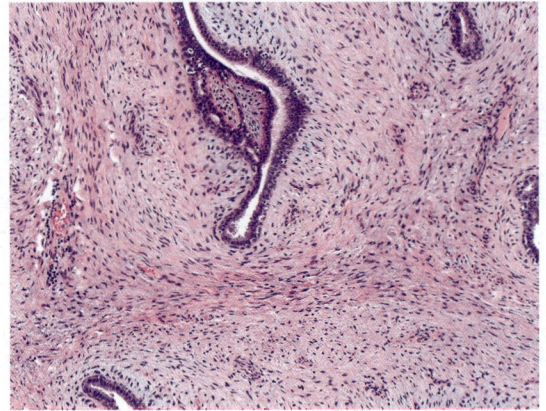

Figure 16-7 The nonspecialized stroma of this conventional fibroadenoma appears especially cellular. Differences in the degree of eosinophilia and the orientation of the collagen bundles and the location of the small blood vessels allow one to distinguish the two types of stroma despite the similarity of their cellular densities.

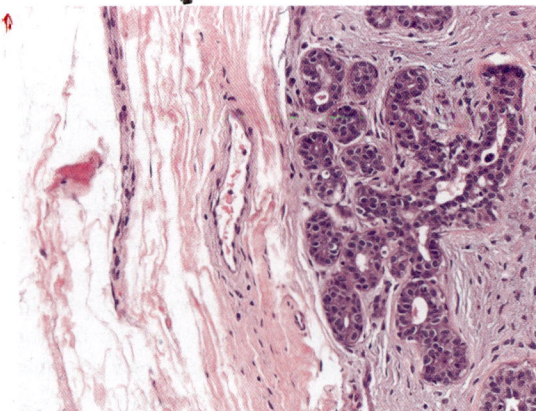

Figure 16-8 A thin rim of attenuated nonspecialized stroma separates the proliferating specialized fibroblasts and entrapped lobule from the adjacent adipocytes.

Characteristics of the Stroma

The neoplastic fibroblasts appear small and bland, but they vary in the details of their cytologic characteristics. Many have small, spindly nuclei composed of homogeneous and dark chromatin, whereas others possess larger, oval nuclei containing granular chromatin and tiny nucleoli (Fig. 16-9). The fibroblasts sit in abundant intercellular matrix, which sometimes compresses their nuclei into irregular, angulated shapes. The density of the fibroblasts and the composition of the intercellular matrix vary from case to case. Some of this variation results from inherent differences among the cases, but much of it reflects varying levels of involution, a phenomenon that takes place in all fibroadenomas but unfolds at different rates in different tumors. During this regressive

Figure 16-9 The fibroblasts of this fibroadenoma vary in cytologic characteristics. Some have small dark nuclei, whereas others possess larger and paler nuclei.

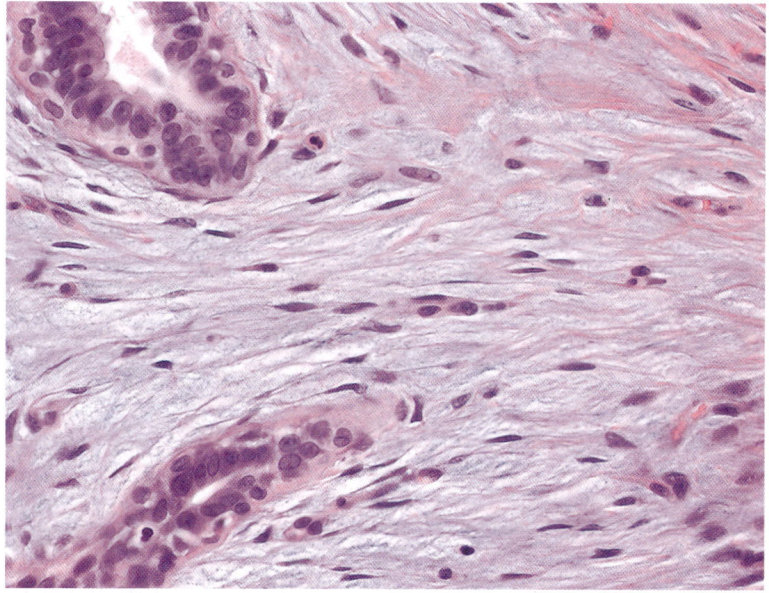

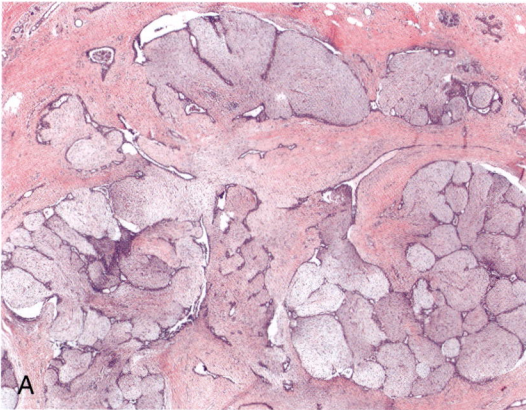

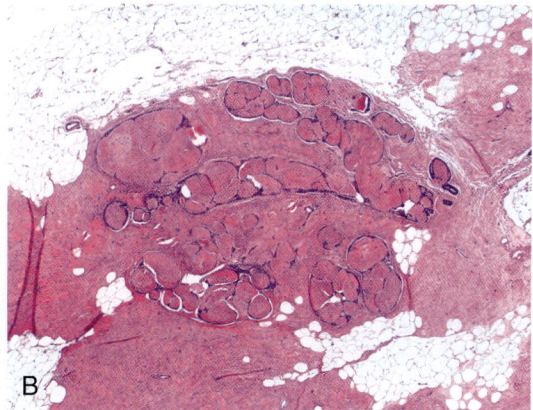

Figure 16-10 A, This fibroadenoma from a young woman contains abundant myxoid stroma. **B,** In contrast, the stroma in this fibroadenoma from a postmenopausal woman consists entirely of dense collagen.

process, the tumor cells disappear, collagen replaces the myxoid material of the stroma, and the glands shrink. Thus, tumors from women in the second and third decades of life usually have a stroma rich in fibroblasts and myxoid ground substances, whereas those from women older than 40 years contain few stromal cells and abundant collagen (Fig. 16-10).

Involution seems to begin in the stroma farthest from the canaliculi (Fig. 16-11), but the multinodular structure and three-dimensional complexity of fibroadenomas limit the diagnostic utility of this point. Nevertheless, this process takes place so predictably that one should view any deviation from the expected pattern with suspicion. For example, it would seem quite unlikely for a fibroepithelial tumor that has been excised from a woman beyond

the age of fifty years and that contains a cellular and myxoid stroma to represent a fibroadenoma. Exceptions to this generalization do occur. For instance, one can occasionally encounter fibroadenomas with cellular, myxoid stroma in women in their forties and in postmenopausal women taking ovarian hormone replacement therapy, but such cases occur only uncommonly.

Although the extent of involution varies from one fibroadenoma to the next, the process occurs fairly uniformly in an individual tumor; thus, the stromal characteristics of a single fibroadenoma usually appear similar throughout. The density of fibroblasts and the composition of the stroma seen in one low-power field resemble those of stroma seen in most other low-power fields (Fig. 16-12). Striking variations in the cellularity of the stroma or the nature

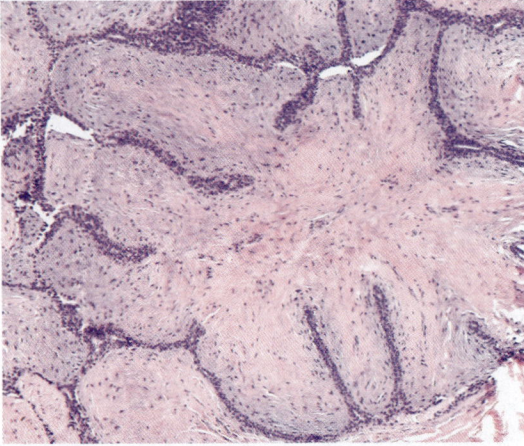

Figure 16-11 The phenomenon of involution has altered the stroma of this conventional fibroadenoma. The tissue farthest from the epithelium appears less cellular and more collagenous than the stroma next to the canaliculi.

of the intercellular matrix argue against a diagnosis of fibroadenoma. Pathologists must take particular care if one part of a fibroepithelial tumor looks like an involuted fibroadenoma and another portion has a cellular stroma; this constellation of findings suggests that a new process has developed in the setting of a preexisting fibroadenoma (Fig. 16-13). Contrary to this generalization, certain uncommon fibroadenomas, especially those from women in the third and fourth decades of life, show striking regional variation in the extent of involution (Fig. 16-14). If other features of such a tumor point to the diagnosis of fibroadenoma, then it seems safe to overlook such variability of stromal characteristics.

Adipose tissue never forms a substantial component of a fibroadenoma. Rarely, one can find a few adipocytes within the nonspecialized stroma at the periphery of the nodule or entrapped between coalescing nodules (Fig. 16-15). Even more rarely, small bits of adipose tissue accompany the vessels that run

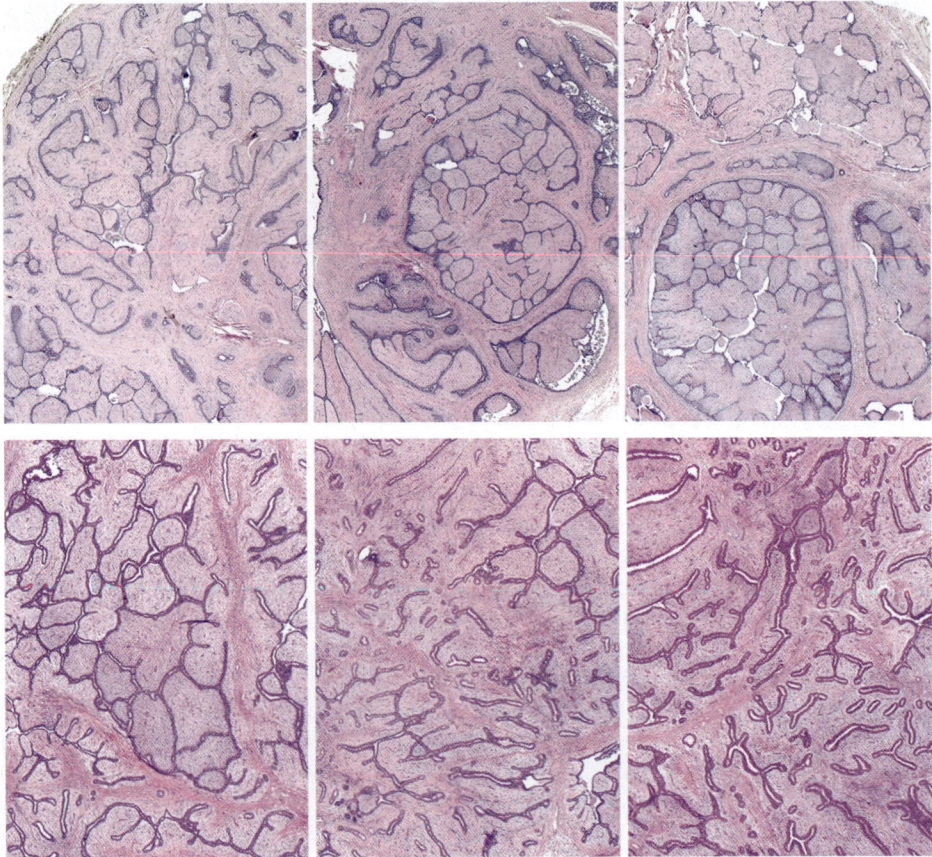

Figure 16-12 The three fields of a single conventional fibroadenoma are shown in the top row and three fields from a second fibroadenoma in the bottom row. Although the stroma in the lower fibroadenoma appears more myxoid and more cellular than the stroma in the upper, the fields illustrate the consistency in the characteristics of the stroma and in the density of the glands throughout each tumor.

Figure 16-13 A, One portion of this fibroepithelial tumor looks like a young fibroadenoma, but the remainder appears inactive. One does not expect to observe such pronounced variation in the characteristics of a conventional fibroadenoma, so such an appearance requires an explanation. **B,** A phyllodes tumor (*right*) has emerged from a conventional fibroadenoma (*left*). Contrast the cellularity of the stroma and the caliber of the glands in the two regions.

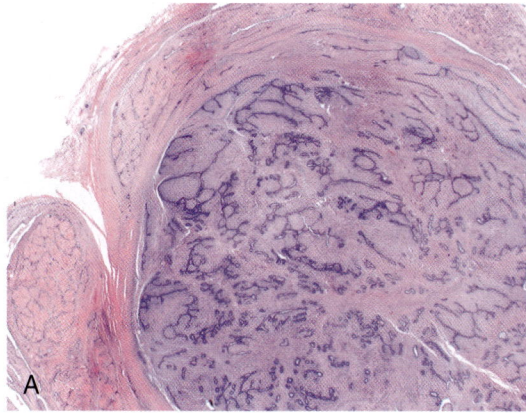

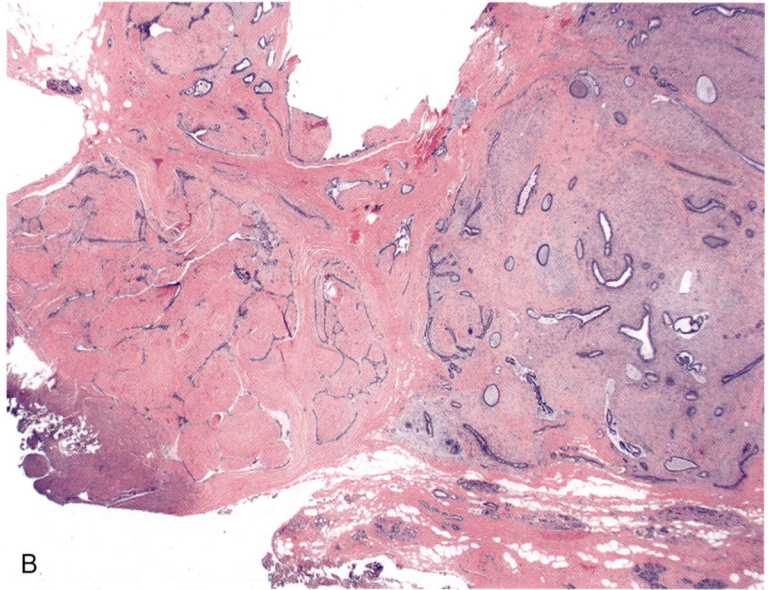

Figure 16-14 This fibroadenoma from a 25-year-old woman contains a region of hyalinization.

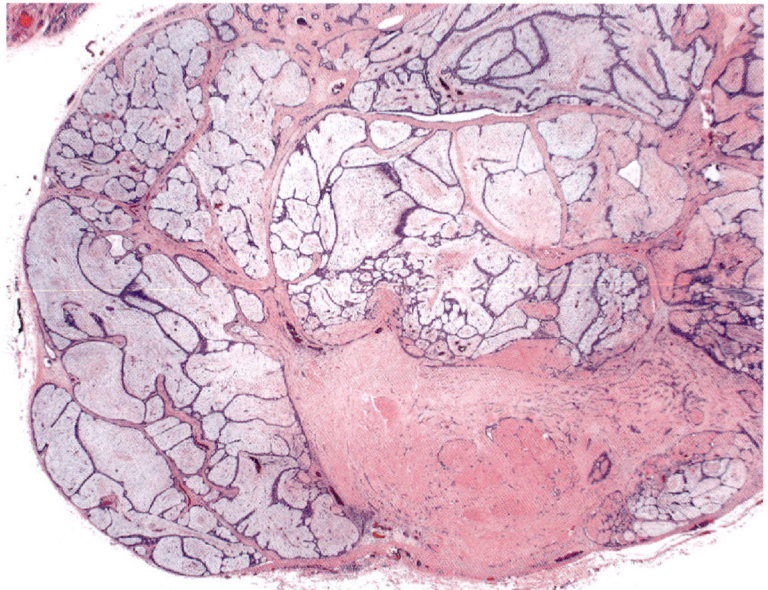

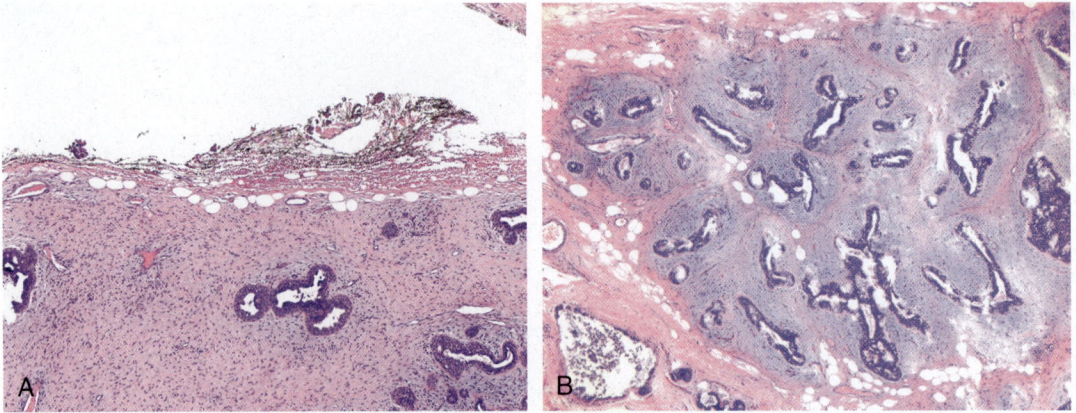

Figure 16-15 A, A few adipocytes have become incorporated at the edge of this fibroadenoma. **B,** Proliferating specialized fibroblasts have entrapped a few adipocytes during the early stage in the formation of this conventional fibroadenoma.

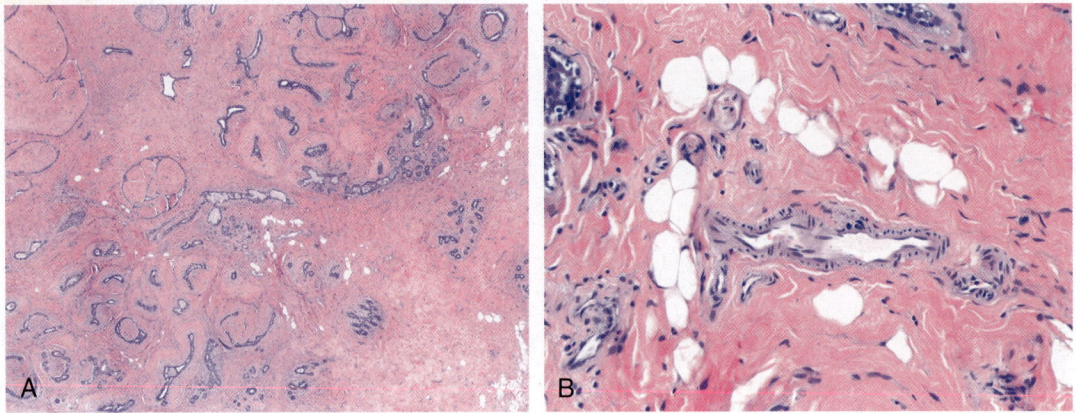

Figure 16-16 A, This conventional fibroadenoma has entrapped an unusually large amount of fat. **B,** The adipocytes accompany the vascular bundles.

within nonspecialized stromal bands (Fig. 16-16). The presence of abundant fat or fat in other patterns or other locations would render a diagnosis of fibroadenoma unlikely. One could legitimately wonder why fibroadenomas so consistently lack adipose tissue. The question does not have an obvious or widely accepted answer, but it might relate to the composition of the underlying mammary parenchyma. Most fibroadenomas arise in women in the second or third decade of life, when fibrous connective tissue makes up the majority of the nonspecialized stroma. Perhaps this abundance of fibrous connective tissue and relative paucity of adipose tissue account for the lack of fat within most fibroadenomas.

Characteristics of the Glands

Because distortion of terminal duct–lobular units in a fibroadenoma goes hand in hand with their incorporation into the tumor, one should not find normal lobules within the lesion. A few lobules near the edge of a fibroadenoma sometimes look only slightly distorted (Fig. 16-17), but the presence of completely unaltered lobules deep within a mass does not usually fit with a diagnosis of fibroadenoma. Furthermore, the distortion of the lobules takes place in a characteristic way and gives rise to either or both of two histologic patterns. The intracanalicular pattern, the more common of the two, consists of long, narrow canaliculi that arch over the surfaces of the stromal nodules (Fig. 16-18). History has obliterated the origin of the term *intracanalicular*, but it seems to reflect the 19th-century view that fibroadenomas represent a type of fibroma and the belief that the neoplastic stromal nodules project into glands (canaliculi), thereby compressing them into tubules of narrow caliber. The less common *pericanalicular* pattern consists of regular, round, open canaliculi

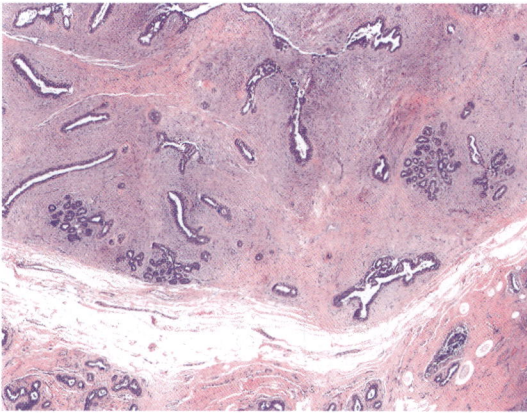

Figure 16-17 One can recognize a few lobules, which appear only slightly altered, at the edge of this conventional fibroadenoma.

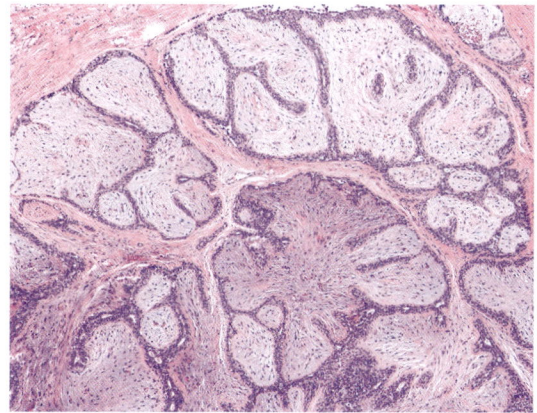

Figure 16-18 Proliferation of neoplastic specialized fibroblasts has distorted the ductules and acini of these terminal duct–lobular units to produce the typical intracanalicular pattern.

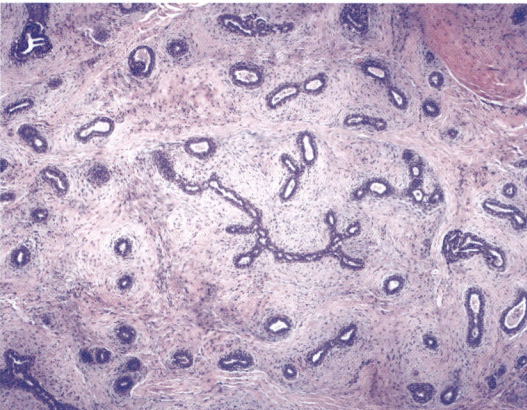

Figure 16-19 Most of the glands in this pericanalicular fibroadenoma consist of round, simply branching tubules, surrounded by concentrically arranged fibroblasts.

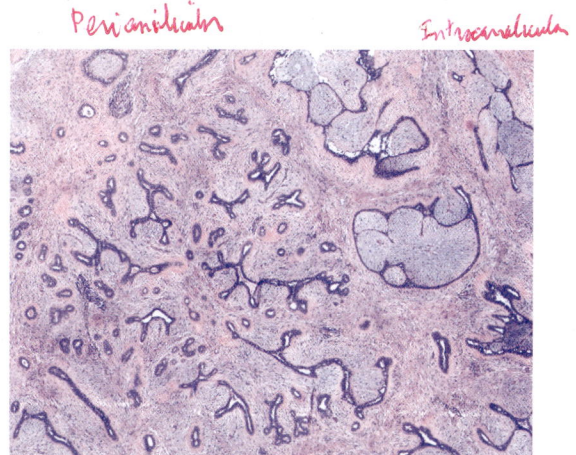

Figure 16-20 This conventional fibroadenoma shows a mixture of the intracanalicular (*right*) and pericanalicular (*left*) patterns.

surrounded by concentrically arranged fibroblasts (Fig. 16-19). We do not have an explanation for the origin of these two patterns, but it might reflect different developmental states of the underlying lobule. The pericanalicular appearance could arise in primitive lobules, and the intracanalicular pattern might develop from more fully developed terminal duct–lobular units. The two patterns commonly coexist in a single tumor (Fig. 16-20), just as lobules of differing complexity coexist in a single patient. The different histologic appearances do not foretell different clinical behaviors.

The canaliculi of an intracanalicular fibroadenoma have uniform, narrow calibers, and the juxtaposition of the luminal border of cells on opposite sides of the canaliculi at somewhat regular intervals gives the lumens a beaded appearance (Fig. 16-21). The canaliculi of a pericanalicular fibroadenoma look

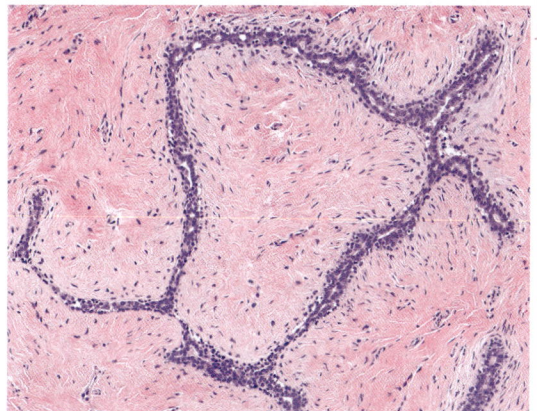

Figure 16-21 The canaliculi showing the intracanalicular pattern have narrow calibers. Juxtaposition of the epithelial cells on opposite sides of the lumen creates a beaded appearance.

like round, regular tubules of uniform diameter. Dilation of the canaliculi, which causes those of an intracanalicular tumor to lose their beaded appearance and those of a pericanalicular fibroadenoma to appear larger than expected, should alert the observer to the possibility of another diagnosis. The luminal cells lining the canaliculi of fibroadenomas appear inactive (Fig. 16-22). They have small oval nuclei, granular chromatin, small nucleoli, and minimal apical cytoplasm. The presence of luminal cells that look more active also raises questions about the accuracy of a diagnosis of fibroadenoma.

Although fibroadenomas contain distorted terminal duct–lobular units, these tumors usually do not display the benign processes that commonly affect lobules. Conventional ductal hyperplasia and apocrine metaplasia, two of the most common components of fibrocystic disease, for instance, rarely involve fibroadenomas. Two artifacts that commonly occur in fibroadenomas display superficial resemblances to ductal hyperplasia. Tangential sectioning of the curving contour of canaliculi (Fig. 16-23) simulates the stratification of hyperplastic ductal cells, and so does the accumulation of dislodged fragments of epithelium (Fig. 16-24). One must take care not to confuse these situations with genuine ductal hyperplasia. Conventional ductal hyperplasia does involve fibroadenomas in certain

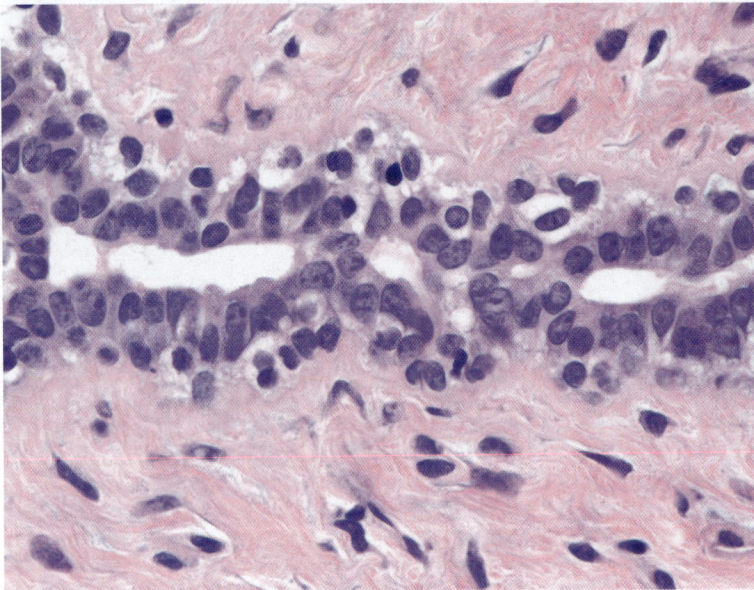

Figure 16-22 The epithelium of a conventional fibroadenoma consists of small, inactive-looking luminal cells and inconspicuous myoepithelial cells.

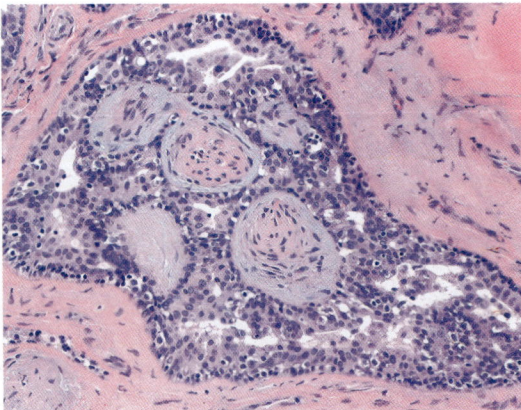

Figure 16-23 One should not confuse the artifact produced by off-center sectioning of the epithelium of a curving canaliculus with genuine epithelial hyperplasia.

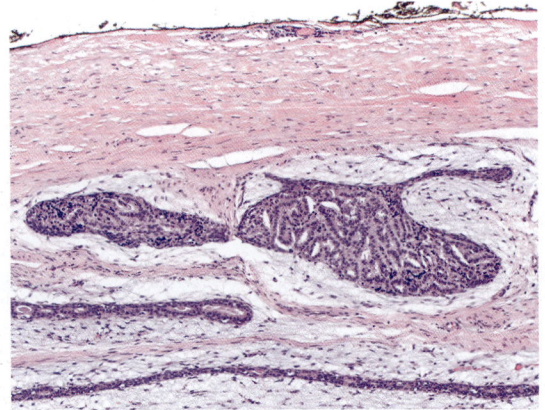

Figure 16-24 The telescoping of dislodged epithelium within the canaliculus of a fibroadenoma has produced an appearance superficially resembling that of ductal hyperplasia.

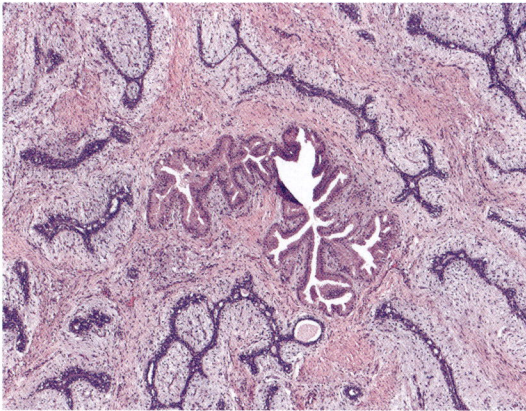

Figure 16-25 This otherwise conventional fibroadenoma harbors a small focus of apocrine metaplasia, and the tissue outside the fibroadenoma displayed pronounced apocrine metaplasia.

Box 16-1

Findings uncommonly seen in conventional fibroadenomas:

- Heterogeneity in the ratio of glands to stroma
- Heterogeneity in the stromal cellularity
- Heterogeneity in the appearance of the intercellular matrix
- Conventional ductal hyperplasia
- Apocrine metaplasia
- Abundant fat
- Unaltered terminal duct–lobular units

uncommon settings. First, the epithelium lining the developing ducts of girls in their mid-teens usually consists of several layers of cells, and the epithelium of a coexisting fibroadenoma can appear similar and slightly hyperplastic. Second, one could observe conventional ductal hyperplasia in a fibroadenoma when the tissue outside the fibroadenoma also shows extensive hyperplasia. These unusual situations notwithstanding, the presence of hyperplastic epithelium within a fibroadenoma should make one reconsider this diagnosis. Apocrine metaplasia, too, occurs only uncommonly in conventional fibroadenomas. Like ductal hyperplasia, apocrine change can involve a fibroadenoma when apocrine metaplasia involves the breast extensively (Fig. 16-25). In other situations, the presence of apocrine cells in a fibroepithelial tumor should prompt one to entertain a diagnosis other than fibroadenoma.

Summary

Conventional fibroadenomas arise from the neoplastic proliferation of specialized stromal cells. The growing mass of fibroblasts draws glands and nonspecialized stroma into it in a way that gives rise to an organized internal structure and an orderly and consistent relationship between the stroma and the glands. The stroma consists of bland fibroblasts embedded in an extracellular matrix that varies from myxoid to collagenous. The entrapped glands appear distorted in characteristic patterns, and the cells lining the canaliculi look inactive. Deviations from these generalizations would give a pathologist reason to consider diagnoses other than fibroadenoma (Box 16-1).

PROBLEMS IN THE DIAGNOSIS OF FIBROADENOMAS

Conventional fibroadenomas do not tax the diagnostic skills of any pathologist, but the classification of unusually cellular tumors and those containing complex glandular tissue can trouble even the most experienced observer. Distinguishing fibroadenomas from low-grade phyllodes tumors always poses a problem, and this difficulty arises regularly in the evaluation of tumors from women older than 40 years.

Uncommon Tumors Classified as Fibroadenomas

According to many pathologists, the spectrum of fibroadenomas includes two uncommon fibroepithelial tumors as well as the classic tumor already described: neoplasms lacking the leaflike growth pattern characteristic of a phyllodes tumor but composed of cellular stroma, and tumors containing especially abundant glandular tissue that displays a range of fibrocystic changes. Tumors in the first group go by the names *cellular fibroadenoma* and *juvenile fibroadenoma*. Pathologists often find these cases especially difficult to categorize, and three factors contribute to their difficulties. First, investigators do not agree on the subclassification of these lesions. Many pathologists regard all such tumors as a single type of fibroadenoma; other observers recognize distinct subtypes. Second, the literature does not demonstrate a consistent usage of the terms *cellular fibroadenoma* and *juvenile fibroadenoma*. Certain writers use these diagnoses synonymously, whereas others apply them to lesions with specific histologic characteristics. The third factor accounting for confusion stems from the uncertain pathogenesis of these lesions. Some examples do not seem to represent noninvasive neoplasms of specialized fibroblasts, as the name *fibroadenoma* suggests. Instead, such cases display characteristics more in keeping with either hamartomas or phyllodes tumors. Purists would refrain from using any variation on the term fibroadenoma to refer to lesions that do not look like benign neoplasms of specialized stromal fibroblasts. With acknowledgment of the variation in the classification of these tumors and the inconsistency in the usage of these diagnostic terms, and with the issue of pathogenesis set aside for the moment, the following discussion reviews the histologic characteristics of the members of this group using the most commonly used terminology.

When used most precisely, the diagnosis *juvenile fibroadenoma* refers to a rare, distinctive type of fibroepithelial tumor seen most commonly, but not exclusively, in adolescent girls. Although the term juvenile fibroadenoma suggests that the tumor represents a type of fibroadenoma, the former differs from the latter in three respects. First, the extracellular matrix typically consists of collagen rather than myxoid ground substances. Second, the stromal cells grow in a pericanalicular pattern instead of the intracanalicular configuration, which characterizes most conventional fibroadenomas. Finally, the epithelium usually displays florid conventional ductal hyperplasia. These deviations might make one question the classification of such examples as a type of fibroadenoma. It seems more likely that they arise as a malformation of breast tissue and thus might represent a form of nodular hyperplasia or a hamartoma. Whatever their pathogenesis, one must not classify these tumors as phyllodes tumors because of the cellularity of their stroma or the presence of ductal epithelial hyperplasia.

The use of the term *cellular fibroadenoma* varies widely. Many pathologists avoid it completely, others use it interchangeably with the term *juvenile fibroadenoma*, and still others still seem not to recognize the term as a genuine diagnosis and use it only as a description of an otherwise conventional fibroadenoma in which the stroma appears unusually cellular (Fig. 16-26). Equally commonly, pathologists apply this diagnosis to lesions showing characteristics of both fibroadenoma and low-grade phyllodes tumor. Because of this wide variation in use, it seems best not to use the term cellular fibroadenoma as an unqualified diagnosis unless all concerned have agreed on an exact definition of the term.

The second type of uncommon fibroepithelial tumor usually classified as a type of fibroadenoma comprises one in which the glandular tissue appears abundant and shows fibrocystic or other proliferative changes. In 1994, Dr. Dupont and colleagues[1] introduced the term *complex fibroadenoma* and defined it as one in which the glandular tissue exhibits cyst formation, sclerosing adenosis, epithelial calcification, or papillary apocrine hyperplasia. Because all four of these processes occur so rarely in conventional fibroadenomas, one could question the rationale for classifying tumors of this type as a variety of fibroadenoma. On what grounds would one postulate a biologic link between complex fibroadenomas and conventional fibroadenomas? Hamartomas and fibroadenoma variants, on the other hand, regularly show these changes. It might make more sense to regard the complex fibroadenoma as a type of hamartoma or a fibroadenoma variant. Uncertainties about the precise classification of these benign tumors should not

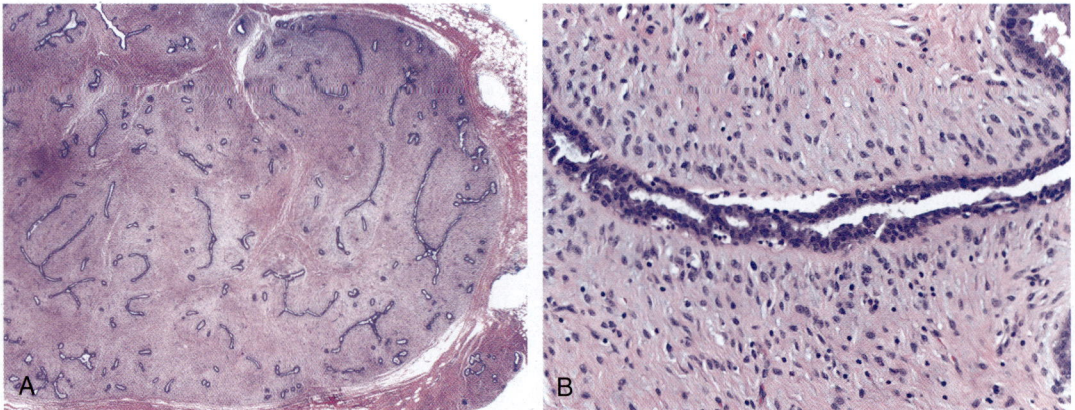

Figure 16-26 A, The fibroadenoma has the structural and glandular characteristics of a conventional fibroadenoma. **B,** Because the stroma appears cellular, certain pathologists would classify it as a cellular fibroadenoma.

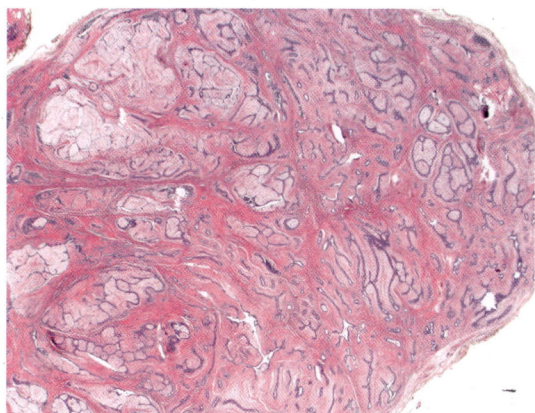

Figure 16-27 This fibroadenoma presented in a 48-year-old woman. All the histologic features fit with the diagnosis of fibroadenoma, so that diagnosis seems appropriate.

eclipse these writers' finding that patients with complex fibroadenomas have a threefold higher likelihood of development of invasive breast cancer than women without such tumors.[1]

The Diagnosis of Conventional Fibroadenoma in the Older Woman

As a rule, fibroadenomas do not arise in women older than 40 years. The tumors do come to clinical attention at this age or even later, of course. A radiologist might detect one on a patient's first mammogram, for example. Nevertheless, well-documented cases in which a fibroadenoma actually developed in a woman beyond the fourth decade of life remain very few. Fibroadenomas resected from women older than 40 years usually show advanced involution. They consist of densely collagenous stroma and atrophic glands. One must think particularly carefully before making the diagnosis of fibroadenoma for a fibroepithelial tumor that appears in a woman older than 40 years and is composed of cellular myxoid stroma. Changes in hormonal balance, especially the administration of compounds with estrogenic properties such as ovarian hormones, digitalis, thyroid hormone, and certain herbal remedies, can stimulate the growth of a fibroadenoma, and such a tumor would have the myxoid, cellular stroma seen in a conventional fibroadenoma. Many women in their perimenopausal years consume such products, and this practice occasionally causes an inactive fibroadenoma to resume growing. Pathologists would do well to search for an explanation such as this before rendering a diagnosis of fibroadenoma for an enlarging mass in a woman beyond the age of 40 years. On occasion, the clinical history does not contain a reasonable explanation for the appearance of a fibroadenoma during the perimenopausal years (Fig. 16-27). If all other features of the lesion fit, one can make the diagnosis of fibroadenoma, nevertheless.

Reference

1. Dupont WD, Page DL, Parl FF, et al: Long-term risk of breast cancer in women with fibroadenoma. N Engl J Med 1994;331:10-15.

Selected Readings

Demetrakoloulos NJ: Three-dimensional reconstruction of a human mammary fibroadenoma. Quarterly Bulletin of Northwestern University Medical School 1958;32:221-228.

Dupont WD, Page DL, Parl FF, et al: Long-term risk of breast cancer in women with fibroadenoma. N Engl J Med 1994;331:10-15.

Fekete P, Petrek J, Majmudar B, et al: Fibroadenoma with stromal cellularity: A clinicopathologic study of 21 patients. Arch Pathol Lab Med 1987;111:427-432.

Foster ME, Garrahan N, Williams S: Fibroadenoma of the breast: A clinical and pathological study. J R Coll Surg Edinb 1988;33:16-19.

Oberman HA: Breast lesions in the adolescent female. Pathol Annu 1979;14(Pt.1):175-201.

Pike AM, Oberman HA: Juvenile (cellular) adenofibromas: A clinicopathologic study. Am J Surg Pathol 1985;9:730-736.

17

Myxoid Fibroadenoma

DEFINITIONS AND CLINICOPATHOLOGIC CHARACTERISTICS

Myxoid fibroadenomas consist of distorted glands embedded in fibrous connective tissue that typically appears especially loose and contains abundant, pale, blue-gray extracellular matrix. Like their conventional counterparts, myxoid fibroadenomas originate around the tiny glandular structures, where bluish-gray mucin accumulates in the specialized stroma (Fig. 17-1). Because of the distinctive, myxoid appearance of the stroma, pathologists have come to refer to this type of tumor as *a myxoid fibroadenoma*.

The choice of this name seems ill-advised for three reasons. First, it suggests that myxoid fibroadenomas represent a variety of conventional fibroadenoma, an unlikely suggestion because the two lesions differ in their most fundamental property: myxoid fibroadenomas arise from the overproduction of extracellular matrix, whereas conventional fibroadenomas represent a proliferation of specialized fibroblasts. Myxoid fibroadenomas would therefore seem more closely related to myxomas of soft tissue than to fibroadenomas. Second, myxoid fibroadenomas can lose their myxoid nature entirely. With the passage of time, collagen comes to replace the myxoid extracellular matrix, leaving pathologists in the uncomfortable and counterintuitive position of referring to a mass containing dense collagen as myxoid. Third, the stroma of genuine fibroadenomas sometimes contains copious myxoid ground substances. Applying the term myxoid fibroadenoma to the myxoma-like lesion precludes the use of the diagnosis to refer to a conventional fibroadenoma with myxoid change, a usage that seems both more intuitive and more natural. Nevertheless, the term has become well established, and writings in the literature do not suggest that this usage will change any time soon.

Myxoid fibroadenomas tend to arise in women in the fifth or sixth decade of life but also develop in younger women. Mammography does not seem to detect myxoid fibroadenomas as consistently as it discloses conventional fibroadenomas, so many myxoid fibroadenomas present as palpable masses or as lesions detected by magnetic resonance imaging but not seen on a mammogram. Macroscopic examination usually reveals a well-defined nodule, sometimes lobulated, that is composed of tissue often described as mucoid, shiny, or translucent. Myxoid fibroadenomas occur in the familial condition known as Carney's syndrome, which comprises cardiac and cutaneous myxomas, melanocytic schwannomas, pigmented cutaneous lesions, and proliferations of endocrine tissues. Most patients with myxoid fibroadenomas do not have the other lesions of Carney's syndrome.

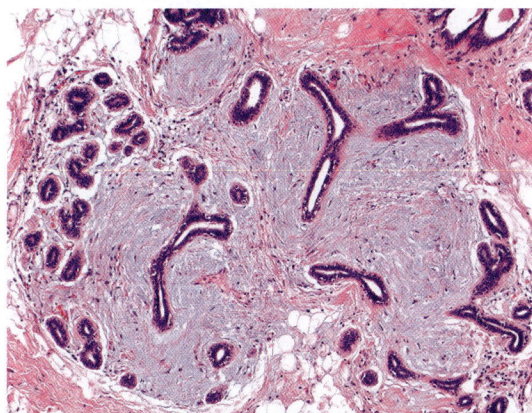

Figure 17-1 The accumulation of myxoid ground substances has created this tiny myxoid fibroadenoma.

HISTOLOGIC CHARACTERISTICS

Accumulation of myxoid material in the specialized stromal compartment, dissection of the myxoid material into the stroma, and distortion of the

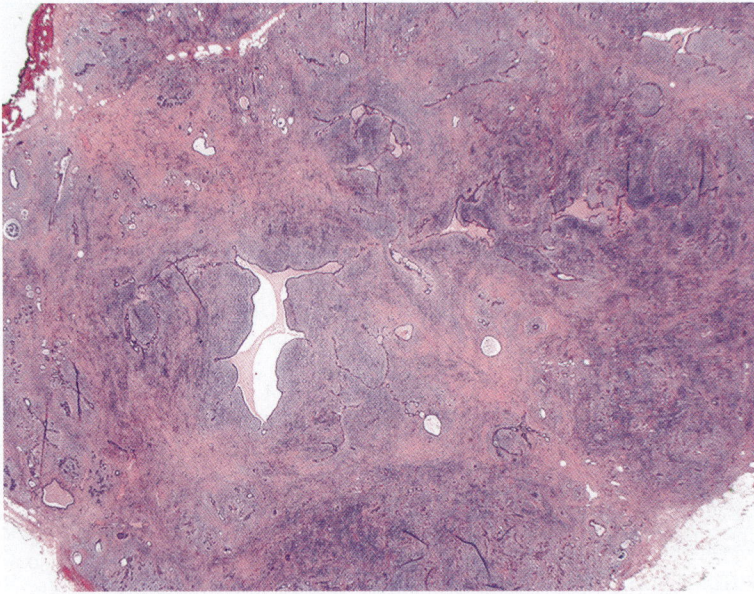

Figure 17-2 The internal structure of this myxoid fibroadenoma does not appear as clearly defined as that shown by most conventional fibroadenomas.

entrapped glands in irregular patterns characterize myxoid fibroadenomas.

Although myxoid fibroadenomas do not represent a type of genuine fibroadenoma, as the name would suggest, the two entities do share a few histologic characteristics. Like conventional fibroadenomas, myxoid fibroadenomas occupy the specialized stromal compartment and contain entrapped, preexisting lobules, ducts, and nonspecialized stroma. Moreover, the nodular accumulation of ground substances seen in myxoid fibroadenomas can give the entrapped glands an arching configuration. This appearance resembles the intracanalicular pattern seen in most conventional fibroadenomas. Finally, myxoid fibroadenomas undergo the same process of involution that takes place in conventional fibroadenomas. As time advances, dense collagen replaces the myxoid ground substances, and the characteristics of the stroma change. At this point, however, the resemblance between the two lesions ends. Myxoid fibroadenomas differ from conventional fibroadenomas in internal structure, contour, the cellularity of the stroma, the frequency with which they contain fat, and the histologic characteristics of entrapped glands.

Structure of the Mass

Although myxoid fibroadenomas have the same multinodular structure that conventional fibroadenomas have, the former may not display this organization as clearly as the latter (Fig. 17-2). It sometimes requires careful inspection to appreciate the internal structure and multinodular arrangement of a myxoid fibroadenoma. This difficulty arises because the accumulation

of mucin can obscure the nodular architecture in different ways. In tumors containing extreme amounts of extracellular material, the internal bands of nonspecialized stroma become so attenuated that one can barely identify them (Fig. 17-3). One might observe only delicate wisps of collagen or small blood vessels marking the locations of the nonspecialized stroma, which partition the mass into nodules (Fig. 17-4). In cases characterized by more modest mucin production, the extracellular material tends to dissect between bundles of collagen and through lobules, instead of distorting them as the proliferating fibroblasts of a conventional fibroadenoma do. This mucin dissection causes the bands of nonspecialized stroma to appear frayed and indistinct, and the internal structure of the tumors thereby becomes blurred (Fig. 17-5).

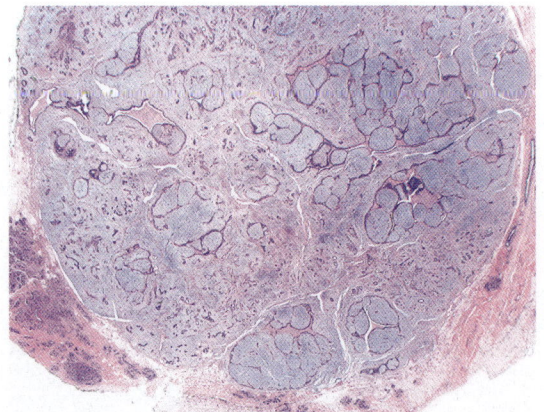

Figure 17-3 The abundance of myxoid material makes it difficult to identify the internal bands of nonspecialized stroma in this myxoid fibroadenoma.

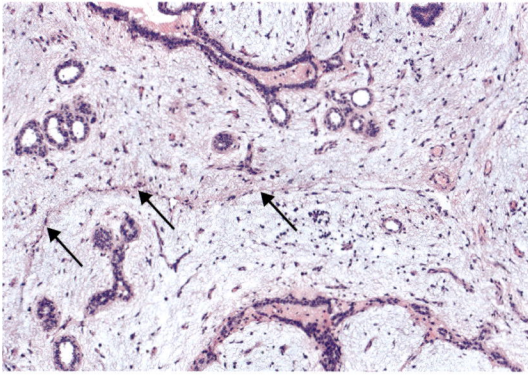

Figure 17-4 The nonspecialized stromal bands have become so attenuated that they appear as slender strands of collagen (*arrows*) associated with small blood vessels.

The characteristics of the periphery of myxoid fibroadenomas can differ from those of commonplace fibroadenomas in several aspects. First, unlike the proliferative fibroblasts of a conventional fibroadenoma, which almost never penetrate the adipose tissue, the myxoid material sometimes directly abuts the fat (Fig. 17-6). The juxtaposition of myxoid ground substances and adipocytes probably reflects the tendency of the gelatinous, myxoid substances to dissect through the peripheral rim of nonspecialized stroma that surrounds these tumors. The same phenomenon would explain the penetration of the myxoid material into uninvolved breast parenchyma and the resulting indistinct margin. The contours of myxoid fibroadenomas often appear lobulated (Fig. 17-7), unlike the smoothly arching perimeter of a conventional fibroadenoma. This appearance may reflect a less forceful manner

Figure 17-5 Dissection of myxoid ground substances among the collagen bundles of the nonspecialized stroma obscures the internal structure of a myxoid fibroadenoma.

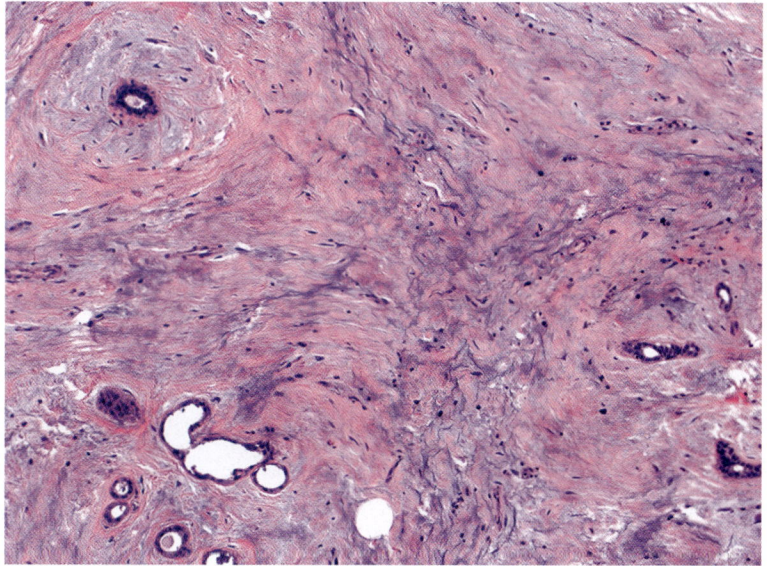

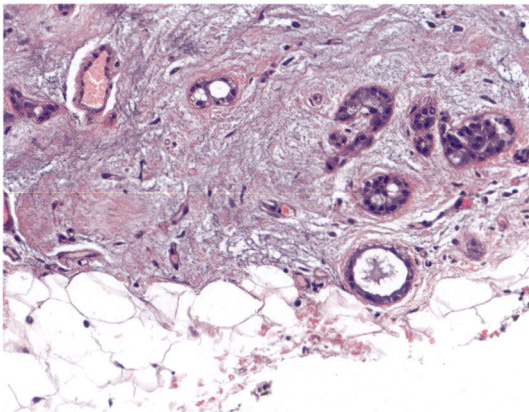

Figure 17-6 The myxoid ground substance of myxoid fibroadenomas often penetrates the nonspecialized stroma and infiltrates the adipose tissue.

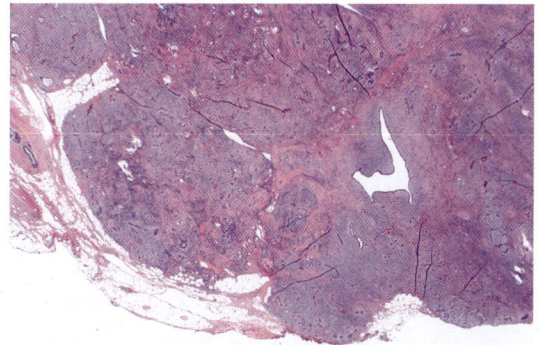

Figure 17-7 The borders of myxoid fibroadenomas often appear more bosselated than the borders of conventional fibroadenomas.

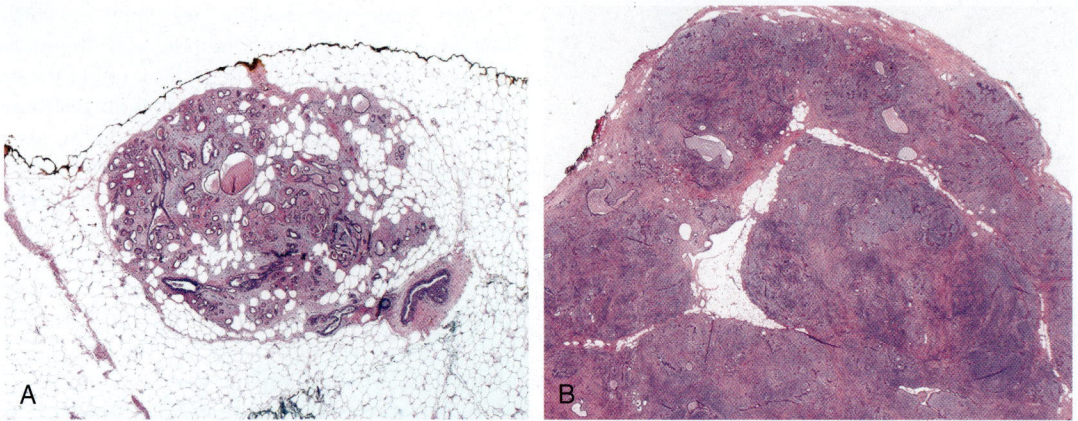

Figure 17-8 A, An early stage in the formation of this myxoid fibroadenoma illustrates the entrapment of fat within the lesion. **B,** As a myxoid fibroadenoma grows, adipocytes often remain trapped within the mass.

of expansion, in which the growing mass incorporates peripheral lobules slowly, thereby allowing them to form bosselations on the surface of the nodule. Such a gradual process of enlargement could also explain the observation that myxoid fibroadenomas frequently incorporate adipocyte tissue (Fig. 17-8), which conventional fibroadenomas rarely do.

Characteristics of the Stroma

Because myxoid fibroadenomas do not apparently represent fibroblastic neoplasms, their stroma displays a lower density of fibroblasts than the stroma of conventional fibroadenomas. The stroma of myxoid fibroadenomas consists of just a few small spindle cells. They possess small, bland nuclei and float in a sea of pale, blue-gray, extracellular mucin (Fig. 17-9). This myxoid material, rather than fibroblasts, accounts for the bulk of the mass. The presence of an unambiguous proliferation of fibroblasts would argue against the diagnosis of myxoid fibroadenoma and would lead one to prefer a diagnosis such as conventional fibroadenoma or phyllodes tumor with myxoid stroma.

Despite the reference to myxoid material in the name of this lesion, the presence of myxoid ground substances does not establish the diagnosis of myxoid fibroadenoma, nor does the absence of this material exclude the diagnosis. Conventional fibroadenomas, hamartomas, and phyllodes tumors can all have an abundance of myxoid material in their stroma (Figs. 17-10 to 17-12), and so can papillomas.

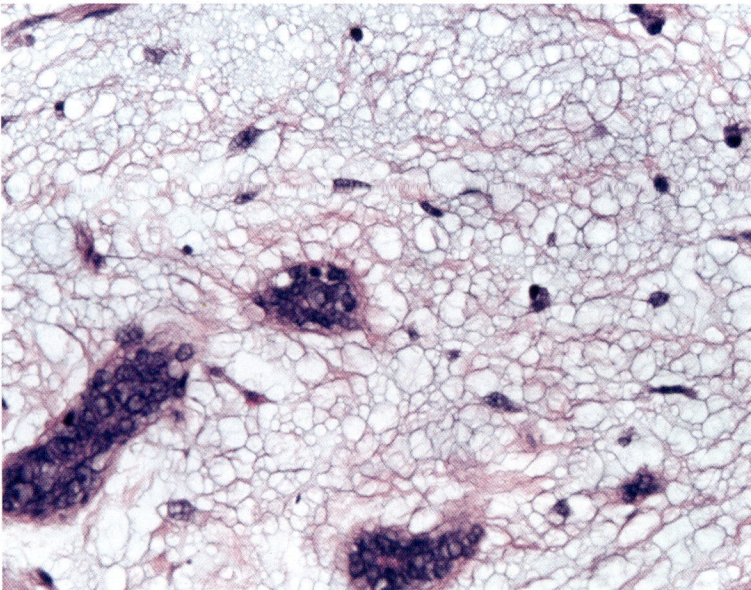

Figure 17-9 The stroma of this myxoid fibroadenoma consists of just a few stromal cells and capillaries embedded in a sea of myxoid material.

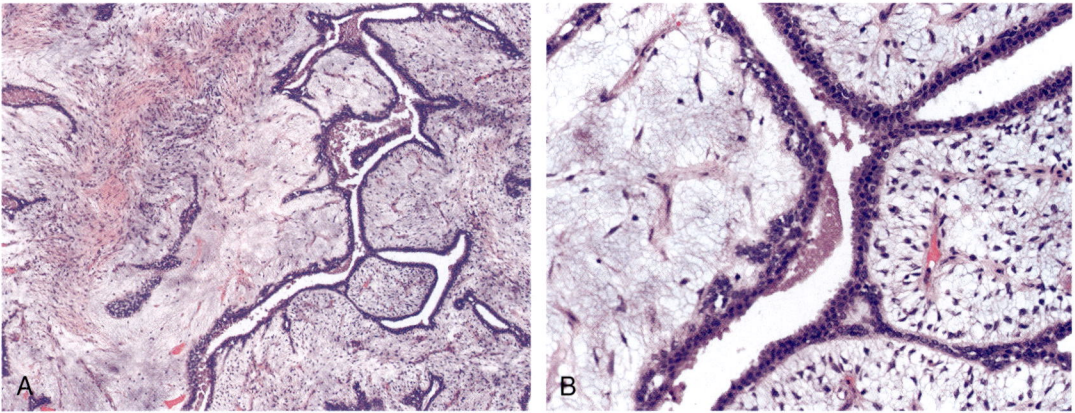

Figure 17-10 A, This conventional fibroadenoma contains a region in which the stroma appears especially myxoid. **B,** High magnification allows one to contrast the cellularity of the two regions.

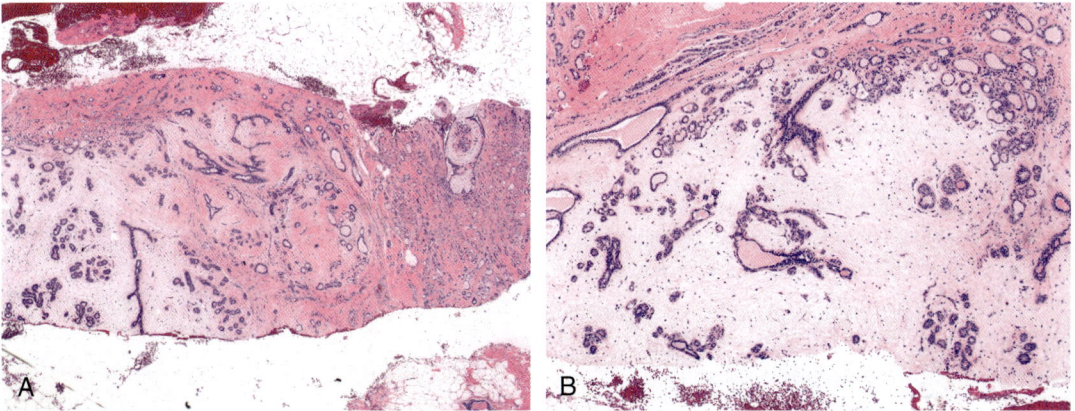

Figure 17-11 A, This core biopsy specimen of a hamartoma shows prominent myxoid change in a portion of the tissue. **B,** High magnification illustrates the accumulation of pale, myxoid ground substances.

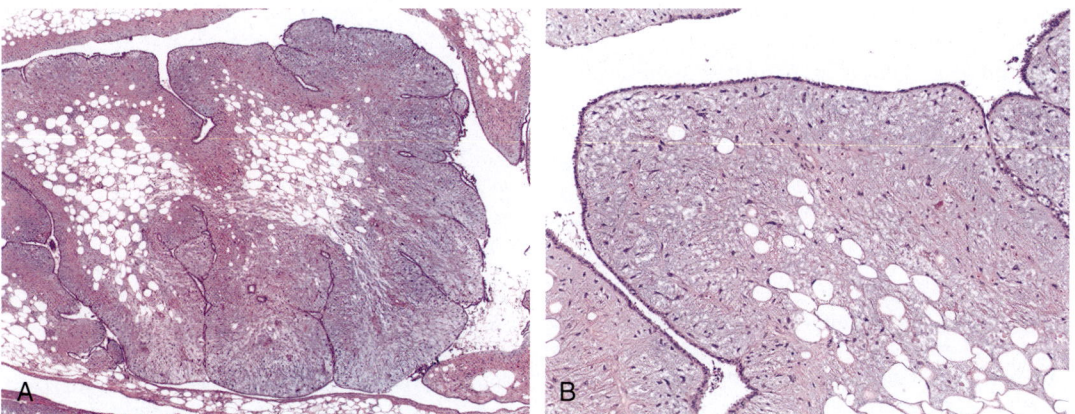

Figure 17-12 A and **B,** This phyllodes tumor has especially myxoid stroma.

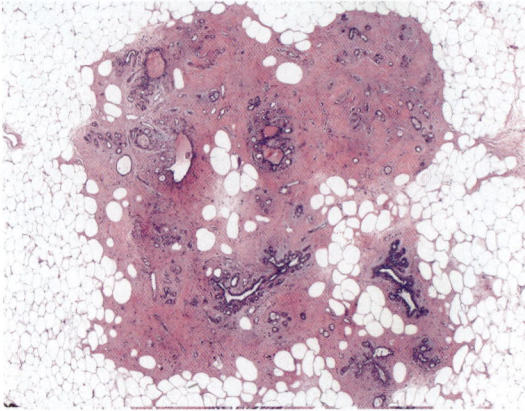

Figure 17-13 Collagen has replaced most of the myxoid material in this myxoid fibroadenoma; nevertheless, other characteristics allow one to recognize the nature of the lesion.

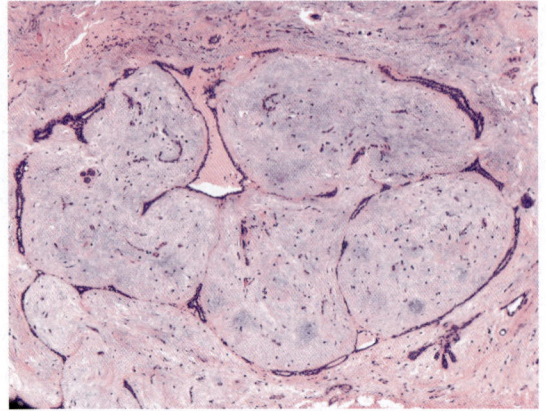

Figure 17-14 The myxoid ground substances in this myxoid fibroadenoma distorts glands to create the intracanalicular pattern seen in conventional fibroadenomas.

Attention to other histologic findings allows pathologists to differentiate these masqueraders from genuine myxoid fibroadenomas. With the passage of time, myxoid fibroadenomas undergo involution just like conventional fibroadenomas (Fig. 17-13). Although the disappearance of this extracellular material eliminates one of the most distinctive features of the lesion, the structural properties of the mass and the architectural characteristics of the glandular tissue persist, and these features allow one to establish the proper diagnosis.

Characteristics of the Glands

The terminal duct–lobular units trapped within a myxoid fibroadenoma become distorted in the same ways as those in a conventional fibroadenoma. Certain glands have the compressed caliber and arching configuration characteristic of the conventional intracanalicular pattern (Fig. 17-14); others have the round, open profiles of the pericanalicular pattern (Fig. 17-15). The two patterns typically mingle (Fig. 17-16), and one probably observes the pericanalicular pattern relatively more frequently in myxoid fibroadenomas than in conventional fibroadenomas. In general, the extent of lobular distortion of myxoid fibroadenomas seems less pronounced than that of usual fibroadenomas. Certain lobules appear only slightly altered, and one can often easily appreciate the underlying lobular architecture of the others. Thus, the presence of easily recognizable lobules within a mass does not argue against the diagnosis of myxoid fibroadenoma. The canaliculi of a conventional fibroadenoma do not look proliferative, nor do those of a myxoid fibroadenoma; in fact, the canaliculi of myxoid fibroadenomas

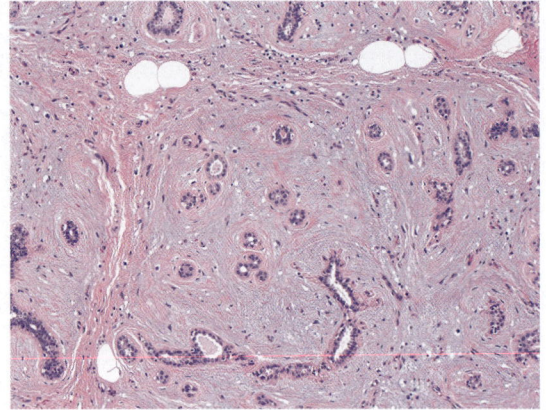

Figure 17-15 The accumulation of myxoid ground substances in this myxoid fibroadenoma has produced a pericanalicular pattern.

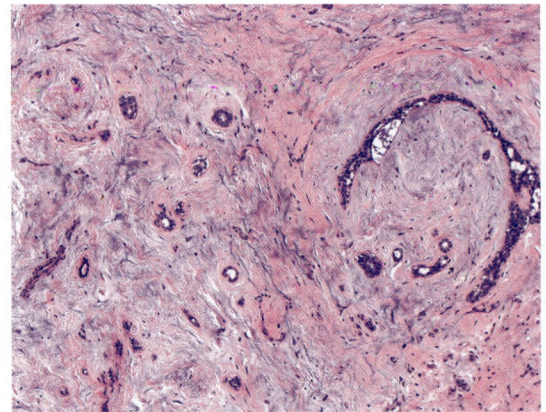

Figure 17-16 The intracanalicular and pericanalicular patterns of glandular distortion mingle in this myxoid fibroadenoma.

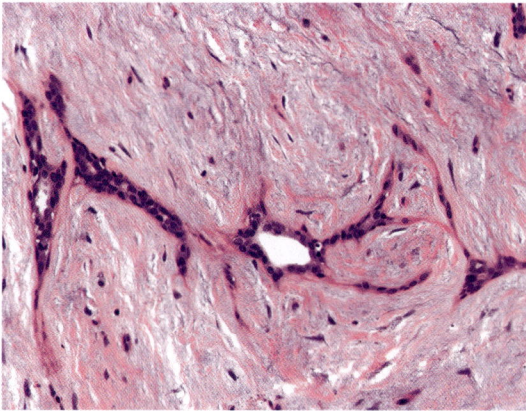

Figure 17-17 The glands of a myxoid fibroadenoma appear compressed. The myoepithelial cells look attenuated and spindly, and the basement membranes appear especially eosinophilic.

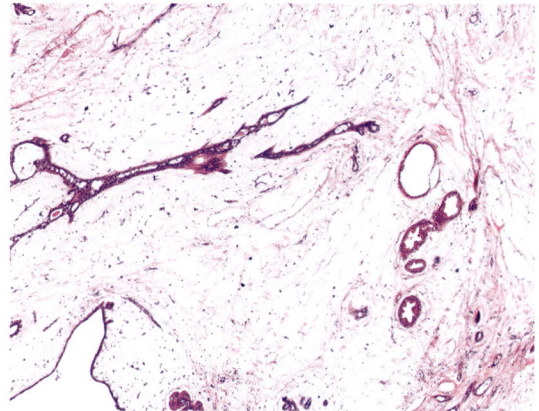

Figure 17-18 This myxoid fibroadenoma contains a focus of apocrine metaplasia.

typically appear atrophic. They have attenuated and spindly configurations with slitlike or even inapparent lumens, flattened luminal cells, long and spindly myoepithelial cells, and thick and brightly eosinophilic basement membranes (Fig. 17-17). The characteristics of the glandular tissue sometimes bring to mind those of sclerosing adenosis, and one wonders whether myxoid fibroadenomas have a propensity to develop from this background.

The epithelium lining the glands of a myxoid fibroadenoma consists of cuboidal or flattened luminal cells and inconspicuous myoepithelial cells. One does not see conventional ductal hyperplasia in myxoid fibroadenoma any more frequently than one observes it in conventional fibroadenomas, but apocrine metaplasia frequently alters the glands of myxoid fibroadenomas (Fig. 17-18).

Summary

Myxoid fibroadenomas originate from the production of myxoid ground substances by stromal cells of the specialized stromal compartment. Permeation of this material between collagen bundles of the non-specialized stroma often blurs the internal structure of the mass. The stroma consists almost entirely of

mucopolysaccharides and contains just a few stromal cells. The accumulation of these ground substances distorts the engulfed glands to produce patterns reminiscent of those of a conventional fibroadenoma. The epithelial cells appear inactive or even atrophic (Box 17-1).

PROBLEMS IN THE DIAGNOSIS OF MYXOID FIBROADENOMA

The diagnosis of myxoid fibroadenomas should not cause problems. Pathologists need only to remember that the presence of abundant myxoid ground substance itself does not establish the diagnosis of myxoid fibroadenoma; one must also observe the characteristic stromal and glandular changes. Thus, conventional fibroadenomas with especially myxoid stroma display a proliferation of fibroblasts not seen in myxoid fibroadenomas, and the glands of the former usually do not exhibit the apocrine metaplasia or the adenosis so commonly seen in the latter. Phyllodes tumors with myxoid stroma usually form obvious fronds, and other regions of the tumors demonstrate proliferation of stromal cells. Hamartomas, too, can show myxoid changes in their stroma, but the glandular architecture of a hamartoma appears disorganized and malformed. Consideration of these aspects of a myxoid tumor should allow the pathologist to classify it correctly.

Selected Reading

Carney JA, Toorkey BC: Myxoid fibroadenoma and allied conditions (myxomatosis) of the breast: A heritable disorder with special associations including cardiac and cutaneous myxomas. Am J Surg Pathol 1991;15:713-721.

Box 17-1

Histologic attributes of myxoid fibroadenomas:

- Accumulation of extracellular matrix
- Minimal proliferation of stromal cells
- Bosselated perimeter with frequent incorporation of fat
- Common presence of apocrine change

18

Phyllodes Tumor

DEFINITIONS AND CLINICOPATHOLOGIC CHARACTERISTICS

During the first half of the 19th century, Johannes Müeller introduced the term *cystosarcoma phyllodes* to refer to an unusual type of fleshy tumor characterized by the formation of leaflike fronds projecting into cystic spaces. Unlike fibroadenomas, phyllodes tumors are potentially aggressive neoplasms that enlarge progressively, can invade adjacent structures, and sometimes recur after enucleation; rare tumors metastasize. Despite many years of study, pathologists have not learned to predict the clinical course of cystosarcomas. Because of this inability, certain writers advocate the use of the noncommittal term *phyllodes tumor*, which they then subclassify as low-grade or high-grade. Such an approach eliminates the potential for the odd-sounding diagnosis *benign cystosarcoma*, which one frequently encounters when the traditional classification scheme is used.

Like fibroadenomas, phyllodes tumors originate from fibroblasts of the specialized stroma; however, the properties of the stromal cells in these two lesions differ. The neoplastic fibroblasts of phyllodes tumors have the potential for unlimited and invasive growth and the ability to stimulate the proliferation of entrapped glands, attributes not possessed by the more restrained stromal cells of fibroadenomas. Moreover, the fibroblasts of phyllodes tumors do not seem to depend as heavily on the glandular tissue for their survival as the neoplastic cells of fibroadenomas do. The stromal cells of certain phyllodes tumors can form large masses completely lacking glandular elements, a phenomenon referred to as *stromal overgrowth*. This independence from the mysterious but powerful influences of the glandular tissue gives the neoplastic fibroblasts of such tumors the ability to metastasize.

Phyllodes tumors usually originate in preexisting fibroadenomas, so phyllodes tumors tend to afflict women about 10 years older than women with fibroadenomas. The tumors often manifest as fleshy masses that are somewhat larger than the typical fibroadenoma and contain cysts into which protrude leafy stromal nodules; however, these classic features do not appear in all cases. Large phyllodes tumors and those of high grade can exhibit necrosis and hemorrhage.

All phyllodes tumors have the potential for local recurrence, although most never realize this potential even if only enucleated. When a phyllodes tumor does regrow, it often appears more aggressive than the original, and subsequent recurrences tend to look even more aggressive. Thus, the malignant potential of phyllodes tumors typically unfolds as time passes, and only rare ones ever develop the capacity to metastasize. Unlike the primary tumors, metastatic foci do not contain mammary glandular tissue. The absence of breast glands indicates that the stromal cells have finally become completely independent of the glandular tissue. Despite this independence, metastatic deposits often flourish near epithelial surfaces. This propensity suggests that the tumor cells still derive some benefit from a close proximity to epithelial cells.

HISTOLOGIC CHARACTERISTICS

Heterogeneity of the histologic characteristics, disorganization of the tissue components, and dominance of the stroma over the glandular tissue characterize the phyllodes tumor.

This aggressive counterpart of the conventional fibroadenoma arises from specialized fibroblasts that differ from those of conventional fibroadenomas in two properties: the ability to invade surrounding tissues and the ability to stimulate the proliferation of the entrapped epithelial cells. Cells with these attributes seemingly evolve from the fibroblasts of a

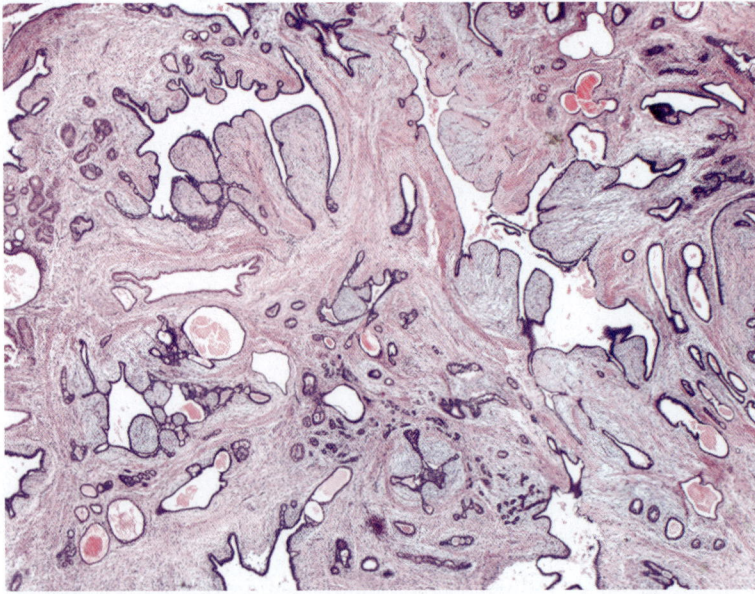

Figure 18-1 The structure of this phyllodes tumor appears variable and haphazard. The proportions of glands and stroma and the configurations of the glands differ from one region to the next.

conventional fibroadenoma, and as the neoplastic fibroblasts of the phyllodes tumor overrun the underlying fibroadenoma, a mass showing regional variation in structure, stromal characteristics, and glandular features emerges. This variability represents one of the most distinctive characteristics of phyllodes tumors. Other, equally important diagnostic features are a disorganized and disorderly relationship between the stroma and glands and a dominance of the stroma over the glands.

Structure of the Mass

Phyllodes tumors lack a consistent structure. The histologic characteristics of the stroma and glands typically differ from one region to the next, and so does the relationship between these components (Fig. 18-1). In certain areas, the proliferating fibroblasts of the phyllodes tumor remain confined to the specialized stromal compartment (Fig. 18-2); the architecture of such regions resembles the structure of a fibroadenoma. More commonly, the neoplastic fibroblasts grow without regard to either stromal compartment; they overgrow regions of the preexisting fibroadenoma, obliterating its organized structure and they invade the adjacent mammary tissues (Fig. 18-3). This invasion of the mammary parenchyma leads to the haphazard incorporation of minimally altered lobules and adipose tissue within the phyllodes tumor (Fig. 18-4). Besides invading the underlying tissues, the fibroblasts of phyllodes tumors sometimes stimulate the growth of the entrapped glands (Fig. 18-5), and this stimulation causes the incorporated ducts to branch irregularly and

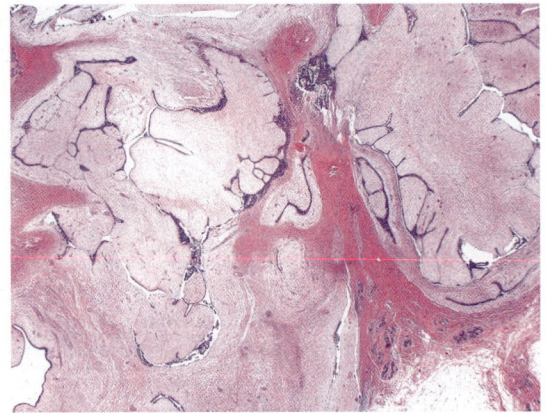

Figure 18-2 Growing in the specialized stromal compartment, the neoplastic fibroblasts of this phyllodes produce an intracanalicular pattern.

to give rise to lobules with irregular and complex configurations (Fig. 18-6). Thus, the usual phyllodes tumor comes to consist of poorly organized and variably arranged stroma and glands, disorderly in appearance and haphazard in arrangement (Fig. 18-7).

The presence of leftover remnants of the fibroadenoma also contributes to the variability in the structure of phyllodes tumors (Fig. 18-8). These fragments display the well-behaved structure of a fibroadenoma, and the organized pattern of these regions contrasts with the unruly appearance of the phyllodes tumor. The persistence of these benign elements can confuse pathologists unfamiliar with the phenomenon.

Figure 18-3 In the upper right corner, the neoplastic fibroblasts of this phyllodes tumor expand the specialized stromal compartment; near the center, the fibroblasts invade the adjacent fat and entrap adipocytes. Remnants of the preexisting fibroadenoma appear in the left.

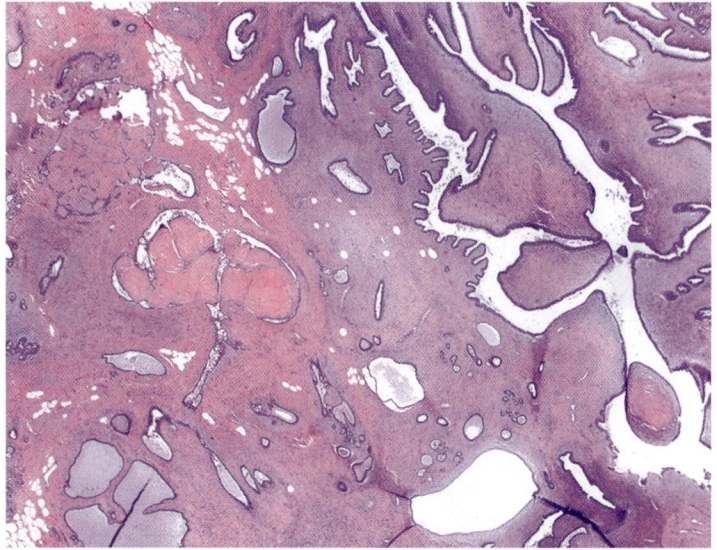

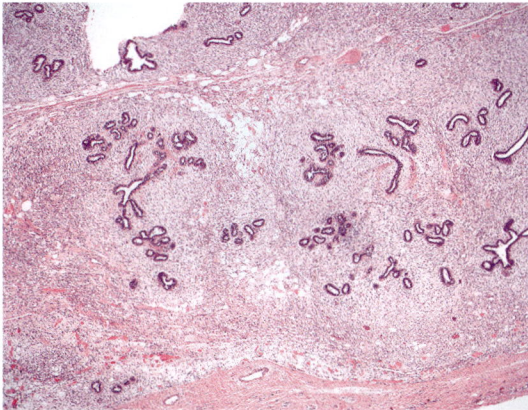

Figure 18-4 The fibroblasts of this particularly invasive phyllodes tumor have overrun the mammary parenchyma, engulfed lobules without altering them greatly, and infiltrated the fat.

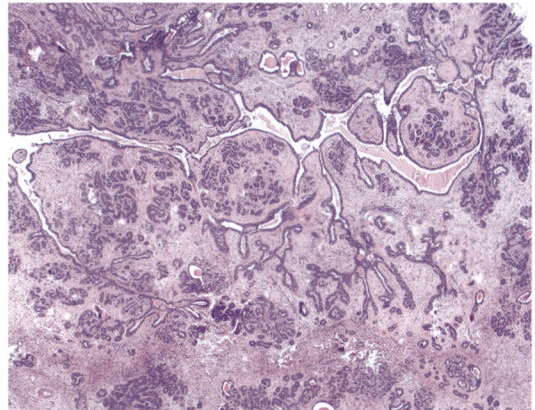

Figure 18-5 This phyllodes tumor shows irregular branching of ducts and disorderly enlargement of terminal duct–lobular units.

Figure 18-6 In this phyllodes tumor, poorly formed lobules with odd configurations have sprouted from the small ducts.

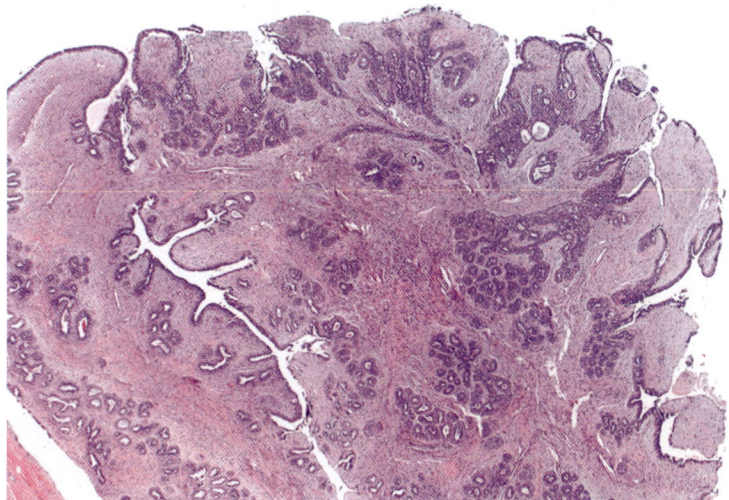

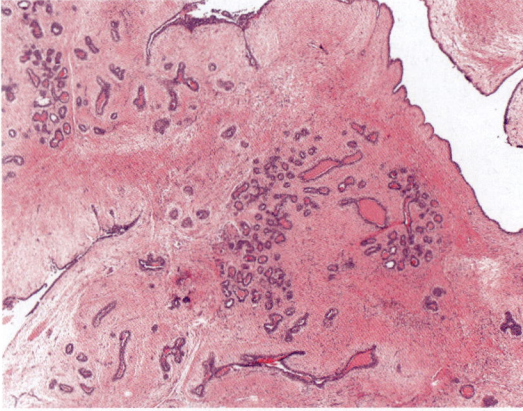

Figure 18-7 This phyllodes tumor demonstrates variability in structure and an inconsistent and disorderly relationship between the stroma and glands.

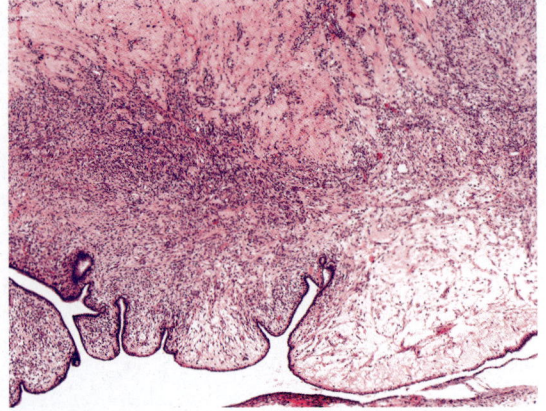

Figure 18-9 Even in this one small region, the stroma of this phyllodes tumor varies in cellularity and in the composition of extracellular matrix.

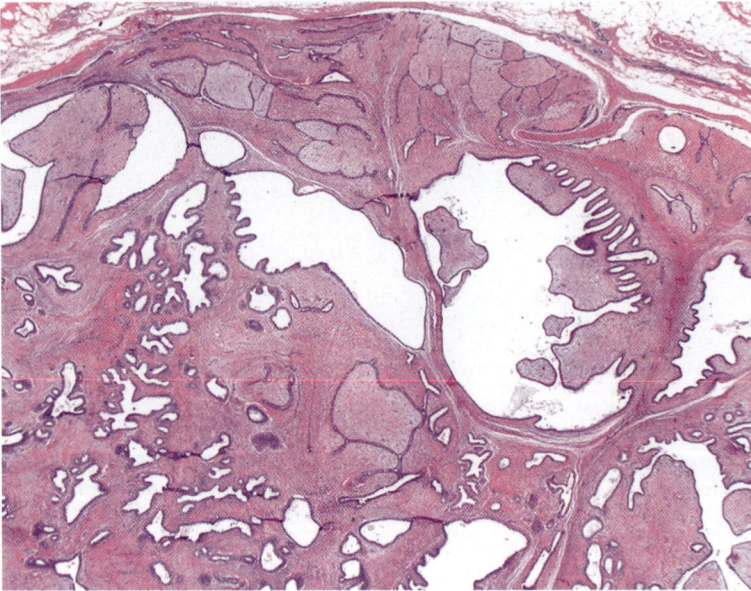

Figure 18-8 The tissue at the top represents the remnants of the fibroadenoma from which this phyllodes tumor originated. The orderly arrangement of the tissue components in the fibroadenoma contrasts with the irregular and disheveled structure of the phyllodes tumor.

If one mistakenly regards these two regions as components of a single neoplasm, one will not know whether to classify it as a fibroadenoma or a phyllodes tumor. Rather than taking this approach, pathologists should recognize that the mass contains both fibroadenoma and phyllodes tumor and that this coexistence of lesions reflects the birth of the phyllodes tumor from a preexisting fibroadenoma.

Characteristics of the Stroma

Just as the structure of a phyllodes tumor often varies within a case, so, also, do the properties of the stroma (Fig. 18-9). Many descriptions of phyllodes tumors stress stromal hypercellularity as a defining characteristic, but the density of the fibroblasts of phyllodes tumors varies greatly both from tumor to tumor and within many individual examples. Rare phyllodes tumors have stroma no more cellular than that of a conventional fibroadenoma, whereas others look as cellular as a high-grade sarcoma; however, most exhibit a stromal density between these extremes (Fig. 18-10). This wide variation in the density of stromal cells and the overlap between the cellularity of low-grade phyllodes tumors and that of fibroadenomas limits the value of this feature in the analysis of fibroepithelial tumors except in the most extreme cases. Thus, one cannot exclude the diagnosis of phyllodes tumor for most tumors composed of hypocellular stroma (Fig. 18-11), nor does a finding

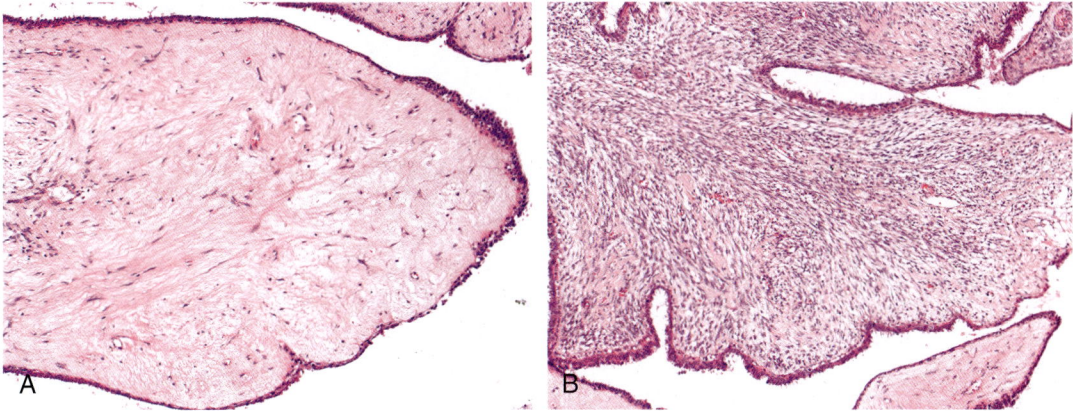

Figure 18-10 The cellularity of the stroma of a phyllodes tumor varies from case to case. The tumor depicted in **A** has hypocellular stroma, whereas the one shown in **B** has hypercellular stroma. **C,** The tumor seen in this photomicrograph illustrates the degree of cellularity seen in a typical phyllodes tumor.

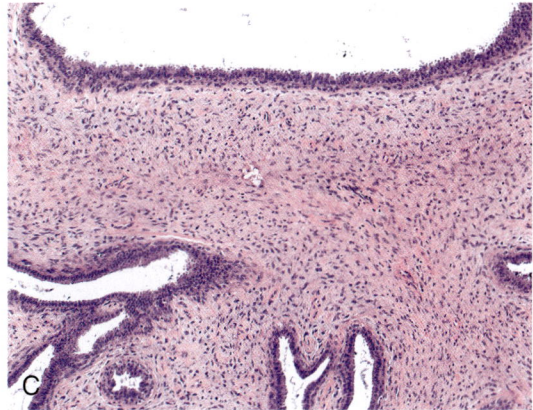

of modest hypercellularity establish the diagnosis of phyllodes tumor. Although the presence of highly cellular stroma strongly favors the diagnosis of phyllodes tumor instead of fibroadenoma, this finding occurs only rarely. Haphazard variation in the extent of stromal cellularity, on the other hand, represents a more commonly encountered and a more reliable finding. Many phyllodes tumors have areas of increased stromal density merging with regions containing fewer fibroblasts (Fig. 18-12); consequently, a fibroepithelial tumor composed of stroma of inconsistently variable cellularity almost always represents a phyllodes tumor.

The nature of the extracellular matrix of phyllodes tumors also encompasses a wide range. It usually contains faintly blue, myxoid ground substances and frequently contains some amount of eosinophilic collagen (Fig. 18-13), but the proportions of these two substances vary. Most commonly, myxoid substances accumulate in small pools between the fibroblasts and collagen bundles. In certain rare cases, though, the myxoid material so dominates the picture that the stroma resembles that of a myxoid fibroadenoma (Fig. 18-14). In other

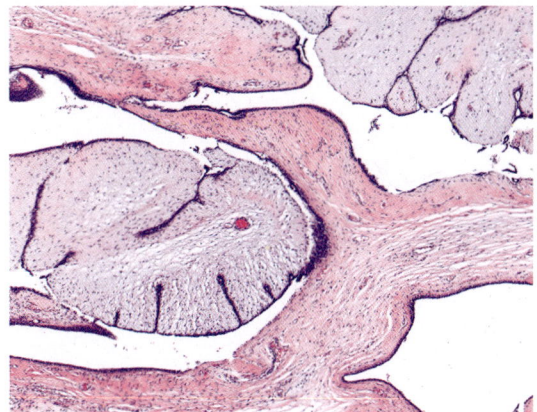

Figure 18-11 The stroma of this phyllodes tumor does not appear hypercellular.

uncommon examples, the extracellular material consists entirely of dense collagen (Fig. 18-15). Like other attributes of the stroma, the nature of the extracellular matrix usually varies in different regions of the tumor, and the presence of a disorderly

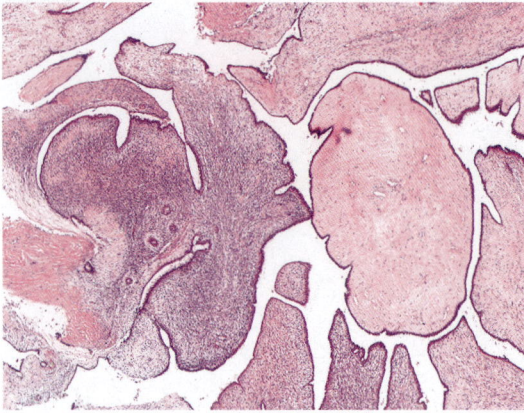

Figure 18-12 This phyllodes tumor displays pronounced variation in stromal cellularity.

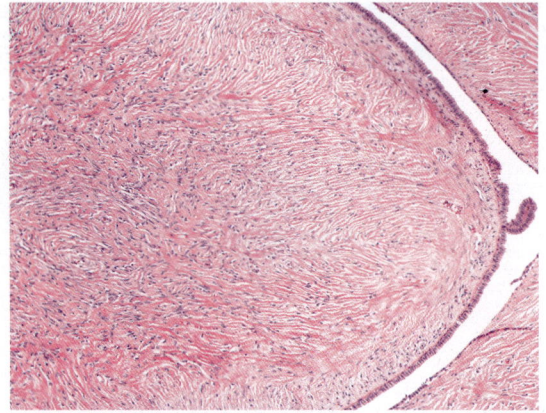

Figure 18-15 The extracellular matrix of this phyllodes tumor consists entirely of collagen.

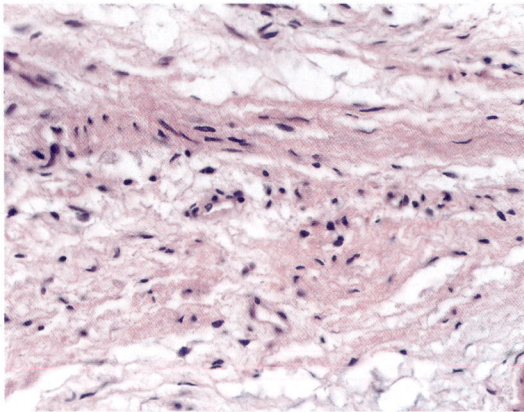

Figure 18-13 The extracellular material in this phyllodes tumor consists of collagen interlaced with faintly blue, myxoid material.

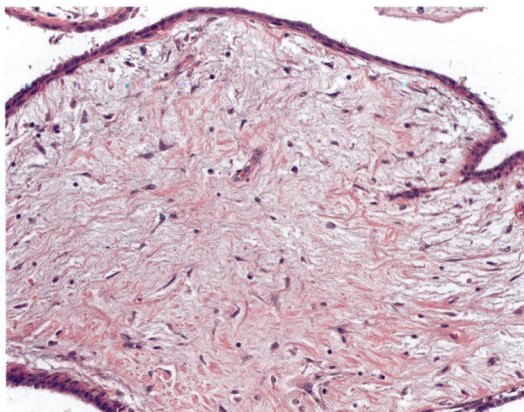

Figure 18-14 The myxoid quality of the stroma of this phyllodes tumor brings to mind the appearance of the stroma of a myxoid fibroadenoma.

mixture of different types of matrix in a fibroepithelial tumor would lead one to favor the diagnosis of phyllodes tumor.

The cytologic attributes of the neoplastic fibroblasts differ from case to case. The cells of high-grade phyllodes tumors look as anaplastic as those of other high-grade sarcomas (Fig. 18-16), but such cases occur quite uncommonly and do not pose diagnostic difficulties. The fibroblasts of lower-grade phyllodes tumors appear small, bland, and uniform. The tumor cells of the usual phyllodes tumor possess plump, oval nuclei, granular and slightly pale chromatin, and small nucleoli; less commonly, the nuclei have spindly shapes and homogeneous, dark chromatin (Fig. 18-17). In both situations, the neoplastic tumor cells do not show the variation in cellular characteristics seen in the fibroblasts of fibroadenomas. Instead, the tumor cells of phyllodes tumors seem to constitute a single neoplastic population, and this uniformity offers a subtle clue favoring the diagnosis of phyllodes tumor over fibroadenoma.

The tumor cells of phyllodes tumors may exhibit mitotic activity, and many writings emphasize the importance of this finding in establishing the diagnosis. This emphasis seems misplaced, because the mitotic rate of phyllodes tumors varies as widely as the other characteristics of the stromal cells. One finds mitotic figures readily in certain clear-cut phyllodes tumors, but only in small numbers in others. Thus, one cannot rely on the absence of division figures to exclude the diagnosis of phyllodes tumor. The presence of mitotic figures in a fibroepithelial lesion carries more significance. Benign fibroepithelial lesions do not display noticeable mitotic activity, and those rare fibroblasts in a fibroadenoma that do divide usually sit close to a canaliculus. Thus, the presence of mitotic figures, especially those located

Figure 18-16 The stroma shows marked cellularity, and the stromal cells appear anaplastic.

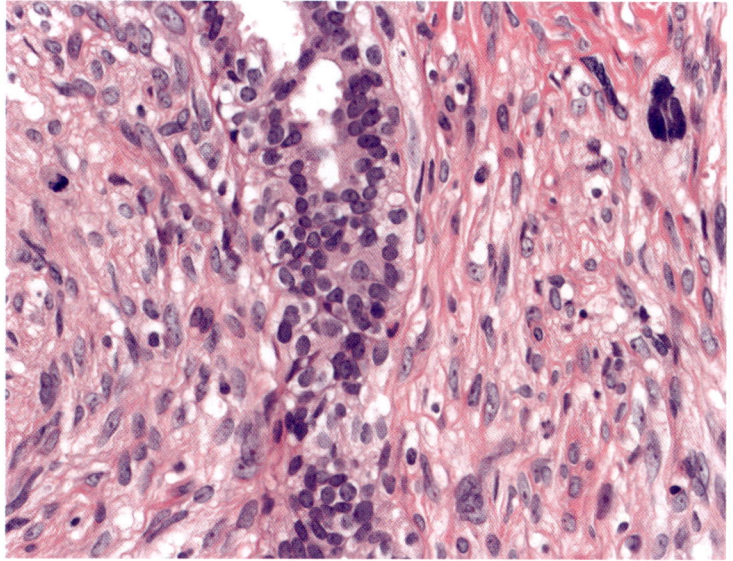

Figure 18-17 The fibroblasts in **A** have slightly enlarged nuclei, granular chromatin, and small nucleoli, whereas the cells in **B** have small, dark nuclei.

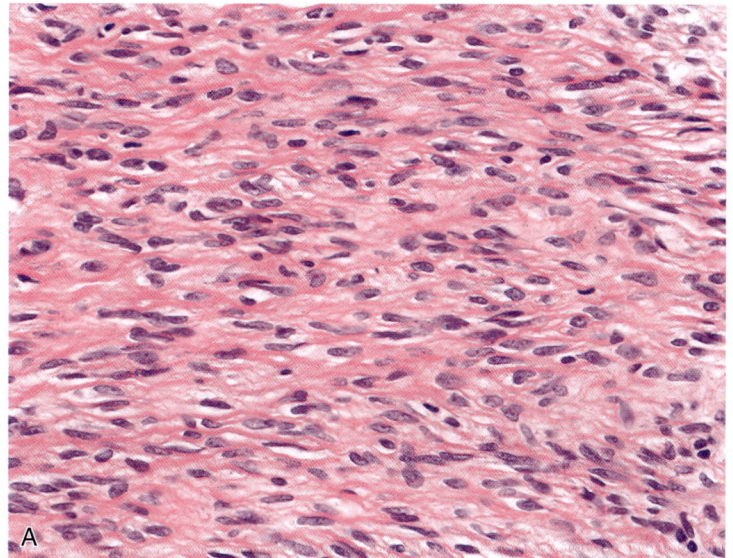

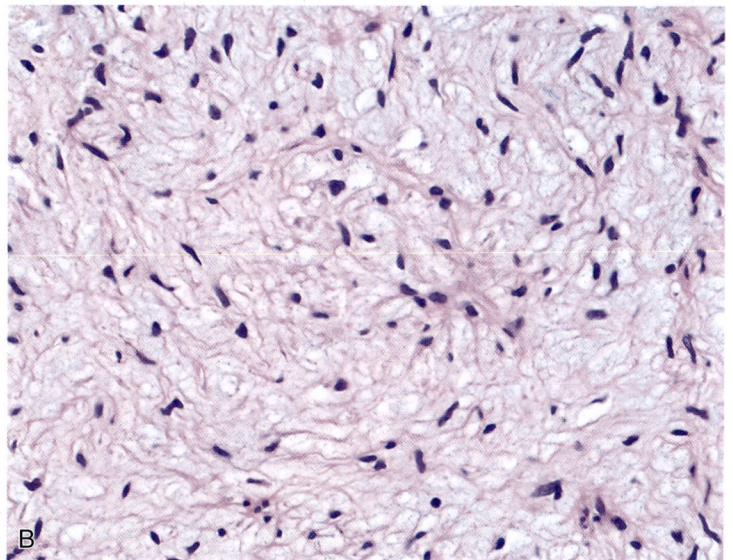

A

B

far from the glandular tissue, should strongly suggest the diagnosis of phyllodes tumor.

The stroma cells of phyllodes tumors can exhibit any type of mesenchymal differentiation. Most commonly they assume fibroblastic or myofibroblastic qualities. Those showing fibroblastic properties have long, slender shapes and aggregate to form fascicles. Myofibroblastic differentiation produces the appearance of pseudoangiomatous stromal hyperplasia. The neoplastic fibroblasts form anastomosing, slitlike spaces that resemble capillaries, and the collagen takes on a bright, eosinophilic hue. In certain phyllodes tumors, such foci display the characteristics of conventional pseudoangiomatous stromal hyperplasia (Fig. 18-18); in others, the pseudoangiomatous alteration displays a fascicular pattern, in which the myofibroblasts look more closely packed and the vascular spaces less obvious (Fig. 18-19A). One occasionally encounters a peculiar form of pseudoangiomatous stromal hyperplasia in which the small stromal cells create a dense pseudovascular network among

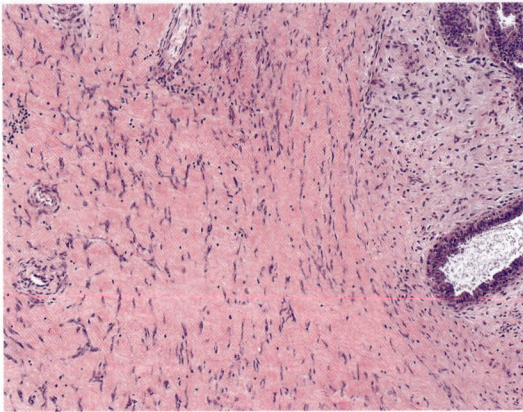

especially small bundles of collagen (Fig. 18-19B). One rarely observes pseudoangiomatous changes in the stroma of fibroadenomas, so the presence of this type of alteration in a tumor of specialized stroma should strongly suggest the diagnosis of phyllodes tumor. When the pseudoangiomatous pattern dominates, the diagnosis of nodular pseudoangiomatous hyperplasia enters the differential diagnosis.

Besides showing fibroblastic and myofibroblastic qualities, the stroma cells of phyllodes tumors can exhibit lipomatous, chondroid, osseous, and vascular differentiation, and the appearance of these mesenchymal tissues can range from completely benign to obviously malignant. The presence of benign-appearing adipose tissue or, more rarely, cartilage can create diagnostic confusion, because it introduces hamartoma and pseudoangiomatous stromal hyperplasia as possibilities in the differential diagnosis. The presence of a characteristic pattern of distortion of the glandular tissue or findings such as stromal atypicality and invasion of the surrounding parenchyma by the stromal cells would favor the diagnosis of phyllodes tumor rather than hamartoma or pseudoangiomatous stromal hyperplasia.

Occasional phyllodes tumors harbor a large number of plasma cells in their stroma. Other fibroepithelial lesions contain plasma cells, too, so the mere presence of such cells does not offer diagnostic guidance. Nevertheless, prominent aggregates of plasma cells like the one pictured in Figure 18-20 most often occur in phyllodes tumors.

Like the other attributes of the stroma of phyllodes tumors, the ratio between the amounts of stroma and glands differs from one area to the next. Certain fields consist of equal quantities of glands and stroma; in others, the stroma predominates (Fig. 18-21). An individual fibroadenoma usually maintains a constant fraction of glands and stroma,

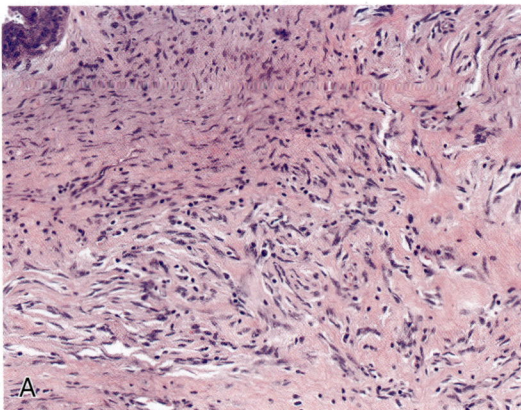

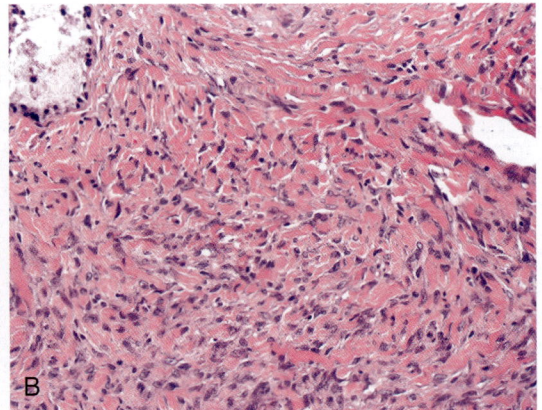

Figure 18-18 The stroma of this phyllodes tumor shows the typical pattern of pseudoangiomatous stromal hyperplasia.

Figure 18-19 A, The pseudoangiomatous stromal hyperplasia in this phyllodes tumor exhibits a fascicular pattern. B, The stroma of this tumor exhibits a pseudoangiomatous-like appearance characterized by tiny bundles of eosinophilic collagen and many myofibroblasts.

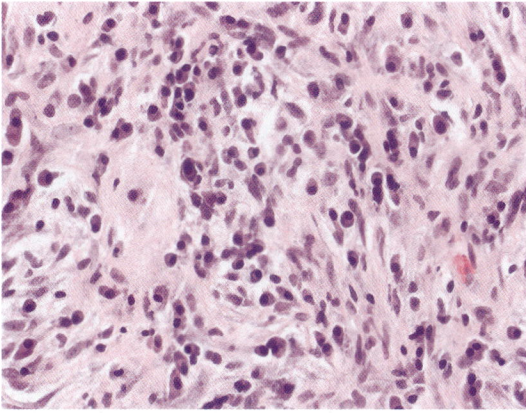

Figure 18-20 A large number of plasma cells congregate in a small region.

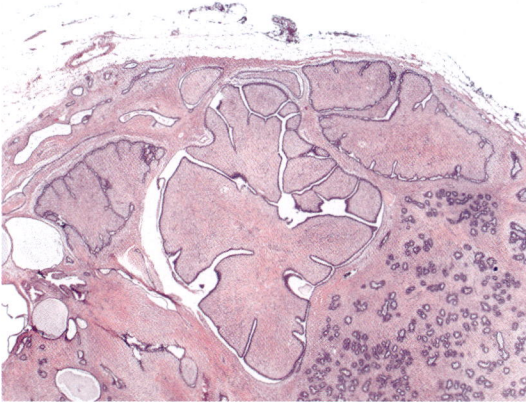

Figure 18-21 This phyllodes tumor displays regional variation in the ratio of its glands and stroma.

so the ratio of these two elements does not differ much from field to field. Marked regional variation in the proportions of stroma and glands of a fibroepithelial tumor should lead one to consider the diagnosis of phyllodes tumor.

Characteristics of the Glands

The glandular tissue entrapped within a phyllodes tumor usually varies in its architecture and in the appearance of its epithelium. The configuration of the entrapped ducts and terminal duct–lobular units depends on the manner of growth of the neoplastic fibroblasts. The fibroblasts of most phyllodes tumors grow partly within the specialized stromal compartment, so the glands often exhibit either an intracanalicular or a pericanalicular configuration, more commonly the former. Proliferation of the epithelial cells lining the glands causes the latter to dilate and to branch; consequently, the glands become irregular in their contours and disorderly in their architecture (Fig. 18-22). Most phyllodes tumors also grow by direct invasion of the mammary parenchyma. In this process, terminal duct–lobular units become incorporated into the tumor without coming to display either an intracanalicular or a pericanalicular architecture (Fig. 18-23). The appearance of these entrapped lobules differs; some appear encased by the neoplastic fibroblasts, whereas others show penetration of the lobules by the tumor cells and dispersion of the ductules and acini. Thus, the glands within a phyllodes tumor typically vary in their architecture and in the pattern of their deformation. This variation in glandular architecture should always make one consider the diagnosis of phyllodes

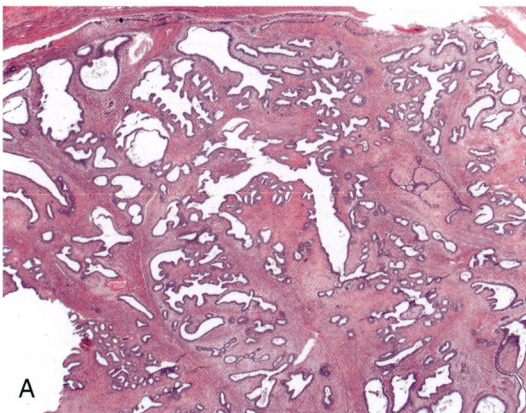

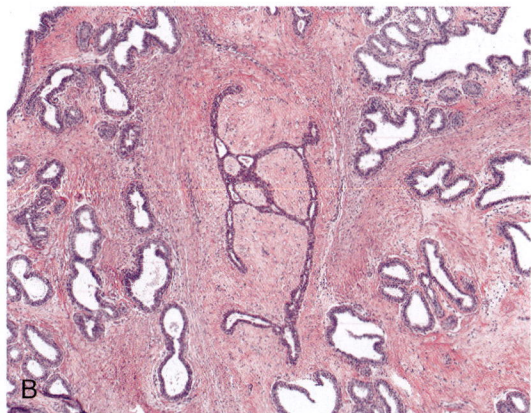

Figure 18-22 A, The glands of this phyllodes tumor have irregular contours and dilated lumens. **B,** Contrast the irregular profiles and dilated lumens of the glands of the phyllodes tumor with the smooth, graceful outlines and compressed lumens of the canaliculi in the residual fibroadenoma situated in the center.

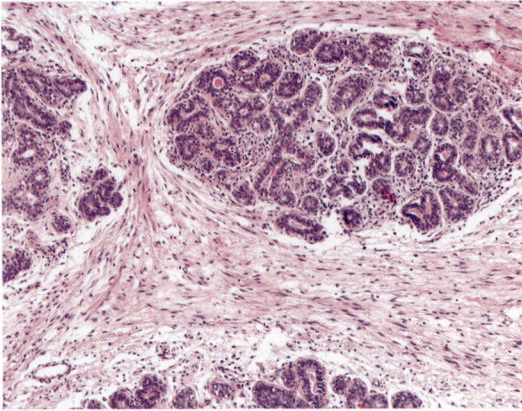

Figure 18-23 The neoplastic fibroblasts have surrounded and engulfed this lobule, trapping it within the tumor but not distorting it.

tumor, especially when one observes minimally distorted lobules permeated by neoplastic fibroblasts.

Virtually all writings about the histologic characteristics of phyllodes tumors emphasize the formation of leaflike stromal fronds projecting into distended, cystic spaces, the phenomenon that inspired this tumor's original name. Two popular misconceptions surround this phenomenon. First, many pathologists believe that the diagnosis of phyllodes tumor requires the presence of stromal fronds. The typical phyllodes tumor does grow in this way, of course; however, many bona fide phyllodes tumors have only minimal frond formation, and some none at all. Thus, one cannot require the presence of stromal fronds to make the diagnosis of phyllodes tumor. On the other hand, one does not observe well-developed fronds in lesions other than phyllodes tumors, so the presence of these distinctive stromal nodules virtually guarantees this diagnosis.

To maintain the diagnostic significance of the leaflike growth pattern, one must adhere to a strict definition of a *frond*. It should display the following characteristics. First, the structure in question must have a considerable size. One should not overinterpret the small stromal nodules that can form in fibroadenomas as the fronds of a phyllodes tumor. Second, the structure should look like an expanding region. Finally, the shape of the stromal mass should differ from the shape of the space housing the nodule. Slight widening of the canaliculi of a fibroadenoma can create the illusion of a frond protruding into a space, but the stromal nodule conforms to the contour of the space and therefore does not qualify as a genuine frond. Figure 18-24 illustrates a genuine frond and examples of artifactually created frondlike structures. One must take particular care

when examining specimens obtained during a core biopsy, because handling of the specimen can cause fragments of a fibroadenoma to resemble the fronds of a phyllodes tumor (Fig. 18-25).

The second misunderstanding regarding the stromal fronds of a phyllodes tumor ascribes their formation to the proliferation of the neoplastic fibroblasts. The creation of a frond does require proliferation of the stromal cells; however, it also requires the creation of a space into which the frond can protrude, and the generation of such a space depends on proliferation of the epithelial cells. As the epithelial cells multiply and grow in a single layer, they enlarge the diameters of the affected canaliculi and thereby form the cysts into which the stromal nodules protrude. Without this epithelial cooperation, the fibroblastic proliferation could never create a frond.

This epithelial proliferation manifests itself in two ways besides the formation of cysts. First, it alters the configurations of the canaliculi. Instead of exhibiting the narrow calibers, arching shapes, and beaded contours characteristic of fibroadenomas, the canaliculi of a phyllodes tumor enlarge, branch in irregular and complex configurations, and do not appear beaded. Second, the proliferative state of the epithelial cells alters the cytologic characteristics of the epithelial cells and sometimes their architectural characteristics. The luminal cells often appear larger than those seen in a fibroadenoma, and the former contain larger nuclei, larger nucleoli, and more cytoplasm than the latter (Fig. 18-26). One can observe epithelial mitotic figures. Although the epithelial cells often grow as a single layer, they can display stratification and the formation of conventional ductal hyperplasia (Fig. 18-27). Such regions of ductal hyperplasia can demonstrate cytologic atypicality of a reactive type (Fig. 18-28). Thus, the presence of epithelial proliferation in a fibroepithelial tumor should prompt one to consider the diagnosis of phyllodes tumor (Box 18-1).

Summary

Phyllodes tumors represent potentially aggressive neoplasms derived from cells of the specialized stroma. Most examples arise from preexisting fibroadenomas; however, rare phyllodes tumors develop from hamartomas and others seem to originate de novo. The ability of the neoplastic stroma cells to invade surrounding cells and to stimulate the growth of the glandular tissue leads to variability in the internal structure of the mass, in the ratio between the amounts of the stroma and glands, in the histologic characteristics of the stroma, and in the structure of the glands (Box 18-1).

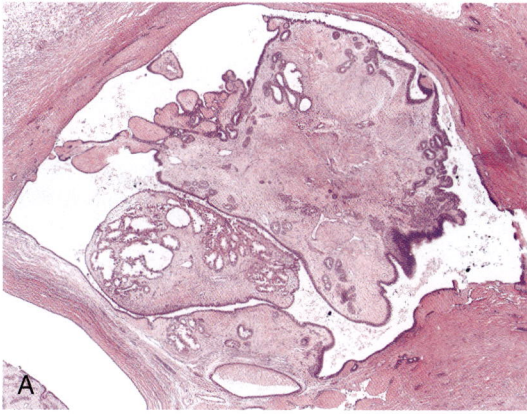

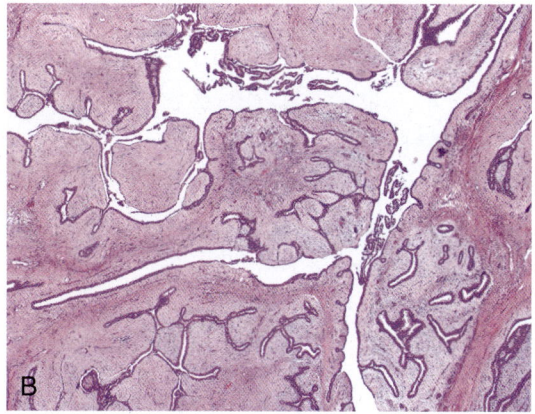

Figure 18-24 A, This structure represents a genuine frond. It appears large and expansile, and its configuration differs from that of the space housing it. **B,** This structure, which superficially resembles a frond of a phyllodes tumor, arose as a result of stretching of the tissue of a conventional intracanalicular fibroadenoma. **C,** Widening of the canaliculi of this fibroadenoma has created a few small stromal nodules protruding into the dilated canaliculi; however, such structures do not represent genuine fronds.

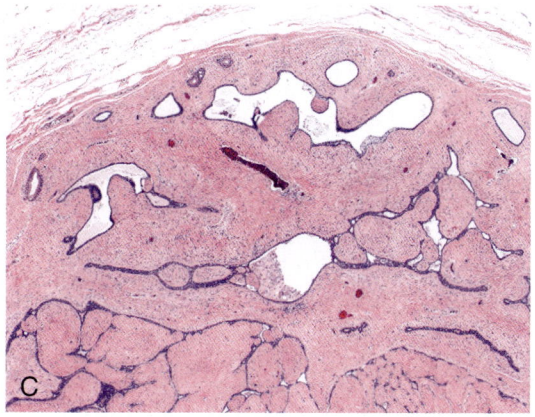

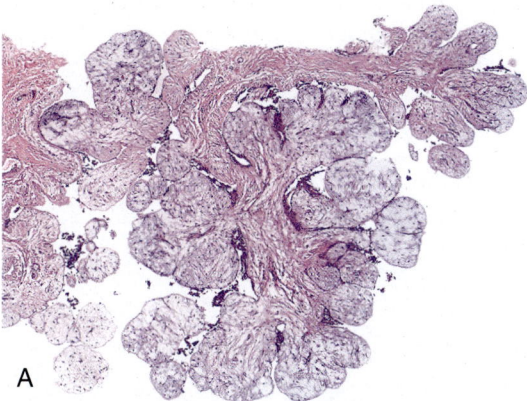

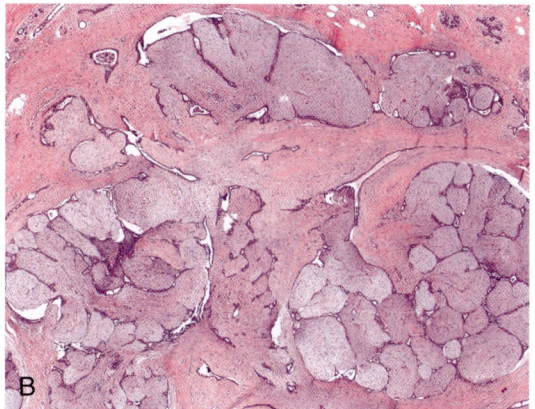

Figure 18-25 A, This fragment of a fibroadenoma removed during a core biopsy seems to form a frond; however, most of the stroma lacks an epithelial covering. **B,** The resected nodule shows characteristics of a conventional fibroadenoma.

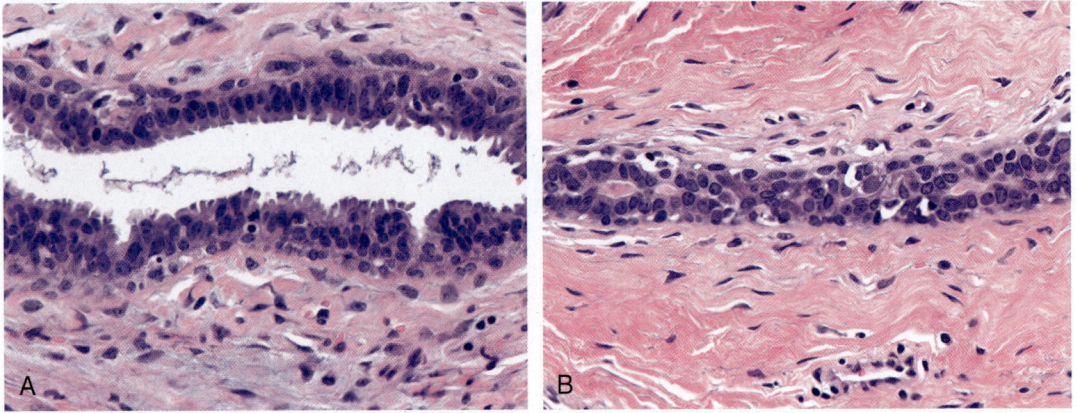

Figure 18-26 A, The luminal cells lining the slightly dilated canaliculus of this phyllodes tumor appear crowded, exhibit tall columnar shapes, and possess modest amounts of apical cytoplasm. **B,** The luminal cells lining the narrow canaliculus of this fibroadenoma have low cuboidal shapes and only a little apical cytoplasm.

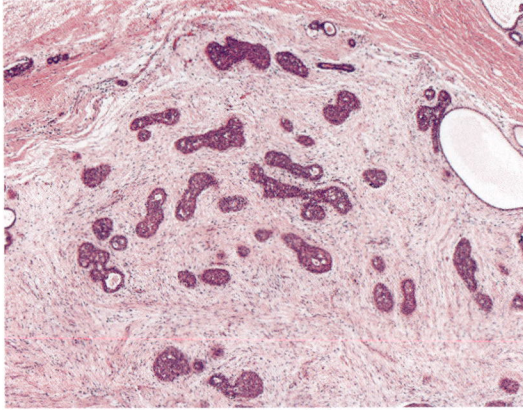

Figure 18-27 The epithelium of this phyllodes tumor exhibits genuine ductal hyperplasia of the conventional type.

Box 18-1

Characteristics of the glandular tissue of phyllodes tumors:

- Variation in its structure
- Disarray in its architecture
- Dilatation of the glandular lumens
- Enlargement and crowding of the luminal cells
- Proliferation and mitotic activity of the epithelial cells
- Reactive cytologic atypia

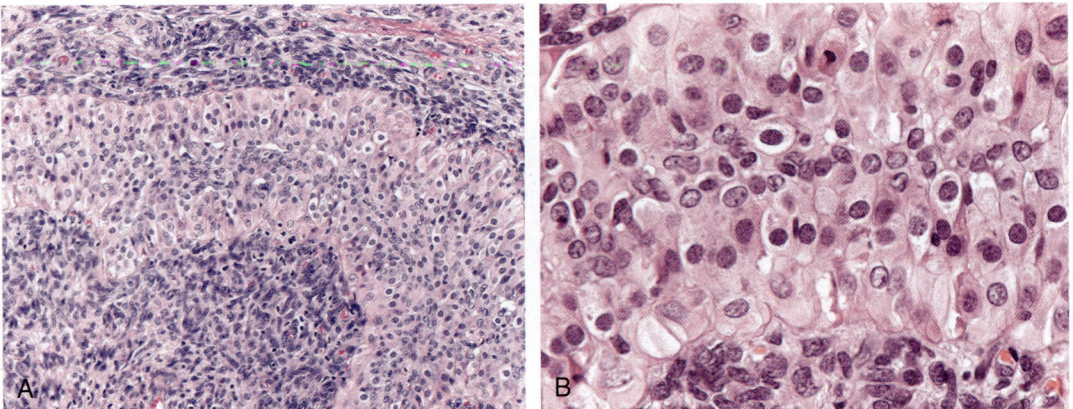

Figure 18-28 A, This phyllodes tumor has provoked an intense proliferation of ductal cells. **B,** The proliferative ductal cells display a reactive type of cytologic atypia.

PROBLEMS IN THE DIAGNOSIS OF PHYLLODES TUMORS

Of all the difficulties posed by fibroepithelial lesions, distinguishing phyllodes tumors from fibroadenomas stands out as the most common and the most troublesome. The points outlined in the preceding chapters should help one separate the typical examples of these two lesions, but borderline cases continue to vex pathologists and so does the analysis of epithelial proliferations within a phyllodes tumor.

The Fibroadenoma–Phyllodes Tumor Continuum

Histologic and demographic evidence suggests that phyllodes tumors usually develop from preexisting fibroadenomas. This hypothesis will surprise many readers, but the practice of surgical pathology provides many examples in which an aggressive lesion apparently evolves from a benign one. Squamous carcinomas of the skin often originate in actinic keratoses, and adenocarcinomas of the colon frequently begin as adenomatous polyps, to cite just two well-recognized examples. Thus, the notion that phyllodes tumors can originate from fibroadenomas does not challenge any long-standing concepts of surgical pathology, and this hypothesis receives support from the frequent intermingling of these two lesions.

From a practical point of view, the presence of regions showing features of a fibroadenoma and other regions exhibiting characteristics of a phyllodes tumor in a single mass can present the diagnostician with two difficulties. First, one must not minimize the importance of the more aggressive-looking regions and make the diagnosis of fibroadenoma. If these latter areas provide the necessary evidence, one should make the diagnosis of phyllodes tumor. The second problem arises when the aggressive portions do not have features required to establish a diagnosis of phyllodes tumor, for we do not have a universally accepted diagnosis for such a borderline case. Certain pathologists employ the term *cellular fibroadenoma* in this situation, but others use the diagnosis in different contexts; furthermore, this term does not seem sufficiently specific to describe a tumor with intermediate characteristics. For now, a descriptive diagnosis such as fibroepithelial tumor with features suggestive of early phyllodes tumor might offer the best choice.

Carcinoma Involving a Phyllodes Tumor

This diagnostic difficulty does not represent a problem in the diagnosis of phyllodes tumors, so it requires only a few comments. Like mammary epithelial cells in other locations, those composing the glands of a phyllodes tumor can give rise to atypical epithelial hyperplasia and carcinoma; however, experience has shown that, unlike fibroadenomas, which occasionally harbor carcinoma, phyllodes tumors rarely do so. To analyze an epithelial proliferation within a phyllodes tumor, one should use the diagnostic criteria and the approach established for proliferations occurring in normal ducts and terminal duct–lobular units, remembering that the ductal hyperplasia that develops in phyllodes tumors can appear especially florid and can demonstrate reactive atypia. Thus, one should generally refrain from making the diagnosis of low-grade ductal carcinoma in situ involving a phyllodes tumor unless the histologic evidence appears so overwhelming that one cannot escape it.

Selected Readings

Grimes M: Cystosarcoma of the breast: Histologic features, flow cytometry analysis, and clinical correlations. Mod Pathol 1992;5:232-239.

Keelan PA, Meyers JL, Wold LE, et al: Phyllodes tumor: Clinicopathologic review of 60 patients and flow cytometric analysis in 30 patients. Hum Pathol 1992;23:1048-1054.

Lu YJ, Birdsall S, Osin P, et al: Phyllodes tumors of the breast analyzed by comparative genomic hybridization and association of increased 1q copy number with stromal overgrowth and recurrence. Genes Chromosomes Cancer 1997;20:275-281.

Noguchi S, Yokouchi H, Aihora T, et al: Progression of fibroadenoma to phyllodes tumor demonstrated by clonal analysis. Cancer 1995;76:1779-1785.

Norris HJ, Taylor HB: Relationship of histological features to behavior of cystosarcoma phyllodes: Analysis of ninety-four cases. Cancer 1967;20:2090-2099.

Powell CM, Rosen PP: Adipose differentiation in cystosarcoma phyllodes: A study of 14 cases. Am J Surg Pathol 1994;18:720-727.

Reinfuss M, Mitus J, Duda K, et al: The treatment and prognosis of patients with phyllodes tumor of the breast: An analysis of 170 cases. Cancer 1996;77:910-916.

Seijo L, Sidhu J, Mizrachy B, et al: Malignant phyllodes tumor of the breast: A report of four cases with associated fibroadenomata. Int J Surg Pathol 1995;3:17-22.

Ward RM, Evans HL: Cystosarcoma phyllodes: A clinicopathologic study of 26 cases. Cancer 1986;58:2282-2289.

19

Hamartoma and Fibroadenoma Variant

DEFINITIONS AND CLINICOPATHOLOGIC CHARACTERISTICS

Mammary hamartomas consist of disorganized collections of mammary tissues (ducts, lobules, fat, fibrous connective tissue, and smooth muscle). Most contain both glandular and stromal components and therefore belong to the family of fibroepithelial neoplasms. The participation of both epithelial and mesenchymal tissues in the origin and growth of hamartomas distinguishes them from both conventional and myxoid fibroadenomas as well as from phyllodes tumors, which represent lesions of specialized stroma with entrapment of non-neoplastic glands. Hamartomas typically afflict women of childbearing age, especially between ages 30 and 50 years; however, one occasionally encounters such a tumor in a postmenopausal woman. The lesion most commonly occurs singly, involves the left breast more commonly than the right, and occasionally recurs after resection. Macroscopic evaluation reveals a well-defined nodule. The tumors vary in appearance depending on composition. Those with abundant fat contain soft, yellow regions; others look homogeneous and tan or white.

In his 1979 textbook *Problems in Breast Pathology*, Dr. Azzopardi[1] briefly discusses the characteristics and classification of an uncommon lesion composed of glands and cellular collagenous stroma. He provisionally classified it as a variant of fibroadenoma, but he left open the possibility that it might have a different pathogenesis. The lesion has received little attention in the ensuing three decades, so it remains as poorly understood as it was then. Despite Dr. Azzopardi's inclusion of the word *fibroadenoma* in his term for this lesion, its histologic characteristics do not suggest a pathogenesis in common with the conventional fibroadenoma. The glands of a fibroadenoma variant

do not resemble the altered lobules of a fibroadenoma, nor does the collagenous stroma of a fibroadenoma variant look like the specialized stroma that gives rise to fibroadenomas. In fact, the histologic characteristics of fibroadenoma variants bring to mind those of a hamartoma rather than a fibroadenoma, and the fibroadenoma variant might, in fact, represent one type of hamartoma.

HISTOLOGIC CHARACTERISTICS

Disproportionate growth of tissue components and disarray of mature mammary tissues stand out as the consistent attributes of hamartomas and fibroadenoma variants. Hamartomas and fibroadenoma variants both consist of disorderly but mature mammary tissues. In neither does the architecture of the tissue components or their relationship to each other duplicate the characteristics of the normal breast; thus, neither lesion looks like an alteration of preexisting, normally formed breast tissue. Instead, both hamartomas and fibroadenoma variants have the appearance of malformations. Because of this fundamental similarity, the lesions share several microscopical characteristics.

Structure of the Mass

Hamartomas consist of well-defined nodules formed from mature mammary tissues. The masses commonly display a clear-cut border and usually compress the surrounding parenchyma. Fat, nonspecialized stroma, specialized stroma, glands, and vascular structures compose the mass (Fig. 19-1). The anatomic organization of these components can mimic the structure of normal tissue so closely that one might mistake a hamartoma for normal mammary parenchyma.

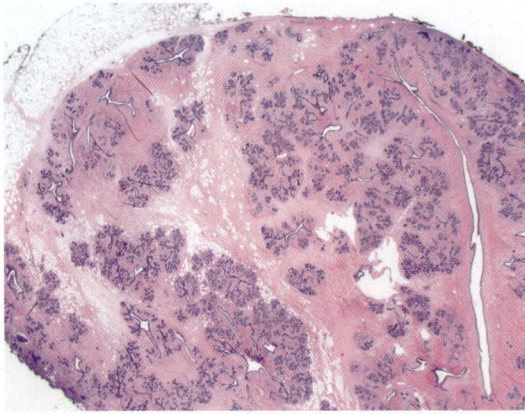

Figure 19-1 This hamartoma consists of ducts and ill-formed lobules embedded in stroma containing fibrous tissue and fat.

The recognition of the presence of a discrete nodule excludes the latter possibility, and detailed examination reveals the disorganization of the neoplastic components of a hamartoma. To illustrate the malformation and disorganization of the tissues in a typical hamartoma, consider the lesion pictured in Figure 19-2, which depicts a discrete nodule composed of "ducts" and "lobules." The "lobules" seem disproportionately more numerous than the "ducts" and do not seem to cluster around the "ducts" as they do in normal mammary tissue. Furthermore, many of the "lobules" appear too large. Figure 19-2B depicts several of these "lobules" or glandular clusters. Although they superficially resemble genuine lobules, they do not appear discrete. One cluster flows into the next, and it is difficult to define the "lobule" to which certain "acini" belong. These aggregates of glands also lack the proper internal structure: One cannot recognize an intralobular terminal ductule, and the stroma surrounding the glands, although bluish in hue, does not display the loose cellularity characteristic of specialized stroma. The stroma in the hamartoma pictured in Figure 19-2C has not differentiated to form zones of specialized stroma, nonspecialized stroma, and fat; instead, the different

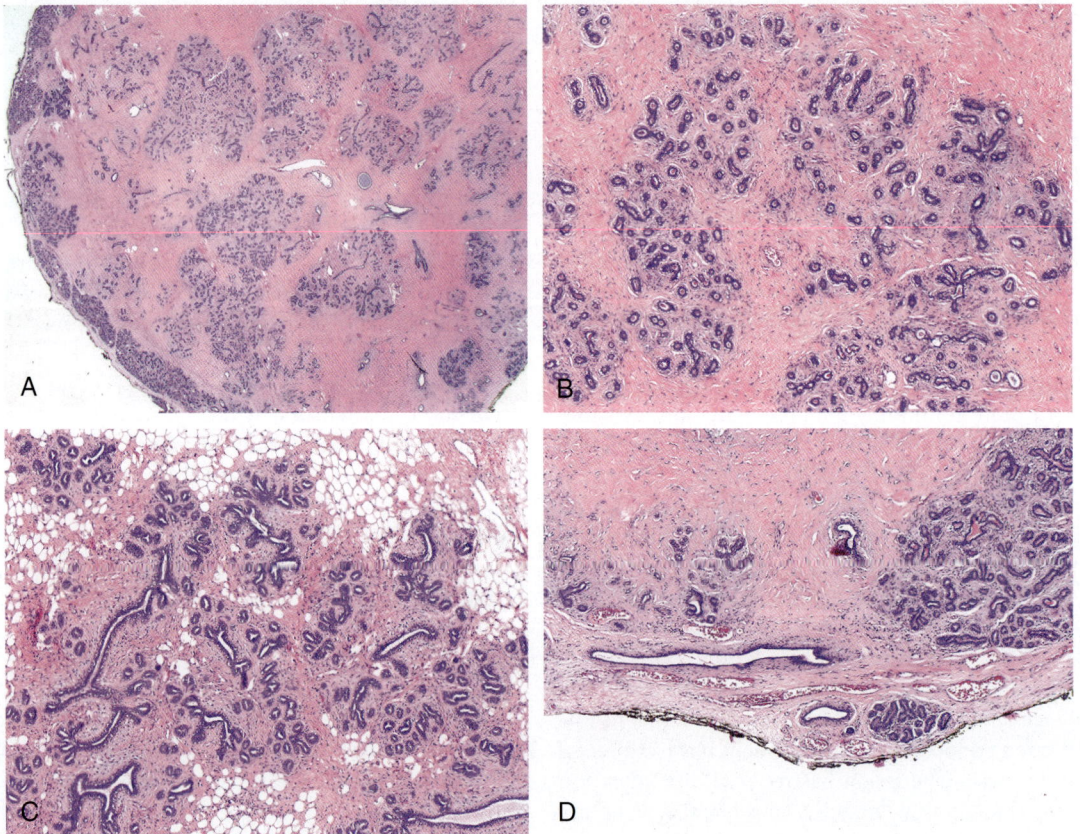

Figure 19-2 A, The number of "lobules" in this hamartoma appears disproportionate to the number of "ducts," the "lobules" and "ducts" do not display the proper architectural relationship, and certain of the "lobules" look much too large. **B,** The "lobules" do not appear discrete, and the fibrous tissue within them does not display the loosely cellular properties of genuine specialized stroma. **C,** Fat intermingles with the fibrous connective tissue. **D,** The capillaries appear malformed, and they run too close to the glandular tissue.

types of connective tissue mingle. Like the glands and stroma of a hamartoma, the blood vessels can appear malformed. The dilated capillaries at the edge of the lesion shown in Figure 19-2D, for example, appear too large in caliber and course too close to the glandular tissue.

Despite the variability in structure and composition of hamartomas, certain patterns of organization recur. In one of the more common ones, the center of the mass consists mostly of sparsely branching ducts embedded in collagenous fibrous connective tissue, and small ducts and their associated ill-formed glandular clusters occupy the periphery of the mass (Fig. 19-3). The center of such a tumor often contains one or two blood vessels of an unusually large caliber or an odd configuration. This orga-nization recalls the structure of the normal mam-mary gland, in which ducts predominate in the center, lobules occupy the peripheral zone, and vas-cular structures run in the subareolar tissue. To emphasize this similarity in structure, writers have referred to this pattern of hamartomas as a *breast within a breast*. In a second common pattern, the hamartoma consists almost entirely of small, branching ducts and lobules supported by fibrous connective tissue and fat in varying proportions (Fig. 19-4). The existence of these different patterns suggests that the cells giving rise to hamartomas differ in the potential for tissue organization. Cells with the ability to form an entire breast would give rise to the *breast within a breast* pattern, whereas those capable of forming only small ducts and lobules

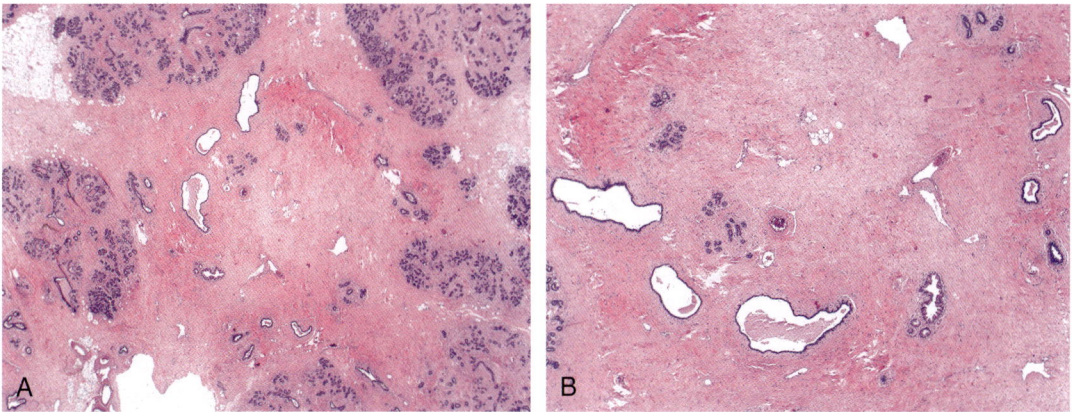

Figure 19-3 A, This hamartoma illustrates the pattern known as *breast within a breast*. The lobule-like structures occupy the periphery of the mass, whereas duct-like structures dominate in the center. **B,** One sometimes finds a large artery in the middle of this type of hamartoma.

Figure 19-4 This hamartoma displays the organization of the lobular type of hamartoma. Slender bands of fibrous tissue subdivide the glandular tissue into smoothly contoured, compact units. Capacious vessels course through the fibrous tissue bands.

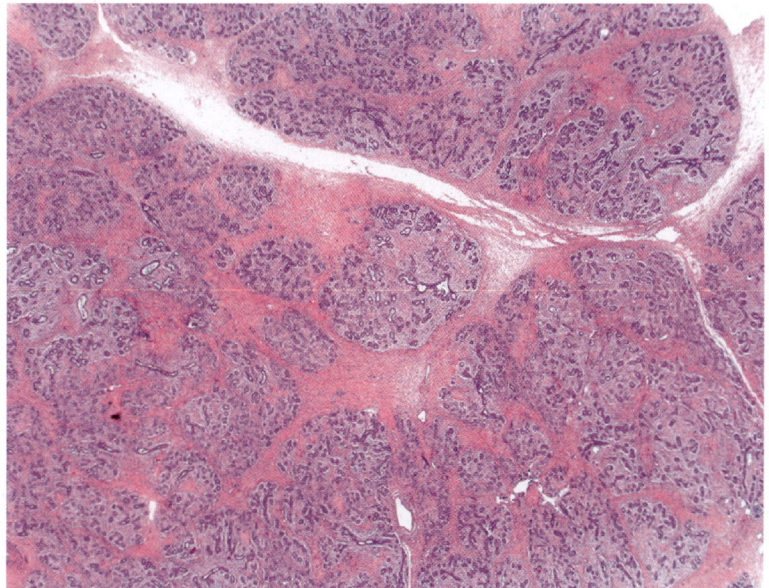

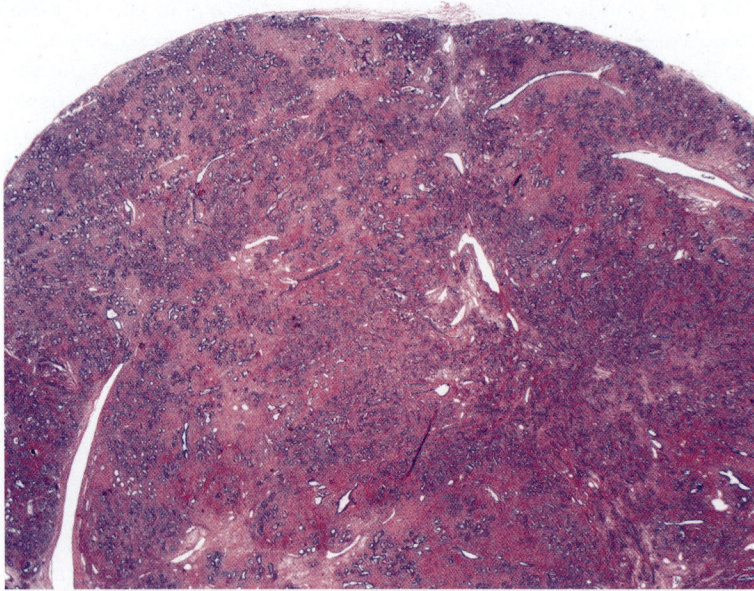

Figure 19-5 This fibroadenoma variant has a well-defined border and consists of aggregates of small glands growing in a collagenous stroma.

would produce the second pattern. Cells with intermediate growth potential would form hamartomas with a mixture of patterns.

Fibroadenoma variants, too, consist of disorderly glands and poorly formed "lobules," which tend to appear large and overly complicated. They sit in fibrous connective tissue that lacks a clear differentiation into specialized and nonspecialized breast stroma (Fig. 19-5). These features overlap with those of hamartomas so much that one might regard the two lesions as the same.

Characteristics of the Stroma

The stroma of hamartomas consists of any of a variety of mesenchymal tissues; often, several types of stroma coexist. Usually one sees dense fibrous connective tissue recapitulating the appearance and distribution of nonspecialized stroma and myxoid fibrous connective tissue surrounding clusters of glands. Fat often mixes with the dense fibrous connective tissue, but the adipocytes do not follow the course of small blood vessels as the fat cells of fibroadenomas do. Instead, the adipocytes of hamartomas mingle haphazardly and indiscriminately with the stromal fibroblasts (Fig. 19-6). Pathologists have used *adenolipoma* for hamartomas in which fat forms the dominant type of stroma and *chondrolipoma* for the rare hamartoma in which the stroma contains mature hyaline cartilage.

Like the supporting tissues, other elements of the stroma sometimes appear disorganized or malformed.

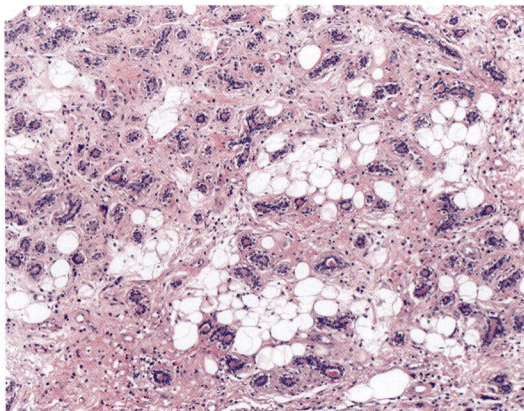

Figure 19-6 The stroma of this hamartoma consists of disorganized fat and fibrous connective tissue.

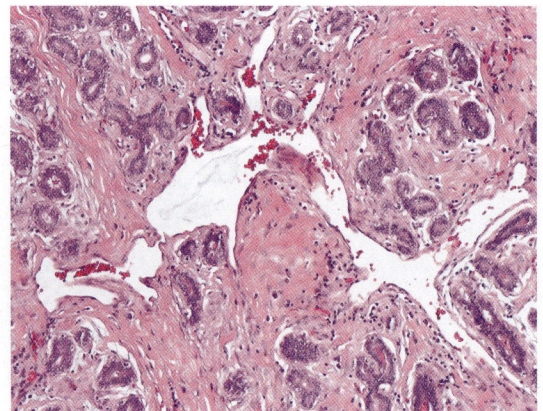

Figure 19-7 The capillaries in this hamartoma appear unusually large; they sit very close to the acini and exhibit an unexpected configuration.

Many hamartomas contain odd blood vessels, for example. Small arteries or veins of an unusually large size sometimes traverse these nodules, and the capillaries in many examples appear capacious, irregular in their branching pattern, and malpositioned (Fig. 19-7). Long, slender, and serpiginous thin-walled vessels, apparently lymphatic vessels, seem to divide certain hamartomas into lobules (Fig. 19-8). Even the lymphoid tissue can look aberrant. One might find plasma cells straying from their proper location in the specialized stroma and mingling with the adipocytes (Fig. 19-9).

The stroma of fibroadenoma variants contains numerous fibroblasts, abundant collagen, and interspersed lymphocytes, plasma cells, and mast cells (Fig. 19-10). Fat does not form a conspicuous component of the stroma of fibroadenoma variants. The coexistence of numerous fibroblasts and abundant collagen stands out as an unusual combination of findings and provides important evidence to support the diagnosis of fibroadenoma variant. The stroma of young fibroadenomas often appears as cellular as the stroma of fibroadenoma variants, but the extracellular matrix of the former consists

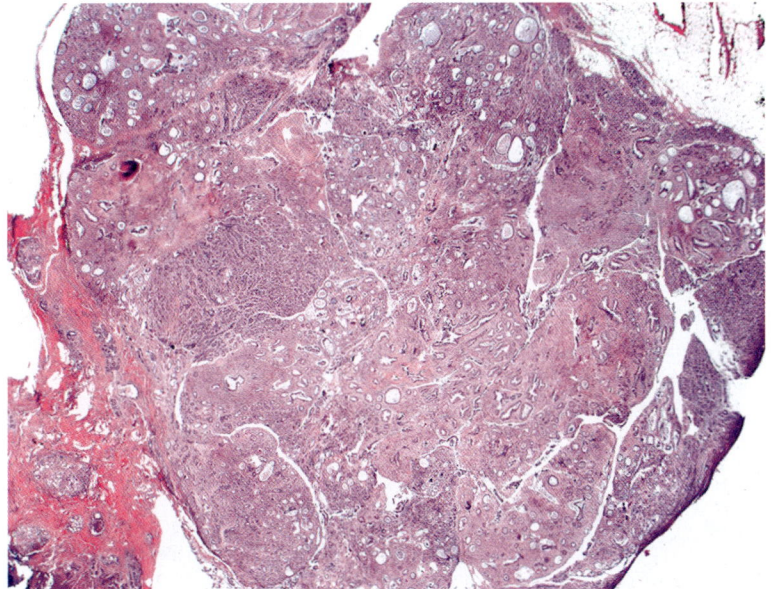

Figure 19-8 This hamartoma appears segmented by serpiginous, thin-walled vascular channels.

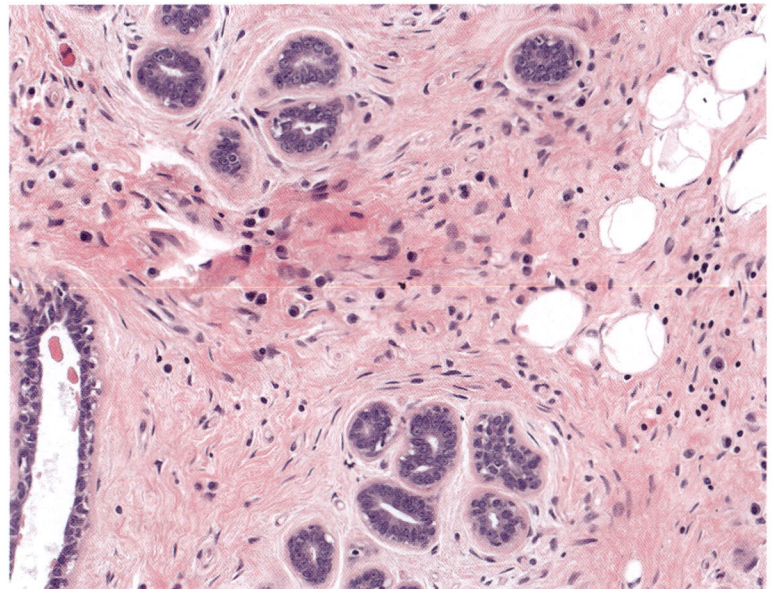

Figure 19-9 The plasma cells seem to wander from their home near the glands and into the fat.

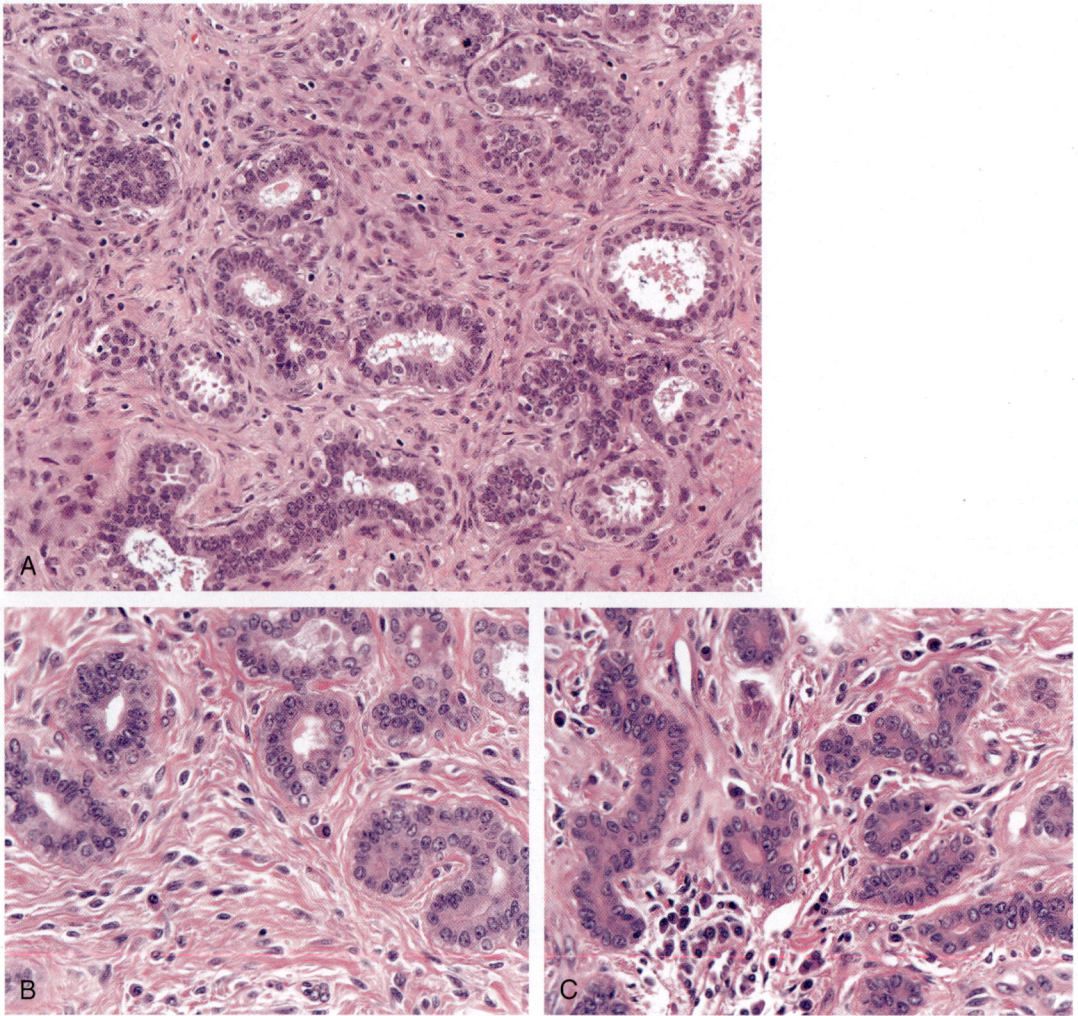

Figure 19-10 A and **B,** The stroma of this fibroadenoma variant consists of many fibroblasts and eosinophilic collagen. **C,** The stroma contains many plasma cells, which can form clusters.

of bluish myxoid ground substances rather than the eosinophilic collagen of the latter. Hyalinized fibroadenomas contain abundant, dense collagen, but their stroma lacks fibroblasts. Thus, the characteristics of the stroma of fibroadenoma variants differentiate these tumors from fibroadenomas. Like fibroadenoma variants, phyllodes tumors typically have a cellular stroma that shows varying levels of collagen deposition; however, the stroma of most phyllodes tumors contains myxoid ground substances as well as collagen. Furthermore, most phyllodes tumors do not have the abundant glands arranged in complex formations seen in fibroadenoma variants.

Characteristics of the Glands

The glandular tissue of a hamartoma can exhibit a wide range of appearances. In the most deceptive examples, the glands can simulate normal terminal duct–lobular units almost perfectly. More commonly, the glands exhibit variation in size and complexity, ranging from small and primitive to large and overly complicated. The epithelium lining the glands does not differ from normal epithelium.

The epithelium of the glands of fibroadenoma variants often appears active. The luminal cells look enlarged and possess large, round nuclei; pale granular chromatin; and prominent nucleoli (Fig. 19-11). Apocrine metaplasia and ductal hyperplasia frequently involve the glands (Fig. 19-12).

Summary

Both hamartomas and fibroadenoma variants represent malformations of mammary tissue. They consist of disorganized collections of mature glands and mesenchymal tissues (Box 19-1).

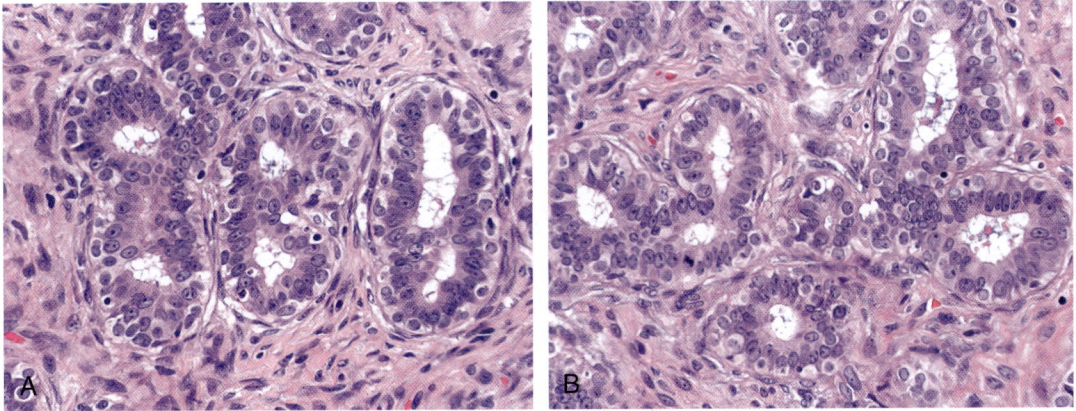

Figure 19-11 A, The luminal cells of this fibroadenoma variant contain large nuclei and nucleoli of a uniform and modest size, and the myoepithelial cells appear prominent. **B,** The luminal cells contain mitotic figures.

Box 19-1

The characteristics of fibroadenoma variants, which may represent a distinctive type of hamartoma:

• Cellular and collagenous stroma
• Abundant, poorly organized glandular tissue
• Frequent presence of fibrocystic changes

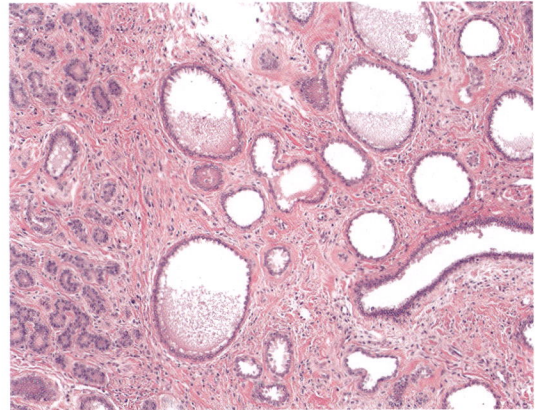

Figure 19-12 The glands of a fibroadenoma variant often exhibit apocrine metaplasia and cyst formation.

PROBLEMS IN THE DIAGNOSIS OF HAMARTOMAS AND FIBROADENOMA VARIANTS

Pathologists familiar with these entities should not find their diagnosis difficult. One might mistake either one for a fibroadenoma or a nodule of pseudoangiomatous stromal hyperplasia, but neither error would pose a serious problem. An occasional phyllodes tumor seems to originate in a hamartoma (Fig. 19-13). The presence of cellular stroma and the formation of fronds allow one to recognize this situation.

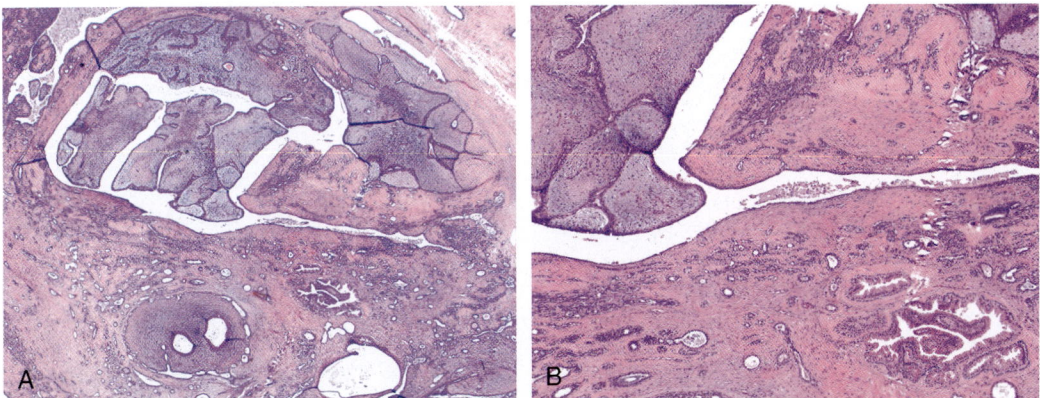

Figure 19-13 This nodule composed of disorderly glands looks like a hamartoma in **A,** but nodules of stromal cells form frond, as seen in **B,** which indicate the emergence of a phyllodes tumor.

Reference

1. Azzopardi JG: Problems in Breast Pathology. (Major Problems in Pathology, vol 11.) London, WB Saunders, 1979.

Selected Readings

Arrigoni MG, Dockerty MB, Judd ES: The identification and treatment of mammary hamartoma. Surg Gynecol Obstet 1971;133:577-582.

Azzopardi JG: Problems in Breast Pathology. (Major Problems in Pathology, vol 11.) London, WB Saunders, 1979.

Daya D, Trus T, D'Souza TJ, et al: Hamartoma of the breast, an underrecognized breast lesion: A clinicopathologic and radiographic study of 25 cases. Am J Clin Pathol 1995;103:685-689.

Fisher CJ, Hanby AM, Robinson L, et al: Mammary hamartoma: A review of 35 cases. Histopathology 1992;20:99-106.

Jones MW, Norris HJ, Wargotz ES: Hamartomas of the breast. Surg Gynecol Obstet 1991;173:54-56.

Linell F, Ostberg G, Soderstrom J, et al: Breast hamartomas: An important entity in mammary pathology. Virchows Arch [A] 1979;383:253-264.

Oberman HA: Hamartomas and hamartoma variants of the breast. Semin Diagn Pathol 1989;6:135-145.

20

Pseudoangiomatous Stromal Hyperplasia

DEFINITIONS AND CLINICOPATHOLOGIC CHARACTERISTICS

Pseudoangiomatous stromal hyperplasia arises from the myofibroblasts of the nonspecialized stroma. Multiplication of these stromal cells engulfs the underlying glandular tissue and thereby produces a biphasic appearance. Thus, pseudoangiomatous stromal hyperplasia, like fibroadenomas and phyllodes tumors, represents a stromal proliferation with entrapment of lobules; however, unlike the other two tumors, which arise from specialized fibroblasts, pseudoangiomatous stromal hyperplasia is an alteration of the nonspecialized stroma. This type of stromal hyperplasia almost always accompanies the epithelial proliferation seen in the early phase of gynecomastia; it occurs commonly as small, poorly defined, and clinically inapparent foci in breast tissue showing fibrocystic changes; and it occasionally forms a discrete mass. Pseudoangiomatous hyperplasia frequently coexists with hamartomas and phyllodes tumors, complicating their histologic appearances.

Pseudoangiomatous stromal hyperplasia affects women during their reproductive years and postmenopausal women receiving hormone replacement therapy. Although benign, the lesion sometimes recurs, and extremely rare cases seem to document the evolution of pseudoangiomatous stromal hyperplasia to myofibroblastic sarcoma.

One usually discovers pseudoangiomatous stromal hyperplasia during histologic study, but occasional foci manifest as well-defined rubbery masses similar in appearance to fibroadenomas.

HISTOLOGIC CHARACTERISTICS

Orderly expansion of the stromal compartments, especially the nonspecialized stromal compartment,

and exaggeration of the entrapped glandular tissue represent the themes of pseudoangiomatous stromal hyperplasia.

Structure of the Mass

Like fibroadenomas, nodular masses of pseudoangiomatous stromal hyperplasia display a consistent and organized structure (Fig. 20-1). The process begins in the nonspecialized stroma, where myofibroblasts proliferate and give rise to an anastomosing network of slitlike spaces. This alteration enlarges the nonspecialized stromal compartment and entraps ducts and lobules, but it does not disturb the relationships among these tissues. The pseudoangiomatous nonspecialized stroma forms bands coursing among the ducts and lobules, and the specialized stroma stands out as uniform cuffs encircling the glandular tissue and separating it from the pseudoangiomatous

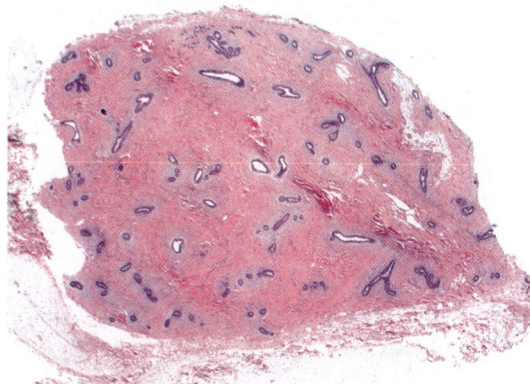

Figure 20-1 Nodular pseudoangiomatous stromal hyperplasia has a uniform distribution of the glands and a consistent ratio of glands to stroma.

stroma (Fig. 20-2). These features resemble those of simple type I lobules. The specialized stroma appears especially prominent, and the myxoid ground substances within it abundant. The intimate spatial association of the changes in the two types of stroma suggests a cause-and-effect relationship between them (Fig. 20-3).

Lobules trapped within the altered stroma appear enlarged both in overall dimension and in the diameter of the acini within them. Furthermore, the architecture of the lobules often looks simplified; they usually consist of sparsely branching tubules widely separated by the altered stroma (Fig 20-4). The intralobular stroma does not commonly exhibit pseudoangiomatous changes; when it does so, however, the alteration usually seems to begin in the center of the lobule (Fig. 20-5). With complete involvement, dense, eosinophilic collagen and myofibroblasts replace the specialized stroma (Fig. 20-6). The arrangement of the collagen bundles and the pattern of the myofibroblasts do not resemble those of a permeative process. The myofibroblasts do not seem to invade the lobule; instead, the appearance suggests a transformation of the intralobular stromal cells into a pseudoangiomatous pattern. Despite this tendency to respect the architecture of lobules, the myofibroblasts sometimes infiltrate the peripheral adipose tissue (Fig. 20-7).

Just as fibroadenomas hyalinize, so, also, do nodules of pseudoangiomatous stromal hyperplasia. The deposition of dense collagen and the dropout of

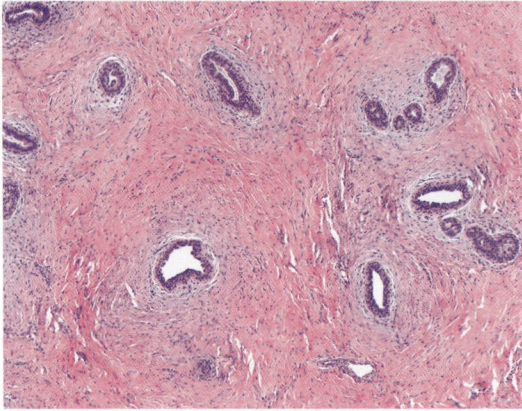

Figure 20-2 The glandular structures appear enlarged. The specialized stroma looks cellular, contains abundant myxoid ground substances, and uniformly cuffs the glandular tissue. The nonspecialized stroma exhibits the pseudoangiomatous change.

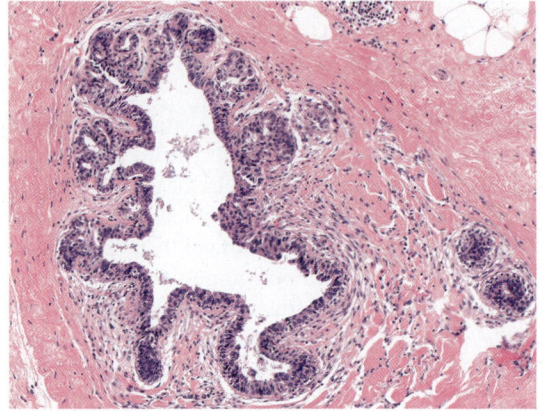

Figure 20-3 The specialized stroma surrounding this duct appears prominent and cellular in the region abutting the pseudoangiomatous stromal hyperplasia.

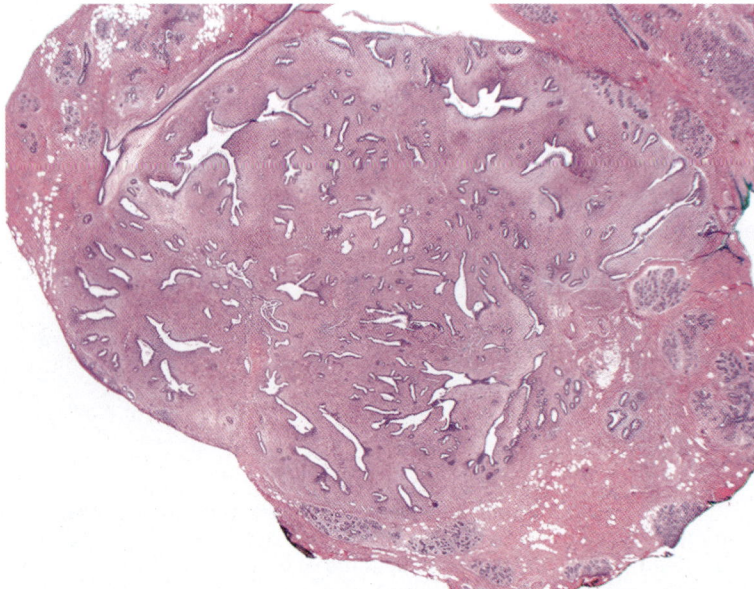

Figure 20-4 The pseudoangiomatous stromal hyperplasia has enlarged and simplified the lobules and has distended the acini within them. Compare those in the center of the field with uninvolved lobules at the periphery.

Figure 20-5 The interior of this lobule exhibits pseudoangiomatous changes.

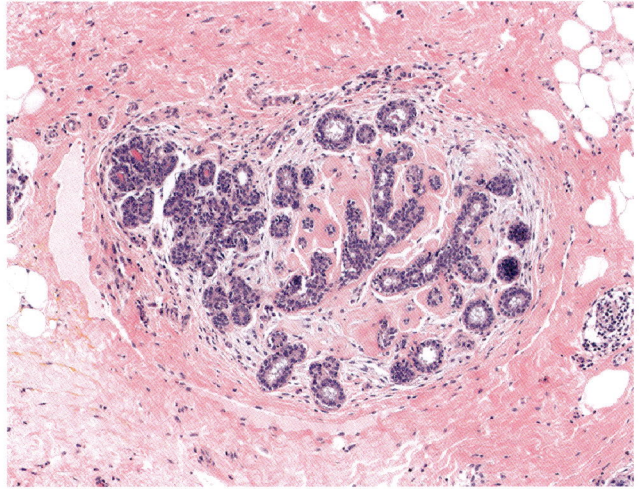

Figure 20-6 Pseudoangiomatous stroma has completely transformed the specialized stroma of this lobule.

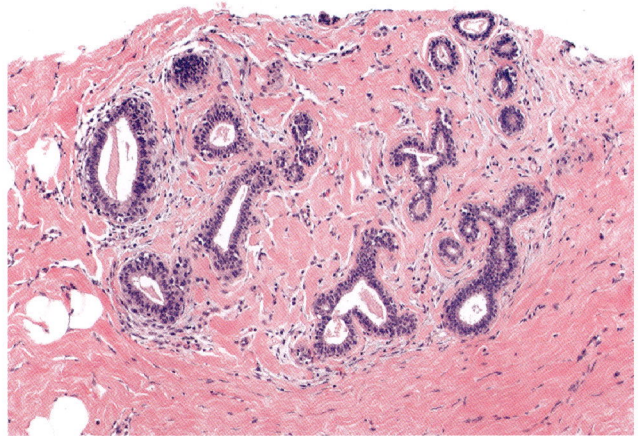

Figure 20-7 The myofibroblasts at the edge of this nodule of pseudoangiomatous stromal hyperplasia infiltrate the adipose tissue.

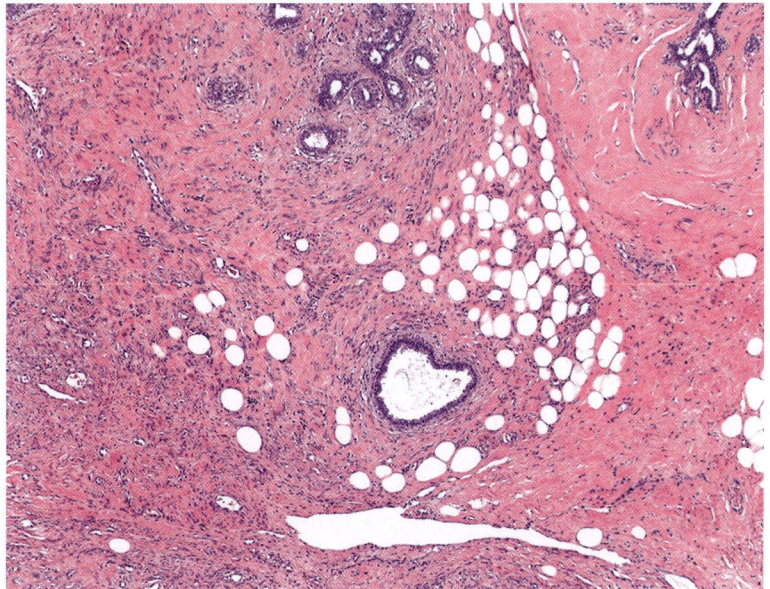

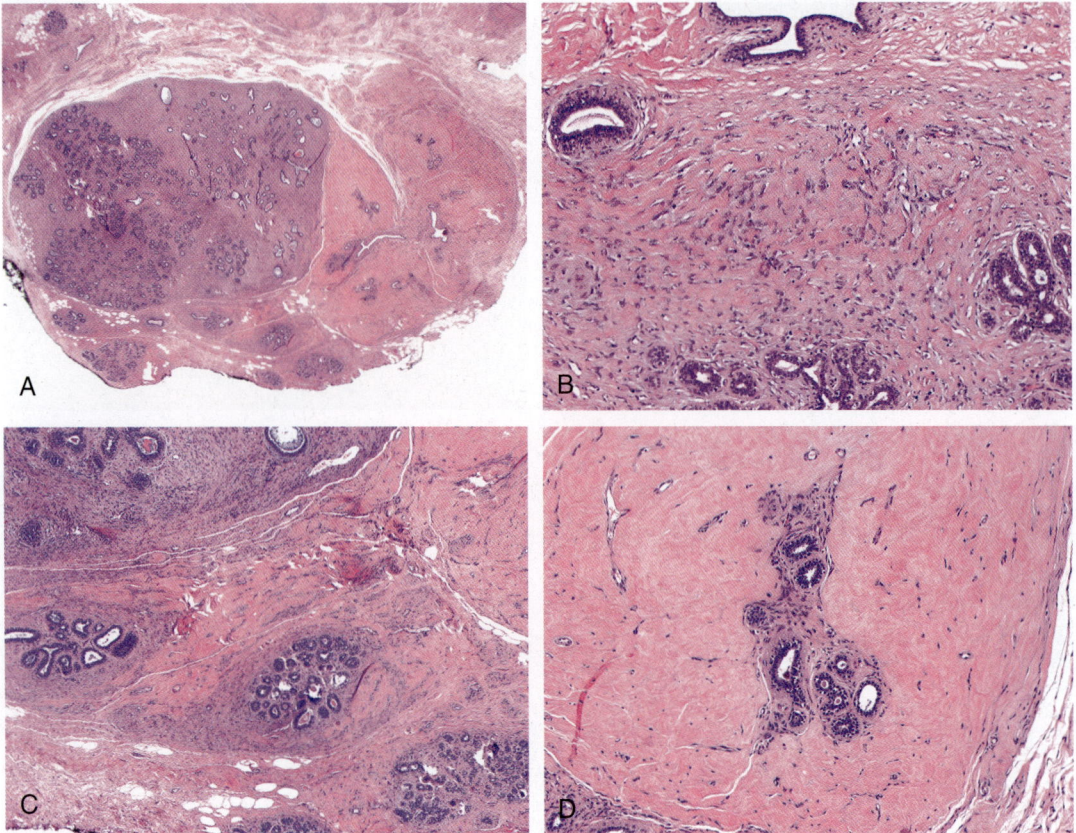

Figure 20-8 A and **B,** Most of this well-defined nodule demonstrates the stroma characteristic of pseudoangiomatous stromal hyperplasia. **C** and **D,** One region demonstrates collagen deposition in the cellular stroma, and another shows hyalinization of the stroma. Rare myofibroblasts and only a hint of a pseudovascular pattern remain in the latter region, and the entrapped lobule appears larger and more robust than one would expect, considering the extent of stromal hyalinization.

stromal cells alter the appearance of the stroma, but these processes do not change the structure of the mass (Fig. 20-8). Despite the hyalinization of the connective tissues and the atrophy of the glandular component, one can still appreciate the expansion of the nonspecialized stromal compartment, the prominence of the specialized stroma, and the relative enlargement of the glandular units.

Characteristics of the Stroma

The stroma of nodular pseudoangiomatous stromal hyperplasia consists of active-looking myofibroblasts that possess obvious, faintly blue cytoplasm and small, pale nuclei (Fig. 20-9). The cells typically form a meshwork of pseudovascular spaces, but they can also grow as compact fascicles that do not form channels, the *fascicular* pattern. The intervening stroma consists of collagen, which often appears especially eosinophilic. The specialized stroma of the proliferative lobules looks

more prominent than usual: It displays an increase in myxoid ground substance and, possibly, fibroblasts (Fig. 20-10). Because of this prominence of specialized stroma, one could confuse nodular pseudoangiomatous stromal hyperplasia with both a fibroadenoma and a phyllodes tumor. Careful inspection of a case of nodular pseudoangiomatous stromal hyperplasia shows that the specialized stroma forms uniform zones, each of the same modest dimension, encircling the lobules and ducts and that myofibroblasts of the nonspecialized stromal compartment account for most of the proliferative stromal cells. Besides creating slitlike spaces, myofibroblasts sometimes form a thin, diaphanous meshwork around the small and thin-walled blood vessels that run in the nonspecialized stroma (Fig. 20-11). The number of small vessels in this compartment seems increased; thus, pseudoangiomatous stromal hyperplasia involves a genuine proliferation of blood vessels as well as the creation of pseudovascular spaces (Fig. 20-12).

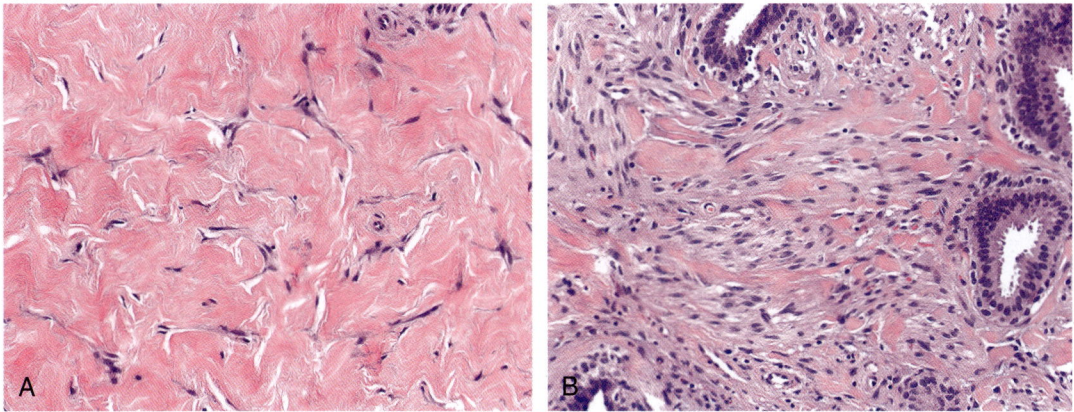

Figure 20-9 A, The typical myofibroblasts of pseudoangiomatous stromal hyperplasia have obvious, bluish cytoplasm and oval, dark nuclei, and they form anastomosing, slit-like channels. **B,** In less common examples, the myofibroblasts form fascicles, and only a few cells create spaces.

Figure 20-10 The specialized stroma forms uniform cuffs of myxoid tissue.

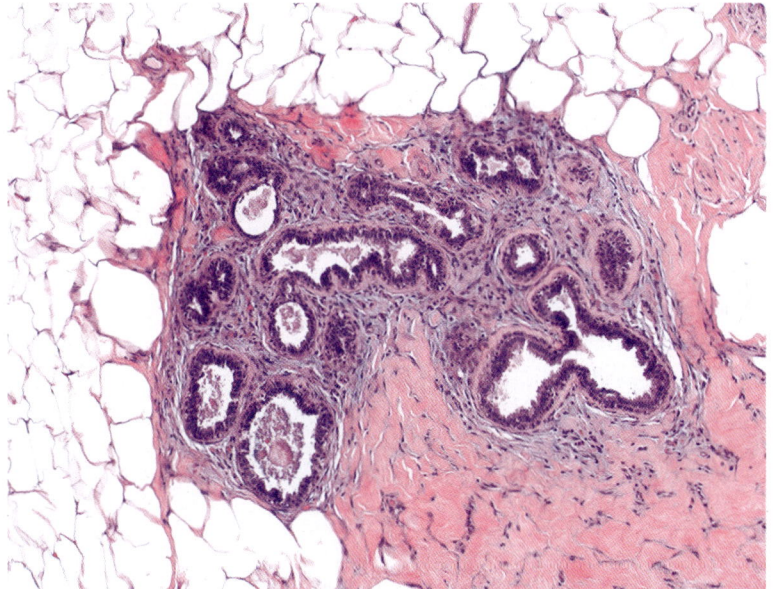

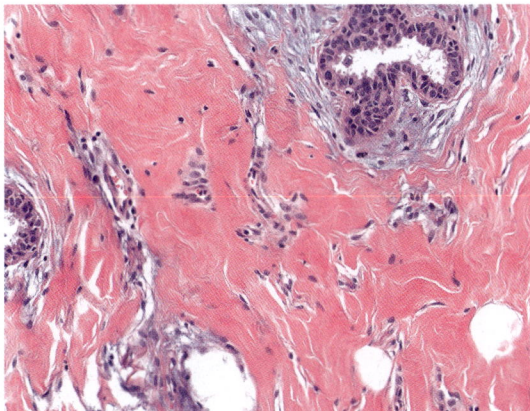

Figure 20-11 A thin sleeve of myofibroblasts surrounds small blood vessels.

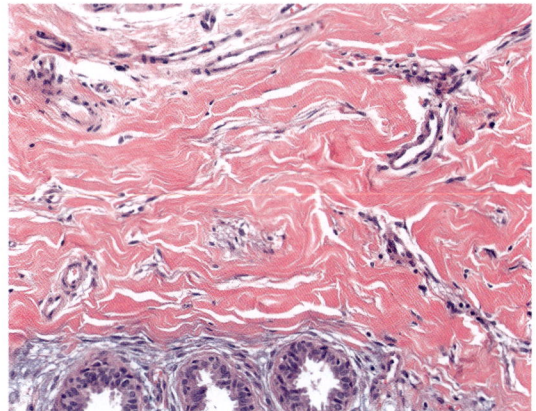

Figure 20-12 Note the prominence of the genuine small vessels in the nonspecialized stroma of pseudoangiomatous stromal hyperplasia.

Characteristics of the Glands

Terminal duct–lobular units within nodular pseudoangiomatous stromal hyperplasia enlarge. Because this growth affects the glands rather uniformly, one may not appreciate the extent of ductal and lobular hypertrophy until one contrasts the size of the glands within the nodule with the diameter of those outside the mass (Fig. 20-13). Such a side-by-side examination also shows the enlargement of the acini. The epithelium lining the acini can have either of two different patterns of proliferation. More commonly, the epithelial proliferation takes the form of conventional ductal hyperplasia (Fig. 20-14). The ductal epithelial proliferation in certain examples of pseudoangiomatous stromal hyperplasia looks especially prominent, and sometimes the proliferative cells look atypical (Fig. 20-15). The level of epithelial proliferation and the unusual cytologic characteristics understandably bring to mind diagnoses such as atypical ductal hyperplasia and ductal carcinoma in situ; however, pathologists should remain cautious about rendering either diagnosis in the setting of pseudoangiomatous stromal hyperplasia. Most often, the cytologic changes reflect a reactive rather than neoplastic phenomenon. Pseudoangiomatous stromal hyperplasia does not immunize the glands from involvement by carcinoma in situ, of course, but these lesions coexist so infrequently that one must observe obvious and typical changes before making the diagnoses.

In the second pattern of epithelial proliferation that one sees in foci of pseudoangiomatous stromal hyperplasia, the luminal cells of the acini form a single layer, enlarging and distending the acini without filling them (Fig. 20-16). The luminal cell nuclei appear variable in the size and shape, and the cells contain a small amount of cytoplasm. One would

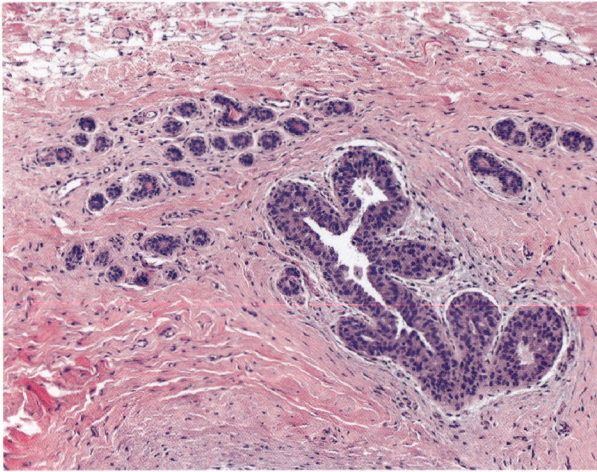

Figure 20-13 The ductule in the lower right looks enlarged compared with those in the lobule in the upper left, and the epithelial cells of the former appear larger and more closely packed than those of the latter.

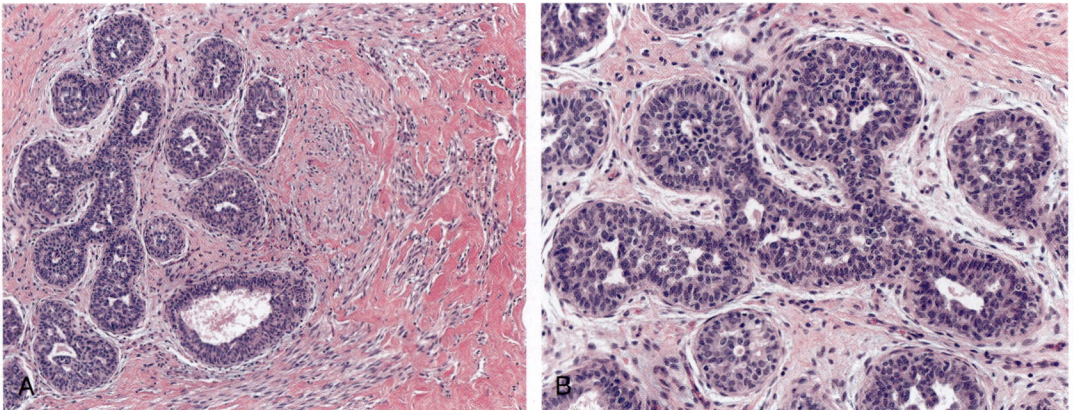

Figure 20-14 A, The lobule entrapped within this nodule of pseudoangiomatous stromal hyperplasia shows florid conventional ductal hyperplasia. B, At high magnification, one can appreciate the benign characteristics of the proliferative epithelial cells.

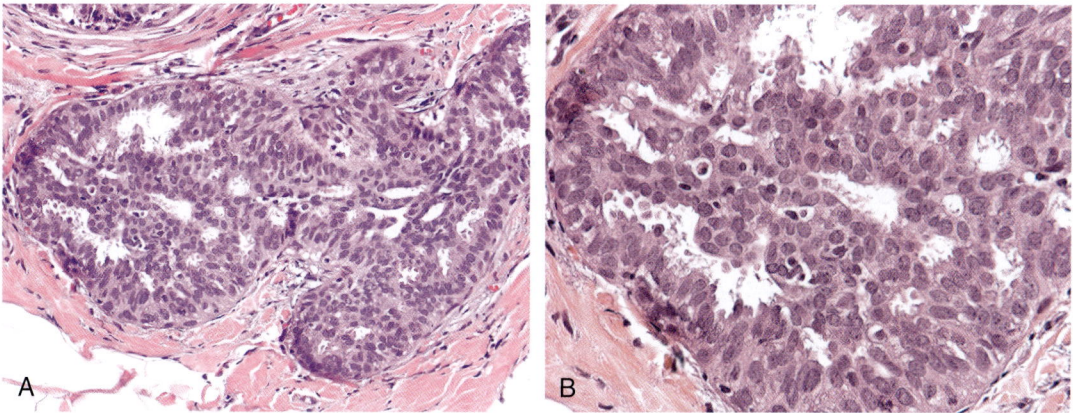

Figure 20-15 A, This focus of pseudoangiomatous stromal hyperplasia shows florid ductal hyperplasia. **B,** Slight enlargement of nuclei and homogeneity of the chromatin make certain epithelial cells look slightly atypical but they merge with similar ones displaying the architecture of conventional ductal hyperplasia, shown **C.**

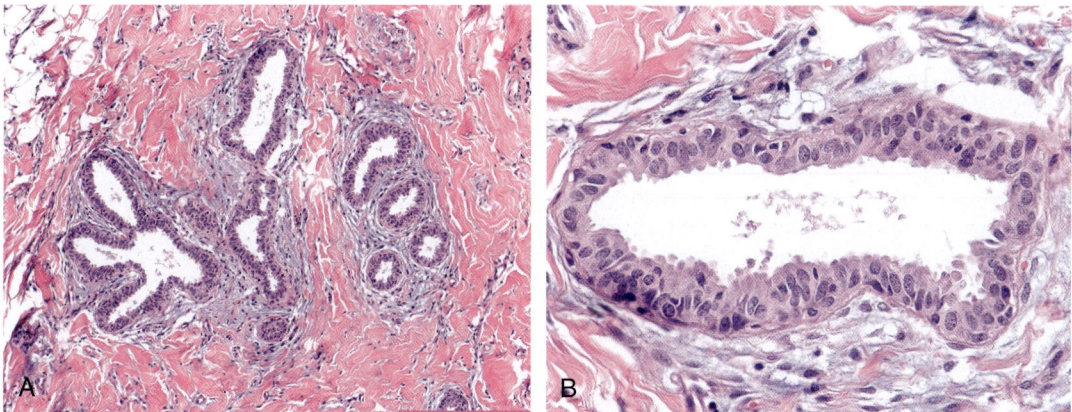

Figure 20-16 A, In this example of pseudoangiomatous stromal hyperplasia, the epithelial proliferation takes the form of a single layer of columnar epithelial cells. **B,** The columnar cells lining the gland in this focus of pseudoangiomatous stromal hyperplasia appear slightly crowded. They have irregular nuclei and small amounts of cytoplasm. **C,** Contrast those characteristics with those of genuine atypical columnar cells, which have uniform, smoothly contoured nuclei and ample cytoplasm.

not ordinarily confuse this form of hyperplasia with carcinoma in situ, but it does superficially resemble flat epithelial atypia. Attention to the size of the luminal cells, the characteristics of their nuclei, and the amount of cytoplasm usually distinguishes between the reactive hyperplasia associated with pseudoangiomatous stromal hyperplasia and flat epithelial atypia.

Summary

Pseudoangiomatous stromal hyperplasia represents an alteration of the nonspecialized stroma that leads to uniform enlargement of the entrapped glands. Although exaggerated in size, the tissue components retain their proper anatomic relationships (Box 20-1).

Box 20-1

Histologic features of nodular pseudoangiomatous stromal hyperplasia:

- Proliferation of myofibroblasts of the nonspecialized stroma in a pseudovascular pattern
- Uniform modest expansion of the specialized stroma
- Enlargement and simplification of the entrapped glands
- Frequent presence of ductal type epithelial hyperplasia

PROBLEMS IN THE DIAGNOSIS OF PSEUDOANGIOMATOUS STROMAL HYPERPLASIA

Lesions with a prominent pseudoangiomatous pattern regularly cause difficulties in classification, because one encounters pseudoangiomatous changes in many breast specimens and in association with many other lesions. This type of change occurs commonly in phyllodes tumors, often in hamartomas, and rarely in fibroadenomas, and pseudoangiomatous stromal hyperplasia sometimes forms a discrete nodule that presents a biphasic picture. Most examples of nodular pseudoangiomatous stromal hyperplasia have distinctive characteristics: a well-defined, smoothly contoured border, a uniform distribution of glands and stroma, homogeneous stroma organized in clearly defined zones of specialized and nonspecialized fibrous connective tissue, and orderly tubular glands. Uncommon cases exhibit features that obscure the diagnosis. The myofibroblasts can grow in a cellular pattern that lacks a pseudovascular architecture, can permeate surrounding tissues in a manner that appears invasive, and can display cytologic atypicality and mitotic activity. Pathologists might have difficulty distinguishing these unusual cases of pseudoangiomatous stromal hyperplasia from phyllodes tumors. The presence of heterogeneity in the composition of a tumor would favor the latter diagnosis, and so would variability in the density of the stromal cells, in the characteristics of the extracellular matrix, in the distribution of the glands, and in the proportions of glands and stroma. One must acknowledge that distinguishing certain cases of cellular and fascicular pseudoangiomatous stromal hyperplasia from a phyllodes tumor may prove extremely difficult.

Selected Readings

Ibrahim RE, Sciotto CG, Weidner N: Pseudoangiomatous hyperplasia of mammary stroma: Some observations regarding its clinicopathologic spectrum. Cancer 1989;63:1154-1160.

Powell CM, Cranor ML, Rosen PP: Pseudoangiomatous stromal hyperplasia (PASH): A mammary stromal tumor with myofibroblastic differentiation. Am J Surg Pathol 1995;19:270-277.

Vuitch MF, Rosen PP, Erlandson RA: Pseudoangiomatous hyperplasia of mammary stroma. Hum Pathol 1986;17:185-191.

Index

Note: Page numbers followed by *f* and *t* indicate figures and tables, respectively. Page numbers followed by *b* indicate boxed material.

[handwritten notes at top: "DCIS vs immature hyperplasia p. 50" / "Collagenous spherulosis 140-143"]

Ductal carcinoma in situ *(continued)*
of apocrine type
high-grade, 90–91, 92f
histologic characteristics of, 90–92, 92f
low-grade, 90–91, 92f
and carcinoma in lymphatic vessels, differentiation of, 75–77, 76f, 77f
cellular polarization in, 10, 11f, 15, 116f
clinical presentation of, 15
cribriform
involving sclerosing adenosis, 233, 233f, 235, 235f
with micropapillary ductal carcinoma in situ, 157
morphologic characteristics of, 140–141, 141t
cytokeratin profile of, 45
detection of, 15
diagnosis of
approach to, 45–46
problems in, 61–83
ductal hyperplasia and, 15–16
glandular differentiation in, 15
in gynecomastia, 81–83, 82f
high-grade, 15
architectural characteristics of, 33
cytologic characteristics of, 33
involving radial scar, 256, 256f
involving stalk of papilloma, 176, 176f
intercellular cohesion in, 114f
intermediate-grade
architectural characteristics of, 33
and conventional ductal hyperplasia, differentiation of, 61–62, 61f, 62f
cytologic characteristics of, 33
involving papilloma, 170, 172f, 179
and papillary carcinoma, differentiation of, 192–193, 192f–193f
in stalk, 174–176, 176f
in irradiated breast, recognition of, 79–81, 79f–81f
lobular neoplasia involving, 139, 139f
low-grade, 26–32
architectural characteristics of, 26–28, 26b
and atypical ductal hyperplasia, differentiation of, 34–35, 35f
cellular polarization in, 10, 11f
characteristics of, contrasted with ductal hyperplasia, 29, 32f
chromatin in, 29, 30f
cribriform, mimics of, 72, 174–175
cribriform spaces and their variants in, 26–28, 26b, 27f
cytologic characteristics of, 29–32, 29b, 29f–32f
cytoplasmic characteristics of, 29, 31f
involving papilloma, 170, 172f
involving radial scar, 257–258, 258b, 259f, 260f
involving stalk of papilloma, 174–176
nuclei in
contours of, 29, 30f
morphology of, 29, 29f
with papillary carcinoma, 188, 188t
regular placement of cells in, 28, 29f
uniformity in, 29, 29b
micropapillary, 203, 207–212
apical cytoplasmic compartments in, 210, 210f, 212f
cellular dimorphism in, 211, 212f
cellular polarization in, 210, 210f

Ductal carcinoma in situ *(continued)*
clinicopathologic characteristics of, 207
with cribriform ductal carcinoma in situ, 157
cytologic characteristics of, 160, 210, 210f, 211f, 212t
definition of, 207
glandular distention by, 212t
extent of, 207, 207f–209f
histologic characteristics of, 207–210
immunohistochemistry of, 211, 212f
and lack of maturation, 210–211, 211f, 212f, 212t
and lobular carcinoma in situ, coexistence of, 207
lumen of glands harboring, contents of, 210, 210f, 212t
micropapillae in
configuration of, 207, 209f, 212t
size of, 207, 209f, 212t
morphologic characteristics of, 212t
nuclear characteristics of, 210, 210f
and tubular carcinoma, coexistence of, 207
microscopic focus of, 35, 35f
nuclear characteristics of, 124, 124f
papillary, mimics of, 72
and papillomas, association of, 161–162
solid
and lobular carcinoma in situ, differentiation of, 130–131, 131f
mimics of, 72
stratification in, 37–39, 38f
Ductal hyperplasia. *See also* Subareolar sclerosing duct hyperplasia
atypical, 33–36, 51, 67
of apocrine type, histologic characteristics of, 90–92, 92f
biologic significance of, 35–36
cytologic atypia without architectural atypia in, 33, 34f
definition of, 33
involving papilloma, 170, 173f, 179
qualitative criteria for, 33, 34f
size criteria for, 34–35, 35f
types of lesions commonly classified as, 35–36, 36f
cytokeratin profile of, 45
diagnosis of, approach to, 45–46
and ductal carcinoma in situ, 15–16
in fibroadenoma variant, 349
flat, and flat epithelial atypia, differentiation of, 42–43, 44f, 45f
with hyperchromatic nuclei, 46f, 47, 47f
immature, 49–51, 49f–54f
micropapillary, 159–160, 203–206
in perimenopausal women, 47–49, 48f, 49f
postmenopausal, 15
in pseudoangiomatous stromal hyperplasia, 356, 356f, 357f
usual (conventional), 15
ancillary characteristics of, 24–25
architectural characteristics of, 16–21, 16b, 16f
with calcifications, 24, 25f
characteristics of, contrasted with low-grade ductal carcinoma in situ, 29, 32f
in conventional fibroadenoma, 316–317
cytologic characteristics of, 21–24, 21f–23f, 24b
cytoplasmic characteristics of, 29

Solid papillary CA ī endocrine differentiate 195

Myoepithelial cells in ductal hyperplasia p.134 Fig 6-43

Histiocytes in papilloma. See Case S10-4682-A4 c̄ cytokeratin stain

Sclerosed papilloma vs nipple adenoma. See S10-4692 Page consult.